Towards Earlier Diagnosis

A GUIDE TO PRIMARY CARE

Keith Hodgkin BM BCh FRCGP FRCP
Previously General Practitioner, Redcar, Yorkshire and Sir Harry Jephcott Visiting Professor in General Practice. Visiting Professor and previously Chairman of Family Practice, Memorial University, Newfoundland, Canada. Visiting Fellow, University of Western Australia.

FOREWORD BY

John Horder OBE FRCGP FRCP FRCPsych
Past President, Royal College of General Practitioners

FIFTH EDITION

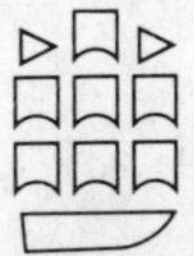

CHURCHILL LIVINGSTONE
EDINBURGH LONDON MELBOURNE AND NEW YORK 1985

CHURCHILL LIVINGSTONE
Medical Division of Longman Group Limited

Distributed in the United States of America by
Churchill Livingstone Inc., 1560 Broadway, New York,
N.Y. 10036, and by associated companies, branches and
representatives throughout the world.

First edition 1963
Second edition 1966
Third edition 1973
Fourth edition 1978
Fifth edition 1985

ISBN 0 443 03131 2

British Library Cataloguing in Publication Data
Hodgkin, Keith
Towards earlier diagnosis.—5th ed.
1. Medicine, diagnosis, for general practice
I. Title
616.07'5 RC71

Library of Congress Cataloging in Publication Data
Hodgkin, Keith.
Towards earlier diagnosis.

Rev. ed. of: Towards earlier diagnosis in primary
care. 4th ed. 1978.
Bibliography: p.
Includes index.
1. Diagnosis. 2. Family medicine. I. Hodgkin, Keith.
Towards earlier diagnosis in primary care. II. Title.
[DNLM: 1. Diagnosis. WB 141 H689t]
RC71.H7 1985 616.07'5 84-7103

Produced by Longman Group (FE) Ltd
Printed in Hong Kong

Foreword

The foreword to the first edition to this book was written by Robert Platt before he became President of the Royal College of Physicians. I liked and admired him greatly, so it is a special privilege to be asked to write the foreword to the fifth edition. It is just as much a privilege to contribute a page to a book which has stood the test of 25 years in what is now a surprisingly competitive field.

Innumerable people have found Keith Hodgkin's book useful during the later stages of learning medicine and as a source of reference in practice. In the fifth edition the essential and characteristic element — Part II — again deals systematically with the early diagnosis of the most important disorders. The product of years of front-line involvement, observation and careful recording has been repeatedly distilled in the light of changing ideas. This time high-risk factors and management options are included as additional aspects of each disorder.

The first part — the philosophy and methods of primary care — is concerned with principles and is for reading. It shares in a world-wide process of reflection about the role of a doctor from whom people seek 'personal, primary, continuing and comprehensive care'. It reveals — and is the more interesting because of — the writer's experience on both sides of the Atlantic.

I know no more stimulating discussion of the general practitioner's job than is contained in the first chapter.

John Horder

Preface to the Fifth Edition

I am surprised and gratified at the continued demand for this book and have carried on the policy followed in the previous four editions.

The text is based on my own experience in practice, teaching and examination being written mainly for trainees, residents and undergraduates who are beginning their primary care experience.

Throughout Part I (Philosophy and Methods of Primary Care) and Part II (A field guide, which describes the wide range of disorders encountered in primary care) I have tried to outline the knowledge and options, for decision making, which the newcomer to primary care must learn in practice.

With this in mind the following additions have been made:

1. *Throughout Part II* for each condition described, I have added sections on:

   a. *High risk factors*: which play a part in diagnosis and prevention.

   b. *Management options*: which include the wide range of therapy, explanations and preventive action that are open to the family doctor.

2. *In Part I* I have rewritten the Chapters on Prevention and the Tools of Practice.

Sections have been added on computers (Chapter 7), Video in the consultation (Appendix VIII) and graphic recording (Appendix IX).

3. Entries have been added in Part II on a number of disorders including Genital Herpes, Cancer, Non-Accidental Injury, Hyperventilation Syndrome, Sexually Transmitted Disease, Contraceptives and many others.

Finally of interest are those clinical sections which have changed little over the years:

— the natural history of most common diseases. Prevalence may change but problems of early diagnosis remain or are more difficult, e.g. measles.

— the clinical pointers which the primary physician uses for early recognition
— the results of observational research, i.e. the descriptions of influenza and common respiratory virus disease, which were based on the collection of virology specimens from 1500 patients over 15 years (Chapter 8 page 176 et seq.)
— the sections on mistakes, misleading features and pitfalls. Undoubtedly we learn from our mistakes but only if we continue to be vigilant of the pitfalls.

1985 Keith Hodgkin

Preface to the First Edition

When I entered general practice in 1949, my first patient was a young telephonist who complained of 'dizzy spells in the busy spells'; my second patient was a short-sighted man who gave a casual history that 'a grey cloud' had recently appeared in the visual field of his right eye. In spite of a long hospital training, I had little idea of how to tackle the first problem and did not realise that the second was an acute eye emergency requiring immediate admission to hospital. This experience illustrates clearly the two main difficulties that arise in the training of a family doctor.

Firstly, many of the common problems of general practice are never encountered in hospital so that the new entrant is forced to learn his job by time-consuming trial and error methods. Even basic principles are of limited use until the doctor is aware of the different emphasis of his new environment, e.g. the simple guide *that common diseases occur most often* cannot be applied until he *knows* the common disorders.

Secondly, the family doctor must have an efficient working knowledge of the early features of a very wide range of diseases. Early diagnosis begins in general practice and the training of good general practitioners is therefore one of the main objects of our medical schools.

I hope that this book will help to bridge the gap between hospital and general practice and to prepare the student (and new entrant to practice) for the altered emphasis and different clinical material.

There are several ways of teaching a very wide subject such as general practice. One is to collect the views of many experts (both specialists and family doctors) and to give perspective to the whole field by careful editing. A simple, though cruder method of giving a perspective view is to describe general practice as seen through the eyes of a single family doctor. By analysis of personal case records, I have tried in a factual way to emphasise those clinical observations that are needed to recognise the early stages of disease.

A perspective picture of the natural history of disease in a general practice has been built up. This view will, I hope, give the student in hospital a better knowledge of those parts of his clinical training that will be useful to him in general practice.

As a medical student when I entered hospital, I was advised to keep records of all the patients whom I encountered. I was taught that clinical records are of greater educational value than textbooks. Since then I kept detailed records of the patients who have come under my care. The analysis, figures and text are based, except where stated, on these personal records.

My aim is to describe how a family doctor works and thinks. I have tried to show how clinical observation has influenced my practice of medicine. I hope that this book will help prospective family doctors to avoid some of the many heart-searchings which I suffered when struggling to modify a hospital training to the extensive needs of a busy general practice.

It is necessary to state the extent of my experience:

Hospital

Student — three and a half years. Records kept of 318 incidents of illness.

Surgical intern — 6 months
Medical intern — 6 months
Paediatric intern — 6 months
Obstetric intern — 3 months
Neurosurgical intern — 3 months

Records kept of 986 incidents of illness.

Morbid anatomy registrar — 1 year. Records kept of 75 post-mortems performed.

Services

Surgeon-Lieutenant in Royal Navy — 3 years. No records kept.

General practice

Three years in private practice
Ten years in one NHS practice

Records kept of every incident of illness.

NHS practice is preferred because the relationship between doctor and patient is professionally happier. NHS patients bring their complaints to the doctor at an earlier stage and although this increases the technical difficulties of diagnosis it also increases the effectiveness of treatment.

The NHS practice is situated on an expanding housing estate which accommodates employees of all types, many of whom work in some of Britain's largest steel and chemical industries.

The methods of general practice that are described have been carried out by a family doctor who was responsible for up to 2500 NHS patients. It was found that standards fell off after the 2500 mark was reached. A family doctor may be able to look after more NHS patients if his practice population is:

(*a*) Static.
(*b*) Contains few children and young families.
(*c*) Contains few old people.
(*d*) Includes many patients who consult other doctors privately, as in some large cities.

A rural practitioner spends more time on travelling and a smaller NHS list may be necessary if standards are to be maintained.

Redcar, 1963 Keith Hodgkin

ACKNOWLEDGEMENTS

My thanks are due to all those who have helped with previous editions.

I am especially grateful to my son, Dr Paul Hodgkin, for his many constructive criticisms and to my wife for her continued help and comment. Also to Anne Harvard and Muriel Pounder for help with typing, proof reading and indexing of this edition.

Contents

Introduction — How to use this book

All primary care involves two essential processes:

A. Decision making that is appropriate to the patients' problems.
B. The creation of sufficient rapport with the patient to gain compliance.

A. THE MEDICAL DECISION MAKING PROCESS

Stage One

The doctor must have sufficient relevant clinical knowledge to enable the patient's story to stimulate rapid recall of likely diagnostic alternatives.

Stage Two

As each diagnostic option is considered, further relevant clinical information is recalled which enables the doctor to weigh up the points for and against each alternative. Further questioning and decisions about examination, investigation, diagnosis and management are then considered and assessed.

Part II of this book, based on a single family doctor's experience, summarises the knowledge needed to weigh the options and choices which may face the primary physician during this everyday clinical decision making. This knowledge must be so well learnt that it is instantly recalled and assessed. This allows the doctor to concentrate on Stage Three.

Stage Three

In parallel with the above, largely clinical — previously learnt process, the family doctor must also make rapid accurate assessments of the patient's personality, feelings and motivations.

Rapport and confidence largely depend on the doctor's skill in incorporating these assessments into his/her clinical decision making. This added skill is learned slowly and painfully with long continued practise in practice.

Stage Four

A final choice must be made which encapsulates the course of action that is most appropriate for the patient as a 'whole person'. This can then be explained to, and discussed with, the patient.

B. PATIENT RAPPORT MUST BE ENOUGH TO GAIN COMPLIANCE

If patient compliance is not obtained the time (and money) of both patient, community and doctor are wasted. This is perhaps the most obvious, yet most frequently overlooked fact in primary care.

A simple common example illustrates the wide range of knowledge, skills and attitudes that have to be learnt to integrate these four stages:

EXAMPLE: A 30-year-old married woman with two children says she has had a headache for several weeks.

Stage One

Possible diagnostic options raised in the doctor's mind.

1. Tension headache (see Part II, p. 248).
2. Migraine (see Part II, p. 294).
3. Cerebral tumour/space occupying lesion. (see Part II, p. 276).

Options 1 and 2 are recalled because they are considered most likely. Option 3 is unlikely but is recalled because the doctor knows that it is both serious and easily missed. The doctor's index of suspicion may be raised because previous delays in diagnosis are remembered.

Stage Two

Recall of the relevant information about these three conditions (of the kind given in Part II) guides further questions and actions. Migraine has the most clear cut presentation and the doctor might decide to confirm or refute this diagnosis first by asking for clinical details about — attacks, possible aura, etc. For effective consultation the relevant clinical knowledge about each option must be recalled and assessed in one or two seconds.

Stage Three

While this *automatic* clinical process is going on the doctor is simultaneously considering the patient's personality: Is she a worrier? Has she had tension symptoms before? What are the age of her children? What support does she get from her husband? Is she afraid of a tumour?

These assessments have to be made in parallel with the clinical thinking because they influence further questioning and the doctor's appraisal of the patient's replies. If the patient is afraid of a tumour she is likely to minimise those features of her history which she thinks suggest a tension origin. If she is in need of a confidant as a result of family problems then the remote but serious possibility of a cerebral tumour may become obscured.

Stage Four

If Option 1 — Tension Headache is considered as the likely cause, then good rapport and careful non-threatening explanations must be tailored to the patient's personality. Drug therapy will be of secondary importance.

If Option 2 — Migraine is the cause, drug therapy with careful instructions and consideration of contraindications, may be the first management priority. Explanation will still be vital but can be short and simple.

If Option 3 — Cerebral tumour is considered possible, many complex clinical and emotional alternatives will have to be rapidly considered and weighed: e.g. further consultations for detailed examination, investigation or observation may have to be arranged.
— Explanations: when these are to be given? What is said? To whom they are given? may all raise difficult choices, (see p. 36).
— A detailed knowledge of the patient's supporting family may have to be gained.
— The 'upsets' caused by initiating these actions may, themselves, cause the doctor mistakenly to delay when immediate referral is clinically indicated.

The complex decision making process illustrated above is first learnt by students when taking histories in hospitals. A lengthy routine is developed taking perhaps an hour. The practising doctor must learn to streamline this lengthy consultation process in a flexible but effective way. Two points should be stressed here:

1. Basic routines of history taking must be adequately learnt in hospital before they can be subsequently streamlined and used automatically. Recall of factual clinical knowledge of the kind encouraged by exams, is necessary but not enough by itself.
2. The streamlining and automatic use of basic clinical routines

take time and considerable self-analysis if it is to be effective. *Practise* in *practice* is essential. There is no substitute for this.

This book aims to help the student in this self analytical learning process by outlining the knowledge, skills and attitudes involved.

Part I (pp. 1–144) of the book should be read first. This describes briefly the skills and attitudes needed by the family doctor.

- Chapter 1 outlines the goals and basic job of the primary physician. It stresses the differences between hospital practice and primary care and describes some of the dilemmas which face a doctor when entering general practice.
- Chapter 2 describes how the clinical process of diagnosis and prognosis is adapted from the hospital to the primary situation.
- Chapter 3 describes the family doctor's contribution to prevention and health education, i.e. what is practical in this developing but neglected 'Cinderella' of all modern health care systems.
- Chapters 4 and 5 describe the development and behaviour of the normal individual. These chapters stress the important and practical requirements of what is sometimes called 'Whole person medicine'.
- Chapter 6 is an extension of the two previous chapters and discusses the relationship of the normal individual to the family and community. The wider community networks which the family doctor must know and learn are described.
- Chapter 7 and the appendices outline the tools of general practice which the family doctor must know and learn to use, e.g. the consultation, the hospital, the practice, the use of computers, audit, etc.

Part II (pp. 147–750 comprises the bulk of the book and is the most important part. It is not intended for continous reading but should be used, in practice, as a *field guide*.

After or during any consultation one or two diagnoses can be looked up and the relevant options and decisions can be checked or discussed with a trainer. Family practice encompasses so many such options which are difficult to remember that I frequently use this book as a check list for my own decisions!

THE DIAGNOSTIC VOCABULARY OF PRIMARY CARE

The concept of a *diagnostic vocabulary* helps both to understand and to teach primary care. The questioning of colleagues and the work of Elstein et al (Ref. 1.0) suggest that most practising clinicians, when presented with any patient's complaint, automatically recall from their diagnostic vocabulary about two to four (rarely more) diagnostic possibilities, which they rank in order of probability. This list then guides their further questions and other actions which are aimed at refuting or confirming their initial ranking. As the clinician collects further information the rank order may be changed, or some items on the list replaced. In the primary care setting, few physicians appear to manipulate more than four diagnostic hypotheses at any one moment, but during a long clinical history they may have considered a much greater number of diagnostic possibilities.

The diagnostic vocabulary, used in this way by most clinicians, appears to have the following signficant characteristics:

- It forms the basis of the physician's clinical actions.
- The effective recall and manipulation of this vocabulary is the basis of the physician's skill and is the essential element that students must learn.
- The range of each clinician's working vocabulary is a measure of previous clinical experience. A premedical student starts with a layman's diagnostic vocabulary of perhaps 20 diseases: a family physician of 5 to 10 years' experience manipulates nearly 500. It would be helpful to know the appropriate expected vocabulary size at various stages between these two endpoints.
- The individual items of each experienced physician's vocabulary and the frequency of their usage are specific for the discipline practised by the physician. Both these parameters are identifiable and measureable for any physician. They therefore have significant implications for the teaching and administration of that discipline. Thus a neurosurgeon, obstetrician, and family physician are, in effect, talking different languages, in a way that can be identified.
- 'Disuse atrophy' of a physician's range of vocabulary appears to follow: (a) diminished clinical experience (b) lack of adequate continuing medical education (c) ageing of the physician. Measurements of vocabulary range and frequency of usage could thus be used to assess any physician's post graduate needs.

For trainees the development of this vocabulary provides the basic framework on to which they will hang their changing clinical knowledge for the rest of their practising lives. Appendix VII (p. 710) analyses and lists the diagnostic vocabulary (475 diagnostic labels) used by 10 family physicians.

EXPLANATIONS OF HEADINGS IN PART II

Like any student 'Field guide' each entry or diagnosis has the same format. The different headings provide check lists of the clinical knowledge that is relevant to each diagnostic label.

The Down's Syndrome entry on page 658 provides an example.

AETIOLOGY

Enough information is given to enable the doctor to give an accurate explanation to a patient or relative. In the case of Down's Syndrome the explanation is longer than for many other entries because knowledge of trisomy, translocation and mosaicism may be needed when explanations are given to well read parents.

DIAGNOSTIC RANGE

Information is given about commonness and probability. This information plays a crucial role in the required rapid recall.

In practice the doctor's recall of any diagnosis is related to his/her index of suspicion as well as the likelihood of occurrence, Thus, diagnoses such as cerebral tumour, (see p. 276), appendicitis, (see p. 468), pulmonary T.B., (see p. 147), must be suspected (recalled) much more often than they actually occur. Also in many diseases the doctor may suspect a disease and then decide that another diagnosis is more probable.

For the working family doctor it is important to know how often any diagnostic label should be 'suspected' as well as how often it is considered 'probable'. This information is given throughout Part II wherever possible. Using Down's Syndrome as an example the following rates per 1000 patients per year are given:

Personal: Suspected 2.0. Probable 1.0. *National*: Overall incidence* said to be 1:660 live births making it the commonest malformation in man.

These figures mean that in my personal practice of 2500 patients in any one year I would be looking after two to three patients with Down's Syndrome. The suspected figure of 2.0 would include these cases but indicates that in an additional two to three cases each year, the diagnosis would be suspected but not proven. These additional

**Reminder. Incidence rates:* a measure of morbidity based on the number of new episodes of illness arising in a population over an estimated period. Usually expressed in terms of sick persons per 1000 individuals at risk.

Prevalence rates: a measure of morbidity based on current sickness in a population, estimated either at a particular point in time or over a stated period. Usually expressed in terms of sick persons or episodes of sickness per 1000 individuals at risk.

cases might be (a) if elderly parents had had a negative amniocentesis (b) if the diagnosis had been considered and then abandoned in a new born baby.

Suspected rates always include the probable rates because this combined rate governs the family doctor's recall of the diagnostic label.

Wherever possible National figures for probable prevalence rates are also given. These are usually taken from the National Morbidity Survey (Ref. 0.2) or as in the Down's example, from another reliable source.

CLINICAL POINTERS

These numbered pointers indicate those clinical signs and symptoms which the family doctor must carry in his head and which stimulate diagnostic recall or which guide the doctor's further questioning or examination.

High risk factors, e.g. previous attacks, contact cases or, as in the case of Down's, 'elderly parents' often trigger the doctor's recall and are listed first.

Wherever possible I have analysed my own experience to indicate how often these pointers are present. Thus if a doctor suspects a diagnosis of Down's, a poor Moro reflex (85%) or hypotonia (80%) are more specific pointers than a Simian Crease which is present in only 45% of probable cases. For common diseases such information has been obtained by analysing material from my practice, usually at least 25 cases. For rare diseases, such as Down's syndrome, I have used material from the literature.

THE DIFFERENTIAL DIAGNOSIS

This section further summarises the way in which the family doctor uses these pointers when weighing up likely diagnostic alternatives.

This practical approach is somewhat different from the exhaustive lists in medical textbooks.

INVESTIGATIONS

Providing a quick 'check list' of the investigational options open to most primary physicians.

DURATION AND COMPLICATIONS

These two headings form a basis for the doctor's decisions when preparing the patient for that which cannot be prevented or cured.

The Down's example illustrates the sort of factual information that a family doctor must learn from the literature to help parents.

MISLEADING FEATURES AND PITFALLS

One of the most informative teaching and learning areas. Significantly this section has changed little over the five editions (20 years) of this book. The many failures and mistakes in the Down's example are especially thought provoking.

MANAGEMENT OPTIONS

These have been included in this last edition because the doctor's retention of management alternatives is memorised by linking them to the diagnostic label. For effective practise these options must be available for instant recall.

Management options are then weighed and tailored to the patient's needs.

In the case of Down's Syndrome, amniocentesis may not always be available and the handling of the parents' problems will vary according to their personalities and attitudes.

Every family doctor needs management check lists because important options, e.g. preventive advice, proper explanations, etc., may be 'crowded out' under the pressures of work load.

For quick reference all therapeutic decisions have been related to the appropriate paragraph of the BNF (Ref. 0.1) which provides doctors with an up to date summary of dose, side effects, cross sensitivities and cost.

INDEX

As with any 'field guide' much useful data, check lists, management options, etc., are scattered throughout Part II. Thus the address of the Mentally Handicapped Association is listed under Down's Syndrome and in the references which gives the addresses of other self-help groups in Britain. The index provides a further key to such information.

I would like to add that despite a strong belief in the equality of the sexes I have found it impractical to use the clumsy, bisexual terms 'he/she', 'his/hers', 'himself/herself' etc. I apologise for the many places in the text where I have assumed that he and she are interchangeable.

PART ONE

1

The general practitioner's job

The obligations and objectives of every general practitioner involve two often conflicting but essential elements:

— identify and resolve the health problems of each individual patient;
— deliver an effective medical service to the community as a whole.

Historically doctors have concentrated their efforts mainly on individual patient care. Recently, as governments and communities have become more sophisticated, an increasing need has been recognised for cost-effective community-based medical programmes. These programmes should include prevention, health education and community support services such as home care facilities, day hospitals, etc.

Perhaps the best and simplest definition of the general practitioner's job is that he should provide *personal health care that is primary, continuous and comprehensive*. This basic description can then be expanded to suit the needs of different communities and countries.*

Let us look briefly at the four descriptive elements of this definition.

*The Royal College of Practitioners (United Kingdom) defines the general practitioner as — 'A doctor who provides personal, primary and continuing medical care to individuals and families. He attends his patients in their homes, in his consulting rooms, or in hospital. He accepts the responsibility for making initial decisions on every problem his patient may present to him, consulting with specialists when he thinks this appropriate. He will usually work in a group with other general practitioners from premises that are built for (or modified for) the purpose, with the help of paramedical colleagues, adequate secretarial staff and all the equipment which is necessary. Even if he is single-handed he will work in a team and delegate when necessary. His diagnosis will be composed in physical, psychological and social terms. He will intervene educationally, preventively and therapeutically to promote his patients' health'. (Ref. 1.1)

A. Personal health care
B. Primary care
C. Continuous care
D. Comprehensive care.

A. Personal health care

This implies a close rapport betwen the patient and doctor.

The doctor must be able, with empathy, to see all the patient's problems from the patient's viewpoint. He must attempt to solve these problems, not in terms of a healthy or unhealthy body, but in 'whole person' terms similar to those that he applies to himself or his friends.

If this skill of seeing the patient as a whole person is to be acquired by any physician he must develop an ability to evaluate objectively and with humility his own performance and personal biases. Self-evaluation is the essential foundation of all evaluation and of effective learning.

B. Primary care

Primary care is the care which any community considers should be handled by the doctor of first contact. The essential point here is that the nature and extent of primary care is decided by the community not the physician. Community constraints may be cultural, social or economic. Thus the nature of primary care in different situations will vary greatly. In a sophisticated urban practice a general practitioner will see and treat a wide variety of behavioural problems; at the other extreme in a primitive setting the patients might consult the primary physician about physical illness only and take their psychological problems to the local witch doctor.

Secondary and tertiary care are both based on the hospital. They achieve their considerable results because the doctors in hospital are able to control and manipulate the patient and his environment. The patient has temporarily and voluntarily abrogated his freedom, at the same time granting to the physician a significant licence to intervene.

A major 'flu epidemic illustrates the relative positions. The primary physician must see 10 times the usual number of patients while the hospital limits admission by announcing that all its beds are filled.

The boundaries of primary care in any community are fixed at one extreme by the patients who decide what problems they wish to bring to the profession and at the other extreme by the availability of secondary care facilities. In rural or urban communities which cannot afford the luxury of extensive secondary care, the primary physician has a very wide range of responsibilities which is gladly shared as soon as the appropriate specialist is available. In rich urban communities, lacking a comprehensive service, the position of primary care often becomes confused because the specialist frequently wishes to provide primary care; such care is often neither continuous nor comprehensive. Thus a patient with backache may have to decide whether to see a psychiatrist, an orthopaedic surgeon or a gynaecologist. In this case, if the patient chooses the wrong specialist considerable effort and money may be wasted before the patient is referred to the correct doctor. The system is wasteful in manpower, expensive for the community and leads to an excess of specialists and unsatisfactory *dual care*, with two doctors giving different advice at the same time.

These points are stressed because they cause many misunderstandings about the extent of primary care which is not *absolute* but must always depend on the community served.

'Ambulatory care' is a confusing term which is usually used to refer to patients who walk into hospital. It is unsatisfactory because it is nonspecific and may be used to cover acutely ill moribund emergencies as well as chronically disabled patients who would be best supported and treated in their own homes.

C. Care is continuous

There are several significant effects of continuous care:

- *Data collection is cumulative*. Frequently the doctor knows a great deal about the patient's personality, previous history and background *before* the patient reports. Thus an urgent telephone message at 10 p.m. will state, simply, 'Please come, father is being difficult again.' When linked to the cumulative knowledge in the primary physician's memory this comes to life as a very reasonable and urgent call:

Father is a diabetic who gets violent when he is hypoglycaemic, refuses to take sugar and beats up his long-suffering wife who has many health problems that have followed an atrioseptal defect. Further relevant information is also recalled about many facets of the total family situation.

Thus to an observer, general practitioner history-taking may often appear superficial when, in fact, major clinical decisions are being based on data already known.

This previous knowledge cues the doctor to assess the patients' complaints in a way that is different in hospital where such knowledge is often not available. Prior knowledge does not necessarily help clinical judgements but must always be taken into account.

- Time can be used diagnostically to sift out trivial and serious disease (see Ch. 2, p. 46).
- Long-term feedback about both diagnosis and treatment is available and tends to make the general practitioner circumspect about the achievements of modern medicine. The family physician lives with his mistakes as well as the successes.
- The general practitioner is aware of the patient's active life in home and community.
- The patient and practitioner are dependent on community support services, e.g. home care programmes health visitors, public health nurses, relatives, neighbours, etc.
- The doctor shares the same community and knows its advantages and disadvantages, e.g. which schools are good, which factories have shut and what the local football team is doing.

The patient as well as the doctor must accept the advantages of continuous care. If the difficulties and dangers of dual care are not recognised by the community, patients tend to 'shop around' and it is possible for a patient to get conflicting advice and treatment for the same complaint from several doctors at once.

D. Care is comprehensive

The comprehensive obligations of primary care to patients and community create the main clinical challenge that faces the general practitioner.

This book aims to describe one general practitioner's perspective view of the wide spectrum of knowledge, skills and attitudes that must be integrated by every individual general practitioner who attempts to fulfill these comprehensive obligations.

The young practitioner starting work in any community must acquire and learn to integrate knowledge, skills and attitudes in three main areas.*

*These three areas broadly cover the five areas put forward by the Royal College of General Practitioners: (1) clinical practice — health and disease, (2) clinical practice — human development, (3) clinical practice — human behaviour, (4) medicine and society, (5) the practice. (Ref. 1.1)

Area I Basic clinical knowledge. Has three broad elements:

— The natural history and management of disease (Part II)
— Normal human development (Ch. 4)
— Normal human behaviour (Chs. 5 and 6)

Area II Knowledge and expectations of the society served. Every community is different but the broad principles and dilemmas are discussed. (Chs. 6 and 7).

Area III The tools for the job. The practitioner must be able to use, modify, develop and create the tools he needs. (Ch. 7 and Appendices II, III, IV and V).

The patient's interests can easily become lost in this wide spectrum of knowledge, skills and attitudes. The family doctor must constantly bear in mind that making accurate predictions is the basis of effective primary care. This applies as much to a case of industrial compensation or suspected battering (NAI) as it does to one of cancer.

This account of the general practitioner's job has emphasised the significance of the personal, primary, comprehensive and continuing elements. Specialists and physicians working mainly in hospital may rightly consider that some of what has been said applies also to patient care in hospital. This is true but in any efficient health care delivery system the hospital and primary care elements should aim to have complementary as well as mutually supportive roles.

Figure 1 illustrates the complementary nature of the case material. Table 1 shows the complementary and mutually supportive roles of primary and hospital care.

The complementary nature of primary and hospital care does not mean that the student's hospital training is misplaced or unnecessary. On the contrary, hospital is the one place where a student can get really close to disease and so learn best those principles of clinical medicine which will be his main asset in general practice.

If the complementary aspect of primary care is to be fully understood, the doctor must recognise those dilemmas that create the present challenge of general practice.

The brief summary of these 'dilemmas' underlines the importance of primary care and stresses that considerable changes of present day medical attitudes are needed.

THE MAIN DILEMMAS OF PRIMARY CARE

I. The dilemma of increasing expectations and diminishing returns.

Table 1 Complementary aspects of primary and hospital care

Primary care	Secondary and tertiary (hospital) care
Patient	
Patient initiates and motivates care	Patient voluntarily abrogates many freedoms
Patient freedom high (independent)	Patient freedom relatively low (dependent)
Patient can relate easily to a single doctor	Difficult for patient to relate to one doctor
Patient secure in his own environment	Patient insecure in foreign environment.
Doctor	
Doctor has relatively little control	Doctor control high
Doctors have to be relatively non-directive	Doctors have to be directive
Doctors responsible for a relatively large community of patients	Doctors required to concentrate extensive resources on relatively small numbers of patients
Doctor is 'cued' by prior knowledge of the patient	Doctor has little prior knowledge of patient
Doctor must know the community 'network'	Doctor must know the hospital 'network'
Clinical	
Trivial disease frequent	Trivial disease rare
Serious disease (a) relatively rare (b) presentation confused by presence of non-serious disease (c) clinical presentation undifferentiated and early diagnosis difficult	Serious disease (a) relatively common (b) presentation confused with other *serious* disease (c) clinical presentation more differentiated.
Continuity	
Data collection cumulative	Data collection episodic
Background of patient often known to doctor before patient presents	Doctor often has no prior knowledge of patient's background
Dual care often uncontrolled	Dual care controlled by doctors
Comprehensiveness	
Doctor must know a little about everything	Doctor must know everything about a special area
Patient expects doctor to help with very wide range of problems	Patient expects doctor to help with relatively narrow range of problems
Economics	
Patient responsible for own nursing accommodation and upkeep	Hospital has to be funded for nursing accommodation and upkeep
Relatively inexpensive	*Relatively costly to patient and/or community*

II. The dilemma of inverse care, i.e. that disease is usually correlated with poverty while appropriate support services correlate with affluence.

III. The dilemma of service, i.e. the conflict between community and individual needs.

IV. The dilemma of early diagnosis — early diagnosis is the most difficult.
V. The dilemma of uncertainty, i.e., the need to take decisions based on insufficient data.
VI. The dilemma of change. Every doctor's skill is based on past experiences; changes in the present continually render this experience inappropriate.

A closer look at the nature of these dilemmas indicates the direction in which primary care should develop and underlines the point made by Maxwell (Ref. 1.2) that communities with a strong primary care service tend to develop health care systems that are both cost effective and comprehensive.

I. THE DILEMMA OF INCREASING EXPECTATIONS AND DIMINISHING RETURNS

This dilemma stems from the fact that doctors are continually trying to frustrate a basic natural law — survival of the fittest. The more people we keep alive, the more medical problems arise. Geriatrics and paediatrics are particularly good examples of this dilemma. A spectacular operation for spina bifida on a baby saves a life but presents parents, patients, community nurses and primary care physicians with major problems that may persist for many decades after the original operation.

Thus the United Kingdom spends 5.5% of its GNP on health; USA spends nearly twice this percentage — equivalent to a per capita expenditure of nearly four times that for the UK (Ref. 1.3). Despite this the average British patient appears to get better value for money in most essential areas (Ref. 1.2). Thus there is universal low cost accessibility for *all* socio-economic groups, e.g. preventive services and those for the aged and needy. In contrast, doctors in the USA can earn two to four times that earned by their British equivalent.

We are painfully and slowly discovering that communities can waste a great deal of money if the wrong priorities in health care are encouraged.

Possible methods of resolving this dilemma

Complete resolution of this dilemma is impossible. The best that we can do is to achieve a satisfactory balance between our main priorities and our available resources of manpower and money. To

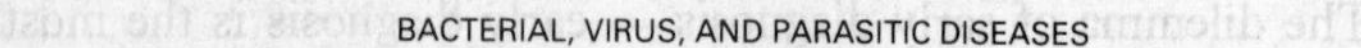

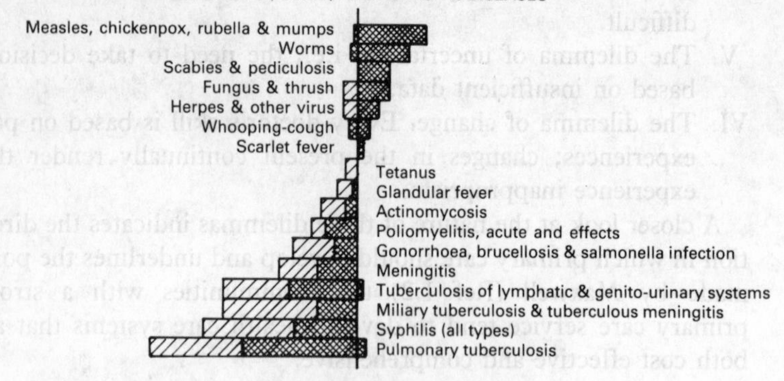

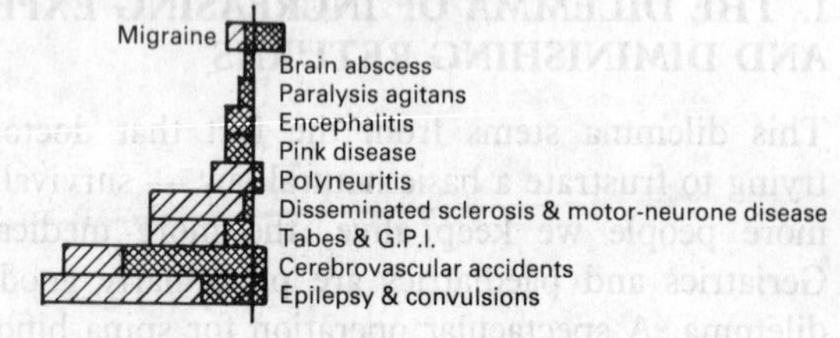

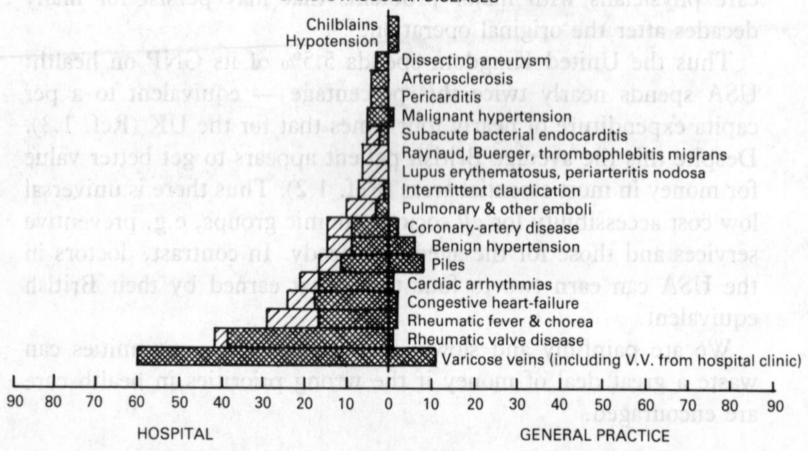

Fig. 1 Examples of my experience in hospital as a student and intern compared with that in one year of general practice as a family doctor.

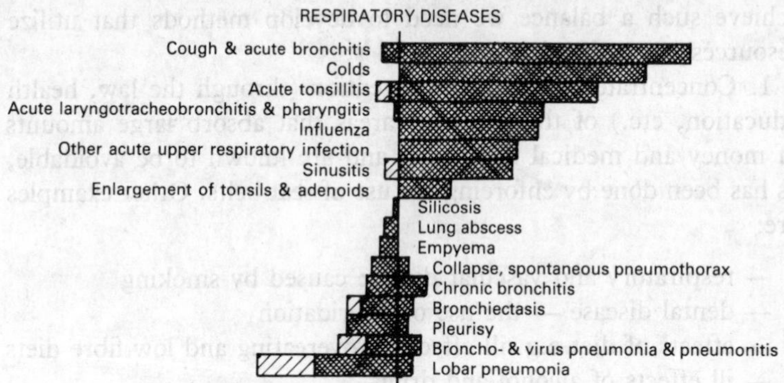
RESPIRATORY DISEASES
Cough & acute bronchitis
Colds
Acute tonsillitis
Acute laryngotracheobronchitis & pharyngitis
Influenza
Other acute upper respiratory infection
Sinusitis
Enlargement of tonsils & adenoids
Silicosis
Lung abscess
Empyema
Collapse, spontaneous pneumothorax
Chronic bronchitis
Bronchiectasis
Pleurisy
Broncho- & virus pneumonia & pneumonitis
Lobar pneumonia

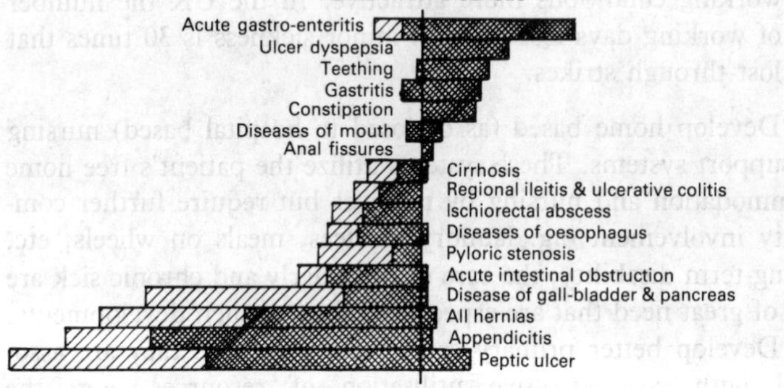
ALIMENTARY DISEASES
Acute gastro-enteritis
Ulcer dyspepsia
Teething
Gastritis
Constipation
Diseases of mouth
Anal fissures
Cirrhosis
Regional ileitis & ulcerative colitis
Ischiorectal abscess
Diseases of oesophagus
Pyloric stenosis
Acute intestinal obstruction
Disease of gall-bladder & pancreas
All hernias
Appendicitis
Peptic ulcer

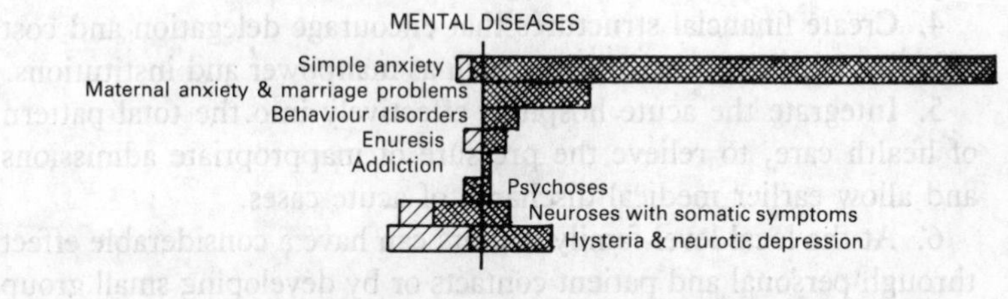
MENTAL DISEASES
Simple anxiety
Maternal anxiety & marriage problems
Behaviour disorders
Enuresis
Addiction
Psychoses
Neuroses with somatic symptoms
Hysteria & neurotic depression

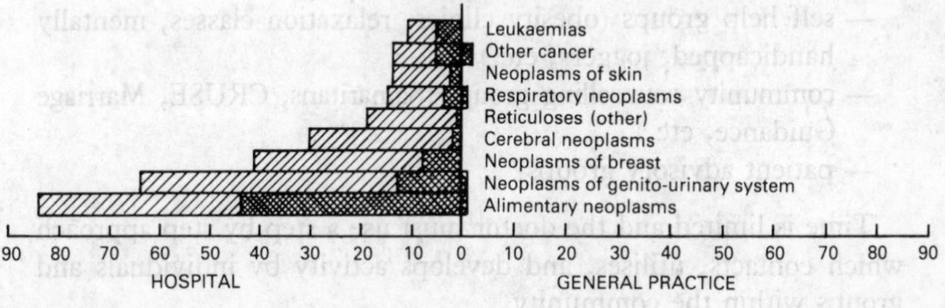
MALIGNANT DISEASES
Leukaemias
Other cancer
Neoplasms of skin
Respiratory neoplasms
Reticuloses (other)
Cerebral neoplasms
Neoplasms of breast
Neoplasms of genito-urinary system
Alimentary neoplasms
90 80 70 60 50 40 30 20 10 0 10 20 30 40 50 60 70 80 90
HOSPITAL
GENERAL PRACTICE

achieve such a balance we need to develop methods that utilize resources most effectively:

1. Concentrate on effective prevention (through the law, health education, etc.) of those disease areas that absorb large amounts of money and medical manpower and are known to be avoidable, as has been done by enforcing the use of seat belts. Other examples are:

— respiratory and vascular disease caused by smoking
— dental disease — the use of fluoridation
— effects of diet e.g. ill effects of overeating and low fibre diets
— ill effects of alcohol and drugs
— prevention of absenteeism due to minor sickness by making working conditions more attractive. In the UK the number of working days lost through minor sickness is 30 times that lost through strikes.

2. Develop home based (as opposed to hospital based) nursing and support systems. These systems utilize the patient's free home accommodation and nursing by relatives but require further community involvement e.g. laundry services, meals on wheels, etc.

Long-term disability, the care of the elderly and chronic sick are areas of great need that are especially suited to such developments.

3. Develop better primary care systems because they are associated with cost effective utilisation of resources, e.g. the community health team is cheaper than hospital care.

4. Create financial structures that encourage delegation and cost effective use of expensive items such as manpower and institutions.

5. Integrate the acute hospitals effectively into the total pattern of health care, to relieve the pressure of inappropriate admissions and allow earlier medical discharge of acute cases.

6. At the local level family doctors can have a considerable effect through personal and patient contacts or by developing small group activities, e.g.

— self help groups (obesity clinics, relaxation classes, mentally handicapped, joggers, etc.)
— community counselling groups (Samaritans, CRUSE, Marriage Guidance, etc.)
— patient advisory groups.

Time is limited and the doctor must use a step by step approach which contacts, utilises, and develops activity by individuals and groups within the community.

II. THE INVERSE CARE DILEMMA

Need for care is greatest when an individual's financial resources are at risk. This applies to rich and poor alike because medical need is maximal when individuals are not earning, i.e. as children, in sickness, pregnancy and old age. For this reason any free enterprise system of health care delivery may fail at times of greatest need.

There are two other reasons why simple market forces fail to produce an efficient service in the health care field:

a. The medical profession has a virtual monopoly position. (Individual advertisement, bargaining and other routine market procedures are discouraged).
b. The 'customer' is dependent on the 'shopkeeper' for assessment of need.

Possible methods of resolving this dilemma

1. Private insurance schemes are only partial solutions.

They have the following disadvantages:

— Poor people rarely have the money or the cultural tradition to support such schemes.
— They are not comprehensive. Thus, many schemes only cover for 'hospital care', as a result, contributors may be admitted for expensive hospital care with only trivial diseases.
— In view of the escalating cost of the health care, premiums must be very large if cover is to be complete.

2. State run and state subsidised comprehensive and compulsory insurance schemes overcome many of these difficulties but still have the following disadvantages:

— May be misused and manipulated by both doctors and patients.
— They tend initially to be open ended; costs escalate, the State tends then to apply non-selective overall ceilings. These often act unfairly and inefficiently.
— The method of payment of doctors and staff who run the service may have many unexpected effects. (See comments below on financial influences.)

III. THE DILEMMA OF SERVICE

In any service, the demand of the individual and the community are often in conflict. This dilemma in simple form arises every time a doctor runs a *busy* clinic; the doctor's ability to provide an effective personal service to each patient conflicts with the wishes of all those patients who are kept waiting while such a service is given.

The 'free enterprise' solution requires that the doctor put up his fees; this will reduce demand and allow the doctor to give more of his time to individual patients. Unfortunately, this aggravates the inverse care dilemma.

This dilemma applies to the doctor's own personal life. The conflicts between the demands of work and family are well known to every doctor. These conflicts may be responsible for the higher rates of divorce, suicide, alcoholism and drug abuse which have been reported for doctors.

Possible methods of resolving this dilemma

1. Delegation. *Definition: Never do a job yourself that can be done as well or better by someone who is paid less*. This basic principle of good business management provides the key to enormous savings in health care costs without corresponding reduction in the standard of service. In Holland and England, most normal deliveries are carried out by midwives, not doctors. The infant and maternal mortality rates of these countries are among the lowest in the world.

Figure 4 (a) (p. 34) shows that 90% of patient contacts can be handled effectively in the community by a family physician. This has been shown by many primary care studies.

Many studies have shown that 20–40% of primary patient contacts can be handled by a properly trained practice nurse.

The intensive Canadian studies of the Family Practice Nurse (FPN) at McMaster have also fully demonstrated the clinical and economic effectiveness of the FPN and shown that the main barrier preventing their widespread use is financial loss to doctors who are paid by fee-for-service (Ref. 1.4).

IV. THE DILEMMA OF EARLY DIAGNOSIS

To be effective a diagnosis must be both accurate and early. Unfortunately, in any disease process, the earlier we make a diagnosis, the harder it is to be accurate. I have tried in this book to show how a general practitioner has attempted to solve this clinical dilemma.

It is sometimes implied that a family doctor's job is largely sociological and that his work is more like that of a social worker than a clinician. Even family doctors themselves will say sometimes that they treat symptoms and not disease. Nothing could be further from the truth, for every action that a family doctor takes should be based on his clinical observations from which he should try as soon as possible to make an accurate forecast, i.e. diagnosis and prognosis.

He must strive to recognise disease in its early stages and should not wait until the classical clinical picture develops. He must learn to act on suspicion, for if he waits for certainty he may delay too long.

Only by concentrating on the goals of prevention and earlier diagnosis will more effective, cheaper delivery of health care be achieved.

Most Western countries spend less than 10% of their total health budget on prevention of disease.

Possible methods of resolving this dilemma

1. Greater emphasis to be placed on preventive medicine by doctors, public health nurses, teachers, in education and the media. A brief glance at the preventative Management Options throughout Part II emphasises the scope for this in Primary Care.

2. Development of wider community diagnostic and support services. Day hospitals for geriatric or psychiatric patients are a good example of this.

3. Extension of present auditing techniques, with greater concentration on the difficult problems of measuring and comparing the outcome of medical activity.

V. THE DILEMMA OF LEARNING TO HANDLE UNCERTAINTY

Each of the four previously discussed dilemmas creates large grey areas with many alternative courses of action.

The experienced general practitioner must be continually able to assess and criticize his own levels of uncertainty. Thus if he tolerates too high a level he will become 'out of date' and refer too few patients; if he is too sensitive he will refer too many and will be unable to make responsible decisions that are in his patients' best interests.

The effective general practitioner throughout his life is restlessly trying to reduce and improve his handling of clinical uncertainty by:

— constant contact with colleagues in general practice
— discussion with specialists

— relevant and continued postgraduate education and reading
— practice activity analysis, audit and self criticism (see Appendix IV, p. 693)
— developing the habit of making rapid checks after each consultation of what has been advised and why.

VI. THE DILEMMA OF CHANGE

Every primary physician's confidence is based on previous experience. Changes in knowledge and attitudes often render such experience out of date. If a doctor does not come to terms with this dilemma he easily becomes blind to the inappropriateness of both his understanding and his counsel.

Two areas of primary care are especially affected by this dilemma:

1. Technical expertise, i.e. new drugs and new techniques are constantly being developed.

2. Changes in lifestyle and community pressures, i.e. attitudes to sex, unemployment, etc.

Changes in the first area are dealt with directly by continuing postgraduate education. Changes in the second area pose a greater difficulty. The doctor must learn to welcome and enjoy solving new and unexpected patient problems.

The doctor should be alert to areas of change.

Areas of change in patient attitudes:

— Changing view about the role of women, sex, marriage and the family
— Changing attitudes to old age, unemployment and ethnic groups
— Increasing demands, by patients, for greater participation in medical decision making
— Increasing patient dissatisfaction with authoritarian medical attitudes, especially in relation to prescribing, health education and the handling of major life events
— Greater demand for preventive and therapeutic counselling.

Areas of change in doctor attitudes:

— Recognition of a greater need to treat the patient as a whole personality

— Recognition that support and comfort to assist the everyday living of patients with prolonged illness is as necessary as relieving symptoms or giving reassurance
— Recognition that it is often counter productive if doctors remain rigidly and emotionally detached from their patients' problems
— Recognition that self audit and self criticism are essential parts of primary care
— Changing attitudes to work and the health care team.

There is a piece-meal approach to many of these problems which is unsatisfactory. Alterations in training based on further research are needed if widespread permanent alterations of medical attitudes are to be achieved.

FINANCIAL INFLUENCES IN PRIMARY CARE

Methods of payment provide one of the most powerful ways of influencing what individuals and professions do. From an administration point of view, management recognises two basic types of payment. (Ref. 1.5)

1. Payment which encourages service to the individual:

— direct payment by patient on a fee-for-service (piecework) basis
— fee-for-service payment by insurance scheme, either private or state (as in Canada and New Zealand).

2. Payment which encourages services to groups as a whole:

— sessional
— capitation
— full-time salary.

1. Direct or item-of-service payment.

Advantages:
- Said to encourage a personalised service.
- High job satisfaction for doctors.
- Patient criticism and participation is greater.

Disadvantages:
- Encourages a disease approach that emphasises care in ill health to the detriment of prevention and health education.
- Patients tend to 'shop around' using inadequate or inappropriate medical knowledge.

- Discourages delegation.
- Encourages doctors to collect where population is greatest. Thus, in big cities, specialists can support themselves doing general practice while they establish themselves in consultant practice. Big cities may then have an excess of specialists to the detriment of other areas.
- Service is open-ended and decisions about number of items required for any incident of illness are difficult to establish and are in the hands of the profession. This may be a good thing but is open to misuse from overservicing.

2. Payment which encourages service to a group as a whole — sessional, capitation and full-time salary.

Advantages:

- Encourages delegation and the Community Health Team approach.
- Encourages prevention and health education.
- Encourages community support services and systems that keep patients in the community and out of hospital.
- Salaries can be adjusted to achieve better distribution of doctors.
- The population cared for by any family doctor is known. This has dramatic effects on the ability to specify rates of all kinds, on research, on measurements of outcome and ultimately on the effects of prevention and priorities.

Disadvantages:

- May discourage a personalised service.
- No financial incentive for doctors who perform extra items of service. Patients may be underserviced.
- Discourages patient participation in decisions.

Reduction of costs by different methods of payment

Diagrammatic models of the two largest items in any health care budget help to demonstrate the way money can used to influence the quality of health care delivery.

These two items are: 1. salaries
2. cost of running hospitals and other institutions.

Each of these areas can be represented diagrammatically as a pyramid or hierarchy (Fig. 2) in which the elements at the top are relatively few and costly while the elements at the base are universal and free.

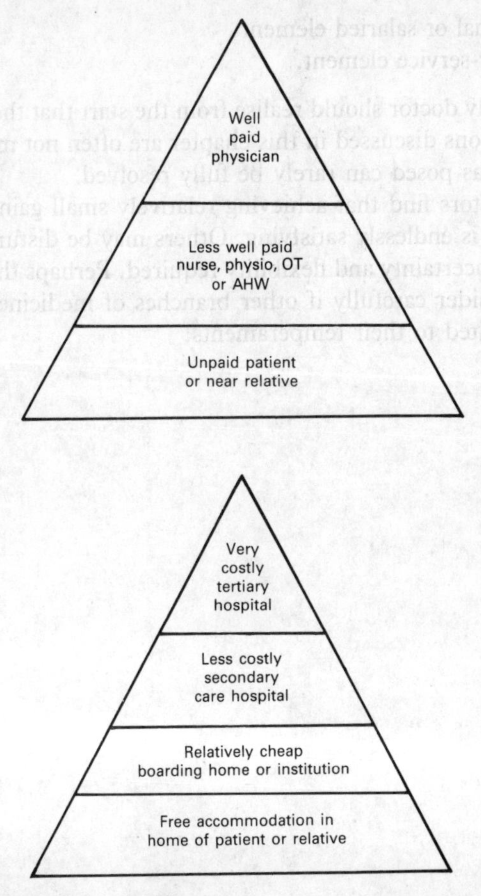

Fig. 2 Pyramids of costs in health care

Clearly, if *effective* medical care can be kept close to the bases of both pyramids, the savings could be considerable. It is unfortunate that any fee-for-service system of payments encourages the concentration of care near the top of the pyramid. Thus delegation is discouraged and expensive institutional beds of all kinds may be kept filled for poorly defined financial reasons.

A satisfactory delivery of health care has yet to be achieved. It would seem that the salaries of all health care personnel (including doctors) should include three elements:

— pension and retirement plans combined with repayment of training expenses

— sessional or salaried element
— fee-for-service element.

The family doctor should realise from the start that the objectives and obligations discussed in this chapter are often not met and that the dilemmas posed can rarely be fully resolved.

Most doctors find that achieving relatively small gains in such a varied field is endlessly satisfying. Others may be disturbed by the degree of uncertainty and flexibility required. Perhaps these doctors should consider carefully if other branches of medicine might not be more suited to their temperaments.

2

Diagnosis and prognosis in general practice: the diagnostic process

'It is, in my opinion, a most excellent thing for the physician to practise forecasting.'

— Hippocrates

Diagnosis and prognosis are the doctor's forecast of what is likely to happen. As Hippocrates realised, prediction is the most important clinical skill that a doctor can develop.

This cannot be too strongly emphasised. All too frequently clinicians regard their diagnoses as absolute; such an attitude prevents the doctor from improving his clinical practice by checking his predictions. Follow-up procedures tend to be either delegated or omitted. Diagnostic predictions are rarely sufficiently certain to justify such omissions.

The whole natural world is repetitive. Man is constantly identifying and re-identifying repetitive patterns so that he can predict future events to his advantage. We call this 'learning to use our experience' and for convenience and ease of communication we name each pattern.

Once named, these labels are built up to form a vocabulary to which we link further facts for future recall (see Introduction).

DIAGNOSIS AND PATTERN RECOGNITION

Recognition of disease is similar to the recognition of faces. Thus if we are looking for a friend in a crowd we need just the right amount of information — not too much, not too little and, most essential, we need to have been sensitised previously to the friend's facial characteristics. To know three salient early features about a disease is often more helpful for recognition purposes than to remember three pages of text. On the other hand, in every case we need enough clinical information from the patient to generate in our mind two or three relevant diagnostic hypotheses which we can then test by further data collection.

PREVIOUS SENSITISATION

As with faces, even when we have just the right amount of information, recognition is greatly assisted if we have seen the pattern before.

As in looking for a needle in a haystack, it is essential that we know (a) the salient features of the needle and (b) a great deal about the appearance of the hay.

All this adds up to one simple fact — effective diagnostic pattern recognition can only be learned in context. This is as true for primary care as it is for radiology or pathology.

DIAGNOSIS AS A HYPOTHESIS

In general practice our diagnostic terms have a strongly anatomical flavour and it is essential that we counter this bias by attempting whenever possible to relate our diagnostic labels to the pathology which underlies disease. Pathology is the common denominator of all diagnostic labels; diagnoses such as old age, chill, abdominal pain, headache and 'not surgical' are best avoided. GPs often have to be satisfied with diagnosis at anatomical level, e.g. 'bronchitis' or 'tracheitis', but this should not prevent them continually striving to achieve the greater clinical accuracy of diagnosis at the pathological level, e.g. 'Influenza A virus infection.'

Fifty years ago, before a distinction had been made between angina pectoris and myocardial infarction, only angina was recognised — a diagnosis which gave the doctor some idea of the likely course of events. The invention of the cardiograph led to the recognition of myocardial infarction and the doctor was able to predict the course of events with greater accuracy. The doctors had invented a new diagnosis but not a new disease.

We often talk about a provisional diagnosis; this is a repetition of terms since every diagnosis is provisional and it is only our intellectual arrogance which assumes that our knowledge is so complete that diagnosis and disease are synonymous.

It is clear that a diagnosis is a hypothesis and therefore a scientific approach is possible. In a scientific experiment we begin by clearly stating our hypothesis of the predicated course of events — we then observe the actual course of events. Finally we test the accuracy of our hypothesis by comparing the predicted with the observed results. Exactly this process is used by doctors when making a diagnosis.

As soon as we have questioned and examined a patient, and are about to take further action, i.e., order special investigations or treatment, we should state clearly on the patient's notes our diagnostic reasons for action. At every subsequent contact with the patient we can then test or modify our original diagnostic hypothesis according to the observed facts. I also like to emphasise all such diagnostic reasons for action by (a) circling them and (b) keeping them to the right side of the record (see p. 131).

This rule of writing down at all times our diagnostic reasons for all actions taken forces a doctor to think logically and act scientifically. In general practice it makes a tremendous impact on our standard of medicine.

The medical record is converted from a memory aid into a basic clinical tool capable of analysis and comparison. The record over the years will collect a sequence of clinical predictions; as time passes triumphs and failures become apparent and the card will be seen as a vital part of clinical integrity that can be used for teaching and research.

Nature has provided us with a surprisingly comprehensive 'early warning system' of symptoms and signs, yet these are at best indirect and only rarely correlate exactly with a particular disease process.

The following example is taken from a practice population of 20 000 N.H.S. patients cared for by 10 doctors in northeast England (Ref. 2.1). A prospective study over a period of 9 months, showed that 351 adult patients reported recurrent symptoms of indigestion, i.e. heartburn, epigastric pain and nausea. 117 had been previously investigated and the presence of already established disease was confirmed. A further 144 complained of the three cardinal symptoms usually associated with a duodenal ulcer, i.e. epigastric pain, relief by food or alkalis, and periodicity. The remaining 90 patients had vague dyseptic complaints that were not specific for any particular disease process. Of the 144 patients with symptoms suggesting a duodenal ulcer, detailed barium studies, etc. revealed that a duodenal ulcer could be demonstrated in only 54, gastric ulcer was responsible for symptoms in three patients, reflux oesophagitis (or hiatus hernia) in 17, cholecystitis in three and in 67 patients radiological investigation failed to reveal any cause of symptoms.

A Venn diagram (Fig. 3) illustrates the diagnostic difficulties facing the clinician in such a situation.

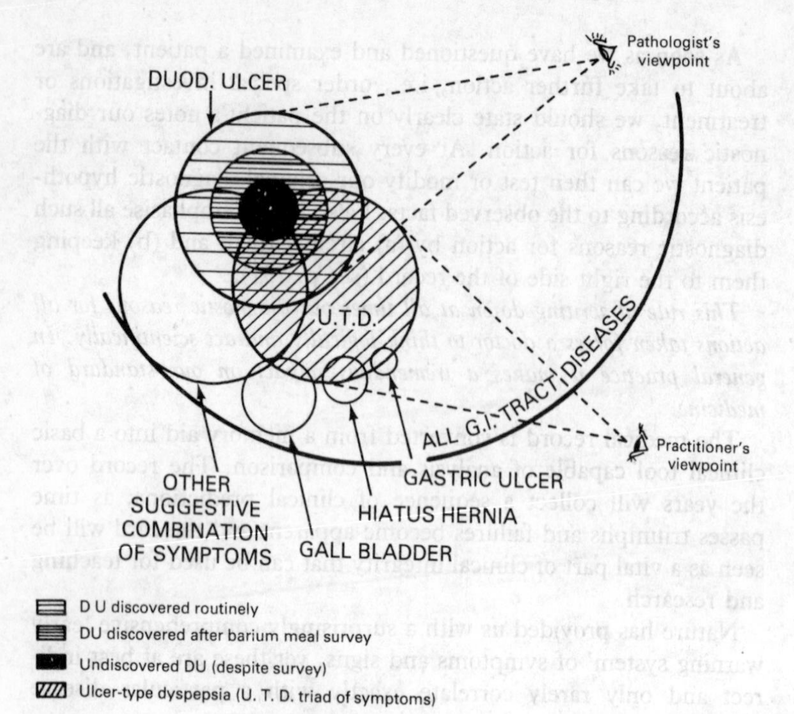

Fig. 3. Venn diagram illustrating the overlapping problems of diagnosis that relate to the diagnosis of duodenal ulcer.

We can see that a number of situations may arise in patients with a duodenal ulcer. There may be

— no symptoms at all
— vague secondary symptoms that are reported incidentally, i.e. heartburn
— primary symptoms that suggest a duodenal ulcer
— symptoms that suggest another disease.

This already complex situation may be further complicated because (a) in any of the above situations the ulcer crater may not be radiologically demonstrable, (b) other disease such as gastric ulcer, reflux oesophagitis or gall bladder disease may all sometimes produce the primary symptoms that suggest the presence of duodenal ulcer.

In such a situation it is not difficult to see why accurate diagnosis is so hard to achieve and why the repeated checking of diagnostic predictions is so essential. In the example just cited the doctor will learn most about the diagnosis of duodenal ulcer if he follows the 67 patients with suggestive symptoms and normal radiological findings. Follow up of the 117 patients already known to have an ulcer will teach him little about diagnosis although he will learn much about treatment and management.

A still further difficulty arises because patients may consciously or unconsciously distort symptoms. Thus patients who are afraid of cancer may either exaggerate or 'play down' their symptoms according to their personality or present fears.

All these variables make early diagnosis a very complex affair. It is easy to see why accurate, early diagnosis by computer or by the patient is likely to remain impractical for a long time.

Diagnostic predictions and the necessary follow-up checks should be recorded and retrievable. A simple method of record-keeping involving these steps is described on page 130 *et seq*.

Figure 1 demonstrates the different clinical material encountered in hospital and general practice. Figure 4a shows that in one year two doctors in northeast England made 13 755 diagnoses on 5767 NHS patients, 11.5% (1602) were referred to hospital specialists for further investigation, 20% (2746) were investigated by the general practitioners themselves, 68.5% (9407) were dealt with on a clinical basis alone. Figure 4b shows the spectrum of diagnoses used by these doctors.

The sifting of the small proportion of serious disease from this large mass of morbidity can be regarded as a two stage distillation process, i.e. primary stage in the community, secondary stage in the hospital. The general practitioner must use comparatively crude, quick, simple methods to provide the hospital with a suitably refined distillate. The hospital can then apply its own skills and complex techniques of diagnosis.

> EXAMPLE: In 20 years of practice I have encountered 12 patients with proven cerebral tumour; subsequent analysis revealed that in every case I had initially diagnosed the headache as a *tension headache*. I diagnose tension headache 200 times every year. If I refer every case of tension headache to hospital to exclude cerebral tumour I will clog the neurosurgical department.

The primary physician must develop simple but effective methods to decide who should be referred for detailed investigation. These methods are described in Part II and later in this chapter.

I propose to describe how the technique of diagnosis as learned by the student in hospital is modified to the needs of general prac-

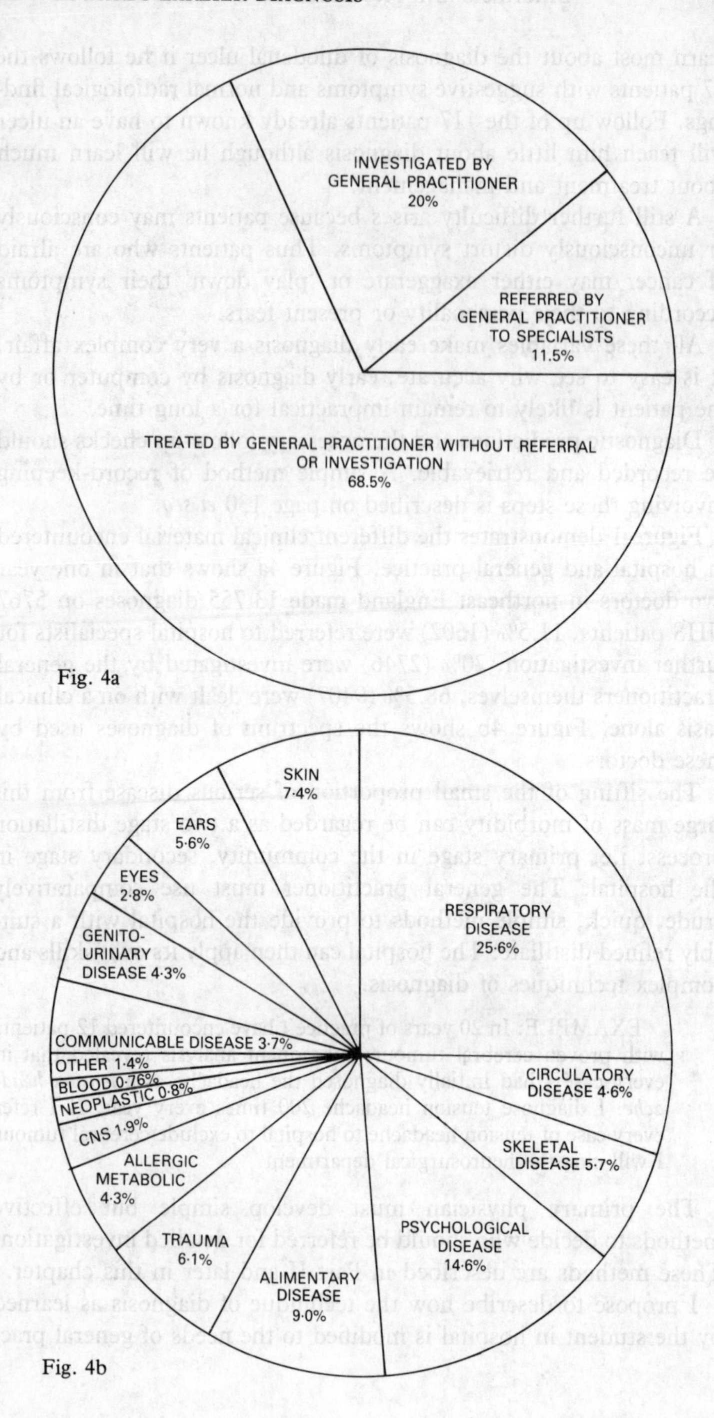
INVESTIGATED BY
GENERAL PRACTITIONER
20%
REFERRED BY
GENERAL PRACTITIONER
TO SPECIALISTS
11.5%
TREATED BY GENERAL PRACTITIONER WITHOUT REFERRAL
OR INVESTIGATION
68.5%

Fig. 4a

SKIN
7·4%
EARS
5·6%
EYES
2·8%
GENITO-
URINARY
DISEASE 4·3%
RESPIRATORY
DISEASE
25·6%
COMMUNICABLE DISEASE 3·7%
OTHER 1·4%
BLOOD 0·76%
NEOPLASTIC 0·8%
CNS 1·9%
CIRCULATORY
DISEASE 4·6%
SKELETAL
DISEASE 5·7%
ALLERGIC
METABOLIC
4·3%
TRAUMA
6·1%
PSYCHOLOGICAL
DISEASE
14·6%
ALIMENTARY
DISEASE
9·0%

Fig. 4b

tice. Before this is done it is essential to discuss the doctor's obligations to the patient when he makes a diagnosis.

DIAGNOSIS AND THE PATIENT — THE DOCTOR'S OBLIGATIONS

When a patient brings a problem to a doctor, the patient automatically gives the doctor a 'licence to intervene'. To understand the physician's obligations that are inherent in this transaction the following examples are helpful.

Let us suppose that you are standing beside a busy road when a man steps out in front of an oncoming car. You knock the man down, causing severe bruising, but prevent a serious accident. The stranger thanks you for your timely intervention. If the car is 200 metres away and you take identical action on the off chance of preventing a possible accident, the man may quite justifiably sue you for assault.

In the first example you are allowed considerable licence to intervene for two reasons:

1. Your predictions of serious consequences are both relevant and accurate
2. A serious accident is clearly prevented.

In the second example you are given no licence to intervene because:

1. Your predictions of serious consequences are uncertain and your consequent actions appear inappropriate
2. A life threatening situation is not imminent.

In medicine, the patient is less aware of both the risks and the predictive ability of the doctor's diagnosis. There is, therefore, a deep obligation for every doctor to relate his actions to his degree of predictive certainty about both prognosis and severity.

Doctors should remember that making a diagnosis does not automatically entitle them to intervene. In psychosocial areas, in some areas of geriatrics, paediatrics and surgery where diagnoses have a low predictive ability, the doctor is wise to be very circumspect before moving from data collection and non-directive counselling into the area of active intervention.

Clear discussion and explanation of all diagnostic issues with patients helps to ensure that the doctor recognises his obligations to all patients in this very significant area.

THE IMPORTANCE OF EARLY DISCUSSION AND EXPLANATION

A great many criticisms of the profession such as those raised by patients' associations, in the media and by Illych (Ref. 2.2) stem from the doctor's failure to give explanations and involve patients in discussion.

The family doctor should develop the habit at the end of every consultation of ensuring that rapport and interaction has been sufficient to:

— foster free discussion
— encourage the patient to ask questions
— allow full explanation.

With a little practice this can be done both quickly and well. Self-analysis of consultation using video (Appendix VIII) helps to eliminate some of the common pitfalls:

— the patient feels hurried by all the non-verbal signals, suggesting pressures of work load, which are put out by the doctor and staff
— the doctor's explanations are not tailored to the patient's needs, e.g. too patronising, too complex
— unexplained jargon is used to deter the patient from asking further questions
— apparent verbal encouragement is accompanied by simultaneous non-verbal discouragement, e.g. the doctor asks 'Any questions?' as he gets up to end the interview
— a prescription is given to the patient as a substitute for listening, explanation or discussion with the doctor
— the doctor fails to give an adequate explanation to the patient because he has not adequately faced up to his own uncertainties
— an authoritarian approach is used by the doctor when a non-directive one would be more appropriate.

THE TECHNIQUE OF MAKING A DIAGNOSIS

As his knowledge of disease and patients increases, the student learns to modify his basic routine to the stream-lined methods of the experienced doctor. He discovers that a surgeon only occasionally examines the chest of his patients and that physicians may omit a rectal examination. He learns this new technique by imitating each specialist in turn; often he is unaware of the principles underlying his changed methods. The friendly banter between physician and surgeon may even encourage him to think that the surgeon's omission is slipshod or the physician's failure to 'put his finger in' is due to fastidiousness. He does not realize that both surgeon and physician are following the same stream-lined method in which the patient's answers to questions guide them steadily towards the diagnosis.

Making a diagnosis involves two distinct mental processes.

1. Thinking of the diagnostic possibilities
2. Mentally working through the possibilities to see which fits the clinical facts.

In the streamlined diagnostic method the doctor takes the patient's history in such a way that it leads him to a small group of three or four possible diagnoses which he then tests or eliminates by examination and special investigation.

EXAMPLE: A patient complains of cough. French's index of diagnosis lists 93 possible causes of cough and is still not complete. No doctor can mentally work through this list. The doctor therefore obtains further information, i.e. duration of the cough and age of the patient, and so reduces the possible diagnoses.

A 50-year-old man with a cough of:

— five day's duration suggests a cold, 'flu' or acute bronchitis
— five week's duration suggests a bronchogenic carcinoma or pulmonary tuberculosis
— five years' duration suggests a smoker's cough, chronic bronchitis or bronchiectasis.

By using his knowledge of the natural history of disease, the doctor has reduced a large list of possibilities into small manageable groups of three or four possible hypotheses that can be tested.

Primary care physicians use three types of information to solve their patient's problems:

1. *Routine clinical information about the patient's complaints.* This is essentially the data base of the standard medical record and is equivalent to the subjective and objective elements of Weed's SOAP format, i.e. *S*ubjective data (history), *O*bjective data (physical examination and special investigations), *A*nalysis (diagnostic predictions and hypotheses) and *P*lan (management).

2. *Background knowledge of the patient, family and community.* In the continuous context of primary care this information is collected over many years and is of tremendous value to the general

practitioner. (An easily learnt quick method of recording background information is described in Appendix IX, p. 728).

3. *Natural history of common disease entities Part II*

(a) Age and sex distribution of disease.

(b) The commonness and geographical distribution: the commonest diseases occur most often; the rare symptoms of the common diseases are commoner than the common symptoms of the rare disease.

(c) The clinical pointers that enable us to recognise each disease: of these 'high risk factors' are often crucial.

1. OBTAINING ROUTINE CLINICAL INFORMATION ABOUT THE PATIENT'S PROBLEMS

The basic plan for obtaining and using this information involves the routine history taking procedure known to every student:

A. Gaining rapport and maintaining confidence
B. History of patient's present complaint
C. Systems or functional enquiry
D. Physical examination
E. Special investigation
F. Medical record.

A. Gaining and maintaining the patient's confidence

— listening, understanding and showing concerned interest
— knowing your job
— explaining your thoughts and actions in terms understandable to the patient.

This fundamental part of all consultations is all too often taken for granted. Patients want to have confidence in their doctor and every contact should increase this. Many factors (discussed on p. 118) are involved, but the most important is that the physician should make it clear that he is glad to see his patients. In return patients will place their faith and confidence in the doctor.

B. History of the patient's present complaints or problems

When a student first takes a medical history he may find that the patient's story bears little resemblance to the clear-cut histories given in lecture demonstrations, because the patient has little idea which symptoms are medically significant. The doctor must learn to distil the significant factors from the patient's story and from the clinical findings. He must learn to put aside some features and elaborate others.

ON SELECTION OF THE SIGNIFICANT SYMPTOMS

The crux of taking a history lies in the choice of symptoms which the doctor elaborates. If he chooses a symptom of little significance he may reach a wrong conclusion and will certainly waste time. It is possible for two doctors to interview a single patient and to obtain different histories because they have elaborated different symptoms.

The art of history-taking can only be learned by experience, but a few rules can be given about selection of the significant symptoms for elaborations.

- Elaborate those symptoms for which there is objective proof, e.g. haemoptysis or rash.
- Elaborate those symptoms which are localized to a specific organ or part of the body, e.g. cough, diarrhoea or pain.
- If two or more symptoms bear an obvious clinical relationship, e.g. haemoptysis and cough, further elaboration of both is indicated.
- Elaborate any symptom which is known to have a special diagnostic significance because it is specific evidence of a serious diasease, e.g. diplopia or convulsion.
- Put temporarily aside symptoms which are vaguely defined or which are known to arise in many diseases, e.g. dizziness, listlessness, anorexia in children, headache, etc.
- Put temporarily aside symptoms which obviously arise from causes not related to the main complaint and which can be dealt with separately, e.g. toothache in a patient with dyspnoea.

A symptom which the doctor has *put temporarily aside* may in fact be significant. For example, the symptom of headache may have been regarded as vague, ill-defined evidence of mental tension. The systematic enquiry may later reveal unexplained loss of appetite or diplopia. The possibility of a space-occupying lesion in the skull is raised and the headache becomes a significant localizing symptoms. The doctor should ensure that (a) all the symptoms are *recorded* — this keeps them constantly before his notice; (b) an *explanation* of all the symptoms is given to the patient at the end of the consultation — this reassures the patient and ensures that the doctor has explained all the symptoms in his own mind.

ON ELABORATION OF THE SYMPTOMS SELECTED

This skill is the unique and essential element of the medical interview which requires long practice and continued updating if it is to be effectively used.

All students learn the seven steps of symptom elaboration. BASTARD provides a useful mnemonic check list.

*B*odily location, site and radiation
*A*mount, i.e. severity of pain or quantity of sputum
*S*tart, nature of onset, etc.
*T*iming i.e. duration, frequency and duration of attacks
*A*ggravating *A*nd *A*lleviating factors
*R*elated symptoms
*D*escription of symptom. Sputum frothy, coffee ground, etc.

Students should learn that this structured cross questioning technique may be threatening to the patient. It differs from open ended facilitating questioning which encourages the patient, increases rapport and can be used to obtain background information about personal and emotive areas.

The structured technique is like a game of tennis while open-ended questioning techniques are like steering a canoe down a river.

The patient's answers to the doctor's structured catechism generate two or three diagnostic hypotheses in the doctor's mind which in turn influence the further direction of the catechism as the physician atempts to confirm or refute the different diagnostic possibilities. This point is stressed because although the primary and secondary physicians use the same questioning methods they must each learn to manipulate different sets of diagnostic hypotheses. The primary physician requires an intimate knowledge of the natural history of common diseases in epidemiologic terms, i.e. age, sex, geographic distributions, etc.

The position is further complicated because during such deliberately structured questioning, the patient frequently gives a clear 'lead' into a sensitive personal area and the doctor then may be wise to abandon the above structured catechismal format and use the less threatening open-ended 'listening' approach.

C. The systems enquiry (also functional enquiry)

It is not uncommon for patients to omit symptoms because they do not realise that they are significant. The object of the systems enquiry is to prevent such omissions. Every doctor must develop his own systematic questioning. My own check-list includes questions about the following:

— headache
— listlessness
— weight (+ alcohol consumption)
— appetite, nausea and vomiting
— cough (+ smoking habits)
— chest pain
— shortness of breath and oedema
— abdominal pain
— micturition: nocturia, frequency, dysuria
— bowel function: diarrhoea or constipation
— menstruation: regularity, duration, discharge and contraception
— any medications not previously mentioned.

If an extensive physical examination is indicated by the patient's history, some doctors like to wait and apply the systematic questioning to the system which they are examining. This saves time but can lead to omissions if the doctor decides not to do a detailed examination.

The systematic enquiry is applied to most cases in hospital, but the general practitioner deals with much that is trivial or obvious and in these cases the systematic enquiry is pointless. The family doctor must learn by experience when he can safely dispense with it.

A good rule is to apply the full systematic enquiry when serious, febrile or psychological disease is suspected.

At a single interview a patient may complain of several symptoms from unrelated causes. This is often confusing and the practitioner must learn to decide rapidly how many disease processes he is dealing with. At the end of the interview every symptom should be recorded, related to a firm or suspected diagnosis and explained.

D. The physical examination

A full examination is indicated when a serious disease is considered; an examination of the part complained of is all that is needed for trivial disorders. It is difficult to lay down exact rules about the extent of the examination in different case, but I find the following guides helpful.

1. Always examine the part or system complained of, e.g. the whole chest is examined of every patient who complains of cough.

2. The diagnoses which have been suggested by the history indicate the systems of the body that should be examined, e.g. when a persistent and continuous headache has suggested the possibility of space-occupying lesion and hypertension, both central nervous and cardiovascular systems are examined in detail.

3. When in doubt, examine more fully. This maxim applies especially when there is need for extra examinations that are slightly outside the doctor's normal routine, e.g. 14-day diarrhoea in an elderly man is considered to be due to enteritis. The possibility of cancer should lead the doctor to perform a rectal or sigmoidoscopic examination. The extra time is rarely wasted and the doubts of both doctor and patient are allayed; the recorded findings may be of use later.

A THERAPEUTIC EXAMINATION

This is indicated when a patient's fear of a particular disease is apparent. The object of such an examination is to reassure the patient, e.g. a young housewife who is due to have her first baby in 6 months develops palpitations and sighing respirations. The simplest way of curing this tension state is to examine the heart, take the blood pressure and then reassure the patient.

Therapeutic examinations frequently reveal unsuspected disease.

When the examination has been completed, the doctor clearly records his diagnostic predictions. He can then decide if further investigation is indicated or if he can consider management.

E. Special investigation

These should always be related to the diagnostic hypotheses that are to be tested and should not be performed on the off chance that they may reveal an abnormality.

F. The medical record

Medical record systems often leave much to be desired. This is especially noticeable when patients first report to a general practitioner. In Britain unlike many other countries previous records are available but can take weeks to obtain. The relevant information is usually buried in a mass of words and paper. Simple, easily available summaries with clearly stated relevant diagnoses and treatment may, on occasions, be life-saving but are, unfortunately, a rarity.

These failures will only be corrected when the profession ceases to pay lip service to the importance of the record and accepts the simple truth that good medicine cannot be practised without logical, well-kept practical records, in which diagnostic predictions and problems are clearly stated and related to clinical findings and managerial decisions.

The development of the problem-orientated record for hospital practice, although time-consuming, has been a great advance, but no really satisfactory similar instrument has been developed for the continuous, comprehensive situation of general practice. This problem is further discussed under the heading 'Tools of General Practice' in Chapter 7 p. 126 *et seq*.

II. BACKGROUND KNOWLEDGE OF THE PATIENT, HIS FAMILY AND COMMUNITY

This includes the patient's previous medical history, family history, social history and a working knowledge of the patient's community and cultural origins.

Much of this knowledge the primary care physician should have acquired *before* the patient presents. This process of absorbing background knowledge occurs naturally as the interested general practitioner 'soaks up' information about his patients and the community in which he works.

An adequate record of previous illnesses with clearly ringed diagnostic predictions or problem list saves time and prevents mistakes.

When a patient is seen for the first time, I like, if possible, to obtain information about the following:

1. Date of birth, sex, marital status, occupation and religion.
2. Previous medical history. A single question about previous hospital admissions or investigations usually provides the doctor quickly with all the past medical information he requires. In some instances I may ask further questions about specific diseases such as tuberculosis or venereal disease; but at this stage such specific questions may worry and deter rather than encourage the patient.
3. Family size with details of pregnancies, miscarriages, etc.
4. Family history. Details about health of parents, siblings, children, etc. with special reference to relevant diseases such as tuberculosis, diabetes, hypertension, cancer. etc.

Obtaining background information is essentially a social, facilitating skill which can be likened to taking a canoe down a river. The patient sets the pace with the doctor occasionally guiding the direction. The information is often only indirectly related to the patient's presenting complaints. Direct questioning about any patient's personal life can be counterproductive in many situations and should be integrated into the main history with empathy.

The use of background information is of tremendous importance to the general practitioner for two reasons:

— It frequently provides vital information of direct clinical relevance, e.g. a chest X-ray was normal one year ago.

— It tells us what sort of person the patient is, e.g. is he going to exaggerate or minimise his complaints?

Diagnosis of disease may be compared to the recognition of birds. The student of ornithology will learn to recognise a rook or crow in an aviary. He will see a large black bird with a white beak. If he finds a dead rook he can name it from a textbook picture. If, however, the student goes out into the field with an ornithologist he will find that the problems of recognition depend upon a different set of circumstances. The field-worker will indicate a small black dot flying in the distance and will identify it as a rook. His reasons for his apparently arbitrary statement would be: (a) it is one of a flock and he knows that rooks are gregarious; (b) it is sunset and rooks always fly home to roost at this time; (c) there is a rookery in the nearby trees.

It is apparent that the physical appearance of the bird played little part in its recognition.

The family doctor uses his background knowledge of *high risk factors* in the practice in a similar way. For example, the doctor is asked to visit John Smith and Petula Clutterbuck. No details are given, but it may be possible for the experienced family doctor to forecast accurately that John has measles and Petula has follicular tonsillitis. The doctor's reasons, based on previous knowledge, might run like this: John is 6 and Petula 8; both mothers are sensible people and would not call the doctor unnecessarily; a febrile illness is therefore suspected; it is the height of summer and only two febrile illnesses are likely — acute follicular tonsillitis since it is little affected by seasons, and measles because there is a small epidemic in the Catholic school; John's parents are Catholics and he has almost certainly been in contact with measles; Petula had a bad attack of measles 2 years ago and her brother had scarlet fever 3 weeks ago.

The use of background information and high risk factors makes diagnosis quicker and more accurate and greatly increases the interest of the family doctor's work.

The above example also illustrates the family doctor's use of his knowledge of the natural history of disease to sort out the likely diagnoses. One difficulty about background information is that it is often personal, private or dependent on insight. Relevant personal information may be given in an offhand way or concealed under a cover story. Direct questioning may be counterproductive and sometimes the doctor may acquire a useful piece of background information that is not relevant until several years later. These problems are dealt with later when discussing the consultation (see Ch. 7).

III. THE NATURAL HISTORY OF COMMON DISEASE ENTITIES

This information is the general practitioner's working capital of clinical knowledge and represents a diagnostic vocabulary of about 500 clinical templates for recognising common disease entities. This vocabulary is built up, streamlined and remembered over the many years in which the practitioner trains, first in hospital and then in general practice. Part II of this book represents the distillation of such clinical knowledge over 20 years of primary care. The structure, perspective and emphasis is different to that of more formal textbooks. (See Appendix VII for table of 475 diagnostic templates used in my practice.)

A simple example of the way that a physician uses this clinical vocabulary is illustrated by the physician's subconscious thought process in the first few seconds of almost any primary consultation. As the patient is shown through the door, the doctor observes a young man; without thought the doctor dismisses perhaps two-thirds of his vocabulary of 500 possible diagnoses, i.e., all diseases unique to women plus all degenerative diseases and all diseases that mainly occur in childhood. When the patient says he has come about a pain in his shoulder the field of diagnostic hypotheses is further narrowed, and so on.

It must be stressed that only about half of the primary physician's working diagnostic vocabulary is obtained from hospital experience. A knowledge of the 'extra' 250 diseases must be acquired in the primary setting itself because these diseases are rarely encountered in hospital.

MODIFICATIONS OF DIAGNOSTIC TECHNIQUE IN GENERAL PRACTICE

1. The use of time as a diagnostic tool

Hospital experience teaches a student to interview, examine and diagnose patients. A high proportion of hospital patients may have serious disease and the doctor can justifiably order complex investigations. In general practice the proportion of trivial disease is high, and widespread application of hospital diagnostic techniques is often unjustified.

> EXAMPLE. During four consecutive years I saw 6258 patients with recent cough of trivial or transient origin and 111 patients with recent cough of serious origin. The ratio of trivial to serious disease was 57 : 1 — a much higher ratio than in hospital.

The dividing line between serious and trivial disease is not always clear and for this reason figures can only be approximate, but Table 2 indicates the size of the problem in my practice.

In general practice the majority of patients with diarrhoea, headache or cough of short duration have trivial disease. A very small number of patients will, however, be starting a serious disease such as colitis or cancer. In most instances the family doctor uses time

Table 2 Ratio of functional or trivial causes to serious causes

Symptom	Trivial cause	Serious Cause
Diarrhoea	100	1
Headache	65	1
Cough	57	1
Hoarseness	55	1
Constipation (many cases of simple constipation are never reported)	40+	1
Listlessness and fatigue	25	1
Lower abdominal pain	20	1
Passage of blood per rectum	20	1*
Dyspnoea	10	1
Haemoptysis	7	1
Dysphagia	3	1
Haematuria	2	1**
Chest pain	2	1
Haematemesis	1	2
Upper abdominal pain	1	3***

*Piles have been regarded as a trivial cause.
**If calculi and benign papilloma are regarded as trivial causes this ratio becomes 65: 1.
***Ulcer dyspepsia has been regarded as a serious cause.

to solve this problem because he cannot get everyone fully investigated.

The doctor identifies the likely trivial causes and knows how long they should persist. He tells the patients what to expect but stresses firmly that they must return if the symptoms have not cleared up in the predicted time; he need not mention why he is saying this. The length of time the practitioner waits will be decided by the natural history of the possible serious disease suspected. He may wait a few hours or several weeks.

Symptoms like dysphagia or haematuria with comparatively low ratios of trivial to serious causes are little problem because likelihood of serious disease is sufficient to justify immediate full investigation of *all* patients.

2. The evaluation of clinical signs

When I was an intern in a cardiovascular unit I considered myself an expert on heart murmurs. Now my opinion is of little value because I listen to so few abnormal hearts and can less accurately identify an early diastolic heart murmur. The family doctor accepts that some hard-won clinical knowledge may be lost — he concentrates on those physical signs that help him in his everyday work.

3. The specificity of signs

Listening to an infant's chest gives little information about the lungs. Assessing the degree of respiratory distress is more accurately done by looking for rib retraction, counting respiratory rate and observing colour.

4. Assessment of signs — their accuracy and usefulness

Medical training teaches a student to assess physical signs. Accurate assessment requires constant practice: a family doctor may be expert at assessing the redness of a baby's eardrum but finds it difficult to judge the significance of an equivocal plantar response.

5. The time needed to elicit a physical sign must be justified by the issues at stake

Thus a family doctor may willingly spend 20 minutes examining a baby's abdomen for a pyloric tumour or intussusception but will rarely attempt to map out the dissociation of heat and pain sensation.

A physical sign or test may be specific, easily assessed and quick, but it is not used if it is superfluous or seldom influences the doctor's diagnostic decisions, e.g. Von Graefe's lid lag sign of exophthalmos, or a rectal examination in suspected appendicitis in a child when the doctor has already decided to admit the patient to hospital.

The general practitioner must learn from experience how full an examination is indicated in different patients. He must be prepared to discard tests that do not help him, but must never abandon the principle that examination is a vital part of medical practice.

He modifies his methods of routine examination and learns to assess the significance of clinical pointers to suit the needs of a busy general practice.

6. The importance of examining the patient at home in his/her environment

Students are rarely taught the importance of examining the patient in his environment, e.g. the *daily living assessment*, examining the ability of an arthritic to get out of bed or into the bath. Such examinations frequently reveal much more than any formal physical examination. (For details see Appendix VI, p. 707).

7. The importance of the extra witness

In many situations vital information and help can be obtained from husbands, close relatives, teachers, etc. The extra effort involved is rarely wasted.

3

Vulnerability, high risk groups and prevention

'Prevention is better than cure.' Few cliches are so obvious and yet so difficult to put into practise.

Two practical steps underly all prevention:

1. Vulnerable or high risk groups must be identified
2. Simple cost-effective methods of protection must be available or developed.

The first involves detailed accurate predictions covering a wide range of risks inherent in diverse human activities.

The second requires extensive detailed research to define what means are effective and the cost of protection.

Despite the obvious advantages, most developed countries spend less than 10% of their health budgets on preventive activities.

Definitions of terms commonly used

Primary prevention means removing the cause of disease as has been done with smallpox or is possible with smoking.

Secondary prevention means early detection of disease at presymptomatic levels, e.g. hypertension or carcinoma of cervix.

Tertiary prevention is the management of established disease to prevent complications or serious effects.

Screening is a form of secondary prevention and is often prefixed with the word *presymptomatic*. A high risk group is identified and then requested to attend voluntarily for appropriate examination or tests which will identify early presymptomatic disease. An age/sex register is often essential for identification (See Appendix II, p. 686).

Case finding is a form of presymptomatic screening which uses an opportunistic approach. The doctor examines or tests a patient for a condition such as hypertension when the patient is attending for another reason. Effective case finding is based on the fact that 70% of any practice population reports every year and over 90% report within 3 years and that many of the remaining 10% are 'known about' or visited coincidentally.

Reception staff are trained to pick out and 'flag' high risk groups when the patients' records are assembled for any clinic. An age/sex register can greatly assist flagging and checking for omissions.

PREVENTION AND PRIMARY CARE IN PRACTICE

There are four administrative levels of prevention. Family doctors have a significant contribution at each level:

- I National
- II Community
- III Practice
- IV Consultation — *This is the main level of input by the family doctor (see disease entries throughout Part II.)*

I. PREVENTION AT THE NATIONAL LEVEL

National schemes of prevention cover those areas where protection is known to be cost-effective and compliance can be obtained by legislation and/or financial incentives.

The following provide the main examples in Britain.

A. PREGNANCY — ANTENATAL AND POSTNATAL CARE

The oldest and most effective scheme; it is now taken for granted, in training and practice, as a fundamental part of primary care. Appropriate financial incentives are available for participants and doctors. Much evaluative research at primary and secondary levels has shown its undoubted benefit and cost/effectiveness.

Practical points for the family doctor

1. Concentration of resources. Antenatal and postnatal care requires planning and discussion at practice level to ensure efficient utilisation of local and practice resources and staff. Estimates of clinic loads and simple time-studies combined with staff discussion reveal that many antenatal routines can be effectively delegated or shared. The obstetric responsibility of several family doctors can be concentrated in the hands of one doctor who is prepared to learn and maintain the relevant expertise.

2. Compliance. Inadequate patient co-operation and compliance failures should be continually monitored, discussed and remedied at practice or consultation levels. This can be computerised in a big practice.

3. Health education in parallel. The advent of relaxation and motherhood classes with the involvement of fathers, has taught family doctors that in the antenatal and postnatal phases, couples are receptive to a wide range of health education, even those that may be outside the immediate antenatal issue. Advice on diet, smoking, exercise, etc. is often acted on and maintained with an enthusiasm that is difficult to engender at other times.

The doctor should be able to organise such valuable health education in a way that does not absorb large amounts of doctor time.

4. *Staff and educational facilities* may be available to the doctor from the local health authority.

5. *Health Visitors* are trained in prevention and provide an excellent service which is often under-utilised by both doctors and patients.

B. IMMUNISATION PROGRAMMES

The elimination of polio, smallpox and diptheria by immunisation is of undoubted value. As further routine immunisation programmes are developed, their cost-effectiveness is relatively easy to assess and apply. Rubella in pregnancy: 10% of mothers are probably still at risk. Active case finding is therefore indicated.

Whooping cough, rubella, measles and tetanus should be routine.

Selective immunisation of specific high risk groups can be considered in tuberculosis, influenza A, mumps, hepatitis, enteric fever, yellow fever, cholera and other diseases for which effective, cheap immunisation is available.

Financial incentives to encourage immunisation programmes by family doctors have only been partially successful.

Practical points for the family doctor

1. Routine immunisation programmes are usually initiated at the practice level at the postnatal visit by either doctor or health visitor.
2. Patients may also be sent for by local authority computer.
3. Compliance. Surprisingly in many communities immunisation levels for Polio, Diptheria, whooping cough, etc., are still too low.
4. The family doctor should monitor and remedy the failure rates in his or her practice. An age/sex register or small computer may be of assistance.
5. Co-operation with the local authority and health visitors is essential.

6. The parent of every baby in the practice should have a card containing reminders of next appointment, etc. This can be kept as a permanent record when the child is older.

C. CONTRACEPTION AND PREVENTION OF PREGNANCY

The demand for such services comes from the groups most at risk. Those who campaign against these services are often not, themselves, in a high risk group. The demand is recognised at a national level and in Britain the patient services are subsidised. National Family Planning services often supplement or replace the services provided by the family doctor.

Practical points for the family doctor

1. A short course of special training in the various methods is indicated for most family doctors.
2. Special family planning Clinics in a practice may lead to more effective utilization of resources.
3. The responsibility of maintaining expertise for running the service can be delegated to one doctor (partner) on behalf of a larger group or partnership, but every family doctor should maintain a working knowledge of the advantages and disadvantages of all methods (summarised in table 31, page 576).
4. Compliance is the responsibility of the patients.
5. Cost to the patient. In Britain the cost is largely borne by the State. In countries where this is not the case, the inverse/care law (p. 21) may complicate the choices put to the patient.
6. Counselling of patients is especially indicated when there are ethical difficulties e.g. the possibility of termination for a girl under 14. In such cases non-directive discussion of all the options may help both doctor and patient.

D. INDUSTRIAL AND OCCUPATIONAL HAZARDS AND PROTECTION

Protection against the hazards of work are a large and specialised part of preventive medicine. The patient is often better informed than the family doctor.

Emotional reactions to disability and compensation vary considerably according to the personality of the injured individual and his/her handling by management, union and doctor.

Practical points for the family doctor

1. The family doctor has clear obligations to the working patient:
   - to protect and advise about risks at work,
   - to treat and rehabilitate any injured patient and enable early return to healthy living and working,
   - to safeguard the patient's rights and interests. In some instances this may mean pointing out that compensation might be available and in others explaining the possible psychological and financial dangers of a long and fruitless quest for it,
   - the family doctor should avoid making value judgements or allocating blame.
2. The family doctor should make a careful record of the patient's description of any accident or injury at the time of first reporting. This prevents distortion later. The patient should be advised to ensure that the accident has been recorded at work and to obtain the names of any witnesses of any accident.
3. The family doctor is the one person who can encourage the patient at an early stage to discuss objectively all the advantages and disadvantages of compensation. Later it may be more difficult for the patient to decide what is best.
4. The family doctor may also have to advise an injured patient to (a) consult their trade union, (b) consult the CAB or the appropriate DHSS pamphlet (N.1.2. and N.1.5), (c) obtain legal advice.

E. SEAT BELTS AND CRASH HELMETS TO PREVENT INJURY

These provide good examples of prevention at a national level which is effective but requires little action from the primary physician.

Such protective legislation may take a community many years to achieve but once legalised it is then taken for granted. Many improvements in housing, sanitation, diet, social security, care of children and the elderly come into this category. Smugness about what has been achieved should not blind doctors as individuals about areas where further protective legislation is needed (see p. 20).

II. PREVENTION AT COMMUNITY LEVELS

Prevention at community level is the province of the community physician and may involve both local legislation and incentives.

Help varies according to the funds available and local conditions, i.e. urban, rural, industrial, etc. The enthusiasm and drive of a region's community physician may be crucial.

Practical points for the family doctor

Good relations with the community physician should be fostered. Perhaps inviting him/her to a practice meeting to discuss

- — problems of prevention in the area
- — the regional status of national schemes of prevention
- — the regional health education facilities (a) health education literature, posters, etc. for health centres, etc. (b) health education officers — are there any? What are their local functions? will they visit your practice to talk to patients and staff, etc?
- — the regional status of voluntary prevention schemes in the area, e.g. Family Planning, Samaritans, Cruse, Marriage Guidance, sex education in schools, etc.
- — any special areas of prevention that are being developed locally
- — other regionally organised supporting services, home helps, meals on wheels, etc.
- — local disaster arrangements (rail, road, air, flood, pollution, nuclear, defence etc.)

III. PREVENTION AT THE LEVEL OF PRACTICE ADMINISTRATION

This is practical when all partners are co-operative and if premises are suitable and available.

Many changes involving practice management and cost have to be agreed, (see Table 3).

Three main operational methods are used:

1. The special clinic approach. A high risk group is encouraged to attend a special clinic. Well baby or cervical smear clinics or Weight Watchers, are examples. Compliance depends largely on the interest and background of patients and the enthusiasm of the doctor.

2. Presymptomatic screening approach. Using an age/sex register all members of a particular high risk group are offered, on a voluntary basis, an appropriate examination or series of tests. All women aged 25–55 might be offered a cervical smear.

Non-compliant patients can be re-circulated;

3. The opportunistic case finding approach. Before patients report, the record of those in a particular high risk group are flagged to remind the doctor seeing the patient to perform the required examination or tests. A great deal of opportunistic health education can also be extremely effective if fed into routine antenatal, post natal, well baby or other similar clinics.

PRACTICAL POINTS ABOUT PREVENTION AT PRACTICE LEVEL

1. Special clinic approach. The main disadvantage is that it only protects a small well motivated, usually well educated, and often least vulnerable, section of the community. It is extremely useful where one partner has a special enthusiasm.

2. Wilson's 10 criteria should be satisfied if screening is to be considered for any condition:

- (i) The condition must have serious consequences.
- (ii) Full knowledge of the natural history.
- (iii) There must be a recognisable latent or presymptomatic stage.
- (iv) Adequate proof that the disease can be modified by achieving earlier diagnosis and treatment.
- (v) An agreed policy on the selection of patients for treatment.
- (vi) Adequate, easily applied, cheap screening tests capable of accurate diagnosis in the early presymptomatic stage. These tests must not give too many false positive or false negative results.
- (vii) The test and treatment should be acceptable to the population.
- (viii) The cost of case finding should be realistically related to the cost of orthodox care.
- (ix) The screening programme, if successful, must be continuously applied.
- (x) Facilities for treatment as well as diagnosis must be available.

The number of diseases that adequately fulfil these criteria is small and some of these, e.g. deafness in children, are relatively rare.

3. Presymptomatic screening versus case-finding. Table 3 compares the advantages and disadvantages of the screening and case-finding approaches. A brief study of this Table shows that for

Table 3 Advantages and disadvantages of presymptomatic screening and case finding.

	Presymptomatic screening	Case-finding
Population at risk	Must be known beforehand, i.e. age/sex register required	Need not be known beforehand as is opportunistic.
Cost	May be considerable, postage, staff, etc.	Small or negligible
Co-operation of partners	Required	Not essential
Patient compliance	Many high risk groups are reluctant to comply, e.g. age, obesity, alcohol may act as a deterrent. Even with repeated reminders least vulnerable patients usually most co-operative	Compliance easier because patient already at clinic for another reason
Doctor's time	Concentrated at one or two special clinics	Spread in small amounts over many routine consultations
Delegation of screening duties	Relatively easy. A nurse can take swabs or BPs	Delegation may be difficult if nurse not available
Repeat checks of positive tests	May require lengthy explanations and reassurance	Repeat examinations or tests rarely disturb patient
Treatment of positive cases	Compliance may be poor as patient feels well	Treatment (and full explanation) are combined with treatment for another disorder already recognised by patient. Compliance usually good
Continuous application of programme	Programme must be repeated or re-started every few years	Can be continued automatically
New or experimental programmes	Require full justification and explanation to group selected	Explanation usually quickly accepted

most purposes the case-finding approach is more cost-effective than the screening approach.

4. Community support services and advice at local level. Many communities as in Britain have provided (free of charge) a great many such services which are of enormous help to the family doctor

and benefit to the community. The Health Visitor service, sheltered housing for the elderly, cervical smears, etc. (ch. 7 p. 142).

5. A known (denominator) population at risk. As in Britain, Denmark or many isolated communities, this denominator provides a unique advantage for the primary care team. Omissions can be identified while standards and indices of health can be applied to the whole community at risk. This makes the measurement of outcomes easier and more accurate.

6. The potential for prevention at the practice level using the primary health care team is great but requires considerable changes in the attitudes of both doctors and medical schools.

7. The following are usually considered cost-effective, presymptomatic secondary prevention programmes suitable for primary care at practice level.

A. Carcinoma of Cervix (see p. 547)

Secondary prevention using routine cervical smears has been shown to be effective. Should be practised routinely by all family doctors on a screening or case finding basis. In Britain state finance should cover costs. All women aged 35–55 should have a cervical smear every 3–5 years. Note: Recent work suggests that the incidence rates are increasing in younger women. Practice screening and case finding programmes must be modified accordingly.

B. Hypertension and cardiovascular disease (see p. 343)

Presymptomatic control of hypertension (Ref. 16.1) is of proven value. 50% of all strokes and 25% of all myocardial infarcts are said to be preventable. It should be practised by all family doctors on a screening or case-finding basis.

C. Carcinoma of breast (see p. 534)

Presymptomatic secondary prevention is of possible but not yet of proven value. Early diagnosis is achieved by (a) teaching patient how to perform regular palpation, (b) thermography, (c) mammography.

D. Developmental screening

Regular monitoring of developmental defects especially: intellect; hearing; vision; motor skills. A useful extension of the well baby clinic. The number of defects identified may be small but the incidental educational benefit of regular visits, may be of great value to parents.

E. Screening of the elderly

Regular monitoring of the elderly. Opinions differ about the relative merits of the screening over case finding approach. Our experience confirmed that of Freedman (Ref. 3.1) who found no special advantages of screening.

F. Health education programmes

The special clinic approach in which attendance is dependent on the interest and enthusiasm of the patient can be applied in many areas, e.g. giving up smoking, losing weight, exercise programmes, Marriage Guidance, classes for retirement, relaxation, motherhood, etc.

The special skills of the Health Visitor are crucial in this area.

IV. PREVENTION AT CONSULTATION LEVEL

The skilled family doctor is in a unique position to provide a great deal of secondary and tertiary prevention in the course of everyday consultation. Most of the diagnostic headings throughout Part II have an entry under 'Preventive Management Options'.

Two skills have to be learnt sufficiently well to enable their automatic incorporation as part of everyday consultation:

1. *Preventive clinical thinking*. Awareness of high risk factors and vulnerable groups leads the family doctor to both early diagnosis and prevention. Almost any entry in Part II demonstrates the way these two items are linked; conditions as different as hypothermia in the elderly (p. 664), scabies (p. 201) and simple anxiety (p. 243) provide examples of this linking of diagnostic pointers and preventive options.

2. *Prevention at consultation level must be opportunistic*. This applies to management as well as case-finding. Thus 2 minutes spent explaining the dangers of smoking to an expectant primipara may lead to permanent compliance while 10 minutes trying to persuade an unemployed 40 year old to give up cigarettes may be totally counter-productive.

The skills of 'appropriate preventive opportunism' must be learnt early through practise, and then updated throughout the doctor's working life.

Thus, the combination, in an adult patient, of the two pointers — fever and recent return from overseas, might raise the following possibilities in the doctor's mind:

— enteric fever — because of previous experience
— Legionnaire's disease — because of a recent medical article
— AIDS — because of a recent television programme.

A by-product of such preventive opportunistic thinking is that it increases patient rapport and encourages 'whole person medical attitudes'.

In many instances preventive options may be dismissed as inappropriate or counter-productive but the family doctor must learn first to recall the alternatives and then either act on them or reject them on sound clinical patient-based grounds.

Three important large areas of prevention are often only practical at consultation level.

A. Prevention requiring alterations of patient life style.
B. Prevention involving psychological problems and changes of behaviour.
C. 'Plugging the gaps' created by any patient's failure to comply with prevention organised on a community or practice level. For instance, it has been shown that patients who ignore appointments for cervical smears have a higher incidence of cervical carcinoma than those who complied after one request.

A. PREVENTION REQUIRING ALTERATIONS OF LIFE STYLE.

Life style changes are difficult to achieve. Several factors must be present if compliance is to be obtained and if advice is not to be counter-productive:

Practical points

1. *The patient must clearly make the decision.* A 'whole person' approach is therefore essential.

2. The patient must be given full understanding of the pros and cons.

3. The personality of the patient must be considered. The fatalistic or the elderly may not want to be bothered.

4. Creation of fear or use of an authoritarian or patronising approach by the doctor is avoided.

5. An opportunistic approach by the doctor is crucial. *But the doctor should guard against the 'lazy option' of never identifying suitable opportunities.*

6. Group therapy may achieve greater compliance than individual counselling.

7. The following life style changes are commonly attempted in primary care:

- *Dietary changes and exercise* in relation to prevention of obesity, ischaemic heart disease, osteoarthritis, diabetes (type II), peripheral vascular disease, essential hypertension, constipation, varicose veins, duodenal ulcer, piles, diverticulosis and cancer of bowel and breast (for details see Part II).
- *Smoking avoidance* may have to be advised in relation to the prevention of chronic respiratory disease of all kinds, cancer of lung, during pregnancy and possibly hypertension.
- *Alcohol avoidance* (see p. 259).
- *Prevention of accidents in the home*. Advice about electric fittings, flexes, fire guards, gas taps and pills may be both timely and productive when home visiting involves the very young and the very old.

B. PREVENTION OF PSYCHOLOGICAL AND BEHAVIOURAL DISORDERS

The affection and support that is given to every individual by relatives, friends and acquaintances protects vulnerable personalities from many of the common psychological (behavioural) disorders. Tension state (p. 246), attempted suicide (p. 257), misuse of drugs (p. 261) and depression (p. 255) provide examples.

Disease or changes in a patient's role or life style may isolate a vulnerable personality from this protection and help to precipitate one of the many psychological and behavioural problems listed by age in Table 5 (p. 110). The doctor is consulted and is often in a position to counsel and support such individuals in ways which help them to adjust to their new roles and regain confidence in themselves. (This is discussed in greater detail in Chs. 5, 6 and 7).

Practical points

1. The doctor may have to provide supportive (often non-directive) counselling for a wide diversity of role changes; many are

listed in ch. 5 (p. 83). The dying patient is discussed on pp. 92, 207, and 607 provides an example in detail.

2. In most such situations the doctor will be uncertain what is best for the patient. The doctor must be sensitive to possible need and then explore what the patient as a 'whole person' wants. Such exploration is usually non-directive and non-threatening.

3. The doctor's own personality and previous experience will govern both understanding and wise handling of the patient's problems.

4. 'Therapeutic listening' may be all that is needed. Practical solutions are usually opportunistic or tailored to the patient's situation. Such solutions will rely on human relationships, not drugs.

5. The community psychiatric nurse may provide valuable help.

C. 'PLUGGING THE GAPS' OF FAILED COMPLIANCE

This is an administrative necessity for most preventive programmes. It is best achieved at consultation level.

Practical points

1. Receptionists can be trained to 'vet and flag' records before any clinic. Thus children who have not been immunised or a woman who should have had a smear can be picked up with little trouble.

2. Computer programmes to assist this process have been developed.

4

The development of the normal individual

Accurate early diagnosis requires that the doctor recognises immediately any clinical abnormality. He must therefore have a working knowledge of the normal.

This involves knowledge of two variables:

A. the range of normality (see Figs 56 and 57, p. 684)
B. the changes that occur in normal development.

For details of both these variables see Appendix IC and ID (p. 683) also Refs. 0.4, 4.1 and 4.2.

A. THE NORMAL INDIVIDUAL

The concept of normality is a mental trick that allows each individual to relate himself to his group. 'Am I normal?' is a question of great importance to all of us. The desire of each individual to conform, physically and mentally, to his own group, is deeply and instinctively felt by everyone.

The objective observer soon realises that there is no such thing as *absolute normality* and he compromises by making reasonably accurate assessments, i.e. ranges of normality, standard deviations from a mean, etc.

We, as doctors, must attempt to know the normal ranges of individual variation for two purposes: (1) to enable us to recognise early any physical or mental abnormalities; (2) to allay when possible the patient's fear of being different.

Throughout this book, the word 'normal' refers to the group of individuals included in the general concept of the *normal range*.

Doctors recognise two forms of comparison with the normal:

1. Measurable comparisons. Reasonably objective accurate estimates of the physical variables, e.g. temperature, pulse, height, weight, etc. Many such normal ranges of measurements have been produced for the doctors' benefit. The general practitioner need not

necessarily carry such figures in his head provided those that he is likely to require are easily available (Ref. 0.4).

2. Clinical comparisons. Subjective assessments of clinical observations that are difficult to measure. Such assessments can only become accurate through personal experience and active practice. Thus an experienced doctor might regard the behaviour of a wife who talked about her dead husband as if he were still alive as being 'normal' if this occurred as part of a bereavement reaction but suggestive of serious mental disorder if this behaviour started several years after the husband's death.

B. NORMAL DEVELOPMENT

The practitioner must also acquire a knowledge of those developmental changes that are 'normal'. He learns much of this in his hospital training but he will need to supplement this knowledge considerably when he finally starts general practice (see Appendix I). The advice and help of the Health Visitor is invaluable.

The following is a check list of those areas of developmental change that are useful to a general practitioner.

The newborn baby

1. Routine physical check of heart, lungs, abdomen, genitalia, skull, skin, spine and limbs
2. The normal range of measurements — weight, length, head circumference (Fig. 56).

Babies (7 days old–1 year) (Refs. 4.1, 4.2 and Fig. 57)

1. Normal physical milestones and their normal variations
2. Normal emotional milestones and their normal variations
3. Normal rates of weight gain and growth
4. Normal feeding habits — breast and bottle
5. Simple feeding difficulties due to poor sucking, sucking with tongue over teat, difficulties due to nasal blockage, too small a teat hole, failure to allow air replacement in a single-ended bottle, etc.
6. Normal variations of appetite, vomiting and bowel habits
7. Minor skin variations — rashes, moles and birthmarks

8. Common parental worries that lie within the normal range — tongue tie, umbilical hernia, phymosis, squints in first few weeks of life, babies that 'sleep all the time', babies that 'never sleep'.

Toddlers and preschool children (1–5 years) (Refs. 0.3, 4.1, 4.2 and Fig. 57)

1. Normal physical milestones
2. Normal emotional milestones
3. Range of normality for weight and height
4. Range of normality for walking, talking and eating
5. Sphincter control
6. Skeletal changes in spine and lower limbs — leg bowing, intoeing, mild knock knees, flat feet, etc.
7. The effects of immunisation
8. The common causes of sleeping problems
9. The effects of sibling jealousy
10. Motor skills (Denver chart, Appendix ID and Ref 4.1)
11. Normal variations of speech, hearing and vision.

School children (5–12 years)

1. Ranges of normality for weight and height.

2. Frequency of respiratory and other infections in first 3 years at school. Most children report 5–15 respiratory infections in this period and parents often require reassurance that this is not unusual.

3. The emotional effects on the child of backwardness, rejection, parental fecklessness, parental laziness, parental selfishness and parental emotional conflicts. These may be extremely difficult to assess but the practitioner is often the only person in a position to give any accurate opinion.

4. Intellectual tests of ability. The practitioner must have a working knowledge of their uses and limitations although he will usually refer the child to a psychiatrist or educational psychologist if these tests are indicated. Dyslexia is an important and easily overlooked example (see p. 271).

Adolescence (13–19 years)

Most general practitioners have surprisingly little contact with teenagers and their knowledge of the normal range of physical and emotional development in this age group may be limited. Practitioners are therefore often wise to refer problems early. Experimentation is probably the underlying drive of this age group. Normally the teenager's experiments, although often outwardly rebellious, help to provide the developing individual with self-confidence. The practitioner will only tend to see those patients in whom the experimentation has produced harmful or antisocial consequences. These consequences may include unwanted pregnancies, venereal disease, homosexual situations, excessive alcohol intake, misuse of drugs, road traffic accidents, acts of violence and delinquency (see Table 5, p. 110). The problems are usually presented to the practitioner by distraught parents and rarely raise difficulties of diagnosis. Often the doctor's only contribution is to refer the problem to other suitably qualified persons.

Unless he has special experience in counselling this group, the family doctor should recognise the benefits of sharing the difficulties of treatment. Many health professionals can help (see Chs 5 and 6).

Adults (19–65)

A knowledge of normal adult physical development is acquired automatically as a doctor trains.

Knowledge of normal adult behaviour is more difficult to acquire and is learned by introspection, general experience and professional medical experience within the community itself. The aspects of adult behaviour that I find relevant to general practice are described in Chapters 5 and 6, page 68 *et seq*.

The menopause (40–50 years)

See page 568.

Retirement and old age (65 years onwards)

This is the time when degenerative disease arises. As the patient ages, these diseases lose their individual characteristics (see Part II) and tend to produce the same problems.

For the general practitioner such problems cover four large and important areas of care.

1. Mobility — walking, stairs, shopping, etc.
2. Self care — dressing, feeding, incontinence, etc.

3. Mental state — memory, orientations, emotions, etc.
4. Social contacts — living alone, relatives, friends, social activities, etc.

A very slight experience of general practice demonstrates the significance of these areas and shows that the causative degenerative disease is often of only secondary relevance.

The family doctor requires an intimate knowledge of these four areas, which forms the basis of much geriatric care. Despite this he should also remember that in old people energetic treatment is not always justified; a detailed knowledge of the patient is also required.

The majority (95%) of geriatric patients are best looked after in their own homes. A small proportion of the remainder (2–3%) — the elderly frail — require relatively little support. This may be in their own home, in sheltered housing or in a modest institution. The remainder comprise a group of patients — the elderly sick — who require more specialised institutional care.

An effective geriatric unit is usually dependent on the following components:

— an assessment sub-unit which ensures that every patient's capacity is correctly assessed and that expensive resources are correctly used
— a day hospital and psychogeriatric unit
— a rehabilitation sub-unit through which patients can be rotated as required
— a reservoir of long stay beds for those patients who clearly cannot stay in the community
— adequate community support services for those patients who can be encouraged to stay in their own homes, i.e. sheltered housing, day hospitals, meals on wheels, holiday relief service, etc.

SERIOUS DEVELOPMENT PROBLEMS THAT INVOLVE SPECIALIST ADVICE

A number of developmental problems are in fact very abnormal. Diagnosis is usually not difficult. Most such problems are both disabling and rare and are therefore best referred for specialist advice. A few are described in Part II.

The practitioner should be able to recognise such conditions and know how to get further advice. Beyond this, knowledge need not be great:

— Genetic and genetic counselling problems.
— Major congenital abnormalities, recognisable at birth, e.g. Down's syndrome (page 658) provides a good example. Other instances are: spina bifida, meningomyelocele, ectopia vesica, hydrocephalus, microcephalus, hare-lip, dermoid cysts, talipes and obvious skeletal abnormalities.
— Major congenital abnormalities, not recognisable until they produce obvious progressive symptoms soon after birth, e.g. obstructions of biliary tract, oesophagus or intestines, hiatus hernias, etc.
— Major congenital abnormalities that are slow to appear and sometimes difficult to recognise, e.g. congenital pyloric stenosis (page 466) fibrocystic disease, congenital heart disease (p. 655) congenital dislocation of hip (p. 656), mental retardation (with or without cerebral palsy), megacolon, phenylketonuria, defects of vision or hearing, etc. Some of these problems can be picked up early by screening (see Ch. 3).

5

The behaviour of the normal individual

Much has been written about human behaviour. The account that follows is in no way comprehensive and outlines only those ideas and concepts that I have found helpful.

A doctor is taught that his patients are individuals rather than cases and that he is expected to do more than just diagnose clinical disease and order treatment. He may be required to redirect energies, alter habits and attitudes or adjust values. Before this is possible he must learn to understand and assess the underlying behavioural influences. He must learn to make emotional and social as well as clinical diagnoses. At this point it must be stressed that such problems follow a 'normal distribution' and that therefore the majority will fall within the range of normality. Doctors all too frequently regard behavioural problems in the same way as they regard disease, i.e. as an abnormality. *The majority of behavioural and so-called minor psychiatric problems are so universal that they can be regarded as being within the normal range.*

Normal human behaviour can be considered to involve the interaction of three basic activities:

— Knowing (concerned largely with factual experience)
— Feeling (concerned largely with emotion)
— Striving (concerned with motives and drives).

Each activity is difficult to define and we must often look into ourselves for understanding.

A practical approach to human behaviour requires that we try to understand how these activities are integrated and related.

Knowing (as in diagnosis) is a result of remembering and then matching up (recognising) patterns of previous experience to enable predictions to be made. Action based on these predictions can then be taken — we recognise a rain cloud and take an umbrella.

Feeling requires that we relate ourselves to our pattern of experience. These patterns may affect our relationship with things or people, i.e. annoyance at getting wet if we forget the umbrella or pleasure when we recognise a friend and share our umbrella.

Striving is harder to define but is really the basic drive or motivation that relates what each individual knows and feels to what he actually does. This drive is of three kinds:

— Instinctive, i.e. not related to previous experience — when a baby tries to walk
— Subconscious, i.e. related to a previous 'conditioning' of which the individual is unaware
— Conscious, i.e. related to conscious reasoning as when we take an exam or carry out our job.

In all human behaviour these three drives are present in varying degrees.

If any of these drives lead to action successfully performed the individual feels secure and his self-confidence is increased. Thus we may say that a toddler is walking confidently or we may feel a surge of confidence when we pass an exam. This feeling of confidence will temporarily affect other activities and we feel prepared to tackle anything. There is a *generalisation gradient* — a characteristic of many conditioned responses. Conversely if the drive leads to failure there is loss of confidence and depression.

Children mainly acquire their confidence from emotional security combined with learning and successfully performing finite skills. They learn the meaning of success and failure in terms of finite things such as walking, sport, exams, etc. They will prefer to perform skills at which they are expert and will increase their confidence in so doing; emotional rejection by the family will decrease confidence. As children we learn to orientate ourselves spatially in a physical world by picturing our surroundings and ourselves at the centre. This enables us to move about with logic and precision. Adults from puberty onwards become aware of personal relationships on which our confidence is increasingly based. The adult orientates himself in his personal world by allocating himself a 'role' — competent doctor, good mother, happy husband, good mixer, etc. By successfully performing this role the adult gets his self-confidence. He will identify with the role he feels he is best at and will protect with an immediate often aggressive reaction any attempt to denigrate this role. Thus a mother will react aggressively if I tell her that her children look a bit underfed, similarly a doctor may get aggressive if a patient asks for another opinion. Both statements are attacks on the role view of each individual. To protect their self-confidence individuals are likely to react with aggression, irritation or depression depending on their basic degree of security which in turn depends on their heredity, their education and their previous experience. This somewhat over-simplified picture allows us to look more clearly at a few of the more important emotional and behavioural disturbances that are presented to the general practitioner (see Table 5, p. 110).

Anxiety (and worry) can be regarded as a normal healthy state of expectancy or watchfulness that relates to a future happening likely to threaten us, our family, or group. Patients request treatment for anxiety because it is unpleasant, not because it is abnormal.

It must be stressed that anxiety often improves an individual's performance and is usually an essential ingredient of most successful enterprises.

Fear follows anxiety when the future happening seems in imminent danger of occurring.

Terror and panic represent blind illogical actions that follow excessive fear when no attempt is made to relate these actions to a previous pattern of experience.

Reassurance occurs when the individual is enabled to insert a barrier between himself and the threat. The barrier may be physical or temporal, e.g. when patients seek reassurance that they've not got cancer — the patients come for reassurance that they are not going to die *soon*, not that they are not going to die at all. This principle is important when handling patients with any fatal disease because it is often possible for the doctor to allow the patient (if the patient wishes) to realise the truth and yet at the same time to insert the hope of a long barrier of reassuring time between the threat and its fatal outcome.

A more complex form of barrier is used in the adult world of personal relationships — self-deception. We all live in varying degrees of 'fool's paradise'.

Indecision or even paralysis as well as anger and aggression are immediate and instinctive reactions towards any threat to our self-confidence or to our 'role picture' of ourselves.

Depression follows failure and like elation (and physiological inhibition) may show a generalisation gradient and affect other related activities.

Guilt — also a feeling of failure — is usually felt by an individual who considers that he has failed to fulfil his role adequately. This internal feeling of guilt has nothing to do with guilt in the legal sense. A daughter who has sacrificed her life to looking after an old mother is likely, when the mother dies, to feel far more guilty than the daughter who has done little or nothing for her mother.

These concepts are an essential part of 'whole person medicine' because they illustrate how emotional security and self-confidence protect individuals and that the affection, friendship, recognition and concern of others protects every individual from the destructive effects of insecurity.

I propose now to discuss certain further concepts that I have found helpful about the mind:

- — the subconscious
- — thresholds of awareness
- — stress, insecurity and other disturbing influences
- — 'role' theory

and then to describe in greater detail some of the common emotional patterns encountered in general practice, e.g. anxiety, aggression, depression, guilt, etc.

In this way I hope to show how a family doctor makes and utilises emotional as well as clinical predictions (diagnoses).

SUBCONSCIOUS MOTIVATIONS

At the start of this chapter we suggested that there were three kinds of motivations for action — instinctive, subconscious and conscious.

The practitioner can do little to influence instinctive reactions and is not expected to do more than comment on a patient's conscious motivations. By contrast the patient's subconscious motivations are important to the doctor for two reasons:

- — Subconscious attitudes can sometimes be modified and often utilised
- — The patient's unawareness of motivation makes it essential that the doctor should have some understanding.

In almost every consultation the practitioner will find that he is being given subconscious leads by the patient. A wife will tell the doctor that there is nothing worrying her, but a quivering lip or the constant twisting of a button will belie this statement.

Applications to practice

The doctor must learn to recognise, understand and handle these subconscious motivations:

1. RECOGNITION

The practitioner recognises the statement with subconscious implications because the emphasis is wrong — the statement does not 'ring true'. The 'belle indifference' of the hysteric and the person who 'protests too much' are classic examples.

The diffident under-emphasised approach normally begings: 'By the way . . .', 'While I'm here . . .', 'I hope you don't mind if . . .', 'I think I've probably come unnecessarily . . .'. A matter of clear importance to a patient is left till the last or even denied. Such patients are sounding out their own as well as the doctor's willingness to discuss the subject.

Diffidence of this sort usually indicates that the patient feels insecure; this may be just in relation to the doctor or it may reflect a wider insecurity.

Overemphasis of statements usually means that a patient feels rejected or threatened in some way, e.g. that the doctor is not taking their complaints seriously enough; thus a patient will say aggressively that a pain has been upsetting him continuously since he was last seen several months before. If the doctor points out tactfully that he previously asked the patient to report if the pain did not improve, the patient may then give a less aggressive more accurate description of a pain that is clearly intermittent.

Both emphasis and underemphasis represent different types of insecurity in the patient and must therefore be handled with encouragement. Any irritation shown by the doctor is likely to be counterproductive.

The cliché phrase. Every one of us has faults or insecurities that we wish to gloss over. We often find a pat phrase or cliché that does this for us. The doctor can often recognise both phrase and motivation:

'I'm not much of a scholar like' probably indicates a deficient education.

'Better call you early than be sorry later' means that the patient knows the call is late and is not very sorry.

'I can forgive but I can't forget' means I've not yet forgiven.

'They've never wanted for a thing' probably means that a family have been given only what their mother wants.

'While there's life there's hope' said by a near relative usually means that they've not really faced the possibility of death.

After a week or so in practice most doctors will have discovered the underlying meaning of the following:

'I'm not one who bothers the doctor unnecessarily'
'It's not the money but the principle that matters'
'I didn't come to you earlier because I was afraid I had cancer'
'I'm not one for complaining'

Non-verbal clues to subconscious motivation are possibly of greater importance than the verbal. We are probably unaware ourselves of many such clues. Recently I watched a number of consultations with Dutch general practitioners: although unable to understand what was said I could estimate with considerable accuracy the personality of the patient and the relationship between patient and doctor.

2. UNDERSTANDING

Correct understanding and diagnosis of subconscious reactions is essential. We all have subconscious reactions and if we look at these we discover that our motive is often to protect a basic source of self-confidence. Most patients draw their self-confidence from five areas of activity (see also Ch. 6 and Appendix IX uses the Familygram to record confidence areas):

— Marriage and sex
— Family and immediate group relationships
— Hobbies, leisure and wider social relationships
— Work and job
— Finance and material status.

If the practitioner suspects subconscious motivations he should unobtrusively explore the patient's activities in these five areas.

A foreman reported palpitations of 10 months duration. He admitted that his job was a responsible one and gave him great self-confidence. The patient insisted that the increased responsibility had nothing to do with his symptoms. Despite this, after a suitable pause further questions revealed the significant information that the patient's new and responsible job had also started 10 months previously. This would suggest that the job *was* a causative factor and that 'holding it down' was especially important to the patient's confidence.

3. HANDLING

All of us (doctors and psychoanalysts are no exception) paper over the cracks in our psychological walls. Despite the teachings of the psychoanalytical school the general practitioner will find that many subconscious human reactions are both protective and normal.

The practitioner can learn much that will allow him to help his patients but he is wise in the majority of cases not to force open discussion of subconscious motivations. It does not help an inadequate man to be told that his subconscious reactions are due to his inadequacy; if a wife has subconsciously turned a blind eye to her husband's infidelity it may not help her to be told that this is the cause of her symptoms. The consultation should be kept at the indirect subconscious level for as long as the patient wishes. Most such reactions will be 'normal' and the problems are best solved by the patient. The family doctor only occasionally need show that he has recognised a subconscious motive and should not be too obvious in his exploration of such tender areas. When all these skills of diagnosing (and handling) of normal problems have been learned, the doctor is in a position to recognise the abnormal. In clearly abnormal cases he will instigate more postive treatment and will be grateful for the help of psychiatrists, psychoanalysts, social workers, neighbours, etc.

Handling the diffident patient with a relatively low self-esteem requires a different approach to that for the overconfident individual.

The diffident, insecure patient lacks confidence in many areas and anything that is said may be misconstrued. Thus the patient says her baby is bottle fed and even a non-commital 'mmm' from the doctor is likely to be felt by the patient to be a noise denoting disapproval. Encouragement for these patients is best given by good eye contact and a single encouraging head nod.

Such patients tend to be discouraged by:

— verbal comments of all kinds by the doctor
— telephone interruptions, etc.
— direct questioning about personal areas
— overconfident behaviour by the doctor.

The doctor can be much less circumspect with the overconfident patient who is usually less sensitive to both verbal and non-verbal influences. Most patients, however, when they visit the doctor, tend to feel insecure initially.

4. RECORD

The graphic method described in Appendix IX (p. 728) provides a quick, easily learnt record which allows recall of a patient's suspected motivations. Despite their obvious subjectivity, assessments of such motivations affect every doctor's decisions. Subsequent recall is therefore essential.

Mistakes and pitfalls

1. The doctor fails to appreciate that his or her own behaviour is as deeply shaped by subconscious motivations and partially acknowledged feelings, as the patient's. It is only too easy to allow these submerged biases to influence how we react to patients.

2. A common misunderstanding arises because all patients are afraid of suffering from 'imaginary disease'. The patient comes to the doctor for reassurance and after examination or investigation is told that there is nothing wrong. The patient takes the doctor's statement literally and assumes that the doctor is saying his symptoms are imaginary or that he has wasted the doctor's time.

3. The doctor attempts reassurance but shows irritation or undue haste, and the patient's subconscious insecurity is increased.

4. An insecure patient mistakenly feels the doctor is being critical — a frequent misunderstanding with mothers.

5. The doctor himself shows his insecurity by reacting aggressively to a patient's aggression. The doctor-patient relationship inevitably deteriorates.

6. The doctor feels uneasy when emotions are expressed by patients and is afraid of showing emotion himself. Both reactions are understandable, in a professional situation, but are often counter-productive. As doctors we should not be afraid of using our natural feelings of empathy as a legitimate part of our professional interactions with patients.

7. The doctor tries to explore a 'protected area' of a patient's subconscious and the patient feels this is unjustified. A Catholic patient might feel that an unrequested discussion of birth control was unwarranted. An attractive 30-year-old woman once told me that she changed her doctor because even at the most trivial consultations he made her feel that her symptoms were due to difficulties in her sex life.

8. One of the most frequent mistakes that practitioners make arises because the doctor has failed to realise that the patient

subconsciously wants something that the doctor is not able or prepared to give. There is a wide range of such situations. They are so common that if there is any difficulty with a patient the doctor should always ask himself. 'What did the patient *really* want from me?' The doctor must be aware of a patient's underlying subconscious needs even if they cannot always be fulfilled (Ref. 5.1). Otherwise the actions of both doctor and patient will appear irrational to the other and both will become needlessly frustrated. A few common examples:

The patient wants an explantation for a symptom — the doctor says that no serious disease is present but does not explain the symptom.

The patient wants an organic illness as a face-saver — the doctor cannot find one.

A mother wants reassurance about her handling of a child — the doctor tells her that she is worrying needlessly.

The doctor tells a diffident patient who lacks confidence — 'Pull yourself together' or 'It's up to you'.

A patient who overvalues himself and uses illness to bolster up his role view of himself — the doctor refers him to a psychiatrist or tells him his complaint is psychogenic.

Any patient who has an ulterior motive or is using his illness to influence his relationships with other people — the doctor tells the patient that he has no organic disease.

Those fortunately rare patients who because of some past experience with doctors subconsciously resent the whole medical profession. Such patients may subconsciously manipulate different medical opinions or situations in a quite unnatural way. Whatever the doctor says or does is likely to be wrong.

THRESHOLDS OF AWARENESS

The concept of the subconscious requires also that there is a level of consciousness. This level we take for granted but tend to regard as fixed. A little example reveals that this level far from being fixed is very variable:

If the reader considers for a moment the pressure of his shoes on his feet, he will simultaneously become conscious of this pressure; before, he was unaware of the sensation.

We all know that it is possible to forget a pain or headache when we are excited only to become aware of it again when we are bored.

Anxiety, boredom, depression, fatigue, illness, apprehension and insecurity all appear to lower an individual's thresholds to symptoms — especially pain. A vicious circle is set up because awareness of a symptom may lead to anxiety with further lowering of thresholds. The sense of helplessness in the face of any chronic symptom will lead to a similar vicious circle of awareness and lowered thresholds.

Thresholds can be raised by excitement, interest, group activities and drugs. Thus the practitioner may be able to help a patient both by removing the cause of a symptom and by raising the patient's threshold to it. Many self-help groups increase the patient's confidence. The group support appears to increase the patient's feeling of control and raises thresholds of awareness. This effect is seen in many hospices and cancer self-help groups. Doctors have much to learn from such groups.

Thresholds to pain vary considerably in different ethnic groups and in different individuals as studies of women in labour show.

Probably closely related to a patient's threshold of awareness is the threshold for taking action, i.e. reporting to the doctor, as is shown by the following study from this practice.

A random sample of 200 adult patients, under our continuous care for 12 years, was analysed to assess the number of incidents of disease reported to the doctor during this time. The patients could be divided into three groups of about equal size (Table 4) according to the frequency with which they reported disease. Analysis revealed that the frequent attenders reported more minor complaints than the other two groups. The reporting rate for an

Table 4

Group	Number of patients in the sample	Number of patients with influenza A serologically positive	Percentage of serologically proven influenza in each group
Rare attenders (0–19 incidents)	65	10	15.5
Medium attenders (20–29 incidents)	56	8	14.3
Frequent attenders (30–120 incidents)	79	12	15.2
Total	200	30	15.0

acute febrile disease such as influenza by contrast was identical for all three groups.

A further study from this practice revealed that the incidence of post-herpetic neuralgia was significantly higher in the group of frequent attenders than in the other groups.

Applications to practice

1. The practitioner must make allowances for different thresholds of awareness in different patients before he can achieve an objective assessment of a symptom. Thus if a patient attributes a chest pain to heart trouble it may feel more severe than if the pain is attributed to a knock.
2. The concept of thresholds provides a useful and realistic explanation that may help the patient as well as the doctor to understand the nature of some symptoms associated with anxiety.
3. The practitioner may be able to help patients by advising group activities that raise thresholds of awareness — a job, a holiday, an evening out, etc.
4. Many symptoms associated with depression probably arise because of the lowered threshold of awareness.

STRESS AND UNRESOLVED CONFLICT

As with physical disease emotional problems have two components:
— The precipitating cause (the seed)
— The patient's personality (the soil).

It is often said that stress causes psychoneuroses. This is rather like saying that resistance stops an aeroplane going faster — a true statement — but when an aeroplane's wing is being designed we have to know what is meant by resistance. Is it the pressure that is built up in front of the wing or is it the suction (i.e. absence of pressure) that occurs behind it? Similarly, the hypothesis of stress does not help in dealing with the practical problems of psychoneurosis. Many patients develop tension states when they are unemployed; they start a job and their symptoms disappear although the job has presumably added to the stress of life. Are we to say that the causative stress is boredom, i.e. absence of stress? As soon as reasoning takes this kind of turn we are wise to reconsider our position.

An unmarried teenage girl complains that she is feeling listless, tired, weepy, irritable and cannot sleep. Systematic enquiry reveals nothing abnormal — her periods are regular and she denies missing a period. A pregnancy test is sent off without the patient being aware of its purpose. At the subsequent interview in 10 days time when the test is positive, the girl admits that she has missed 2 periods and is afraid of pregnancy but disapproves of termination. She is persuaded to discuss and face her problems and make arrangements about the baby. As soon as these steps have been taken the tension symptoms disappear. She will probably go through the strains of childbirth without further symptoms of tension. What caused the symptoms of tension? Not physical or social problems, because these should have been maximal at term. Not fear or guilt, because her symptoms did not start until 2 periods had been missed. Once she had faced up to her problems and made her decisions, although she still had to face the world and childbirth, her tension symptoms disappeared. It was the failure to face her conflicts and not the conflicts themselves that caused the tension symptoms.

All too often a family doctor is powerless to help the internal conflicts of his patients.

> EXAMPLE. A mother of four children — a devout Catholic — develops tension symptoms because she feels that she no longer loves her husband. If the doctor explains that her conflict is due to fear of further pregnancy and not loss of affection, he may well precipitate a guilt reaction that will increase the resentment against her husband.

Because the term stress can refer to almost any precipitating cause it is unsatisfactory and should, if possible, be avoided.

If we look carefully at the so-called psychoneurotic behaviour patterns that are presented to the practitioner we often find that there is an unresolved conflict which involves the patient's role or status. This conflict in turn undermines confidence, lowers thresholds of awareness and allows many tension and behavioural symptoms to 'surface'. The unmarried girl in the above example had to face the conflict of roles between 'teenage daughter' and 'unmarried mother'.

Internal conflicts that involve patients' roles (mental images of themselves) are so common that it is necessary to elaborate the concept of roles.

INTERNAL CONFLICT, THE CONCEPT OF 'ROLES' AND SELF-CONFIDENCE

When discussing the ambiguous term 'stress' I pointed out that I found it was more helpful to think not of the stress but of the possible unresolved conflicts in a patient's life. We all of us want both to have our cake and eat it. Thus the privileges of a new role are happily accepted. Frequently, however, the inherent obligations of the role have not been fully faced. The unresolved conflict which follows may cause loss of confidence and tension symptoms whose origins the patient only partly understands.

To understand the nature of many such unrecognised internal conflicts the concept of role-playing and role-identity is helpful. If a patient comes to me as a doctor he expects me to behave in a certain way, while I expect him to undergo examination or questioning about many personal subjects that would be considered rude in any other situation. We have allocated to each other the respective roles of doctor and patient. We both play our parts and life is easier because we can, within limits, each predict the behaviour of the other. Occasionally two individuals may have different views about a role, as when a patient comes into the consulting room smoking or when a doctor uses a patient to teach students. Usually, however, society allocates our role and we play it happily without thought. The following is an example of internal reactions that may follow a conflict of roles.

> EXAMPLE. A conscientious 23-year-old housewife married to a schoolmaster reported increasing but intermittent headaches with loss of sleep and occasional dizziness. Examination of the nervous and cardiovascular systems failed to reveal evidence of organic disease. The patient was tentatively questioned further about her family relationships. She had no children but was spending much of her day travelling 5 miles to help her mother. She was unable to see much of her husband. The husband was very sympathetic but the patient felt guilty. The doctor pointed out that she had a greater obligation to her husband than to her mother and that it might be better for everyone if she did less for her mother and more for her husband. She was obviously glad to do this and her symptoms settled.

In this example role theory would suggest that there was an unrecognised unresolved conflict between the patient's desire to play the role of the *good daughter* and that of the *good wife*. The conflict was internal and entirely dependent on the patient's own internalised views of herself and her role.

A little introspection reveals that we create an internalised view of our own physical world. This allows us to find our way about and co-ordinate our movements geographically.

In a similar way we build up an internalised picture of our role in relation to our personal world, this helps each of us to predict and interpret the actions and emotions of others with a minimum of explanation.

There are, however, three special characteristics of this role that are of tremendous importance to the practitioner:

1. We mind very much what other people think of us. As we have seen, self-confidence — that essential driving force that we all collect so assiduously and protect so aggressively — is largely derived from our successful performance of our role.

The internalised 'role view' that each adult individual has of himself must be a 'success story' if he is to maintain his self-confidence. We mind what other people think of us because our peers are the ultimate judge of our success and therefore our source of confidence and drive.

2. An adult individual will start to play a new role; if he feels he has done this successfully his self-confidence increases and as a result he becomes dependent on the new role, which may be that of a successful doctor or soldier but can also be that of a successful delinquent or a successful invalid. The individual with the chip on his shoulder achieves a relative feeling of success by denigrating the efforts of others or by magnifying his own problems.

> EXAMPLE. The very recently qualified doctor at first feels he is still a medical student, but after 2 or 3 weeks he/she may be upset, aggressive or get a new suit if a patient mistakes him for a student — he has become 'hooked', probably for ever, on his new role as a doctor. Because self-confidence is involved an individual's internalised role picture of himself tends to be rosy. This means that in susceptible individuals fear of failure alone may by itself cause an internal conflict with psychoneurotic symptoms, e.g. examinations.

3. Because success is judged by our peers and not by ourselves we tend to picture our roles in general terms that allow each individual to define his/her role in delightfully vague, often illogical or hypocritical ways. Thus the good citizen will be horrified at killing his fellow man but if he changes his role to that of the good soldier he may kill without question. For this reason most people, including doctors, discover that they worry most about those of their mistakes that are going to be apparent to their colleagues or others. Through the ages wars, torture and much cruelty has been

perpetrated in the name of love. Role theory provides an explanation of this illogical behaviour. Similarly it explains much of the illogical, difficult and resentful behaviour of patients who have been subjected to accidents, long periods of sickness or unemployment, etc.

Applications to practice

1. Depression, apparently unexplained anxiety, tension symptoms and acts of aggression may all be useful pointers to internal conflicts involving the patient's self-confidence or internalised role view of himself.
2. Unobtrusive exploration of the five delicate areas (marriage, family, friends, job and status) that provide our self-confidence is indicated.

The reader should study Table 5, p. 110 which indicates some of the many effects of insecurity and loss of confidence. Appendix IX describes a graphic method of recording such insecurities.

3. The general practitioner is one of the few uninvolved individuals who may see patients when they are in the process of changing roles. Occasionally we may be able to influence a patient in the vital few weeks before the new role has become an impregnable basis of the patient's self-confidence, i.e. before the patient has become addicted to the new role. Once addiction has occurred, influencing or altering the role will be extremely difficult.

Compensation cases are a good example. The doctor's natural inclination is to wait and hope that the patient will not raise the question of 'compo'. Usually by this time the patient has become fully hooked on his new role of 'injured individual who deserves recognition'. The general practitioner should therefore raise the question of compensation with the patient immediately an accident arises. He should ensure that any accident has been properly recorded in the official works accident book and the witnesses' names properly entered. The doctor should, at the outset, identify with the patient and underline the danger of getting a chip on his shoulder about compensation. From the start he should encourage the patient in the idea of getting back to work as soon as possible and point out the fact that if the patient has a good case he is likely to fare better financially if he returns to his working role as soon as possible. Few better examples can be given to illustrate the need for early *emotional* as well as *clinical* diagnosis.

Some important examples of role changes in which the doctor may be involved:

Retirement — the patient has difficulty finding a new role
The death of a spouse
The menopause
The mother whose family have all left home (the 'empty nest')
The start of a long chronic illness
The start of any illness or accident in which money or family relationships may be involved (disablement, compensation cases) etc.
When an elderly patient becomes housebound or confined to bed
When a daughter discovers she has to look after her aged parents
When a younger sibling achieves a marked success
When aged parents die and a daughter has to live on her own
When a young mother who wants a family aborts
When a middle-aged mother who already has a large family becomes pregnant
When a patient becomes unemployed or redundant
When any adult begins to develop a chip on his shoulder
When a teenager leaves school and cannot get a job (a major social disaster)
When a teenager goes to university
When a teenage girl starts taking the 'pill'.

New roles are automatically accepted on leaving school, starting a new job, on marriage or parenthood. Most roles are accepted willingly. It may take longer for the reluctant individual to accept a fresh role, i.e. the daughter who has a conflict between job, parents and home; once individuals are involved actively in a role it will eventually be incorporated into their internalised view of themselves.

4. The theory of role identity helps to explain the common but puzzling behaviour pattern when an individual can have complete belief in a role which appears quite illogical to an unbiased observer (doctor), e.g. the hypochondriac, the patient who feels *entitled* to a few days off work, or the teenage "drop out."

5. We allocate roles to others as well as ourselves. This again leads to problems in relationships. Thus a family may label one member 'clever' and another 'clumsy'. Doctors use similar labels often detrimentally — 'problem patient', 'neurotic', 'frequent attender'. These labels can cause suffering and may do considerable

harm by interfering with an individual's acquisition of confidence. When used by doctors about patients such labels may relieve our feelings but often prevent us from seeing the real individual.

Role theory helps us to understand many behavioural problems. It also helps the doctor in two other ways:

- It often shows the doctor how best to encourage and support a patient during a period of change
- A change of role may alert the doctor that a particular patient is vulnerable.

ANXIETY AND WORRY

Anxiety is a normal, healthy, state of expectancy or watchfulness that relates to a future happening likely to threaten the individual's family, security or position in society (role). Anxiety is thus a normal emotion that is often an essential ingredient of many successful activities. It is unpleasant and may interfere with an individual's activities and relationships. Patients therefore want to be rid of it. For the doctor, anxiety is an emotional pointer and symptomatic treatment can be just as ill-advised with anxiety as it can be with abdominal or chest pain.

The clinical features of anxiety are described on page 243.

Applications to practice

1. Simple worry about a medical matter. There is a simple threat to the patient's security and provided the patient has confidence in the doctor, simple reassurance is all that is required in most instances.

2. The patient is anxious but fails to recognise the causes; this failure increases the patient's anxiety and may even lower thresholds sufficiently to uncover other symptoms. The patient's unawareness of the cause is often protective because he does not wish to increase his insecurity by admitting to himself the reasons for his worry. Any situation in which an individual has left one role and not yet acquired confidence in his new role may produce this situation, e.g. promotion syndrome, tired housewife syndrome, etc.

3. Some patients, as a result of heredity, education or intractably difficult emotional relationships, may have a permanently lowered threshold to anxiety, e.g. the housewife who has a mother or a mother-in-law permanently on her back. These individuals may be frequent attenders at the surgery. The doctor probably helps these

patients by being available but should not always expect to achieve radical cures.

4. The practitioner's best guide to the assessment of anxiety is previous knowledge of the patient.

EXAMPLE. A happily married 40-year-old, financially-secure fitter who rarely visited the doctor suddenly reported an attack of acute dyspnoea (sighing type). Full examination was negative and the doctor was able to predict correctly that symptoms were due to anxiety following the sudden death (heart attack) of a friend at work.

5. An awareness of our own anxieties — as the doctor — is equally necessary, e.g. 'Am I reacting to that appendix I missed last week?' or 'Am I over anxious because this patient's father is a doctor?'.

Misleading features and pitfalls

1. Anxiety and organic illness frequently co-exist. The doctor must always eliminate the possibility of organic disease.
2. The practitioner must learn to recognise *abnormal* fears and phobias which may suggest a psychosis or obsessional neurosis.

REASSURANCE AND FAILURE TO REASSURE

Reassurance can only be achieved if the patient has confidence in the doctor.

Confidence is always elusive and hard to create. Every doctor/patient contact varies but the following help to foster an atmosphere of trust:

The doctor must know his job
The patient must feel that the doctor knows his job
The doctor should give simple accurate explanations that each patient can understand
The patient must feel that the doctor has listened to his story and taken adequate steps to investigate, etc.
Surgery premises should be good and the staff efficient and friendly. (A powerful confidence builder that is occasionally overlooked in otherwise excellent practices.)
The doctor must be aware of the common causes for misunderstanding between doctor and patient

EXAMPLE. An intelligent 50-year-old smoker whose wife died of cancer of the breast 5 years before noticed a chronic shoulder pain. Examination and chest X-ray were normal. The doctor was surprised when the patient was obviously upset and resentful on being told that nothing was wrong. The doctor, because he did not know the cause, had failed to explain the reasons for the patient's pain. Further discussion revealed that the patient felt he was being told that his symptoms were *imaginary*.

The concept of an imaginary disease or symptom is logically a contradiction in terms but this is an emotional not a logical situation. In our society so much has been implied about the *malade imaginaire*, neurosis and needless use of the doctor that a universal contempt for these reactions has been created. It is the practitioner's job to recognise and counter such misunderstandings. Patients tend to treat their bodies as machines, without minds, and explanations of mental as opposed to physical processes must be very carefully given.

Applications to practice

1. The doctor must learn to diagnose 'failed reassurance' early.

2. Some common pointers suggesting possible failure to reassure are:

The patient fails to look reassured and is obviously unhappy at the end of the interview.
The patient continues to question the doctor after an explanation has been given.
The patient brings a relative to the interview. The attitude of the extra parent or a spouse will often alert the doctor before anything has been said at all.
Indirect (or direct) hints that the patient wishes some further investigation or action.
The doctor gets up to terminate the consultation but the patient remains seated!

3. The practitioner must know and understand the many social pressures, community influences and popular misconceptions that may hinder his attempts to dispel simple anxiety. These differ greatly in different communities: within ethnic groups their own beliefs about health and illness have a great effect and must be understood, while in our western society the effects of the mass media must be assessed.

Suggestion and social pressures of this sort may cause anxiety by raising doubts, making the patient feel insecure and causing internal conflicts. Personal events and contacts are a more potent source of suggestion than the vaguer influences of the mass media, but all may be relevant to a patient's anxiety or failure to be reassured.

4. There is a significant difference between reassurance and comfort. Reassurance is often not possible whereas comfort nearly always is. For a patient who has just learnt that he has a serious disease, reassurance may be inappropriate; while it may be deeply comforting to be given the opportunity and time to discuss this new situation with a trusted and knowledgeable doctor.

5. Irritation and asperity shown by the doctor under pressure of work are probably the biggest single cause of failure to reassure.

GUILT

We know from our own experience that guilt usually follows feelings of personal failure. These may be failures of either omission or commission. We feel less guilt on behalf of others and for failures that are clearly not our fault. Guilty feelings may be concealed by aggression, deception or self-deception. All these reactions suggest that here too our self-confidence and internalised role picture of ourselves is closely involved.

A mother who leaves an ill child with a neighbour while she goes to work may feel guilty when she returns home and finds her child worse. She may as a result put in an urgent call to the doctor, who must learn to diagnose and manage the causes of the parental guilt as well as the child's illness.

Patients' upbringing plays a great part in creating their 'role view' of themselves and is therefore responsible for many feelings of guilt both conscious and subconscious.

Applications to practice

1. Patients may have a guilty reaction in the following common medical situations:

- Fear of calling the doctor needlessly, especially at night
- Fear that they have delayed too long before calling the doctor
- When a patient has not done what the doctor suggested
- When a patient feels that he or she has gone against social custom, i.e. the mother who has allowed her children to get hold of some matches or pills.

2. Doctors must learn to recognise their own reactions in the following medical situations:

- When they feel they may have made a clinical mistake
- When patients question the service that the doctor provides
- When they recognise that there is truth in a patient's criticisms
- When a patient's problems are similar to the doctor's own unrecognised problems.

3. Guilty reactions will often lead a patient to distort the facts. A mother giving a history to a hospital doctor may imply that she called the general practitioner earlier than she really did. Similarly the practitioner must resist the impulse to distort the clinical facts to justify admitting a patient to hospital.

4. The doctor will rarely discuss the origins of guilt reactions with his patients but will find that recognition of their origins helps him to deal effectively and unemotionally with their consequences.

AGGRESSION

Aggressive behaviour may arise in doctor or patient. Its origin and effects must be clearly understood.

Aggression is natural, normal and often both protective and constructive, but it may be destructive. For this reason nature has produced a number of evolutionary checks to modify aggressive behaviour between members of the same species. Many such situations have been described: when herring gulls face each other aggressively on the border of their nesting territory each will suddenly turn its head to the right and start viciously tearing up grass; they will then walk away from each other as if nothing had happened. Such activities that allow aggression to be 'worked out' are called *displacement activities*. These observations are extremely relevant to human behaviour. An old Irish doctor from whom I learned much used to say, 'if you feel angry or aggressive towards a patient — convinced perhaps that they have 'deliberately' put in a call at three in the morning for the sole purpose of getting you out of bed — always examine them before you show your feelings.' If this is done the doctor will find that his aggressive attitude melts away as he performs the 'displacement activity' of examination.

Aggressive behaviour is usually an individual's subconscious reaction to feelings of insecurity, inferiority, or any attack on his source of self-confidence. In life as a whole, aggression may be a valuable if somewhat uncontrollable drive in an individual's life. It must be stressed, however, that subconscious aggressive reactions must at all costs be kept out of the doctor/patient relationship for one very simple reason:

Aggressive behaviour either in doctor or patient inevitably causes the distortion of vital clinical, emotional and social information that is presented to the doctor.

If a doctor is aggressive because he feels his clinical acumen is being questioned by a request for a second opinion, the patient is liable subsequently to exaggerate many symptoms to justify the request. If patients feel inadequate they may be aggressive and distort clinical symptoms to justify and explain their failure to themselves.

Occasionally a doctor may deliberately put on a facade of aggression if he thinks this is in the patient's interest. This is not a truly aggressive reaction because it is completely conscious and under control.

Applications to practice

Every practitioner must learn how to remove his own and his patient's aggression from the doctor/patient relationship. Each doctor has his own ways of doing this but all methods basically utilise the following steps:

RECOGNITION

The doctor must learn to recognise aggressive behaviour immediately in both himself and his patients. If action is not taken the interview will rapidly get out of control because both parties increasingly try to achieve different objectives.

ACCEPTANCE OF AGGRESSION

The doctor should make the first move to avoid an 'action and reaction' situation in which aggression escalates to further aggression. The doctor must learn to stifle his immediate reactions by making an examination or by asking the patient for more information.

CONSIDERATION OF THE CAUSES

The doctor must consider the possible underlying causes of the aggressive reaction. Is the patient insecure or afraid of some serious disease? Is he reacting to the doctor, to his staff or perhaps to doctors as a whole? Is there guilt? Is the doctor insecure about his clinical position? And so on.

EXPLANATION OF THE PATIENT
This is really a *displacement activity* that allows the doctor to 'work out' his own aggression which he stifled earlier. The explanation must also help the patient and not set up further aggressive reactions. Thus if a patient wants a second opinion about a headache to exclude the possibility of a cerebral tumour, the practitioner should be perfectly prepared to arrange this. It would be reasonable for the doctor to explain that the chances of finding a tumour are exceedingly remote. If the doctor then added that he considered a second opinion to be a waste of time and money, there might be a further aggressive reaction from the patient that would almost certainly cause exaggeration and distortion of symptoms. The doctor might then react aggressively and be less receptive to the possibility of serious disease.

DISCUSSION
Discuss future constructive action to be taken. This combined action reintroduces the idea in the minds of both parties that they have the same objective — the improvement of the patient's health.

REACTIONS TO REJECTION, INSECURITY AND ISOLATION

Rejection is a frequent by-product of many personal relationships. The individual feels that he has been 'refused admission' to a relationship with either a group or with another individual.

Diffident and insecure individuals are especially prone to these reactions. The insecure individual who overvalues himself will react 'huffily' while the diffident patient who undervalues himself will quietly discontinue the relationship, convinced once again that he and his complaint are of little importance to anyone.

I suspect that many present-day attitudes of our profession create much needless feeling of rejection in patients, yet few other reactions destroy a relationship so rapidly.

REGRESSION

This concept suggests that under certain circumstances individuals may attempt to adapt to new or difficult circumstances by reverting to a behaviour pattern of an earlier less mature phase of life.

This concept is helpful to the practitioner when handling adults as well as children.

Applications to practice

1. Toddlers frequently regress if their security is threatened, e.g. they revert to the 'bottle' or nappies when a younger sibling competes for parental affection.
2. Adversity or feelings of failure may cause adults to regress to a previous more successful role, e.g. the mother who wants to go back to her old job when her new young family are clearly most dependent on her.
3. Adults regress from an independent role to a dependent role when they are ill.
4. Old people may regress from a rigid independence to a role of increasing dependence.

DEPRESSION

Originally the term 'reactive depression' referred to the depressed state which followed some failure or personal catastrophe while 'psychotic or endogenous' depression was used to refer to abnormal states of melancholia of the manic depressive type. It was thought that these two were separate entities. In practice they appear to be opposite ends of a single spectrum. Antidepressant drugs are effective for milder cases of depression as well as the severely depressed 'psychotic' patient.

Major life events and certain social factors appear to be precipitating factors in severe as well as moderate degrees of depression. The work of Brown (Ref. 5.2) suggests that sudden loss by separation or death was a major factor in precipitating depression in certain high risk groups.

He identified the following high risk factors:

— women over 30
— loss of mother before the age of 11
— 3 or more children at home under 14
— absence of a job other than that of housewife and mother
— low income group.

Brown considers that the possible common factor is absence of a close confidant for a woman with an already low level of self-esteem.

Brown's work is not conclusive but is consistent with much about depression that is observed in general practice. Antidepressants — BNF 4.3 (Ref. 0.1) — are useful because they make depression bearable. Supportive friends and confidants probably help to protect vulnerable individuals from developing depressions (see Part II, p. 255).

Applications to practice

1. The similarity between depression and the inhibitory phenomenon described by the neurophysiologists is striking.
2. Much of the 'depression' seen by the general practitioner is likely to be within the normal range, i.e. reactive.
3. Antidepressants (and tranquillisers) undoubtedly help the symptoms of depression but should not be regarded by either patient or doctor as sole cures or preventatives. Patients should be carefully followed up so that patients are encouraged wherever possible to reduce or do without long-term treatment and 'repeat presciptions'.
4. If depression is extreme or prolonged then psychiatric referral is considered.
5. Discussion and counselling aim to increase understanding and self-esteem. Changes of job, life style or social contacts may have to be discussed.

THE DYING PATIENT

There is considerable evidence that our subconscious cannot accept the possibility that those we love (or we ourselves) can die.

> EXAMPLES. Patients with cancer who attended a clinic for radiotherapy know that such clinics are almost entirely for people with cancer yet they appear to avoid applying this knowledge to themselves.
>
> If a patient is told for any reason that he only has a few weeks to live, the doctor may then be surprised to find the patient planning his life for months or even years ahead.

Kubler-Ross describes five different kinds of reaction to the knowledge of death:

— denial
— bargaining
— anger
— depression
— acceptance.

One or all of these reactions can be noted in many patients who are struggling to come to terms with the knowledge that they are about to die. *The stages are rarely consecutive.*

Denial, of which two examples are given at the beginning of this section, is often unconsciously encouraged if the doctor is himself afraid to discuss death with patients.

Bargaining occurs usually when the patient has to take decisions.

Anger is often suppressed by patients but is apparent in their diaries.

Depression. Patients may become withdrawn. Often at this time physical well-being is low. Relatives and doctors help at this stage, not by saying or doing anything, but by being available.

Acceptance. Patients achieve a degree of detachment that clearly helps them to accept that they are about to die. Often this coincides with a period when the patient feels physically well. *As with the other stages, this degree of detachment may not remain.*

Application to practice

1. Investigation reveals that a patient has not long to live. Regardless of what has gone before both doctor and patient subconsciously often wish to avoid discussing the subject. The patient may become increasingly anxious (see also pp. 207 and 677).

2. The doctor must help the patient to face up to the fact of dying in the patient's own way at the patient's own pace.

3. The doctor achieves this by encouraging the patient to ask the vital questions.

Patient (exploring): 'How long am I going to be ill, Doctor?'

Doctor (giving the patient a lead that he can take further if he wishes): 'I think it will be a long illness.'

Patient (still exploring): 'Am I going to get better?'

Doctor (giving another lead): 'The outlook is not as good as we would like.'

At this point if the patient ceases his exploration, the doctor knows that the patient is subconsciously not ready to ask the question 'Am I going to die?'

4. Such non-directive counselling techniques are not always suitable. The doctor must learn to use his knowledge of the background and personality of the patient to judge if a more direct approach is indicated. But in every case the doctor must tread warily between the extremes of the blunt truth that destroys the patient's ability to hope and deception, with loss of trust.

5. Gradually the emotional understanding and mutual respect between patient and doctor increase; both help each other to deal with their own inadequacies.

6. The doctors must always remember that continuing support is essential for both patient and relatives. Extensive or detailed verbal input however true or wise probably helps the physician more than the patient and is sometimes counter-productive.

7. Patients tend to judge doctors by their actions not their words.

8. Where feasible death should be arranged in the patient's home A recent Gallup survey in the United Kingdom showed that

— Perception, by patients and relatives, of pain control was better at home
— Perception, by those involved, of explanation and support from the doctor was better at home
— Few patients or relatives raised the question of terminating life.
— Available community support services were underused.

BEREAVEMENT

The acute feelings of loss that we feel when the death occurs of someone we love demonstrates the way we are tied emotionally to those around us.

Two phases of bereavement are usually observed:

The stage of protest. The stage of protest lasts a few days to several weeks. During this phase patients will say that they have to go through the shock of realisation many times a day.

The stage of acceptance and readjustment. There is a period lasting from several months to 3 years when patients are relearning to look forward to life and to live with their loss.

Application to practice

1. There is often a strong sense of omission and guilt in those close to someone who has died — a result perhaps of our unconscious refusal to accept the possibility of death. The doctor can help sometimes by warning patients that such reactions are very common.

2. The sense of guilt may make some individuals react aggressively — 'This should have been done', etc. These reactions are a part of the stage of protest. The practitioner should always visit relatives after death to encourage discussion and understanding.

3. Unexpected or sudden death, especially in young people, frequently causes similar symptoms in suggestible contacts.

4. A spouse may behave as if the dead partner is still alive. This is not uncommon and should not be regarded as abnormal. The behaviour ceases after a few mouths.

5. The practitioner may be able to help a bereaved relative by praise or by showing his respect for the person who has died.

6. Sleeping pills should be given to bereaved relatives with the greatest caution. Habituation in this situation is all too common.

6

The normal individual and the group

Recently, increasing interest has been shown in the relationship of the individual to the group.

Our present emphasis on the individual may obscure our awareness of important group influences.

'No man is an island, entire of itself' is not a trite quotation but is a significant natural law that governs a great deal of human behaviour.

From an evolutionary viewpoint we see that evolution requires a survival of the fittest *species* not survival of the fittest *individual.* For evolution to have worked through the ages there must have been very powerful influences that have subjugated the interests of the individual to that of the species.

If we look at our own experience of different groups — family, friends, colleagues etc. — we find a repetitive pattern of which we are often unconscious.

- The individual initially receives support from and contributes to a particular group.
- If the amount of giving and receiving are reasonably balanced the individual is likely to gain both security and confidence from this group.
- The strength of an individual's bond (loyalty) with any group will vary according to the amount of both giving and receiving.

Like the chicken and its egg we may find it difficult to say which comes first — giving or receiving — but clearly a strong behavioural force is at work.

Arguments in favour of a powerful bond between the individual and the group come from many sources — ethological, philosophical and spiritual.* But perhaps the strongest arguments are from personal experience, especially those in general practice.

*An interesting parallel to the human situation is that of the bee: the integration of the individual within the group is of such a high order that it is possible to regard the hive as the individual. For many people, religious belief links the individual to the group.

Every day we see the shy toddler drawn like a magnet back to the security of its mother's knees; every day we encounter patients who have been isolated from their group in one way or another and are showing signs of insecurity; every day we encounter individuals who have benefited from increased group contact; practitioners see the inner workings of many marriages — effective and ineffective (most of us have wondered at the forces that keep so great a variety of couples together); every day we are privileged to see, in our patients, the powerful protective bonds of friendship and self-sacrifice at work.

The dilemma of service (p. 21) is another facet of this interdependence of the individual and the group; the managerial grid (Fig. 7, p. 133) is a graphic representation of the same relationship.

ACCEPTANCE AND REJECTION

This is a large area of human activity that plays a considerable part in the lives of our patients.

Every individual needs: (a) to be needed (b) one or more individuals to love.

Acceptance and rejection are two fundamental psycho-social terms that are significant because they embrace the relationship of every individual to his group. They involve a wide range of behavioural patterns that stretch from complicated rituals, e.g. degree ceremonies to the simple non-verbal communicative acts that are the basis of ordinary human contact and politeness — shaking of hands or fists, smiling, etc. These are summarised in Desmond Morris's book *Manwatching*.

A similar wide range of acts of acceptance and rejection can be traced in animal behaviour.

We all have experienced the pleasant and unpleasant effects on ourselves of both acceptance and rejection, but despite this we know surprisingly little about the force itself.

The two terms are useful professionally because of their wide application to human situations and because they allow the doctor to analyse human relationships without introducing emotive value judgements about right and wrong.

Applications to practice

1. In children, total or partial rejection by one or both parents has a devastating effect on the child's confidence at any age. A few of the many pointers that the practitioner should bear in mind are:

- The battered baby
- Failure to thrive
- The excessively quiet or timid child or toddler
- The young child that is unusually affectionate with complete strangers
- The child that regresses
- The mother who always blames the child's behaviour on external circumstances
- The delinquent child
- The child that wanders
- Faecal incontinence in a toddler or school child
- The child who is always brought to the doctor by father instead of mother

Many other common behavioural disorders may be suggestive.

2. In teenagers, acceptance or rejection by different peer groups may have tremendous effects on the individual's subsequent life, e.g. drugs or career.

3. In adults, acceptance, friendship and affection provide a strong protective shield for the average individual against the common behavioural and so-called psychoneurotic disorders. Their positive therapeutic influence should never be forgotten. The influence of a 'suitable confidant' in protecting individuals against depression (mentioned in previous chapter) is a good example.

By contrast, rejection may lead to loss of confidence, aggression or a chip-on-the-shoulder.

The doctor should remember that he is in a powerful position to make patients feel rejected, especially if he implies that a patient is worrying needlessly or not progressing as expected.

4. The whole subject of acceptance and rejection of individuals in relation to their group has far-reaching effects. Unfortunately the practitioner has few yardsticks and will frequently be unaware of the extent or nature of such effects.

5. Society tends to reject the disadvantaged, the unemployed, the disabled, the chronic sick, the aged, and the patient with a colostomy or dying slowly of cancer. The practitioner must counter the subconscious tendency to follow society and likewise reject such patients, for he can do much to alleviate their loneliness, lack of confidence and isolation.

SELF-CONFIDENCE AND THE GROUP

A little introspection reveals that self-confidence provides us with an essential driving force. Everyone hoards and aggressively protects this carefully collected commodity.

With children, confidence is obtained from a combination of love and family security and the successful accomplishment of actions and skills. Rejection by the family, physical disablement, ill health and threats to the individual's total security can all reduce the child's confidence (see Table 5, p. 110).

As each individual becomes mature, personal relationships have an increasing influence. We *give* to a group and picture ourselves as performing a role in relation to it. Our self-confidence depends on our ability (real or imagined) to perform this role successfully. In this way, through the judgement of our peers, we are tied firmly to the group that gives us confidence.

In sport, for instance, skill alone fails to satisfy the individual's need for recognition from his peers. 'Par values' in golf are an ingenious way of relating personal to group performance. The method can be applied to any personal audit of process, e.g. Practice Activity Analysis (see Appendix IV, p. 693). Truly isolated individual activities are very rare.

Much of the general practitioner's work is concerned with individuals who have lost confidence following insecure group relationships. The doctor must learn to explore tactfully those areas that may interfere with the patient's group contacts.

Physical health, physical safety and performance of skills
Social factors that affect security — housing, poverty, unemployment, etc.
Creative activities and the individual's willingness to give as well as receive from the group involved
The individual's social contacts cover four areas, discussed below:

I marriage
II family
III job
IV wider social contracts — friends, recreation, etc.

These steps appear complex; but in practice most physical and social factors are known routinely. Assessment of creative attitudes is unreliable, so the practitioner usually concentrates on the patient's social contacts.

I. MARRIAGE — THE PAIR BOND

We are perhaps wrong to regard marriage as a human institution.

Ethology suggests that its origins lie deeply in our evolutionary past.

A study of penguins showed that 55% of 'unions' remained intact for several successive seasons, 33% were ended by death (or disappearance) of one partner, and 12% ended in 'divorce'. Humans appear to follow a similar pattern.

Most of us can recall the surge of self-confidence that was generated by the discovery of mutual attraction in our first sexual experiences.

For most happily united couples there then follows the deeper self-confidence arising from the bonding commitment of shared activities which involve giving as well as receiving — home, family, holidays, job, etc.

The general practitioner has the fascination of watching individuals (including himself) as they travel on this complex journey that starts with the role of *mutually attracted pair* and progresses with ever-increasing involvement and maturity through the successive stages of family life:

— home creation
— preschool family
— school family
— teenage family
— parents with independent family
— grandparents and grandchildren
— mutually dependent 'Darby and Joan'.

Almost unconsciously the practitioner will find himself making emotional diagnoses by placing individuals into these different categories so that he can predict their reactions and monitor their sources of self-confidence. Over the years the family doctor will subconsciously build up a vital store of such information.

'The Jack-Spratt phenomenon' helps to ensure that man and wife do not have to compete for their self-confidence. Thus mutual attraction appears to be stimulated by characteristics that are complementary. Over the years the practitioner will observe that in many happy marriages a balance is reached as the couples play complementary roles. Thus one partner will be careful, worrying, cautious, the other will be optimistic and 'slap-happy'.

The real experts in this field are those couples who have been happily married for long periods of time.

Discussions with such patients suggest that in many happy marriages over the years powerful pair bonds are created by many interactions besides those of sexual interplay. Such parasexual shared activities appear to include:

— mutual worry, especially about children
— laughing together
— eating together
— cooking and shopping for each other
— the physical closeness of the other partner both in the home and in bed.

This explains the observation of many general practitioners that in the young as well as the elderly, strong pair bonding of affection, tenderness and loyalty can be created despite poor or nonexistent mutual sexual activity.

In such new situations the practitioner may not have previous personal experience to guide him and must be prepared to show understanding and empathy before he can even work out his own attitudes.

Applications to practice

THE FAILING MARRIAGE

1. Marriage and sex are one of the major sources of an adult's self-confidence. This means that:

- Most individuals will be reluctant to recognise the failings in their own marriage.
- Many individual doubts will be raised indirectly or under a 'cover story', *before* the patients have themselves recognised the problem.
- By the time the patient has consciously recognised the possibility of failure the marriage relationship may have deteriorated beyond the point-of-no-return.
- The family doctor, health visitor or primary health team member is often the only person available for early indirect approach. Every family doctor knows this situation — the mother who ostensibly brings a child about a small worry and then 'unloads' a half-recognised marriage problem.
- Because self-confidence is involved the practitioner should be sensitive to the patient's need to keep the interview indirect. This is the time for therapeutic listening and non-directive counselling.

2. From previous contacts the general practitioner often knows

the patient's problems. Sometimes he will need to explore this area unobtrusively (or indirectly at a later interview).

3. At this early stage of partial recognition the doctor must diagnose the various alternatives:

Is the patient airing a minor doubt to a sympathetic ear?
Is the patient subconsciously trying to face a significant problem and is she perhaps in need of a therapeutic listener?
Is the patient shy about a problem that has already been fully faced?

The doctor is wise to let the patient set the pace. He does this by making a non-committal supportive remark which the patient can take further, or by saying 'What do *you* feel about this?' or 'You have quite a problem there'.

Marriage guidance counsellors or others with counselling skills are involved only if the patient wishes this.

4. Many marriage problems will settle if given time. Advice from outsiders is rarely of help. The patient's solutions, however bizarre, are more likely to succeed than a solution provided by an outsider.

5. Once a marriage conflict is in the open, the practitioner may be involved because both parties will want to enlist him on their side. When this happens the doctor should try to reduce the emotional temperature by:

— not taking sides
— getting both parties to consult him together
— encouraging the parties to think constructively about relevant decision making outside the immediate quarrel, i.e. the children, the house, finance, jobs, etc.

6. Even in the most clear cut marriage disagreements the doctor should avoid criticism (either direct or implied) of one partner to another. A man may be a gambler, addicted to drink, violent, hopelessly inadequate with a wife who is full of complaints about her husband; despite this the wife may be deeply hurt or upset by a doctor's criticism of her husband. Such is the strength of the pair bond.

7. The following 'outsiders' or institutions may be helpful in a marriage dispute:

— marriage guidance counsellors
— probation officers
— the law

— priest
— health visitors and district nurses
— relatives and friends.

The practitioner must be careful to watch that he keeps professional confidence and is wise to *record* the full statements of both parties.

II. THE FAMILY — KINSHIP RELATIONS

The general practitioner tends to encounter the failures rather than the successes in family relationships. These he sees from three angles:

a. Different types of family — some types have more problems than others
b. Situations of tension between family members that lead to insecurity, e.g. sibling jealousy, etc.
c. Behavioural patterns (often antisocial) that arise in the insecure member, e.g. enuresis, wandering, etc. (described on p. 269 *et seq.*).

DIFFERENT TYPES OF FAMILY

When the family doctor attempts to assess the possible insecurities that underly a particular behavioural problem he may find the following rough classifications helpful:

• Group I — the large (often low income) family with a well-defined, extended family network. The parents are busy keeping the family fed, clothed and financially afloat. The children learn early that each family member is dependent on the rest. Behaviour problems may be plentiful but tend to occur early and sort themselves out, often helped by the supportive activities of the extended family network.

Such families tend to have a fairly rigid role structure. Husbands are often not expected to do housework or cook and children are cared for mainly by the female members.

• Group II — the nuclear family. Both parents working; few children; activities shared; often separated from near relatives — a common family pattern. Most of these families are free of major behavioural problems, although the parents often worry excessively and may appear to be creating their own difficulties. Family standards are often materialistic and parents may add to their children's difficulties by placing undue stress on educational success.

• Group III — The single parent family. Increasingly common.

The strains on the single parent may be considerable, especially in the first 5 years.

- Group IV — Families suffering unemployment. The problems are numerous and destructive because they all lead to loss of confidence in one or more household members.
- Group V — the family with a rigid, difficult or inadequate father. The mother turns to her children for affection and satisfaction. The father's relationship with his children is often erratic. There may be major behaviour problems in the early years — enuresis, tantrums, wanderings, etc — but most settle eventually.
- Group VI — the family with a mother who is unstable, egocentric or fails to relate adequately to her children; the mother does not appear to get enough pleasure from her family. The chidren demand attention but somehow mother is always preoccupied. The situation may be further aggravated because the mother may also fail to relate to her husband who may become detached from his family and 'married to his work'. Children of such families seem to be in trouble from the start and their problems tend to increase and not decrease as the children get older.
- Group VII — The family from a different ethnic background to the community and doctor. As with class and income, large differences between doctor and patient can create problems of understanding. A knowledge of these different cultural patterns and norms is essential and often gives the doctor a picture of the 'richness' as well as the difficulties of family life in socially and ethnically different groups.

The doctor should always try to treat the family as a whole and not just the individual problem. In practice it is usually extremely difficult for an outsider to alter family dynamics.

SITUATIONS OF TENSION BETWEEN FAMILY MEMBERS THAT LEAD TO INSECURITY

Sibling jealousy. The older sibling usually starts reacting when the younger child is about 9 months old. If the age difference of the siblings is large or if the onset is late, the situation can become intractable.

The favoured child. A mother or grandparent upsets the balance of the family by spoiling one child. Symptoms of insecurity may develop in the siblings. The favoured child may later have difficulties when adjusting to school or life as a whole. As adults these favoured children are often self-centred and easily develop a chip-on-shoulder.

The unloved child. One or both parents may, for a variety of reasons, tend to reject one sibling. This is likely to lead to major behaviour problems in the child who becomes increasingly difficult. A vicious circle of attention seeking is soon set up.

Father-son antagonisms. Often appear when the son is in his teens.

The possessive mother. Some mothers seem unable to let their children live their own lives. This relationship is often associated with psychosomatic disease such as asthma in a child. The problem is also encountered in adults, e.g.:

— The bachelor son dependent on his mother (usually a reasonably stable situation)
— The possessive mother who interferes in the relationship between her son and daughter-in-law
— The unmarried daughter who 'looks after' mother
— The married daughter whose possessive mother lives with or close to her daughter and interferes.

The quarrelling parents. When both parents become more concerned with their differences than with the family that they have in common, their children suffer. Such parents often try to involve the children in their quarrels, with destructive effects.

The doctor should remember the large part played by heredity and that at the present time it is almost impossible to assess the relative effects of the heredity and conditioned (acquired) influences in any family.

Applications to practice

1. The family doctor should make a quick assessment and record (appendix IX) of every family problem in terms of the emotional security and insecurity of each individual in relation to (a) the rest of the family, and (b) the outside world. Increasing the security of one member may cause a relative insecurity in another, curing an alcoholic may upset his wife by reducing the dependence of husband on wife. The doctor must attempt to treat the family as well as the individual member.

2. In most problems his approach will be supportive. He must

— help the parents by listening and showing concern
— treat the individual, often symptomatically
— play for time to enable the individuals to solve their own problems and gain confidence

— refer severe behaviour problems to a child psychiatrist
— enlist the help of a social worker if indicated.

3. The practitioner should distrust personal extrapolations from his own family experiences.

4. The practitioner should be aware of the tremendous long term effects of family influences, especially those during the first 5 years of a child's life.

5. The 'problem family'. Social pointers that may alert the doctor to the presence of 'trouble' in a family include the following:

- Parental pointers:
  - — Unsupported mother (and the much rarer unsupported father)
  - — Mental illness or subnormality in one or both parents
  - — Physical illness in the mother
  - — Repeated, numerous or unwanted pregnancies
  - — Social disadvantage, e.g. unemployment, poverty, race, etc.
  - — Social inadequacy, e.g. alcoholism, father constantly changing or losing job, or previous history of crime
  - — Wilful irresponsibility, e.g. repeated accidents from falls, injuries, burns or accidents with tablets
  - — Apathy in the mother; the doctor gets the feeling that the mother never cares about anything, not even her children
  - — Cruelty or violent behaviour; a dog that 'cringes' at sudden movements of any adult is a good indicator of such behaviour; in such households the children are sometimes abnormally 'quiet'; previous convictions for cruelty
  - — Poverty that is clearly a result of parental inefficiency and not poor wages; the practitioner gains much information about this when he goes to wash his hands at the end of a house call
  - — The presence of an added family burden, e.g. an invalid parent or handicapped child
  - — Recurrent aggressive or antisocial behaviour towards doctor or visiting staff
  - — Trouble with neighbours
  - — Continual change of domicile.

- Environmental pointers:
  - — Unsatisfactory or unhygienic housing
  - — Insanitary surroundings, e.g. caravan sites, slum clearance, etc.
  - — Geographical locality
  - — Unsatisfactory or unhygienic furnishings — the state of floor

covering, walls, paint, etc.; the absence of adequate fireguards.

- Baby or child pointers:
  - — Failure to gain
  - — Unexplained bruises (battered baby)
  - — Inadequate or dirty clothing
  - — Inadequate sleeping accommodation
  - — Persistent crying
  - — Poor hygiene
  - — Children left alone or in charge of other young children
  - — Toddlers who are clearly confined or who continue to suck a bottle or 'dummy' because it is the only comfort that is truly theirs
  - — A baby feeding from a 'propped' bottle.
- Other pointers:
  - — Reports of irregularities from neighbours and relatives
  - — Repeated defaulting from antenatal, paediatric or surgery appointments.

A practitioner may notice a few of these pointers in otherwise normal or 'happy feckless' families but most so called 'problem' families will demonstrate a number of the above characteristics.

6. In our practice the frequency of social problems was:

— Housing problems (6 per 1000 patients per year)
— Geriatric difficulties (5 per 1000 patients per year)
— Occupation (5 per 1000 patients per year)
— Financial mismanagement (4 per 1000 patients per year)
— Major mental problems (3 per 1000 patients per year)
— Neighbours and community relationship (3 per 1000 patients per year)
— Parent — child problems (2 per 1000 patients per year)
— Relatives (2 per 1000 patients per year)
— Unmarried mother (increasing rapidly over recent years).

The figures are only a very rough guide and represent only the major problems. Many are difficult to solve and persist in the practice for several years.

7. For many of these major problems the general practitioner will need some assistance from a social worker or health visitor, etc. This help should be carefully chosen because it may be needed for a long time.

8. Very occasionally removal of one or more members from the family environment may be the only satisfactory solution to a family problem.

9. Any suggestion of physical abuse towards children or other family members requires early recognition, assessment and referral. For details see 'Non-Accidental Injury' (p. 675 *et seq*).

III. THE JOB

For most of us, our job, whether it be that of secretary, mother, industrial worker or doctor, plays a vital role in maintaining our self-confidence. Most doctors have experienced the anxiety, the inability to concentrate, and the vague feeling of depression that follows making a mistake — especially a mistake that is likely to be obvious to our colleagues or patients.

Patients rarely mind being asked about their jobs. Unfortunately if a job is 'going badly' and affecting self-confidence, the patient will be reluctant to admit this. The practitioner may have to take this into account.

Many jobs are boring and repetitive and if the individual cannot give and receive confidence from his 'mates' or peers he turns to other sources.

Application to practice

1. If the doctor considers that the job is responsible for tension symptoms he should explore the patient's job relationships and not the work itself. The following common situations provide good examples of this:

The promotion syndrome (a man from the shop floor is promoted to work with graduates)
The professional man starting a new job
The foreman with a difficult shop steward
The semiskilled worker who is forced to work under a new boss or with fresh 'mates'
The schoolmaster, foreman, etc., with disciplinary troubles.

2. Sometimes the technicalities of a job are too much for an individual. Confidence is lost because the patient is overburdened by responsibility or job expectations that are too great.

3. The devastating effect of unemployment and divorce on self-confidence should never be forgotten.

4. A patient may be doing a job badly because he has an endogenous depression.

IV. SOCIAL AND EXTENDED FAMILY CONTACTS

Hobbies, social contacts, family parties, religious groups, trips, old time dancing, clubs, pubs, bingo, football matches, sport of all kinds, often play a tremendously important part in the giving and receiving of self-confidence and preventing tension states, etc. The impact of television and the mass media in this context is uncertain.

Within most communities there are many supportive groups which can have a tremendous influence on isolated individuals. These include

— ethnic and religious
— service clubs, i.e. Rotaries, Lions, etc.
— activity clubs, i.e. gardening, dog breeding, athletic, etc.
— groups related to a specific disability, i.e. AA, diabetes, etc.

It is the family doctor's job to know and develop contacts with such clubs so that he can put suitable patients in contact with them.

Liking patients and people makes this aspect of one's job amusing, interesting and friendly. Perhaps as general practitioners we should be more systematic and professional about this field of activity that can be so important to our patients. Certainly there is a place for extending the influence and expertise of the occupational therapist into the community. The practitioner should never forget the therapeutic power of giving and receiving friendship.

INSECURITY IN THE COMMUNITY AS A WHOLE

In the family group we have seen that many situations are associated with insecurity, loss of self-confidence and certain types of behaviour pattern. These common behaviour patterns are summarised in Table 5. Similarly in the larger community group it is possible to identify behaviour patterns that are associated with individual situations of insecurity.

In the broad spectrum of normal behaviour, individual reactions tend to gravitate towards two extremes — the diffident and the over confident. The presentation and management of the two extremes is different.

Table 5 *Confidence, Insecurity and Behaviour*. Some common behavioural patterns that may be aggravated by insecurity and loss of confidence.

Age in Years	Confidence gained by	Insecurity and deprivation caused by	Behavioural effect of deprivation that may have to be considered
0–1 Infant	Parental attention — Smiling — Touching — Eye Contact — Cuddling — TLC (Tender, loving, care)	Loss of maternal attention — Maternal job — Husband's demands — Sibling demands — Maternal fecklessness — Poverty Loss of paternal attention Parental Rejection	Excessive crying Feeding problem Sleeping problem Failure to thrive Battering
0–4 Toddler	Praise by parents Attention of parents Successful learned skills — Motor — Speech and Singing — Toileting — Dressing — Helping — Imitating Activities with Parents — Games, Trips, Eating TLC	Another baby Sibling competition Sibling disease Sibling success Parental favourites Parental jobs Parental marriage problems	Tantrums Toilet problems (delay) Speech delay Food fads Negative approach Wandering Rocking Hyperactivity Revolt over dependence Other attention seeking Regression Breath-holding attacks
5–12 Child	Skills successfully performed — Mental — Motor — Creative Praise of adults, i.e. parents, teachers, peers Activities with Parents — Eating, games, trips, holidays, etc. TLC	Sibling success or disease Parental interest is elsewhere — job, etc. Teacher interest lacking Peer interest lacking Parental marriage problems	Enuresis Faecal incontinence Soiling Stealing School phobia Truancy Abdominal pain Vomiting Ill health Revolt Dependence Psycho-somatic disorder

Age in Years	Confidence gained by	Insecurity and deprivation caused by	Behavioural effect of deprivation that may have to be considered
13–19 Teens	Peer opinion Skills successfully performed — Mental — Motor — Creative Sexual success Job success Taking parents for granted	Failure with: — School — Job — Sex — Peer Group Unemployment Fear of future failures Acne	Revolt or overdependence Extreme views and religion Violence Vandalism V.D. Drugs or Alcohol excess Pregnancy (unwanted) Accidents Driving and Road traffic accidents Criminal activities Suicide Psycho-somatic disorders Anorexia nervosa
20–60 Adult	Status of work, job, money, housing, car, etc. Social status with peers, neighbours, leisure, etc. Creative pursuits Successful raising of family	Failure through: — Illness or disability — Inadequate personality — Marital problems — Job demotion — Unemployment Menopause, boredom and 'empty nest' Interfering 'in-laws'	Anxiety and tension Self deception Hysteria Hypochondria Absenteeism Malingering Depression Suicide Divorce and marriage problems Violence and crime Alcohol and drugs
60 + Elderly	Status of past work Successful marriage, etc. Contact with children and, grandchildren Contact with friends of own age becomes increasingly vital	Ill health — physical Mental deterioration Loss of Spouse, bereavement Lack of Social contact Loneliness Financial insecurity Aggressive children	Anxiety and tension Talkativeness Eccentricity Alcohol Depression Paranoia Suicide

Type I. The diffident reactions to insecurity

These include:

Simple self-consciousness (blushing, stuttering, clumsiness, palpitation, etc.) induced by any individual's insecurity in relation to a group

Tension states (symptomatology described on p. 246) induced by such situations as:

— Promotion syndrome — promoted individual not yet accepted by the group

— Tired housewife — isolated from contemporaries in her nuclear home

— Mother and daughter syndrome — strong-willed mother inhibits daughter's confidence, daughter has chronic tension state

— Possessive mother-in-law situation — daughter-in-law is isolated from her own family (her previous source of confidence) and is unable to get confidence from her marriage and develops tension symptoms.

The general practitioner will find that these syndromes and behavioural patterns all have the following characteristics in common:

1. Symptoms, e.g. blushing, tension symptoms, etc. prevent these patients from doing what they want. There is no obvious motive.

2. Attempts to 'master' symptoms consciously, makes them worse. A situation of 'paralysis from analysis' may develop.

3. Symptoms are vaguely described, ill-defined and often reported under a cover story.

4. Patients' insight is good initially, but as insecurity increases confidence is gradually lost, insight disappears and there may be a 'cry for help' gesture. Patients do not mind referral to a psychiatrist and may initiate this.

5. Internal conflicts are often apparent to both patient and doctor.

6. Patients will admit to feeling insecure and lacking in confidence. Such patients easily feel rejected.

7. Patients tend to undervalue themselves in relation to their group.

Treatment is by recognition and encouragement. Often it is successful and rewarding.

Type II. The over-confident reaction to insecurity

These include:

Simple resentment, anger and frustration
Accident and compensation neuroses
Post-concussional syndrome
Munchausen syndrome and the deliberate deceivers
Some severe hysterical syndromes
The chip-on-the-shoulder syndrome — the individual, usually male who blames everything but himself for his own failure, may 'take it out of' his family
The poor-little-me syndrome — usually a woman; may be attractive, often spoilt as a child; self-centred; hard as nails; gets everyone fussing round her
The chronic hypochondriac — may develop from any of the above as life 'closes in' round them in middle age.

In contrast to the type I behavioural patterns the characteristics of this group are reversed:

1. Symptoms allow these patients to do what they want. Thus there is a clear self-motivation that is more apparent to others than to the patient.

2. There is no apparent desire by the patients to 'master' their symptoms.

3. Symptoms are usually definite, clearly defined and often related to a previous organic illness. The patient is possessive about the illness — 'my pills', 'my rheumatism', etc., and can sometimes be observed consciously noting a diagnosis for future use. There is little diffidence about symptoms and major investigations and operations are accepted easily or welcomed.

4. Insight is poor and self-deception may be considerable. Attempts to wean patients of symptoms are resented, as is any suggestion of psychiatric referral.

5. Patients do not admit readily that they lack confidence and tend to hide their insecurity by means of aggression or self-deception.

6. Patients tend to overvalue themselves in relation to their group.

Treatment is usually difficult, often resented by the patient and rarely successful.

THE BEHAVIOURAL GRID

This is a simple 'model' that helps us to understand the nature of the two types of behaviour pattern just described because it relates the individual to the group.

Most individuals tend to gain confidence and drive from their group and may lose it in isolation: most of our important reactions require that we resolve the 'food queue' dilemma — i.e. if food is in short supply and we try to go before our turn the queue will turn against us, while if we always allow others to go first we will starve. In the *normal* individual, therefore, a concern for self is balanced by an equal concern for the group; a similar situation can be observed every time a large crowd leaves an auditorium or room through a single door.

Figure 5 puts this relationship graphically. In any community the majority of normal individuals will be on or near to the line OA. Most of the community will be within the ellipse but as the dotted lines are approached the scatter will become thinner and individuals will be increasingly isolated from the main group. Those individuals lying above the line OA will overvalue themselves in relation to the majority, while those below the line OA will undervalue themselves in relation to the majority.

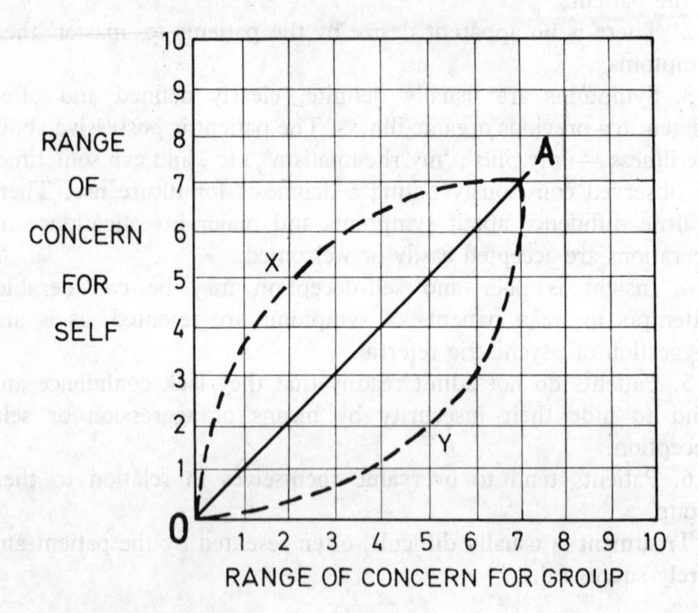

Fig. 5. The behavioural grid

If as a result of heredity, faulty education or circumstances (promotion, mother-in-law, marriage, etc.) any individual becomes isolated on the lower edge of the ellipse, his insecurity and lack of confidence will tend to type I — diffident behaviour pattern. Individuals isolated on the upper edge will show a different pattern of isolation and tend toward type II (over-confident) behaviour patterns. These individuals are reluctant to revalue themselves at a lower level, i.e. move downwards on the grid; this is the reason why the type II behaviour patterns are all so intractable and why their cure involves prevention and education.

This simple model provides insight into some of the circumstances and controllable factors in a patient's life that are associated with what we now vaguely label psychoneurosis.

EXAMPLE 1 — THE TIRED HOUSEWIFE. A teenage girl at 2, 3 does not expect a lot of life or herself but would like to be a good mother. She marries and moves to the isolation of her new nuclear home at point Y (2, 5). The tension symptoms associated with isolated and undervaluation of self start to appear. Cure will involve contact and friendship with a new group through neighbours, school activities, antenatal clinics, a job, an active housewives' association, etc. (point 4, 4 on the grid). Sometimes the patient will regress to 'Mum' at 2, 3 with disappearance of tension symptoms.

EXAMPLE 2 — THE COMPENSATION CASE. A reasonably *normal* steelworker at the position 4, 3 suffers a major works accident and is removed from his usual group contacts to point 4, 2. He becomes the centre of attention in a hospital setting which may even increase his self-importance and he finishes up at the point X (5, 2). After some months the medical profession say he is cured and he is left stranded at X where the vicious circle of isolation and protection of status removes the natural drive to return to his group. Similar patterns of isolation associated with overvaluation of self can be pictured in all the type II behaviour patterns.

The failure of tranquillisers and antidepressants

Looked at in this way it is not surprising that tranquillisers and antidepressants frequently seem so ineffective in both types of behaviour pattern. Their effect may be to numb the individual's feeling of isolation and may hamper his natural drive to return to the group on the line OA.

In the last century gin was perhaps used as we now appear to use tranquillisers.

It is vital that the medical profession study this whole problem more constructively, in terms of the whole person and human group behaviour rather than in terms of disease processes.

The practitioner should look more closely at the protective and therapeutic power of friendship and develop methods of getting isolated and insecure individuals back into group activities within the community. Finance from government, health and social services could profitably be diverted from our escalating drug bill for the purpose of fostering group activities and simple friendship in the community.

7

The tools of general practice

'We trained very hard — but it seemed that every time we were beginning to form up into teams we would be reorganised.
I was to learn later in life that we tend to meet any new situation by reorganising; and a wonderful method it can be for creating the illusion of progress while producing confusion, inefficiency and demoralisation.'

—Petronius Arbiter 210 B.C.

In the previous chapters we have looked at the different kinds of accurate information that the primary physician must learn to collect and use:

— clinical
— emotional
— social and cultural.

We have discussed the practitioner's need to arrange this information so that he can identify and utilise clinical and behavioural patterns.

In this chapter I propose to discuss the tools that enable the general practitioner to collect, organise, store, retrieve and use this information for the benefit of patients.

The main tools to be considered are:

I The consultation
II The hospital and specialist services
III The medical record, methods of recording, information storage and retrieval, computers etc.
IV The practice — staff, premises and communication.
V The social support services available in the community.

Every practitioner must learn to use these tools and must then learn to assess and streamline their use. The quotation at the start of this chapter can easily apply to reorganisation in practice.

The developing practitioner should learn to ask the following questions about any proposed reorganisation:

— will it help patients?

— is it economical for the participants in terms of time and cost?
— does it increase understanding and trust between patients, staff and colleagues? This last question makes the doctor think in terms of personalities; it would be relevant if staff reorganisation was under consideration.

An answer of yes to these 3 questions renders Petronius Arbiter's conclusions (quoted above) unlikely.

I. THE CONSULTATION

The consultation can be divided into the well known nine basic objectives:

S 1. Obtaining the patient's confidence through understanding, empathy, showing concern, by listening and giving simple accurate explanations
2. The reason for the patient's visit
3. Relevant background information including social, family and past history
4. Elaboration of the main complaints (including systems enquiry)

O 5. Physical examination
6. Special investigation

A 7. Diagnosis, prognosis and analysis
8. Accurate recording of findings, action taken, etc.

P 9. Handling, management and treatment.

Theoretically each objective is achieved in logical sequence. In practice each element competes for time and every consultation must be tailored to fit the different needs of each patient. The doctor must learn to be flexible and after reaching objective 2 must make a number of quick decisions about the future conduct of the interview.

The art of consultation can only be learned by constant practise. Consulting techniques can be improved by self monitoring and audio-visual techniques, but ultimately, as with other skills, every aspect should be so well learnt that it is used automatically while remaining accurate and flexible.

The following examples are given to demonstrate some of the different ways in which I might deal with different consulting situations:

• The unknown patient, fresh on my list, with an obvious organic symptom. I would concentrate on objectives 1, 2, 4, 5 and

8 (confidence, history, examination, record) because exploration of organic symptoms is likely to be the quickest way of giving confidence in this instance. Early exploration of emotional relationships may impair confidence by suggesting that the doctor suspects 'neurosis'. By the time objectives 6, 7 and 9 (investigation, diagnosis, treatment) have been achieved much valuable information about 3 (background and relationships) is likely to have emerged.

• The unknown patient, fresh on my list, with a long previous history suggesting either organic or functional disease. I would concentrate on giving confidence (objective 1) by letting the patient talk about objectives 2, 3 and 4 (history and emotional relationships). I would record details (objective 8) freely because the patient will be used to this. I would get the patient back for further interviews to complete objectives 5, 6, 7 and 9 (examination, investigation, diagnosis and treatment). These further interviews could be more actively structured and therefore quicker than the first interview.

• The known patient with an obvious organic symptom. Objectives 1 and 3 (confidence, emotional background) are probably already achieved and difficulties with the remaining objectives are unlikely.

• The frequent attender with chronic or recurrent organic disease. The patient is known. The relationship with the doctor should be clear and easy.

• The frequent attender who is insecure and with indefinite problems. Such patients are probably the most difficult of all to interview for the following reasons:

(i) the patient is diffident and vital information may be given unexpectedly, i.e. during examination
(ii) symptoms can and often are due to serious organic disease
(iii) the doctor considers that he knows all about such patients although the patient may feel otherwise
(iv) the patient very easily feels rejected and this will aggravate his or her insecurity
(v) all objectives 1 to 9 may have to be carried out with tact and care.

Over the years most such patients settle down and the practitioner will often be surprised to discover that a rewarding relationship has developed.

• The patient who is diffident about a problem. The problem is usually only half recognised by the patient and often presented indirectly with a 'lead' or under a 'cover story'. The practitioner is frequently busy but must be prepared to take the interview further for he may not get another opportunity. I would tactfully concentrate on objectives 1, 2, 3, 4 and 5 (confidence, history, background, examination) and leave 6, 7 and 9 (investigation, diagnosis and management) till a later interview. I would record information (8), by using a graphic method (appendix IX) or from memory after the interview. If I was 'under pressure' I would take this interview to the stage at which the patient had recognised her problem and then tactfully terminate it by arranging for examination or investigations at a further interview.

Every patient will be different and each doctor will learn by experience how best to achieve the different objectives. The practitioner should always avoid showing irritation or frustration or appearing in a hurry. Consultations should, whenever possible, be terminated by the patient and not the doctor. If the doctor is forced to terminate a consultation he should do so indirectly, by carrying out an examination or investigation (blood test, etc.) and clearly arranging another appointment.

Questioning techniques and the patient

The following points should be remembered:

1. Good eye contact combined with a slight encouraging nod are the simplest, quickest and most effective way that a doctor can simultaneously encourage the patient and show concern.

Verbal encouragement can easily be misunderstood and often wastes valuable time.

These points become very obvious if consultations are observed or videotaped.

2. Patients naturally expect the doctor to start asking structured questions about their main complaint. This also allows the doctor to assess and plan further steps.

3. From this base the doctor can make any necessary exploratory forays into the sources of confidence and sensitive areas of a patient's life. If the doctor uses an open-ended approach — 'Tell me a bit more about that,' — the patient can go just as far as he wishes.

4. If a diffident patient is upset or if a talkative patient takes advantage of the opportunity then the doctor can unobtrusively return to the structured part of history-taking, i.e. either symptom elaboration, systems enquiry or examination.

In these ways the primary physician can control the consultation and lead the patient into giving a quick, effective story with a minimum of direction and a maximum of encouragement.

Some common emotional interactions

It is seldom stressed that a doctor's assessment of a patient's story and the clinical examination may be greatly influenced by emotional motives ('hidden agenda') in the minds of both patient and doctor. Considerable distortion of clinical facts may arise from exaggeration or underemphasis of clinical findings. The family doctor can only obtain an objective view of the true clinical facts by making allowances for the various causes of distortion.

Some of the common situations which illustrate this everpresent problem are given below.

• Emotional reactions which may cause a patient to exaggerate or perpetuate symptoms:

a. The patient fears that symptoms which he considers important will be ignored by the doctor.

> EXAMPLE. A middle-aged man complained of 6 months' precordial pain. It was noted from the patient's records that he had seen the doctor 2 months previously when systematic questions about chest pain were entirely negative. On being asked why he did not mention the chest pain at the interview 2 months previously, the patient said that he had not wished to bother the doctor. This may have been true, but it is more probable that the patient had subconsciously exaggerated the duration of his symptoms because he was worried about his heart and afraid that the doctor might not examine it.

b. The patient perpetuates symptoms because doctors or relatives have persistently *pooh-poohed* his complaints without giving adequate explanation. Subconscious exaggeration or perpetuation of symptoms is common in patients who have been labelled *neurotic*. If the doctor reacts to this situation without understanding or by telling the patient that it is up to him, the patient may react by further exaggeration and perpetuation of symptoms.

> EXAMPLE. A 16-year-old girl had three convulsions. These were considered to be hysterical. The girl was referred to a physician for a second opinion. An electroencephalogram and full investigation of the nervous system were negative and the specialist bluntly told the girl that she was getting blackouts because she wanted to 'draw attention to herself'. The convulsions continued until the girl was given a full and more sympathetic explanation of the nature of her complaints.

c. The patient is frightened of appearing in the wrong. Exaggeration of symptoms is not uncommon when patients are afraid that they have panicked or put in an urgent call for trivial reasons. If the doctor shows annoyance when dealing with these patients, the exaggeration of symptoms may be further increased. Family doctors themselves experience this natural reaction when they feel the need to justify an emergency admission to hospital.

d. The patient has an ulterior motive. The child or adult who malingers to avoid school or work may exaggerate symptoms; *compensation neurosis* is a more complex example.

- Emotional reactions which may cause patients to minimise symptoms:

a. The patient who is used to discomfort or pain. These patients may wait a surprisingly long time before calling the doctor. Thus, an elderly patient may be deceptively off-hand about the severe pain of a coronary thrombosis or perforated ulcer. Conversely, tough athletes may worry excessively about the most trivial complaints.

b. The patient who gives a responsible job priority over personal health. Foremen, professional and self-employed men are especially liable to play down their symptoms. The prime offender in this group is the young mother with a family to look after.

EXAMPLE. A 22-year-old mother of three put in a call at midnight because her 4-year-old daughter had earache. After dealing with the daughter, I was just leaving when the mother said, 'Oh, by the way, while you're here, Doctor, I'm losing a little . . .' Further enquiry elicited that she was 2 months pregnant with heavy bleeding from a miscarriage and needed immediate hospital admission.

c. The patient who is afraid of serious disease. Obvious complaints are often minimised or ignored by these patients. Every family doctor knows the patient who refuses an X-ray for fear that it may reveal cancer or tuberculosis. It is not uncommon for a woman to wait many weeks before consulting the doctor about a lump in her breast because she is afraid of cancer. Parents or relatives who are responsible for the care of others may feel guilty lest they have overlooked disease. Fear of criticism by neighbours or others may lead to considerable distortion.

EXAMPLE. A mother who was out at work all day left her 4-year-old son in the care of neighbours. On return from work at 5 p.m. she found that the boy had developed a rash and she put in an urgent call. When giving the history she insisted that he had been perfectly well that morning. As the boy had a fully developed classical measles, this was extremely unlikely.

NOTE. Parents with a sense of guilt require careful handling if the doctor is to avoid senseless rows.

d. The patient (or relative) who has a limited medical knowledge — first aid workers and nurses are liable to be overconfident and may distort symptoms unconsciously.

EXAMPLE. A state registered nurse reported one afternoon that her 9-year-old daughter was complaining of abdominal pain. She said that there was no need to call until the following morning as the pain was due to pyelitis from which the daughter had previously suffered. Because we have a practice rule that all patients with abdominal pain are seen as soon as possible, I visited the daughter that same afternoon. A diagnosis of acute appendicitis was made and a gangrenous appendix was removed that evening.

- Emotional reactions which may make the doctor underestimate the significance of clinical findings:

a. The doctor plays down the significance of symptoms because the patient has exaggerated them. This situation of emotional action and reaction is common. Every doctor can think of patients in whom symptoms of organic disease have been mistakenly labelled *functional*.

EXAMPLE. A 40-year-old family man with a previous history of psychoneurosis retired to bed saying that he was getting pains all over and felt dizzy whenever he got up. He complained of pain in his head, chest, back and both legs and claimed that he was unable to move his right leg. After 14 days, in an attempt to reassure the patient that there was nothing wrong, an X-ray of right hip was ordered. By chance the whole pelvis was included in the X-ray and a large sarcoma of the right ischium was noted. Further X-rays revealed multiple secondaries in spine, ribs and skull.

b. The doctor is short of time and accepts the patient's evaluation of symptoms without adequate elaboration.

EXAMPLE. I was called to a family and found the father and two children in bed with typical influenza. After dealing with these three patients I was just leaving when the mother asked if she could have a bottle for her cough. As I was busy with the epidemic, I complied without making further enquiries. Two days later she had developed an influenzal pneumonia.

c. The doctor fails to find objective corroboration of the patient's subjective symptoms. In the early stages of some common diseases, e.g. peptic ulcer or prolapsed intervertebral disc, it is difficult to obtain objective proof of organic disease. The diagnosis depends entirely on the patient's symptoms which the doctor may incorrectly assume are functional.

EXAMPLE. In 20 patients with symptoms of dyspepsia and upper abdominal pain considered to be of functional origin, a follow-up after 4 years revealed that in half, a peptic ulcer had been demonstrated by either a barium meal or operation.

• Emotional reactions which may make the doctor exaggerate the significance of clinical findings:
Most family doctors are short of time and the tendency is to under-estimate clinical findings. The doctor may, however, exaggerate the significance of symptoms when he sees the disease through the eyes of anxious relatives, e.g. when he looks after the children of personal friends. Similarly, if the doctor is suddenly afraid that he has made a mistake, his sense of guilt may make him exaggerate both the significance of clinical findings and the consequences of his mistake.

Applications to practice

1. The doctor will rarely feel satisfied with his interview technique.
2. The doctor should be critical of his technique and always be prepared to study, improve and modify his methods.
3. Patients should always feel that the doctor is glad to see them.
4. Patients should always feel 'accepted' by the doctor, i.e. that he is 'on their side' and that he sees 'their' illness through 'their' eyes. This is why the doctor's own medical experiences are often important.
5. Patients should never feel that the doctor is in a hurry (even when he is).
6. Patients should not be made to feel that the doctor is being critical, patronising or standing in judgement.
7. If the doctor for any reason feels that a show of firmness is needed, this should be done without emotional heat, i.e. the doctor should be sure that he is not releasing his own emotional frustrations and aggressions on the patient.
8. Every doctor's interview technique will be different.

Howard Barrows of McMaster University stresses that there are only four outcomes of any consultation that matter.

- Accurate assessment of all the patient's problems
- An appropriate management plan in terms of payoff, risk and cost
- Efficient, economical use of time
- Rapport must be sufficient to ensure compliance.

If these outcomes are met it should not matter if the doctor asks unusual questions or develops an unorthodox style.

9. Video-tape assessments of consultations provide an excellent tool for analysing and improving consultation techniques. Such assessments are suitable for trainees and experienced doctors. Many established physicians are initially resistant to these rather threatening procedures but soon discover that they are both helpful and rewarding.

Appendix VIII (p. 724) outlines in detail a technique which I have found helpful as a trainer.

II. THE HOSPITAL AND SPECIALIST SERVICES

The hospital service is the most significant influence in the general practitioner's life. It is also the most important weapon available to the primary physician for both diagnosis and treatment. It is vital that he uses it correctly and with discrimination. Over-referral will lead to inefficiency, bottlenecks, long waiting lists and bed shortages; under-referral will mean that his patients are not getting the benefit of the services available. The practitioner's 'dilemma of service', i.e. the qualitative versus the quantitative elements of the service to be provided, clearly operates in this field.

Applications to practice

1. The primary physician must assess the correct balance of referral by getting to know each department available to him. He must learn how to prepare the clinical material to fit the requirements of each specialist. For example warts, minor surgery, casualties, abortions, surgical emergencies in children, obstetric and geriatric problems may have to be dealt with in different ways in different areas.

2. The practitioner should find out if the consultant feels that the service provided is being used correctly.

3. The practitioner should attend postgraduate lectures that demonstrate the developments in different specialities.

4. There is a need for improved communications and greater understanding between the doctors working in the community and those working in hospital. Friendly consultants can often be persuaded to talk at practice meetings or working luncheons in a health centre.

5. The telephone consultation with friendly and appropriate

consultants is a vital tool for all general practitioners, especially those working in isolated areas.

Such a conversation, perhaps late at night, about a possible obstetric or paediatric problem will often save an admission and prevent needless worry.

The rates for hospital referral and investigation in this practice are given in the practice audit figures in Appendix IV (p. 700).

III. THE MEDICAL RECORD AND RECORDING METHODS

In primary care an ideal patient record should fulfil five functions. In order of priority these are:

Priority 1. An *aide memoire* to the recording doctor. Reading the record should remind the doctor of:

— relevant clinical, psychological and social findings
— options considered and predictions made
— decisions taken and action advised.

Priority 2. An indicator to partners and practice staff of decisions taken and action advised by the recording doctor.

Priority 3. Provide data capable of being used to 'audit' the recorder's practice, i.e. follow up, 'random case analysis', etc.

Priority 4. Provide suitable material for teaching and analysis, i.e. for trainees or talks.

Priority 5. Provide data suitable for pilot surveys, retrospective analysis and research.

Unfortunately, few practice records achieve consistently even the first priority.

> EXAMPLE: The following excellent research project was carried out by Dr Alison Leader when a trainee:
> Dr Leader asked 20 trainers to agree on the six most important pieces of information that every record should contain. She then analysed a random sample of 4266 records from the 20 practices to ascertain the percentage of records in which the trainers fulfilled their own criteria. Table 6 gives her results.

Several points should be made about this revealing survey:

1. Many doctors who are accepted by their colleagues as suitable trainers appear to operate with low standards of recording. It is difficult to prove that standards of care and training can be improved by better recording, but it seems likely.

2. What was *actually* recorded is clearly much less than the trainers thought.

Table 6 Analysis of 20 trainer's records.

		Percentage of records that met criteria
Criteria 1	Each record will detail:	
	Patient's Surname	100
	Patient's Forenames (implying sex)	100
	Patient's Date of Birth	98
	(N = 4266)	
Criteria 2	Each record will state patient's occupation:	
	Males (Aged 16–65; N = 1318)	25
	Females (Aged 16–60; N = 1355)	15
Criteria 3	Each record will indicate patient's marital status:	
	Males (over 16 years; N = 1451) Stated explicitly	1
	Females (over 16 years; N = 1730) Stated explicitly	38
	Females (over 16 years; N = 1730) Implied or explicitly stated	63
Criteria 4	Records and correspondence will be organised in chronological order and held together (Treasury tags, etc.)	
	Adequately tagged record cards	18
	Adequately tagged letters	22
Criteria 5	A problem card or similar method of recording significant events will be maintained	7
Criteria 6	When the name of a drug prescribed is recorded the dose and amount prescribed will also be recorded.	
	Note: there was no way of discovering (in this survey) if a drug had been prescribed *without* recording it at all.	
	Dose recorded	45
	Amount recorded	55
	Both recorded	34

3. The records analysed would only be partially successful as an aide memoire to the recording doctor. Few of the records would inform partners in an emergency or help another doctor at a routine consultation; the obvious gaps and lack of consistency of the records would render them of little use for audit, teaching or research.

4. The tactic of asking patients to fill in the gaps left by a record, i.e. 'Did I prescribe two or three yellow tablets a day for you last week?' may have a devastating effect on the patient's confidence in the doctor.

5. Even the simply delegated task of arranging recorded information in chronological order which saves many hours of doctor/consulting time, had not been achieved.

The chief reason for low standards of records are twofold:

• *Lack of time*. Adequate record writing is difficult to abbreviate and speed up. Time spent on recording competes with valuable interview time.

• The discipline of general practice has not yet developed minimum requirements and training procedures for records appropriate to the short 5–12 minute primary care consultation. Interviewing techniques are analysed, taught, discussed and videotaped but the essential 'time slot' for writing the record is overlooked. Family doctors often appear guilty about their failure to examine patients but are rarely guilty about their failure to keep adequate records.

Possible practical solutions

1. Family practice must develop an agreed discipline, to enable brief clear summaries to be recorded during short consultations. This skill would be learnt and adopted by doctors in their early training years when not under work-load pressures. The present haphazard methods of learning inevitably lead to low standards of recording with many omissions.

2. At present the only satisfactory universally applicable method is to create a shortened written version of the process that the doctor has learnt in hospital. This modified record must be streamlined to use only about a sixth of the consultation time, i.e. less than 60 seconds in many instances. This streamlining process requires much personal thought and practise.

3. In the absence of any formal discipline of recording for primary care, each doctor must work out their own effective methods. Appendix IX shows how this has been done by one busy family practitioner and provides a model which illustrates the problems and some possible solutions.

4. Modifying the recording process involves 3 steps:

• List possible items and decide which are essential and must be recorded.

• delegate to secretarial staff as much of the process as possible, e.g. the date of the consultation and arranging reports in chronological order

• develop, practise and perfect, methods of quick recording. This involves using one word summaries, abbreviations, medical shorthand and graphic methods.

Fig. 6 and Appendix IX illustrate some of these methods.

5. Other possible methods of quick recording.

• Dictation. A short record is dictated at the end of each consultation. A secretary then types this into the record later. At first sight this appears a good system, unfortunately the disadvantages outweigh the advantages and few doctors use it:

Advantages:

— A clear legible record is created
— The patient is not aware of the recording process.

Disadvantages:

— The dictation process is not directly related to the doctor's clinical thinking. Vital details may be forgotten and not recorded
— Under work-load pressure the dictation process is left until the end of the clinic or omitted altogether
— Records of home visits are easily omitted
— A considerable 'bottle neck' of patients' records may collect behind an overworked typist
— The process is costly in secretarial time
— Mistakes may occur in the process of dictation and typing
— The dictation process itself takes up doctor consultation time. Skilled summaries using medical shorthand are probably as quick.

• The patient fills in their own data base and complaint proforma. Rarely used because disadvantages are so great:

Disadvantages:

— Requires a high degree of patient medical knowledge and literacy
— The doctor must digest much rigidly structured information which itself takes time
— Hidden agenda and non-verbal overtones are not transmitted to the doctor
— Little, if any, consulting time is saved.

• Micro-computers in the consulting room (see p. 140).

Present Disadvantages:

— Expensive
— Floppy disc memory capacity, limits their use to a few areas only, e.g. antenatal patients
— Present programmes demand greater not smaller usage of doctor consulting time (Continued on p. 132)

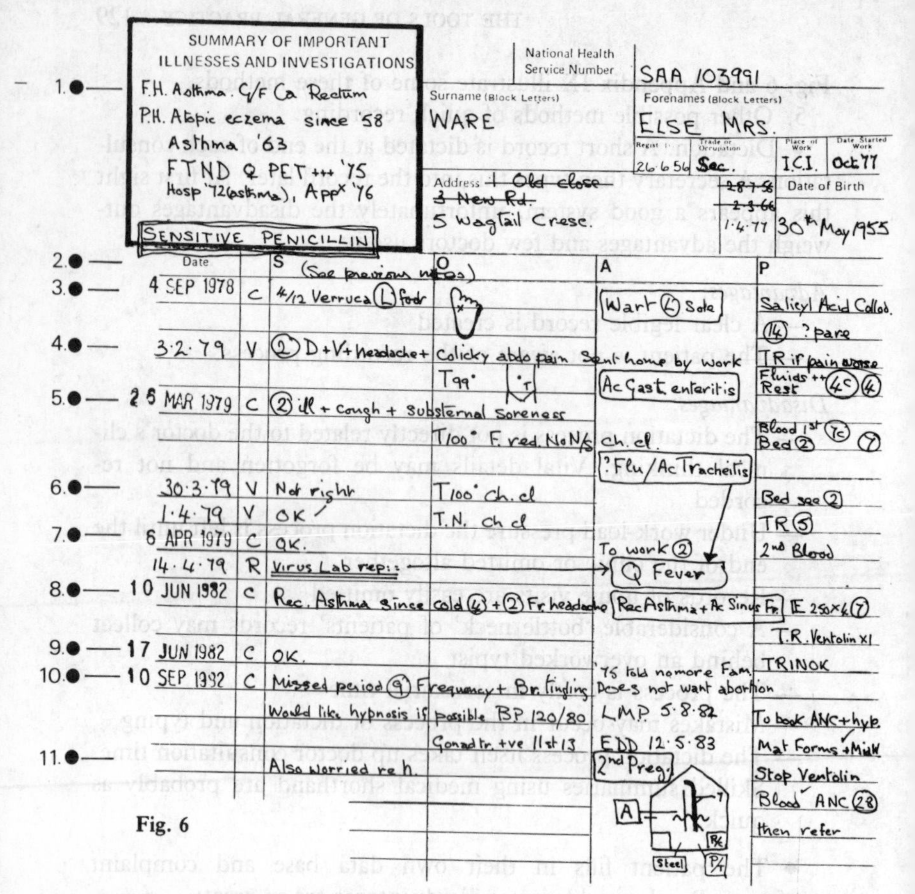
SUMMARY OF IMPORTANT ILLNESSES AND INVESTIGATIONS

1.● F.H. Asthma. C/F Ca Rectum
P.H. Atopic eczema since 58
Asthma '63
FTND ♀ PET +++ '75
Hosp '72 (asthma), App^x '76
SENSITIVE PENICILLIN

National Health Service Number: SAA 103991
Surname (Block Letters): WARE
Forenames (Block Letters): ELSE MRS.
Regn: 26.6.56 | Trade or Occupation: Sec. | Place of Work: I.C.I. | Date Started Work: Oct 77
Address: 1 Old close (28.7.58); 3 New Rd. (2.3.66); 5 Wagtail Cresc. (1.4.77)
Date of Birth: 30th May 1955

	Date		S	O	A	P
2.●			(See previous notes)			
3.●	4 SEP 1978	C	4/12 Verruca Ⓛ foot		Wart Ⓛ Sole	Salicyl Acid Collod. ⑭ ? pare
4.●	3.2.79	V	② D+V+ headache+	Colicky abdo pain. Sent home by work. T99°	Ac Gast. enteritis	TR if pain worse. Fluids ++ Rest ④
5.●	25 MAR 1979	C	② ill + cough + substernal soreness	T/100 F. red. No N/S	ch. cl. ? Flu/Ac Tracheitis	Blood 1st Bed ② ⑦
6.●	30.3.79	V	Not right	T/100° ch. cl		Bed see ②
	1.4.79	V	OK	T.N. ch cl		TR ⑤
7.●	6 APR 1979	C	OK.		To work ②	2nd Blood
	14.4.79	R	Virus Lab rep:		Q Fever	
8.●	10 JUN 1982	C	Rec. Asthma since cold ④ + ② Fr headache		Rec Asthma + Ac Sinus Fr.	E 250×6 ⑦ T.R. Ventolin ×1
9.●	17 JUN 1982	C	OK.			TR IN OK
10.●	10 SEP 1982	C	Missed period ⑨ Frequency + Br. tingling. Would like hypnosis if possible	BP 120/80. Gonad tr. +ve 11st 13	75 told no more Fam. Does not want abortion. LMP 5.8.82 EDD 12.5.83 2nd Preg.	To book ANC + hyp. Mat Forms + Milk
11.●			Also worried re h.			Stop Ventolin. Blood ANC ㉘ then refer

Fig. 6

KEY TO THE NUMBERS IN FIGURE 6

1.● A *running* summary of all important previous illnesses and medical data. The summary is brought up to date by a secretary every time a new page is added to the record. Over the years problem lists tend to get ignored, lost or not up-dated. Even if they are regularly up-dated over several years, they then tend to be overloaded and confusing.

Advantages of the running summary are:

— all relevant information is immediately to hand on the current page of the record
— automatically up-dated
— if the doctor is ringing diagnoses a secretary can be taught which of the ringed diagnoses on the current page need to be carried routinely over to the summary on the new page
— the new page is left sticking out of the file for this to be done after clinic before the record is filed
— over the years this saves many hours of valuable doctor consulting time.

2.● S.O.A.P. (Subjective, Objective, Analysis, Plan) is staggered horizontally, i.e.

S O A P
Subjective information
Objective findings
Analysis
Plan outlined in full on right margin

This ensures that everyone knows *where* to look for information. The Subjective and Objective information are recorded mainly on the Left side and act as an aide memoire, while Analysis and Plan, which summarise the important decisions taken, are *clearly* emphasised by always being on the right side of the page. As in a financial statement, everyone knows what to look for and where to look for it. The subjective and objective data can spill over into the columns on their right, but the column for management is reserved for the recording of management plans only. *Also note how the clear ringing of diagnoses* (*both suspected and provisional*) make sense of the management plans as well as the Subjective and Objective data recorded.

3.• A routine consultation. Note: (a) a secretary has put the date on beforehand with a date stamp, (b) a simple diagram is more accurate and quicker than a description of the site of the wart, (c) the patient has used the term *verruca* but the doctor has used the shorter term wart because it is quicker to write, (d) ⑭ indicates a request for patient to see the doctor at clinic in 2 weeks.

4.• A house call for an attack of diarrhoea, vomiting and colicky pain. Note: (a) temperature of 99°F with tenderness in the left iliac fossa, (b) under 'Plan' the patient has been asked to report if the abdominal pain gets worse or continues, has been given a certificate off work for 4 days, put on fluids and bed rest and asked to report to surgery in 4 days, (c) there is no record that she did report back.

5.• A fresh consultation for an AURI. Two diagnoses are considered possible so both are recorded. If a diagnostic register were being kept both would be recorded as *suspected* diagnoses. Note also that a 7 day certificate off work has been given and a blood test of virology (paired serum) has been taken.

6.• The doctor has been recalled to make a further house call because the patient is still ill.

7.• The patient reports at surgery that she's OK for work, the doctor takes the second sample of blood needed for virology. 8 days later the lab reports that the infection was due to a Q fever, and the secretary — responsible for entering lab reports on the records has also entered a change of the original diagnosis. This change will also be recorded in the diagnostic register.

8.• Patient reports with an acute frontal sinusitis of 2 days duration and 4 days recurrent asthma. She is given one Ventolin inhaler and a 7 day course of erythromycin (E). Antibiotics are always shortened to the capital letter with a double vertical.

9.• Patient is well but asked to report (TR) if there is any more trouble.

10.• Patient reports with second pregnancy. Does not want a termination. After a severe pre-eclamptic toxaemia (PET +++) in 1975 — mentioned in the running summary — she was told she should not have further family. Note: (a) she is told not to take Ventolin while pregnant (b) booked for routine antenatal clinic and hypnotic relaxation.

11.• As patient is leaving she reports that she is worried about her husband. She is questioned about this and the relevant confidential details are recorded on a family gram — see Appendix IX (p. 728).

— Doctor must learn to type
— Doctor may have to summarize records
— Unless research funds are available, dictating a record for later typing is at present probably quicker, cheaper and produces a similar end result.

IV. THE PRACTICE

In our practice in one year (p. 33) 2 doctors dealt with a total of 13 755 different clinical, emotional or social situations: two-thirds (9407) were diagnosed immediately and given simple advice for treatment; a fifth (2746) were further investigated; a tenth (1602) were referred to hospital. The practice size totalled 5767 NHS patients of which over 4000 individuals reported illness during the year.

Several further facts about this information must be emphasised:

1. The figures are similar to those elsewhere in other Western countries
2. The range of problems dealt with was great and included nearly 500 different diagnostic categories.
3. Many different combinations of age, sex, family and socio-economic background were encountered
4. Over 25 different hospital departments were involved
5. Over 40 different community and welfare organisations had to be contacted
6. An average of 5 home visits per doctor were deemed necessary on every working day
7. 24 hour cover was given throughout.

Before an organisation can deal efficiently with this number of problems on a 24 hour basis, two points must be stressed: (1) any system must be flexible to allow for human failings in patient, staff and doctor, (2) no system will be entirely satisfactory. Both these facts have led general practitioners to adopt different ways of working, i.e. single-handed, group practice, health centre, etc.

Every method has exponents and critics. Efficient and inefficient organisation will be found in each type of practice.

The position is further aggravated because in every community there is a large reservoir of unreported morbidity; thresholds of reporting are usually beyond the control of the medical profession and considerable fluctuation may follow changes of social custom, reports in the mass media, etc.

For these reasons one of the main functions of any practice organisation is to provide the primary physician with a network of resources that allows a manageable flow of relevant clinical and emotional information from his community of patients. This in turn will be governed by how the doctor wishes to resolve the dilemma of service.

THE MANAGEMENT GRID AND THE DILEMMA OF SERVICE

The management grid (Fig. 7) is a graphic model that allows us to see some of the major effects of the dilemma of service.

At the two extremes of the dilemma are two types of practice.

THE 10,1 PRACTICE

This type of practice will give a highly personalised service to a few patients.

Advantages: A high quality of service to a few individuals is possible; high job satisfaction for doctors; individual patients are usually satisfied.

Disadvantages: Such a service is impractical for the whole community as it would require many more doctors. Patients can

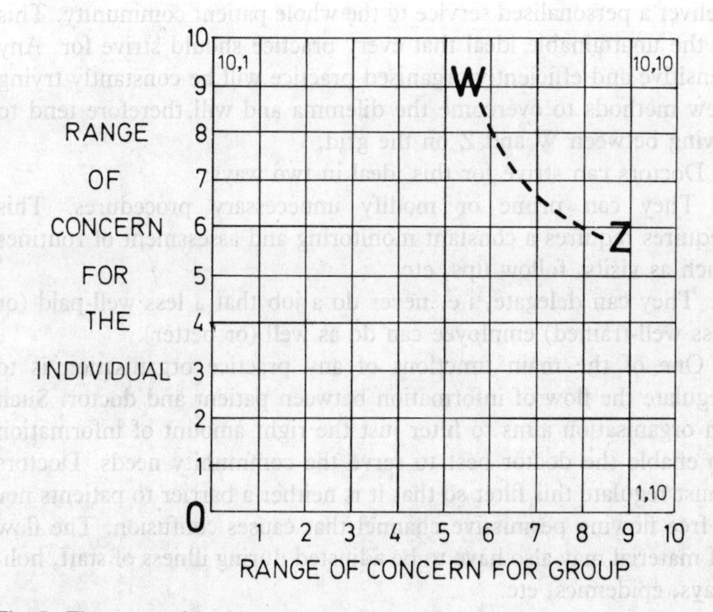

Fig. 7. The managerial grid.

easily become too dependent on the doctor. The doctor finds it hard to delegate and may try to be a 'maid of all work', i.e. type his own letters, remove gall bladders, set fractures, etc., but do nothing very well.

THE 1,10 PRACTICE

This aims to deliver medical care to the whole community, but is impersonal.

Advantages: Deals effectively with large quantities of patients. Community priorities are usually clearly defined and all sections of community receive the same standard of service. Dependence of the patient on the doctor is discouraged. Delegation of the doctor's responsibilities may lead to a wide-ranging service. Receptionists can be taught to perform cardiographs, nurses can be taught how to screen high risk groups, etc.

Disadvantages: Individual patients are less well satisfied because the service may be impersonal. Patients easily feel rejected. Personal or emotional problems may be neglected. Information flow within the necessary large organisation may be inhibited or distorted.

THE 10,10 PRACTICE

This aims, despite shortage of doctors and limited resources, to deliver a personalised service to the whole patient community. This is the unattainable ideal that every practice should strive for. Any sensitive and efficiently organised practice will be constantly trying new methods to overcome the dilemma and will therefore tend to swing between W and Z on the grid.

Doctors can strive for this ideal in two ways:

1. They can prune or modify unnecessary procedures. This requires requires a constant monitoring and assessment of routines such as visits, follow ups, etc.
2. They can delegate, i.e. never do a job that a less well-paid (or less well-trained) employee can do as well (or better).

One of the main functions of any practice organisation is to regulate the flow of information between patient and doctor. Such an organisation aims to filter just the right amount of information to enable the doctor best to serve the community needs. Doctors must regulate this filter so that it is neither a barrier to patients nor a free flowing permissive channel that causes confusion. The flow of material may also have to be adjusted during illness of staff, holidays, epidemics, etc.

An important principle is involved here, for it is the doctor not the patient who decides priorities. If doctors are to serve their whole community they must at the same time safeguard patients' interests and ensure that individual patients do not feel rejected.

Practice resources

The tools that enable the doctor to regulate work and the flow of information and clinical material within the practice are:

A. Staff — receptionists, secretaries, nurses, etc.
B. Systems of organisation — appointments, repeat prescriptions, telephone advice, call systems
C. Interpersonal relationships between members of staff
D. Equipment — dictating machines, 'intercom' systems, etc.

Much has been written about these subjects.

Practical details of many excellent methods and systems have been described. Each method will have different relevance to different practice situations; the readers will find much in the literature to help them deal with their own personal 'dilemma of service'.

I propose only to discuss the relevance of the above factors to *information flow*, because this is so important and because it demonstrates the principles which underly all practice organisation.

A. DELEGATION OF RESPONSIBILITY TO STAFF

If a nurse or receptionist is given responsibility and then refers every little detail back to the doctor, overwork and irritation will follow. The doctor is likely to make mistakes. Conversely, if the receptionist or nurse creates too big a barrier or distorts information, the patient will become upset or frustrated and may well exaggerate symptoms in order to break through the barrier of delegation.

The solution involves

- Clear guidelines delineating the extent of the staff responsibilities and the type of information that must be passed to the doctor (Appendix V p. 702).
- Clear recording of information to be passed on.
- Staff, when dealing with patients, should always avoid the 'direct confrontation' or blunt refusal by tactfully asking for more information. Thus if there is a shortage of appointments the patient should be asked 'Is it urgent?', or 'Could you help

by coming tomorrow?', etc. Telling a patient bluntly that there are no appointments or that the doctor is too busy is likely to produce an aggressive reaction.
- Regular staff meetings in which staff and doctors can discuss problems.
- Staff and doctors in all dealings with patients should learn to safeguard themselves against unexpected or unpredictable developments. Receptionists should encourage patients to report back if worried or if something unexpected happens.

I always end a patient contact by saying, 'Let me know if things aren't right.' Such safeguards and loopholes may be life-saving and will certainly protect the doctor and staff.

B. SYSTEMS AND REGULATORS AFFECTING FLOW OF INFORMATION BETWEEN PATIENT AND DOCTOR

1. Financial. The time-honoured method. The demand for a doctor's services increase; he limits workload by increasing his fees. This method is financially satisfactory for the doctor.

Disadvantages: • Poverty tends to be correlated with ill-health; even the 'well off' can be short of funds when raising a family and in retirement. A patchy delivery of medical care develops in which all sections of the community do not get the same standard of service.

• Considerable distortion of information flow. Poor patients will tend to delay calling the doctor, with disastrous consequences. Rich patients may be overtreated. Thus in a poor community operations for appendicitis will be more often complicated by perforation. In a rich community there may be an increase in the number of normal appendices removed. Sooner or later the community will bargain with the medical profession to ameliorate the defects of this type of system as has been done in Britain.

2. Home visiting. Reveals valuable emotional and socioeconomic information. May be essential if patient is housebound. Patients may prefer to see the doctor in their home.

Disadvantages: Expensive in terms of doctor's time and transport. Clinical examination and investigations in the home are difficult and tend to be omitted or inadequate.

3. Surgery or office consultations provide the most satisfactory form of consultation from the doctor's point of view. If the doctor is short of time, he will inevitably wish to encourage the patient to come to surgery or office.

Disadvantages: Unsuitable for the very ill or bedridden. The doctor may be unaware of home circumstances, i.e. poverty, rigid background, expensive tastes, etc. Patients may dislike coming to the surgery for a number of reasons — distance, cost, weather, publicity, etc. Patients may exaggerate clinical information to justify the request for a visit.

4. Appointments systems. A most potent method of controlling the doctor's flow of work. Like all powerful weapons its effects can 'backfire' if wrongly used (see Table 7).

Disadvantages: Very easily becomes a barrier at periods of peak work-load or doctor shortage. Patients become frustrated and distort clinical information. Staff is under pressure from both patients and doctors; a vicious circle of frustration and aggression is set up between doctor and patient. Patients then use failure to get an immediate appointment as an excuse for their failures to co-operate with the doctor — 'I didn't come because you're so busy, Doctor.' The appointment system is such a valuable regulator of flow that the doctor should see that it helps patients as well as doctor. The system should be frequently monitored to avoid 'appointment hunger'. The doctor should ensure that urgent cases are seen without delay and that diffident or co-operative patients do not suffer at the hands of their more aggressive fellows or the 'dragon at the gate' of the surgery.

5. Practice transportation. In some circumstances it is economical and more effective to arrange unofficial transportation of patients to and from surgery premises. I paid a driver to use my car each week to pick up 6 to 16 old people and bring them to the surgery for a 'social outing' combined with a 2 monthly check-up. This ensures fuller and more regular checks. This system has now been extended to cover other types of patient on a daily basis.

Table 7. Advantages and disadvantages of appointment systems.

Advantages	Disadvantages
— Patient waiting reduced	— Undue delay before getting an appointment.
— Less crossinfection	— Epidemics may block the clinic
— Doctor can adjust work rate	— Some patients unable to book ahead
— Fewer home visits	— Patients without telephones have problems
— Smaller waiting area	— Extra manning of telephone and reception

Any system can be made to work satisfactorily if the doctors and staff are helpful and co-operative.

6. Repeat prescriptions without seeing the doctor. A powerful tool for cutting down the demand for repeat consultations.

Disadvantages: • The issue of prescriptions without consultation may inadvertently encourage dependence or habituation

• Essential follow-up consultations are omitted.

• The system may save doctor time but is probably wasteful and costly in terms of drug usage.

This regulator should be used with great caution. Several simple micro-computer programmes are available which are easy to use and enable the doctor to monitor the system and avoid some of the disadvantages.

7. Telephone advice. Another powerful but two-edged weapon for saving the doctor's time and regulating the flow of information between patient and doctor. Intelligent patients can be taught to save themselves and the doctor much worry and trouble by accurate reporting of clinical situations. Mistakes will be avoided if the doctor

— is aware of his own motives for giving telephone advice instead of consulting
— knows his patients
— satisfies himself that the patient or relative is happy at the end of the conversation
— asks the patient to telephone again if they are worried.

8. Telephone answering services. If these are 24 hour 'manned' and combined with a radio paging system they can save the doctor much time and worry.

Disadvantages: Costly to run and may occasionally lead to loss of confidentiality.

9. Telephone answering machines. Special circumstances may make these machines useful for the doctor.

Disadvantages: Patients dislike them and they may lead to mistakes. Many doctors avoid their use if possible.

10. Emergency Treatment and Deputising Services

Advantages: Allows a hard pressed doctor or partnership time off, especially at night.

Disadvantages:

— Costly
— Continuity of care is interrupted
— More patients are admitted to hospital
— Important information may not be transmitted at the time of an emergency

— All the problems of dual care i.e. advice from two doctors.

11. Rota Systems Several doctors within an area or practice work together to cover different nights, weekends and holidays.

Probably the most satisfactory form of cover available in primary care.

12. Cover by emergency or casualty departments of a hospital

Advantages: Doctor not required to pay for the service. 24 hour cover.

Disadvantages:

— The incorrect use of hospital services
— May overload a useful hospital service
— More hospital admissions likely
— Costly to community
— Cannot be used for long periods of time.

13. Physical barriers. The doctor should be aware of the effects on patients of physical barriers created in the surgery by desks, grills, hatches, etc.

14. Confidentiality of records. A patient may be considerably inhibited if a member of the surgery staff is known personally to the patient. The patient fears the confidentiality of the doctor's record. Reliable and discreet staff are the only solution to this difficult problem which should not deter the doctor from keeping good records.

C. INTERPERSONAL RELATIONS BETWEEN MEMBERS OF STAFF

Defective relations can increase the doctor's work and distort information flow by producing frustration, especially the suspicion that one member of the organisation is doing work that should be done by another.

1. Defective interdoctor relationships usually arise from inequalities (real or imaginary) in one of the three common and shared areas:

— workload
— time off
— pay.

Frustration may lead to poor communication (both verbal and recorded) between partners with consequent inhibition of the flow of necessary clinical information and stimulating clinical discussion.

Regular practice meetings or discussions are the best 'lubricant' between partners.

2. Defective interstaff relationships may lead to similar failures to communicate or record vital information.

3. *Defective doctor/staff relationships* usually arise if the doctors take any member of staff for granted or if they fail to define roles and individual duties with sufficient clarity (see Appendix V). Doctors who are needlessly irritable or blame others for their own mistakes.

These last two situations are unlikely to arise if staff feels free to discuss problems at any time wtith the doctors.

The best method of both preventing and dealing with all these situations is by frequent practice/staff meetings and monitoring (or sampling) the relevant factual data concerning quantity and distortion of information flow, i.e. knowing the number of patients that attend each clinic or doctor and if necessary obtaining objective data about time spent on different activities.

D. EQUIPMENT (Appendix III)

Good appropriate office equipment is essential for information flow within the practice and allows the doctor to control and monitor work load.

A wide variety of fittings and equipment are available. Suitability depends on the nature and size of the practice.

Files. A4 size is the most suitable and should consist of a folder with a place for A4 size sheets that can be tagged together and one or two pockets for loose reports (See Fig. 6 p. 130).

Filing. Wall shelves with pigeon holes are cheapest but occupy a lot of wall space. Filing cabinets are expensive, take up a lot of room and may wear out if overloaded. Carousels take up least space, are extremely efficient but the most expensive.

Typewriters, dictating machines, paging system, office 'intercoms', word-processors and other expensive electronic equipment are essential in any large practice. A visit to any large well run practice will provide the interested doctor with practical information about cost, usage and available models.

Computers in practice. The potential for use of computers in primary care is immense but at present the number of available and useful applications to practice are limited because the disadvantages which have to be overcome greatly outweigh the advantages.

Essentially a computer is a filing system which combines a large (but not unlimited) capacity with the capability of very rapid (but not instantaneous) search and retrieval.

For handling large amounts of variable but easily and accurately classified (measurable) information, a computer is often the ideal tool, e.g. in research, for the financial accounts of large numbers of patients or for monitoring the prescription or cost of drugs.

Any practitioner interested in using a computer should ask himself the following questions:

1. Does the volume of my information justify using such a large filing system?
2. Is the nature of my information easily and accurately classified into variable groups? Age, sex, address, number or length of visits and drugs prescribed are all easily and accurately classified while information about diagnoses or reasons for visits would be difficult.
3. Who is going to type the large amounts of information into the computer filing system and then keep it up to date to justify its use?
4. How much time am I myself prepared to spend defining and classifying information so that it can be fed into the computer's numerous files for subsequent retrieval and use?
5. Who is going to pay for the hardware and programming (software) costs which tend to escalate?

Examples: Programmes which identify the numbers of repeat presciptions issued or which check up on patients who are due for a vaginal smear are suitable for monitoring by computer in most large practices because all the variables are easily classified, i.e. name, address, age, sex, date of previous smear, when next smear is due, whether positive or negative, etc. Similarly there is little difficulty in classifying the numbers, type and frequency of drugs prescribed and to whom the prescriptions were made out. A typist can be paid to create and then maintain such a computer file, because all the variables are easily and accurately classified by a secretary.

By contrast any attempt to put practice records on a computer file presents much greater difficulties requiring constant discipline and work from the participating doctors. No computer filing system will compensate for records which are inadequate and incomplete in the first place. Any interested group of doctors must therefore agree the items which they wish to record and then design an encounter form. This must be filled in consistently by all doctors at every consultation. If this cannot be achieved there is a danger that the doctor's uncertainties will be 'put in'. These uncertainties will then of course 'come out'. At best such output must be disregarded; at worst it is used as data for analysis for which it is unsuitable. The time and thought required is considerable and cannot be delegated to staff. It is often more effective and much less costly for the doctors to improve their standards of written records before they seriously consider computerisation.

Applications to practice

1. Computerisation should only be considered for practice procedures which are repetitive and frequent. Large practices will always find computers more helpful than small ones.

2. The large capacity of a computer's files should be both filled and kept up to date. If a secretary cannot do this the doctors are unlikely to do so. All information filed must be capable of quick, accurate, classification by a secretary.

3. The following three areas of application are at present being developed:

- The monitoring of office procedures, i.e. practice accounts, age/sex registers (Ref. 7.1), immunisations, cervical smears, stock control, monitoring the elderly and other high risk groups. These improve the service to patients and assist staff. They do not at present save the doctor time or money.
- Information packages: drug sensitivities, drug costs, useful addresses, health education printouts for patients and summaries of recent work, etc. are all useful areas which are being developed.
- Applications to the consultation. Mainly experimental at the present time. A programme giving instant reference to the cost, dosage and interactions of drugs based on the National Formulary will probably be soon available.

4. Developing computer use in practice is a fascinating and interesting subject which at present is best regarded as a form of primary care research (Refs. 7.2 and 7.3).

5. Wherever possible visit a practice that is using a computer before buying one yourself. This will allow you to make realistic estimates of costs and possible usage.

V. COMMUNITY ORGANISATIONS

There are many community services and allied professional activities in the community that may help the patient. Most such services are relevant to treatment and not diagnosis. The primary physician should have full understanding of their workings. He should ensure that these organisations are not needlessly used but that his patients get the full benefit of them when indicated.

In our community the following are some of the many resources that are freely contacted for help.

Primary health care team

— Attached practice nurses
— Health Visitor
— Social Worker (including Psychiatric SW)
— Community Ocupational Therapist is sometimes available.

A full team is crucial to effective primary care. Unfortunately, as a result of shortages of community funding or the methods of payment of doctors, the team is rarely complete and may be absent altogether.

LOCAL AUTHORITY

— local Hospice
— ambulance
— home help
— meals on wheels
— bathing services
— baby sitting services
— night sitting service
— play groups
— home laundry (in some areas only)
— chiropody, etc.
— sheltered housing and institutional accommodation for old people, difficult children, etc.
— antenatal relaxation classes.
— family planning
— child psychiatry services

HOSPITAL AUTHORITY

— bed bureau
— occupational and physiotherapy in the community as well as hospital
— psychiatric social worker
— mass X-ray and cervical smear services, etc.
— group therapy classes
— day hospital (geriatric and psychiatric)
— holiday relief services to allow caring relatives to go on holiday

CENTRAL AND OTHER AUTHORITIES

— probation and prison services
— umemployment and youth opportunities programmes
— social services and their welfare departments
— Government training units

— industrial rehabilitation unit
— ophthalmic and pharmacy services, etc.
— welfare and personnel departments of large commercial firms

EDUCATIONAL AUTHORITIES

— schools and university medical departments
— heads of departments, headmasters and teachers
— night schools, training and technical colleges
— boys clubs, etc.

VOLUNTARY ORGANISATIONS

— men's clubs
— housewives' associations
— old people's associations
— Red Cross, Rotarians, Lions, Samaritans, CRUSE etc.
— Citizens Advice Bureau
— Marriage Guidance Council
— many other political and privately financed organisations
— Alcoholics Anonymous; Al-anon and Al-teen groups
— Weight Watchers
— medical associations — diabetic, colostomy, spastic, multiple sclerosis, etc. (addresses are given for UK throughout Part II).

OTHER PROFESSIONS

— priests
— lawyers, etc.
— teachers.

PART TWO

8

Infective and parasitic diseases

Please read the introduction for explanation of figures and analyses.

ADULT PULMONARY TUBERCULOSIS

Classification ICHPPC 011 (RCGP 0020)

DIAGNOSTIC RANGE (incidents per 1000 patients per year)
Personal: Suspected 10.0; Probable 1.0; *National* 0.5 (Ref. 0.2).

AGE INCIDENCE
Adults of all ages who have been infected previously.

CLINICAL COURSE
The classical clinical picture of tuberculosis is now rarely seen in developed countries. Many cases are discovered by X-ray or examination of high risk groups and are symptomless.

CLINICAL POINTERS
1. High risk factors: (a) contact cases; (b) the elderly (c) immigrant patients especially from India; (d) Alcoholics. A high index of suspicion in these groups leads to identification of most cases.
2. Persistent cough. Practice experience: 40% of fresh cases were discovered by X-ray of all patients with cough of 4 or more weeks' duration.
3. Pneumonic illness (especially when associated with pleural pain or effusion). (Practice experience: routine radiological examination of such patients revealed 20 per cent of fresh cases.)
4. Haemoptysis is a significant early sign that always warrants a chest X-ray.
5. Persistent vomiting, anorexia or painless gastric symptoms.
6. Fever of seven or more days duration.
7. Listlessness and anxiety about health — vague symptoms that are easily ignored.

8. Wasting, loss of weight, history of sweats, clubbing of fingers and physical signs at the apex or elsewhere in the lungs are usually associated with tuberculous toxaemia and advanced disease.

9. Associated disease: pleural effusion, fistula-in-ano, erythema nodosum and phlyctenular conjunctivitis may all be early pointers.

INVESTIGATIONS

1. Chest X-ray or minature mass X-ray.
2. ESR — not always raised (See Appendix IB p. 681)
3. Examination of sputum and gastric washings for acid-fast bacilli. This helps to isolate infective cases.

DURATION

Chronic and progressive unless treated.

COMPLICATIONS

Secondary spread to other parts of the body. Death.

MISLEADING FEATURES AND PITFALLS

1. The slow onset of tuberculosis makes the patient anxious about his physical condition. The doctor treats the anxiety and overlooks the pulmonary disease — a very easily made mistake.
2. Gastric symptoms may arise in early pulmonary tuberculosis.
3. A bronchogenic neoplasm may develop in a patient with active tuberculosis.
4. The condition is overlooked in the elderly because symptoms are ascribed to age, bronchitis or congestive heart failure. There is an increasing risk of this in our modern ageing societies.

DIFFERENTIAL DIAGNOSIS

Diseases that may be confused with pulmonary tuberculosis:

Pneumonia

Similar features: elderly patients commonly affected; acute respiratory illness; cough; haemoptysis, fever; pleurisy; rapid respirations.

Distinguishing features: contacts and previous history of chest troubles absent, basal lesions usual; improves with antibiotics; chest X-ray differentiates.

Bronchiectasis: chronic bronchitis

Similar features: elderly males commonly affected; long history of chest troubles, chronic cough; haemoptysis; dyspnoea; fever.

Distinguishing features: cough is productive especially in mornings; radiology and bacteriology differentiate.

Congestive heart failure
Similar features: elderly patients commonly affected; chronic cough; dyspnoea; haemoptysis, loss of weight.
Distinguishing features: causes of heart failure apparent (fibrillation or hypertension); fever absent; basal rales; peripheral oedema; venous back pressure in neck and liver, radiology and E.C.G. differentiate.

Bronchogenic carcinoma
Similar features: persistent cough; haemoptysis; loss of weight; dyspnoea; low fever.
Distinguishing features: history of smoking; contacts and previous chest troubles absent; radiology and cytology differentiate.

Diabetes mellitus
Similar features: unexpected loss of weight.
Distinguishing features: cough absent; thirst; glycosuria and other symptoms of diabetes; chest X-ray and blood chemistry differentiate.

MANAGEMENT OPTIONS

Prevention: (a) Patient education to prevent infection of others; (b) routine BCG immunisation at 12 or 13 years especially in high risk groups; (c) active case finding by doctor especially in high risk groups.

Established disease: (a) Referral for specialist advice about: infectivity, investigation of contacts, correct choice of chemotherapy BNF 5.1.9 (Ref. 0.1) and duration of active treatment, (b) support and education of patient and family at home by practitioner.

PRIMARY TUBERCULOUS ADENITIS (WITH SYMPTOMS)

Classification: ICHPPC 017 (RCGP 0020)

A primary tuberculosis infection with adenitis may arise in neck, lungs or gut.

DIAGNOSTIC RANGE

Few cases are encountered in developed countries.

AGE INCIDENCE

10 to 20 years.

CLINICAL POINTERS

1. High risk factors: (a) contacts; (b) immigrant children.
2. Insidious onset may last 1–4 weeks.

3. Listlessness.
4. Loss of appetite or weight. Babies may fail to gain.
5. Localising signs from the adenitis: a cervical adenitis is obvious; a wheezy cough or abdominal pain may suggest that mediastinal or mesenteric glands are affected.

INVESTIGATIONS
1. Tuberculin test.
2. Chest X-ray may show a primary hilar adenitis or infection.
3. Urine examination excludes non-tuberculous chronic urinary infection.

DURATION
The infection may last many weeks.

COMPLICATIONS
Blood-borne spread may lead to miliary tuberculosis, tuberculous meningitis or osteitis. All these complications are becoming increasingly rare in countries with high standards of living.

DIFFERENTIAL DIAGNOSIS
Diseases that may be confused with primary tuberculous adenitis:

Urinary tract infections
Similar features: insidious onset; listlessness; fever; prolonged course; babies and children liable.

Distinguishing features: pyuria (a single pus-free specimen does not rule out pyuria); tuberculin tests may be negative.

Aspiration pneumonia
Similar features: insidious onset; listlessness; fever; prolonged course; cough; babies and children liable.

Distinguishing features: preceeding respiratory illness persistent adventitious sounds in chest; tuberculin tests may be negative; chest X-ray differentiates.

Subacute cervical adenitis
Similar features: subacute swelling of cervical glands.

Distinguishing features: tuberculin tests may be negative; settles in 10 to 14 days with antibiotics; differentiation occasionally difficult.

NOTE. The coincidental consecutive occurrence of several illnesses may simulate a primary tuberculous illness. Further difficulties also arise because measles or whooping cough may aggravate an underlying primary tuberculous infection — aspiration pneumonia is simulated. Enlarge mediastinal glands also arise in pertussis.

WHOOPING COUGH

Classification: ICHPCC 033 (RCGP 0040)

AETIOLOGY

Haemophilus (*Bordetella*) *pertussis*. In the last 20 years the natural history of this disease has changed — possibly a result of immunisation. At present most infections are mild, but severe infections are increasing in poorly immunised communities.

MODE OF SPREAD

Droplet.

DIAGNOSTIC RANGE (incidents per 1000 patients per year)

Personal: Probable 0.9+; *National* 2.4 (Ref. 0.2) Epidemics used to occur at intervals of 3 to 5 years.

AGE INCIDENCE

The majority of cases (85%) are under 8 years and 40% are under 2 years (Fig. 8).

CLINICAL COURSE (IN MODERATE OR SEVERE CASES)

1. Incubation stage: 7 to 14 days (occasionally longer) — diagnosis rarely possible.
2. Catarrhal stage: 7 to 14 days — diagnosis often difficult.
3. Paroxysmal stage: reaches its height in 7 to 14 days and lasts up to 14 weeks — diagnosis obvious.

In immunised children all or none of these stages may develop.

CLINICAL POINTERS DURING THE CATARRHAL AND PAROXYSMAL STAGES

1. High risk factors: (a) contacts (80%), especially babies under 6 months; (b) debilitated or unimmunised children.
2. Persistent cough (100%): Mainly nocturnal (90%) at first resembles bronchitis; after 7 to 14 days the typical coughing spasm (84%) develops; the spasm makes the child red or blue in the face.
3. Low fever is present early and may persist for the first two or three weeks.
4. Puffiness of eyes may indicate nocturnal cough in children.
5. Vomiting (48%) occurs after a typical coughing spasm.
6. The whoop (40%) is a hoarse inspiratory stridor that starts as the child recovers his breath after a paroxysm of coughing. It usually appears 1 or 2 days after the onset of vomiting. Sometimes babies and very ill or immunised children do not 'whoop'.

INVESTIGATIONS

1. A differential white-cell count reveals an absolute lymphocy-

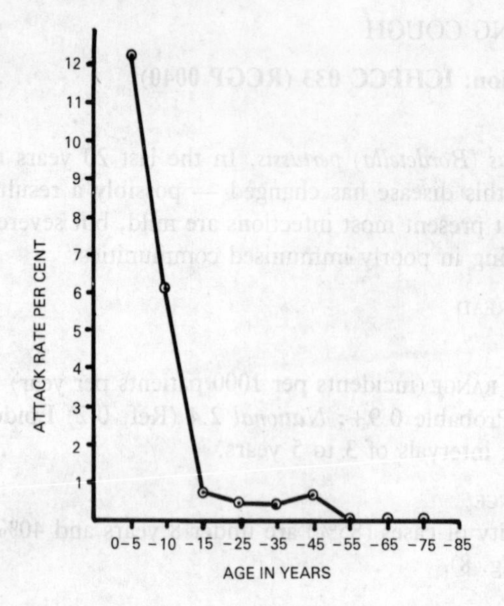

Fig. 8 Whooping cough. Age incidence of 67 consecutive cases

tosis. This test may help if symptoms are atypical or if asthma is suspected.

2. Cough plates for droplet culture are seldom used.

3. Chest X-ray is indicated if chest complications are suspected. Enlarged hilar glands are often noted in uncomplicated cases.

COMPLICATIONS

1. Acute bronchopneumonia occasionally occurs in the first 3 weeks of the disease. Babies are especially liable and may be so ill that cough and whoop are temporarily suppressed.

2. Collapse and basal pneumonitis. Persistent fever and moist adventitious sounds at the affected base become apparent as the disease subsides.

3. Bronchiectasis and chronic lung damage may develop if a collapsed lung is allowed to persist.

4. Rectal prolapse and haemorrhages in nose, conjunctivae and eardrums may result from excessive coughing.

5. Death and serious complications are rare. Babies under 6 months and debilitated children are at risk.

MISLEADING FEATURES AND PITFALLS

1. In an immunised child a mild form of the disease can occur. Vomiting and whoop are absent and the cough clears up quickly.

2. Parents often confuse the hoarse brassy cough of a croup or tracheitis with the inspiratory stridor of the whoop. An accurate description of the cough differentiates.

3. Children (especially babies) who have had whooping cough tend to whoop with any subsequent cough.

4. Whooping cough occasionally occurs after middle age.

5. Hilar adenitis on chest X-ray may suggest other diseases.

6. Adeno-virus infections and early asthma can both cause a persistent nocturnal cough which is easily confused with pertussis.

DIFFERENTIAL DIAGNOSIS

Diseases that may be confused with whooping cough:

Acute Bronchitis

Similar features: persistent nocturnal cough; low fever; children mainly affected; generalised adventitious sounds in chest.

Distinguishing features: contacts absent; cough clears after 7 to 10 days; coughing does not make child red in face or sick; distinction difficult in early stages.

Aspiration Pneumonitis

Similar features: persistent spasmodic nocturnal cough; low fever; children mainly affected. (Pneumonitis may complicate pertussis.)

Distinguishing features: contacts absent; coughing does not usually cause vomiting or whoop; localising adventitious sounds in chest; chest X-ray may differentiate.

MANAGEMENT OPTIONS

Prevention: (a) immunisation advised especially to protect high risk groups — The dangers of the disease are always greater than those of immunisation; (b) isolation of active sufferers, especially from high risk groups; (c) antibiotic cover of high risk contacts occasionally justified.

Established disease: (a) rest; (b) sedatives; (c) avoid actions that precipitate cough; (d) full support and detailed explanations to prepare parents for vital nursing tasks ahead; (e) referral occasionally helpful.

SCARLET FEVER

Classification: ICPHC 034 (RCGP 0045)

AETIOLOGY

Streptococcus pyogenes infections, which cause an allergic rash.

MODE OF SPREAD

Droplet.

DIAGNOSTIC RANGE (i.e. incidents per 1000 patients per year)

Personal: Suspected 5.0, Probable 1.9; *National* 1.6 (Ref. 0.2).

AGE INCIDENCE

The majority (68%) are between 5 and 11 years. Cases over 12 are uncommon.

INCUBATION PERIOD

Two to 4 days. The interval between household contact cases is often longer and may be several weeks.

CLINICAL POINTERS

1. Contacts (55%). Isolated cases often occur.
2. Characteristic rash (100%) a salmon-pink flush affects the whole body except the circumoral region; on close inspection a profuse pinpont papular rash that can be seen and feels like sand-paper (helpful in dark skins).
3. Sore red throat (80% — exudate in 50%): Children under 6 years rarely complain of sore throat in spite of obvious inflammation; the inflamed throat appears 24 hours before the rash.
4. Fever (90%) is often high and may be associated with headache, nausea and vomiting.
5. Tongue is covered with a heavy white fur initially and breath may be offensive. After 3 days the tongue peels, leaving a smooth red strawberry tongue with well-marked papillae.
6. Peeling of the skin starts 3 to 10 days after the rash appears and confirms the diagnosis.

INVESTIGATIONS

Throat swab. At present the disease is so mild that swabbing and serology are rarely used to check diagnosis or exclude carrier states. Blood tests show leucocytosis and a rising Antistreptolysin titre.

DURATION

Five to 10 days. Recurrences may occur but diagnosis may be difficult to prove.

COMPLICATIONS

1. Acute otitis media.
2. Acute rheumatism.

3. Acute glomerulonephritis is becoming more frequent but is still uncommon.

4. A carrier state may persist for long periods.

MISLEADING FEATURES AND PITFALLS

1. Transient neck stiffness (10%).
2. Abdominal pain.
3. Failure to exclude the possibility of rubella or mononucleosis.

DIFFERENTIAL DIAGNOSIS

Diseases that may be confused with scarlet fever:

Allergic rashes
Similar features: rash; circumoral pallor occasionally.

Distinguishing features: fever absent; fauces and tongue normal; allergens absent; peeling of skin absent.

Rubella
Similar features: rash.

Distinguishing features: contacts; occipital lymphadenopathy common; rash more blotchy and not punctate; leukopenia.

MANAGEMENT OPTIONS

Prevention: High carrier rates make this impractical. Occasionally antibiotics may be used to protect contacts at special risk.

Established disease: (a) antibiotics BNF 5.1 (Ref. 0.1) effective in first 3 days but rarely justified unless there is a history of acute rheumatism or otitis; (b) careful explanation to parents vital.

ACUTE POLIOMYELITIS

Classification: ICHPCC 045 (RCGP 0065)

An entero-virus which causes a mild febrile illness similar to an echo or coxsackie infection — non-paralytic polio. In a very few cases it destroys the anterior horn cells of the spinal cord causing permanent muscle paralysis.

AETIOLOGY

Poliomyelitis virus types 1, 2 or 3.

MODE OF SPREAD

Transmission is by droplet through gut or nasopharynx.

DIAGNOSTIC RANGE

No cases encountered in the last 20 years, probably a result of mass immunisation. Any unimmunised individual is at risk. Foreign travel and emigration of disadvantaged poorly immunised population groups is still a potential source of infection.

AGE INCIDENCE

Patients are aged between 3 and 30 years.

CLINICAL COURSE

1. The stage of minor illness or invasion — duration 1 day — diagnosis rarely possible.

2. The preparalytic stage develops after 2 to 5 days and lasts 1 to 3 days — diagnosis difficult.

3. The paralytic stage follows immediately, reaches a peak in 1 to 2 days and is complete within 7 days.

4. The stage of residual disability.

The clinical course is variable; the first stage may pass unnoticed; in other patients the disease aborts after the second stage and the diagnosis remains in doubt.

CLINICAL POINTERS IN THE PREPARALYTIC AND PARALYTIC STAGES

1. High risk factors: (a) contacts; (b) other cases in area; (c) recent visit to endemic area; (d) recent immigrants.

2. Fever — usually high at first.

3. Meningism: back stiffness (inability to kiss the knees) is more usual than neck stiffness.

4. Mental irritability: The patient resents examination.

5. Muscular aches and pains are usually present but arise in many febrile illnesses.

6. Late signs suggesting muscle paralysis include loss of muscle power, lost tendon reflexes and especially persistent pain or tenderness in any group of muscles.

INVESTIGATIONS

1. Lumbar puncture in hospital.

2. A domiciliary second opinion.

COMPLICATIONS

Respiratory paralysis may be suggested by difficult, rapid or noisy breathing. Immediate transfer to a specialised unit is then indicated.

MISLEADING FEATURES AND PITFALLS

1. Minor degrees of meningeal irritation sometimes occur in many febrile diseases.

2. The pain and weakness of paralytic polio may be mistaken for

convalescent influenza — evidence of paralysis is only discovered by examination.

3. The disease is now so rare in some communities that diagnosis fails to be considered.

DIFFERENTIAL DIAGNOSIS

Diseases that may be confused with acute poliomyelitis:

Influenza

Similar features: fever; headache; body aches; signs of meningeal irritation.

Distinguishing features: cough and tracheitis; meningeal signs transient; contacts likely.

Acute exudative tonsillitis

Similar features: fever; headache; pain; signs of meningeal irritation.

Distinguishing features: typical tonsillar exudate; meningism is transient.

Acute rheumatism

Similar features; fever; headache; pain; apparent immobility of a limb.

Distinguishing features: preceding sore throat; articular origin of pain and immobility apparent on examination; onset more gradual than polio; several joints usually affected; no evidence of meningeal irritation.

Bacterial meningitis, and aseptic meningitis

Similar features: fever; headache; backache; signs of meningeal irritation.

Distinguishing features: lumbar puncture required to differentiate; admission to hospital indicated.

MANAGEMENT OPTIONS

Prevention: Maintenance of high immunisation rates vital.
Suspected disease: Referral for investigation and management.

CHICKENPOX

Classification: ICHPCC 052 (RCGP 0075)

AETIOLOGY

The varicella-zoster (VZ) virus capable of producing a protracted carrier state with intracellular latency.

DIAGNOSTIC RANGE (rates per 1000 patients per year)
Personal: Probable 33.0 in an epidemic year. Occasional endemic cases were encountered. The diagnosis was rarely in doubt. Epidemics occur every 2 to 3 years. *National* 4.2 (Ref. 0.2)

AGE INCIDENCE
Children under 11 years (92%) — Fig. 9.

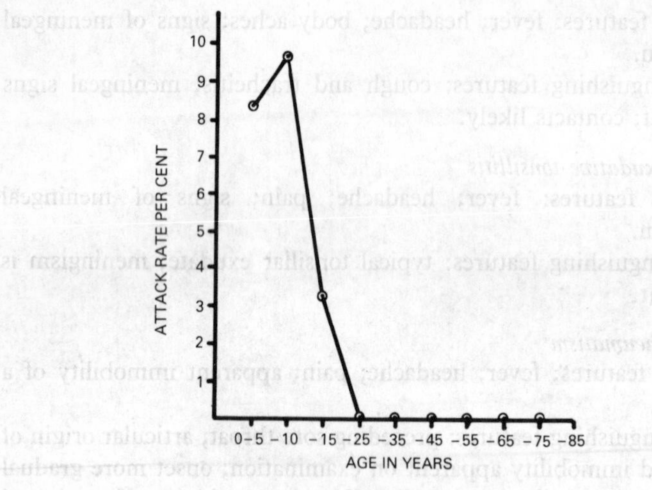

Fig. 9 Chickenpox. Age incidence of 62 consecutive cases.

INCUBATION PERIOD AND INFECTIVITY
Fourteen days. The disease is only infectious in the first 4 days.

CLINICAL POINTERS
1. High risk factors: (a) school epidemic; (b) contact cases (40%); (c) contacts with shingles.
2. Characteristic rash (100%) the individual lesion starts as a discrete red macule (2 mm diameter); in the centre a small papule appears and forms the typical clear vesicle of chickenpox which then breaks and crusts over; often there is a red flare (5 to 20 mm diameter) around the vesicle; the rash takes 2 to 4 days to develop and is often irritable in the early stages.
3. Lesions in the scalp.
4. Low fever.
5. The enanthem (100%): one or two small aphthous ulcers develop on the buccal mucous membrane and palate while the rash is developing.

6. Associated cough is common.

DURATION

Five days. The scabs remain for 14 days but are not infectious.

MISLEADING FEATURES AND PITFALLS

Occasionally the rash is haemorrhagic. The child may be very ill for 2 to 3 days and the probability of encephalitis has to be considered.

DIFFERENTIAL DIAGNOSIS

Diseases that may be confused with chickenpox:

Papular urticaria

Similar feature: vesicular irritable rash affecting trunk and limbs.

Distinguishing features: head rarely affected; no enanthem or fever; urticarial reaction and irritation marked; rash occurs in definite crops.

Scabies, bites and herpes simplex rarely cause confusion.

MANAGEMENT OPTIONS

Prevention: Rarely justified apart from isolation in first four days.
Established Disease: Home nursing; neutral aspirin for irritation.

HERPES ZOSTER (SHINGLES)

Classification: ICHPCC 053 (RCGP 0090)

AETIOLOGY

Varicella-zoster (VZ) virus. Shingles sometimes arises in patients with Hodgkin's disease or cancer and may follow irritation of skin, e.g. deep X-ray therapy. The virus affects one posterior dorsal root ganglion and causes lesions and pain over the corresponding cutaneous segment. The VZ virus like cytomegalo and Epstein-Barr viruses can be carried without causing symptoms, for long periods. Shingles develops when loss of immunity allows the latent virus to multiply.

DIAGNOSTIC RANGE (in rates per 1000 patients per year)

Personal: suspected 4.5, probable 3.4; *National* 4.1 (Ref. 0.2)

AGE INCIDENCE

All ages. The disease is common in the latter half of life. Incidence reaches a peak at 70 years.

CLINICAL POINTERS

1. High risk factors: (a) the elderly; (b) radiotherapy and immune suppression. Contact cases do not occur. Occasionally a teacher with shingles may cause an outbreak of chicken pox in school.

2. Pain (92%) in the affected cutaneous segment may be severe and is usually felt 2 to 14 days before the rash.

3. The characteristic rash (100%) appears unilaterally within the segment of one cutaneous nerve. One (or more) blotchy red patch that resembles a bottle burn is followed in 24 hours by vesicles — sometimes haemorrhagic. The vesicles crust over to heal in 10 to 20 days.

4. Mental depression and malaise (28%). Slight fever is occasionally present.

5. Localised adenitis is often noticed after the rash develops.

COMPLICATIONS

1. Post-herpetic neuralgia (5%). This residual pain is often refractory to treatment especially in the elderly.

2. Corneal ulceration and other eye complications are common when the trigeminal nerve is involved.

3. Motor paralysis may occur especially if facial nerves are affected.

MISLEADING FEATURES AND PITFALLS

Pain in the chest or abdomen several days before the shingles rash may lead to confusion with pleurisy, myocardial infarct or acute abdominal conditions.

DIFFERENTIAL DIAGNOSIS

Diseases that may be confused with herpes zoster:

Herpes simplex

Similar features: neuralgic pain; vesicular rash; local adenitis.

Distinguishing features: onset related to fever or sunlight; pain rarely marked; previous attacks at same site; face usually affected; distribution often bilateral.

Bottle burn

Similar feature: blotchy discoloration at site of acute pain.

Distinguishing features: history; rash does not progress to vesiculation and fades in a few hours.

Chickenpox
Similar features: contact history; vesicular rash; two diseases may occasionally occur together.

Distinguishing features: rash is generalised; vesicles are further apart; rash in mouth.

MANAGEMENT OPTIONS

Established disease: (a) full preparation of the patient for what lies ahead is vital; (b) analgesics BNF 4.7.1 (Ref. 0.1); (c) antivirals (BNF 5.3)

Post herpetic neuralgia: Analgesics. — BNF 4.7.1. Addictive drugs must be avoided.

HERPES SIMPLEX VIRUS (HSV)

Classification: ICHPPC 054 (RCGP 0100)

Herpes Simplex Viruses like varicella-zoster, the Epstein-Barr and cytomegalo viruses are all DNA viruses, capable of producing a protracted carrier state with intracellular latency. There are two types: HSV_1 (oral) and HSV_2 (genital). In both, primary infection is followed by a heavy localised painful vesicular rash affecting the superficial layers of skin and mucous membranes of the infected area, many primary infections are subclinical. The virus lies latent within the infected cells and then often causes recurrent localised secondary attacks which are both painful and infectious.

HSV type 1 infections usually cause lesions of the mouth, face or trunk. It may also cause corneal ulcers, recurrent apthous or ulcers of mouth.

HSV type 2 infections cause lesions in the genital area and vagina. Transmission is usually by sexual contact, though neonates may contract encephalitis from an infected maternal vagina.

HERPETIC STOMATITIS

Classification: ICHPPC 054 (RCGP 0100)

AETIOLOGY

Usually a primary infection of Herpes simplex virus type 1.

DIAGNOSTIC RANGE (in rates per 1000 patients per year)

Personal: Probable 2.5+. The diagnosis was rarely in doubt.

AGE INCIDENCE

Toddlers are especially liable.

CLINICAL POINTERS

1. Oral ulcers, about 2 mm diameter, on the tongue and buccal mucous membrane. They are shallow, numerous and persist for 5 to 10 days.

2. Irritability, crying and restlessness is marked. Pain and difficulty with food lead to considerable disturbance of the toddler's routine.

3. Predisposing factors: any febrile illness, poor household hygiene.

4. Cervical adenitis and fever may occur.

DIFFERENTIAL DIAGNOSIS

Aphthous ulcers of the mouth are identical in appearance but are usually single and occur at any age. These may be manifestations of chronic HSV type 1 infection (see p. 161).

MANAGEMENT OPTIONS

Prevention: General hygiene including sterilisation of feeding bottles and teats — especially if there is a parental history of herpes.

Established disease: (a) soluble aspirin and mouth washes; (b) prepare parents for a difficult 10 days. Antivirals are inappropriate.

Recurrences: See apthous ulcers p. 446.

HERPES SIMPLEX AND COLD SPOTS

Classification: ICHPCC 054 (RCGP 0100)

AETIOLOGY

Herpes simplex virus type 1 infections. A primary infection leads to intracellular latency and further recurrences are likely.

DIAGNOSTIC RANGE RATES PER 1000 PATIENTS PER YEAR

Personal: Probable 11.5+. The diagnosis was rarely in doubt. Most patients give a history of recurrent attacks.

AGE INCIDENCE

All ages, especially the young.

INCUBATION

Not known.

CLINICAL POINTERS

1. High risk factors: (a) parental and other household contacts; (b) history of previous attacks; (c) presence of predisposing trigger stimuli such as fever, sunlight, respiratory illness, smoking and poor household hygiene.

2. Local irritation a few hours before the rash appears.

3. Typical rash (100%): Several vesicles appear in a red patch of skin (1 to 2 cm diamter); after 2 to 3 days the rash crusts over to heal in 5 to 7 days. The face and lips are most commonly affected. Occasionally one or both cornea are infected.

4. Localised adenitis and hyperaesthesia.

COMPLICATIONS

Post-herpetic neuritis: occasional neuritic pains or attacks of hyperaesthesia are felt over the affected cutaneous nerve segment. These symptoms are not always associated with an active recurrence.

Recurrent corneal infections can cause corneal scarring.

MISTAKES AND PITFALLS

Herpetic eye and skin lesions are aggravated by drops (or applications) containing steroids.

MANAGEMENT OPTIONS

Prevention: (a) high standards of household hygiene; (b) protect against trigger factors i.e. avoid smoking and use barrier applications (BNF 13.8.1 Ref. 0.1) before exposure to sun, wind etc.

Active disease: (a) analgesics; (b) general hygiene to prevent spread to others; (c) antivirals effective in first 3 days but these do not prevent intracellular infection (BNF 5.3) Acyclovir eye ointment (BNF 11.3.1) rubbed in at site of irritation will abort recurrences.

GENITAL HERPES

Classification ICHPCC 054 (RCGP 0095)

AETIOLOGY

Herpes Simplex Virus type 2

MODE OF SPREAD

Sexual transmission is usual. Homosexuals often affected.

DIAGNOSTIC RANGE

Many cases are not reported but now said to be the commonest of all sexually transmitted diseases in many urban communities.

AGE INCIDENCE

Mainly teenagers and young adults.

INCUBATION

Two to 12 days.

CLINICAL POINTERS

1. High risk factors (a) Sexual transmission likely (b) known infectivity in contacts (c) homosexual (d) previous attacks.

2. Typical vesicular rash similar to cold spots (p. 162) affecting genitals i.e. penis (tip and shaft), labia, vulva and occasionally inside of vagina.

3. Local pain — often marked and aggravated by intercourse. There may be dysuria.

4. Localised adenitis and hyperaesthesia with malaise and fever.

COMPLICATIONS

Recurrences are likely.

A vaginal delivery when a mother has an active attack may cause a neonatal encephalitis in the baby.

AIDS — a rare associated disease in homosexuals (p. 190).

MANAGEMENT OPTIONS

Prevention: Use condom or avoid intercourse if infection is possiable. Health education (Ref 8.1); See Sexually Transmitted Disease (p. 190).

Established disease: (a) avoid intercourse; (b) antivirals probably ineffective (BNF 5.3 Ref 0.1); (c) analgesics; (d) full frank discussion of future; (e) effectiveness of Acyclovir — BNF 11.3.1 — uncertain.

MEASLES

Classification: ICHPCC 055 (RCGP 0105)

AETIOLOGY

Measles virus is an RNA paramyxovirus.

DIAGNOSTIC RANGE (in rates per 1000 patients per year)

Personal: Probable 40.0 (in epidemic years). 1.0 (after immunisation programme)

National: 4.5 (Ref. 0.2) The diagnosis was rarely in doubt.

AGE INCIDENCE

The disease is unusual in patients over 10 years (Fig. 10). In many Western countries measles has been modified as a result of immunisation programmes. Immunity from mother for first 12 to 15 months.

INCUBATION PERIOD

Fourteen days from contact to rash. The serial interval between household contacts varies from 10 to 15 days.

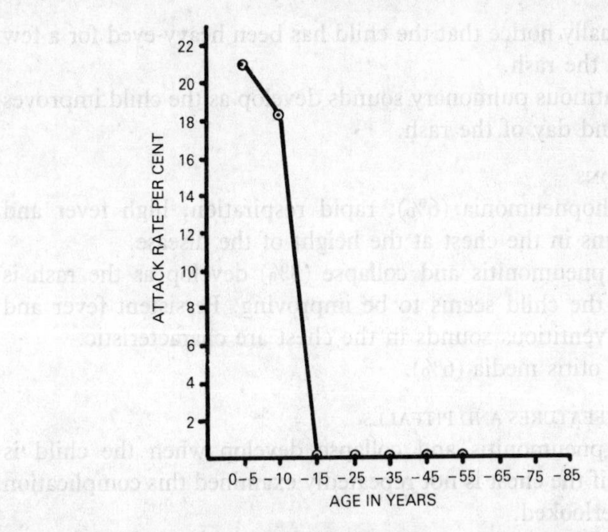

Fig. 10 Measles. Age incidence of 181 consecutive unimmunised cases in one year.

CLINICAL COURSE

1. The stage of incubation — duration, 7 to 10 days.
2. The catarrhal stage — duration 2 to 4 days.
3. The stage of rash — duration 2 to 4 days.
4. The convalescent stage — duration 2 to 4 days.

CLINICAL POINTERS

1. High risk factors: (a) history of contact (95%); (b) patient not immunised; (c) age: 9 months to 10 years.

2. Cough (100%): dry and irritant; in the majority of cases (81%) it starts 1 to 4 days before the rash appears.

3. Fever (95%) is low for 1 or 2 days then before the rash appears the child is very ill and fever is high.

4. Koplik's spots (100%) are found inside the cheek. They usually appear 1 to 2 days before the rash. The spot is a discrete papule 2 mm diameter with a pinpoint fleck of white at its centre. In mild attacks they are few in number but in severe attacks they coalesce to give the epithelium a deep red granular appearance that may be covered with a faint white reticulum.

5. The rash (100%) is characteristic. Starting as discrete maculo-papules 1 to 3 mm diamter, the spots rapidly coalesce to form the typical blotchy measles rash. The rash often starts behind the ears.

6. Photophobia and conjunctivitis: often not obvious but

mothers usually notice that the child has been heavy-eyed for a few days before the rash.

7. Adventitious pulmonary sounds develop as the child improves on the second day of the rash.

COMPLICATIONS

1. Bronchopneumonia (6%); rapid respiration, high fever and minimal signs in the chest at the height of the disease.

2. Basal pneumonitis and collapse (3%) develop as the rash is fading and the child seems to be improving. Persistent fever and localised adventitious sounds in the chest are characteristic.

3. Acute otitis media (6%).

MISLEADING FEATURES AND PITFALLS

1. Basal pneumonitis and collapse develop when the child is improving; if the chest is not repeatedly examined this complication is easily overlooked.

2. Persistent fever for several days before the onset of the rash may puzzle the doctor and the child may be sent to hospital for investigation.

3. Abdominal pain may occur at the time of Koplik infiltration and is occasionally marked. Confusion with appendicitis may then occur.

4. Fever, prostration and malaise are usually extreme. This may surprise physicians whose clinical experience of measles has been limited; a diagnosis of pneumonia and hospital admission may be wrongly entertained.

5. Mild, atypical cases with only a few spots and no cough or Koplik's spots can occur in babies and immunised subjects.

DIFFERENTIAL DIAGNOSIS

Diagnosis is often difficult during the incubation and catarrhal stages, because cough and fever suggest many febrile respiratory illnesses. The diagnosis becomes clear after two to three days when Koplik's spots and then the typical rash appear. Occipital adenitis is common in measles and if Koplik infiltration is slight confusion with rubella may occur.

MANAGEMENT OPTIONS

Prevention: Immunisation at about 15 months.

Established disease: (a) preparation and support of parents essential; (b) Rest, sedatives and cough supressants; (c) antibiotics if protection against bacterial complications is needed; (d) gammaglobulin occasionally justified to abort an attack.

RUBELLA (GERMAN MEASLES)

Classification: ICHPPC 056 (RCGP 0110)

AETIOLOGY
Rubella virus

DIAGNOSTIC RANGE (in rates per 1000 patients per year)
Personal: Epidemic year 60.0; *National* 5.1 (Ref. 0.2)

AGE INCIDENCE
Mostly under 11 years and rarely under 6 months. (Fig. 11).

INCUBATION PERIOD
Eighteen days. The interval between onset in household contacts varies from 11 to 21 days.

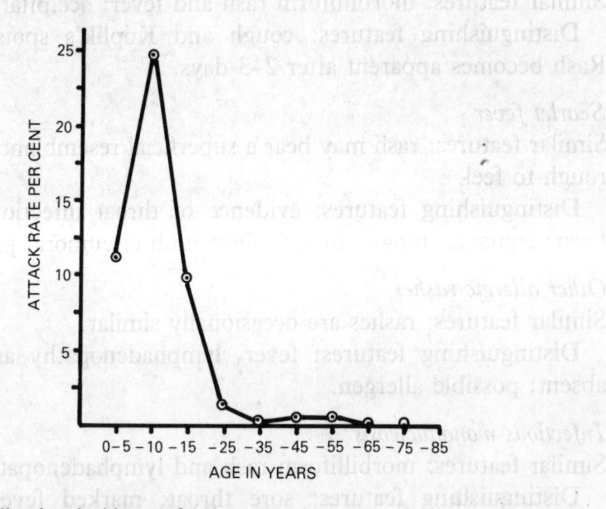

Fig. 11. Rubella. Age incidence of 140 consecutive cases.

CLINICAL POINTERS

1. High risk factors (a) contacts (b) patient not immunised.
2. The rash (100%) is similar to that of measles but the macules are smaller and more discrete. It may last only a few hours and is rarely confluent.
3. Cervical adenitis (90%): posterior cervical, occipital or posterior auricular lymph glands are commonly affected. They are sometimes tender and painful.
4. Systemic disturbance is limited to a slight fever. There is no enanthem in the mouth.

DURATION

Two to 4 days.

COMPLICATIONS

Rubella in the mother during the first 100 days of pregnancy may lead to deafness and other congenital defects of the foetus. Early diagnosis is essential when a pregnant mother is at risk.

Occasionally a transient polyarthritis, peripheral neuritis or carpal tunnel syndrome develops a few days (usually two to ten) after the rash. Children rarely develop these complications.

DIFFERENTIAL DIAGNOSIS

Diseases that may be confused with rubella:

Measles

Similar features: morbilliform rash and fever; occipital adenitis.

Distinguishing features: cough and Koplik's spots; contacts. Rash becomes apparent after 2–3 days.

Scarlet fever

Similar features: rash may bear a superficial resemblance but is not rough to feel.

Distinguishing features: evidence of throat infection and high fever; contacts; tongue furred; flush with circumoral pallor.

Other allergic rashes

Similar features: rashes are occasionally similar.

Distinguishing features: fever, lymphadenopathy and contacts absent; possible allergen.

Infectious mononucleosis

Similar features: morbilliform rash and lymphadenopathy.

Distinguishing features: sore throat; marked fever; enlarged spleen; positive serology and blood picture; young adults usually affected.

MANAGEMENT OPTIONS

Prevention: (a) Ideally all girls should be immunised before they are 14 years. Rubella vaccine should not be given if pregnancy is possible or likely within 3 months. (b) Gammaglobulin given within 10 days of contact protects women who may be pregnant. (c) immunity check of women attending for antenatal and contraceptive advice.

Established disease: (a) Isolation from women who may be pregnant. Consider termination if infection occurs in early pregnancy (b) Symptomatic treatment is occasionally needed.

ACUTE VIRAL HEPATITIS

AETIOLOGY

Several viruses of very different type can cause hepatitis.

— *Hepatitis A virus* has a 2–5 week incubation, is usually spread by faecal contamination, is rarely fatal and causes the majority of cases of jaundice in communities with a good standard of living.

— *Hepatitis B virus* has a 2–3 month incubation, is spread by injection or close contact and is rarer than the A virus. High risk groups include drug addicts, homosexuals and travellers from Asian countries.

— *Hepatitis non-A, non-B* has an intermediate incubation period and is most likely to be spread by transfusion. It is endemic in small numbers in most countries. The virus has not been identified.

— Epstein Barr, Rubella, Cytomegalo- and Adeno-viruses can all occasionally cause hepatitis.

— other causes of painless clinical jaundice which should be remembered are: any haemolytic process, septicaemias, Weil's disease and jaundice from drugs, e.g. the pill, chlorpromazine, etc.

ACUTE HEPATITIS A

Classification: ICHPCC 070 (RCGP 0130)

SYNONYMS

Infectious hepatitis, short incubation hepatitis, MS-1 hepatitis, infectious jaundice.

AETIOLOGY

Hepatitis A virus.

SPREAD OF INFECTION

Probably by faecal excretion of incubating or early cases. Convalescent carriers have not been demonstrated. Infection occurs by the oral route. (Parenteral infection can occur). Most epidemics centre round a particular school, often with noticeably poor hygiene discipline.

Endemic and epidemic cases may arise in an area intermittently over several years to be followed by several years without any cases.

DIAGNOSTIC RANGE (in rates per 1000 patients per year)
Personal: Probable (epidemic year) 12.0, Endemic 1.0, *National* 0.8 (Ref. 0.2).

AGE INCIDENCE
The majority (75%) are school children.

INCUBATION PERIOD
Said to be 14 to 30 days. (The interval between the onset of jaundice in two members of the same household was sometimes as long as 3 months. This suggests the possibility of an intermediate subclinical contact rather than a B virus infection.)

CLINICAL POINTERS
1. High risk factors: (a) household contacts; (b) other school or institutional cases; (c) other district cases; (d) foreign travel; (e) poor lavatory hygiene.
2. Vomiting (80%) starts 1 to 4 days before the jaundice and persists for several days.
3. Anorexia is marked (90%).
4. Abdominal pain (50%) 1 to 2 days before the jaundice. It is generalised, intermittent, and not related to vomiting.
5. Jaundice (70%) shows first on the sclerotics. In the next 2 to 4 days it may deepen and affect the skin after which it gradually fades and vanishes in 10 to 20 days.
6. Bile in urine (80%): 1 to 2 days before clinical jaundice appears, the urine is dark orange or brown and stains clothing.
7. Clay-coloured stools.
8. Low fever (30%).

INVESTIGATIONS
1. Urine: urobilinogen and bile salts. (A simple test: shake the urine and if froth persists and is yellow, bile is probably present.)
2. Liver function and other biochemical tests.
3. Antigen/antibody studies if virus identity is needed.

DURATION
Varies from 7 to 28 days usually a mild disease.

COMPLICATIONS
Permanent liver damage — adults are more susceptible, especially after repeated attacks.

MISLEADING FEATURES AND PITFALLS
1. Abdominal pain may be present for several days before the jaundice.

2. The sclerotics of red-haired children and the elderly may normally appear slightly yellow.

3. True icterus may not be apparent in artificial light.

4. Subclinical cases without evidence of jaundice are not uncommon.

DIFFERENTIAL DIAGNOSIS BEFORE JAUNDICE DEVELOPS

Diseases that may be confused with infective hepatitis:

Acute appendicitis

Similar features: right-sided abdominal pain; low fever and vomiting.

Distinguishing features: pain usually precedes vomiting; tenderness is rarely confined to liver; bradycardia unlikely; differentiation may be difficult and admission to hospital for observation occasionally indicated.

Early stages of any febrile illness in children

Similar features: excessive vomiting, anorexia and fever.

Distinguishing features: the diseases are usually distinguished by waiting 1 or 2 days.

DIFFERENTIAL DIAGNOSIS AFTER JAUNDICE DEVELOPS

Carcinoma obstructing bile duct

Similar feature: painless jaundice.

Distinguishing features: jaundice is steadily progressive; fever absent; gall bladder sometimes palpable; rare in young patients; contact cases absent; biochemical tests.

Stone in bile duct

Similar features: jaundice; fever.

Distinguishing features: pain is usually severe; rare in young patients; biochemical tests.

Severe anaemias

Similar feature: slight painless jaundice.

Distinguishing features: icterus is slight and only slowly progressive; pallor marked; icterus is apparent on face rather than sclerotics; blood and biochemical tests differentiate; urine is normal colour.

MANAGEMENT OPTIONS

Prevention: (a) Investigate institutional sources of infection; (b) Isolate for first week; (c) Improve and check general hygiene of contacts and cases.

Established disease: (a) rest; (b) normal activity resumed when clinically recovered; (c) no special diets.

ACUTE HEPATITIS B

Classification: ICHPPC 070 (RCGP 0130)

SYNONYMS
Serum hepatitis, long incubation hepatitis, MS-2 hepatitis, Australia antigen hepatitis.

AETIOLOGY
Hepatitis B virus.

MODE OF SPREAD
Mainly parenteral following: injections, transfusion, dialysis, tattooing, etc. Hard drug addicts are especially at risk.

Infection by oral route can occur from infected faeces as in hepatitis A infections. 'Gay' communities are at special risk.

Carrier states and sporadic cases can occur. The A virus can also be spread by the parenteral route.

DIAGNOSTIC RANGE
No proven cases encountered in practices under review.

INCUBATION PERIOD
Said to be 2 to 3 months.

CLINICAL POINTERS, etc.
As for Hepatitis A but urticaria and polyarthralgia may occur.

COMPLICATIONS
Cirrhosis, hepatoma and death.

MANAGEMENT OPTIONS
As for hepatitis A.

MUMPS

Classification: ICHPPC 072 (RCGP 0140)

AETIOLOGY
Mumps virus.

MODE OF SPREAD
Droplet.

DIAGNOSTIC RANGE (in rates per 1000 patients per year)
Personal: Epidemic year 50.0. *National* 1.0 (Ref. 0.2). Epidemics

occur every 3 to 4 years but may be modified by vaccination programmes. Occasional endemic cases also occur.

AGE INCIDENCE

The majority (90%) are under 11 years (Fig. 12).

INCUBATION PERIOD

About 18 days. The serial interval between household contacts varies from 14 to 24 days.

CLINICAL POINTERS

1. High risk factors: (a) household contacts; (b) school contacts.
2. Characteristic swelling of salivary gland [100%] — mainly the parotid [75%]. The swelling appears below and in front of the lobe of the ear. The posterior edge of the ramus of the jaw cannot be felt. The submandibular and sublingual glands cause swelling under the jaw giving a moon faced appearance if all three sets of glands are affected.
3. Pain on eating or earache [80%] especially with parotid mumps. The ear drum is not reddened.
4. Redness of the duct orifices of the affected gland and fever are inconstant signs.

DURATION

The swelling lasts for 3 to 5 days. Sometimes the infection spreads from one salivary gland to another over a period of 1 to 3 weeks.

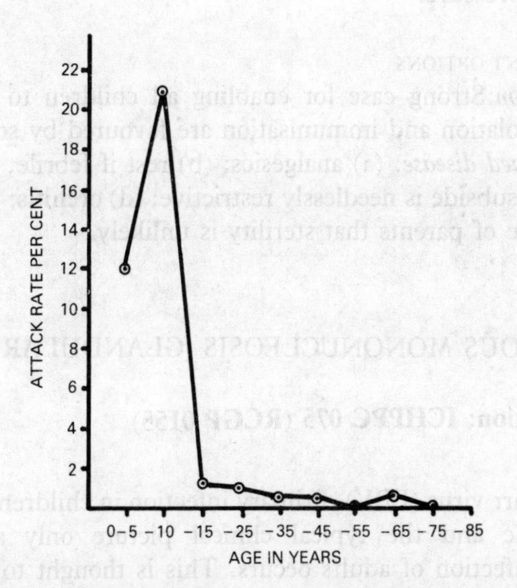

Fig. 12 Mumps. Age incidence of 124 consecutive cases in one year

COMPLICATIONS

1. Ovaries, testicles and pancreas may be affected on the fourth to tenth day of the disease. All these are most likely to arise in adults.

2. Mumps encephalitis on the fourth to seventh day and can occur without salivary gland swelling. Sometimes mumps follows the encephalitis. A febrile illness with restlessness, disturbance of sleep rhythm, headache and meningism during a mumps epidemic suggests encephalitis (two cases in 10 years both were treated at home).

3. Recurrences are very occasionally noted (three in 10 years).

4. Unilateral nerve deafness (1 case in 10 years).

DIFFERENTIAL DIAGNOSIS

Diseases that may be confused with mumps.

Acute cervical adenitis

Similar feature: swelling under jaw or in side of neck.

Distinguishing features: high fever; malaise marked; cellulitis and reddening of skin occur; tenderness marked; other salivary glands not affected; ramus of jaw palpable.

Apical dental abscess

Similar feature: submandibular swelling.

Distinguishing features: dental sepsis evident; affected tooth tender to pressure.

MANAGEMENT OPTIONS

Prevention: Strong case for enabling all children to acquire the disease. Isolation and immunisation are favoured by some.

Established disease: (a) analgesics; (b) rest if febrile; (c) isolation till glands subside is needlessly restrictive; (d) orchitis: steroids and reassurance of parents that sterility is unlikely.

INFECTIOUS MONONUCLEOSIS (GLANDULAR FEVER)

Classification: ICHPPC 075 (RCGP 0155)

AETIOLOGY

Epstein-Barr virus (EBV). Primary infection in children is probably non-specific and the typical clinical picture only arises when primary infection of adults occurs. This is thought to explain the low infectivity of the clinical cases.

MODE OF SPREAD

Direct oral contact. Contact cases and epidemics occur but are unusual in most countries. Infectivity is low but throat washings contain virus for months after an acute infection.

DIAGNOSTIC RANGE (in rates per 1000 patients per year)

Personal: Suspected 1.9, Serological 0.7, *National* 1.3 (Ref. 0.2).

AGE INCIDENCE

Typical clinical picture occurs in adolescents and young adults.

INCUBATION PERIOD

Unknown. Said to be 10 to 14 days in children and up to 50 days in young adults.

CLINICAL POINTERS

1. Onset is of two types:
— Slow; 1 to 6 weeks with persistence of mild symptoms of fever, malaise, headaches, muscle and joint aches and listlessness;
— acute; 2 to 3 days with fever, prostration, headache, and often heavy tonsillar exudate.

2. Systemic symptoms usually include fever (80%), headache, anorexia and listlessness.

3. Enlargement of one or more groups of lymph nodes: the glands are often tender and only moderately enlarged — they may not appear until third or fourth week (50%).

4. Splenic enlargement, often absent (50%).

5. Prolonged but not progressive course. Fever, listlessness and glandular enlargement may last 4 to 16 weeks. The clinical course is usually not severe but convalescence is annoyingly slow. Listlessness may persist for months.

6. Sore throat with or without exudate occurs early (80%).

7. A rubella-like rash and jaundice are said to occur at the time of glandular enlargement.

INVESTIGATIONS

1. Blood count and smear. A high lymphocyte and monocyte count with characteristic atypical cells occurs at end of first week.

2. Serological tests for heterophile antibody (Paul-Bunnell, Monospot, etc.). Titres start rising after fourth to seventh day of illness. In first 10 days only 50 per cent of cases are positive. Later most cases are said to become positive.

COMPLICATIONS

Prolonged convalescence common. Recurrences, encephalitis, and jaundice occasionally develop.

DIFFERENTIAL DIAGNOSIS

Diseases that may be confused with glandular fever:

Acute tonsillitis, cervical adenitis

Similar features: sore throat with heavy tonsillar exudate; fever; adenitis; spleen occasionally felt in children with acute tonsillitis.

Distinguishing features: onset sudden; recovery rapid; blood findings are normal.

Rubella

Similar features: rash; fever and localised cervical adenopathy.

Distinguishing features: onset sudden; duration short; systemic disturbance slight; contact cases; blood findings differentiate.

Leukaemias

Similar features: adenopathy; fever; splenomegaly; onset similar.

Distinguishing features: disease is steadily progressive; blood findings usually differentiate; hospital investigation indicated.

Hodgkin's disease

Similar features: adenopathy; fever; splenomegaly.

Distinguishing features: systemic disturbance usually slight at onset; biopsy and hospital investigation may be indicated. Rare.

Undulant fever (brucellosis) and typhoid fever

Similar features: prolonged fever, rash, and splenomegaly.

Distinguishing feature: blood findings usually differentiate.

History suggesting possible origin of infection.

Secondary syphilis, septicaemias, Vincent's angina, tuberculous adenitis, serum sickness and infective hepatitis

All occasionally enter into differential diagnosis.

MANAGEMENT OPTIONS

Symptomatic treatment only.

VIRUS INFECTIONS ISOLATED FROM PRACTICE

From 1957 until 1973 respiratory diseases were monitored in my practice in Britain using paired sera and, more recently, virus culture. From 1965 to '66 nasal and throat swabs were cultured weekly from four patients with respiratory disease chosen randomly.

Nearly 1500 paired sera and 200 cultures were taken of which less than a third were positive.

Influenza A and B epidemics could be recognised on clinical

grounds, but apart from the exanthemata, the identification of the respiratory viruses on clinical grounds alone was almost impossible.

Even with virological studies it was usually difficult, apart from influenza A and B, to identify any epidemic patterns, reservoir or mode of spread.

The description that follows is based on this material and gives some idea of the difficulties involved in the clinical differentiation of the common respiratory virus infections.

The following points are of interest to primary physicians:

— the picture has not changed much in the 10 years since these studies ended.
— the great numbers and variety of virus diseases which are reported to a single practioner in 16 years.
— the management of all these infections is still largely symptomatic and aims to prevent complications from secondary descending bacterial infections

CLASSIFICATION

Most of the viruses isolated are at present classified under a single heading, ICHPPC 0799 (RCGP 0180). In some instances, e.g., influenza, cold, pneumonia or meningitis, they may be classified under the disease heading.

RHINOVIRUS INFECTION (COMMON COLD VIRUS)

NUMBER OF SEROTYPES: 100+

Many serotypes circulate in a community at one time, but only persist for a few months. Said to be responsible for 40% of all respiratory illness.

(Practice experience: isolations were rare because the mild symptoms did not justify either reporting to the doctor or extensive investigation.)

INCUBATION PERIOD

One to 2 days.

CLINICAL MANIFESTATIONS

1. Sore throat and slight fever may occur on first day.
2. Coryza followed by secondary infection.

HOUSEHOLD ATTACK RATES

High.

DURATION

Three to 7 days.

PARAINFLUENZA VIRUSES

NUMBER OF SEROTYPES: 4
(Type 1 = Sendai strain). All endemic.
(Practice experience: isolations 16; many cases probably never reported or not severe enough to justify virological investigation.)

AGE
Children affected mainly.

INCUBATION PERIOD
Five to 6 days.

CLINICAL MANIFESTATIONS

1. Coryza — frequently present. Pain on coughing.
2. Cough — frequently present; tracheitis, laryngitis and croup common. Wheeze in older children.
3. Sore throat — present in adults and children.
4. Fever — sometimes high (39.0°C) in adults as well as children.
5. Shivering: body aches occurred with fever.

HOUSEHOLD ATTACK RATE
Other householders reported similar symptoms but more than one febrile case in a household was uncommon.

DURATION
Four days in children, up to 10 days in adults.

COMPLICATIONS
Bronchiolitis and bronchopneumonia may occur in young children.

ADENOVIRUS INFECTIONS

NUMBER OF SEROTYPES: 31
(Practice experience: 17 proven cases; endemic and epidemic.)

AGE
Children and adults affected.

CLINICAL MANIFESTATIONS

1. Coryza rarely reported in adults.
2. Cough — usually present; often slight, sometimes associated with substernal soreness.
3. Sore throat — usually marked; occasionally tonsillar exudate noted.
4. Conjunctivitis — not noted in our cases.

5. Fever — usually present. Sometimes as high as 39·5°C in adults.

6. Shivering — a common early complaint.

7. Body aches and headache commonly reported with high fever.

8. Cervical gland enlargement was not noted in any of the adult cases.

HOUSEHOLD ATTACK RATE

Several minor household or localised street outbreaks recorded. Can mimic influenza because sometimes causes two adults in same household to be febrile at same time.

DURATION

Four days in children, up to 10 days in adults.

COMPLICATIONS

In children bronchiolitis and bronchopneumonia sometimes arise.

COXSACKIE A

NUMBER OF SEROTYPES: 24

(Practice experience: no isolations.)

CLINICAL MANIFESTATIONS

Said to cause a febrile sore throat (and sometimes coryza) in all age groups. Also said to cause herpangina.

Exanthems, meningo-encephalitis, myocarditis-pericarditis and pleurodynia all said to occur.

Types A 16, 10 and 5 are said to cause occasional small outbreaks of Hand, Foot and Mouth disease — a mild illness with discrete small vesicles of hands, feet and mouth.

COXSACKIE B

NUMBER OF SEROTYPES: 6

(Practice experience: 12 isolations in four minor outbreaks.)

AGE

Children and adults affected.

CLINICAL MANIFESTATIONS

1. Respiratory symptoms minimal, and confined to a sore throat (one child had exudate) or slight coryza.

2. Fever — marked.

3. Body aches and headaches — common. Causes epidemic

myalgia (Bornholm disease) but this condition was not encountered in this practice.

4. Neurological complications — common; back stiffness frequent; meningism in some cases. Bell's palsy noted in one of our cases.

5. Abdominal pain — noted transiently at the onset in two cases.

6. Evidence of myocarditis-pericarditis, meningo-encephalitis, orchitis and exanthems are all said to occur during the disease.

HOUSEHOLD ATTACK RATE

Said to be high, but although cases appeared all over the region during outbreaks, isolated cases were the rule.

DURATION

Three to 10 days.

ECHO VIRUS

NUMBER OF SEROTYPES: 32

(Practice experience: six isolations from two epidemics.)

AGE

Children and adults.

CLINICAL MANIFESTATIONS

Similar to Coxsackie, Influenza-like illness with high fever cough, tracheitis and body aches noted. One adult had enlarged painful cervical glands. In one outbreak meningism was noted.

Rashes, myocarditis/pericarditis and meningo-encephalitis are all said to occur, but were never experienced in our proven cases.

HOUSEHOLD ATTACK RATE

Proven cases were spread over the region not several in one house.

DURATION

3 to 10 days.

RESPIRATORY SYNCYTIAL VIRUS

(Practice experience: slight — 2 isolations; endemic.)

AGE

Adults as well as children affected.

CLINICAL MANIFESTATIONS

Said to cause epidemics of bronchiolitis in babies. Our cases were afebrile with cough, wheeze and laryingitis and did not occur in epidemics.

INFLUENZA VIRUSES AND INFLUENZA

Classification: ICHPPC 487 (RCGP 2485)

NUMBER OF SEROTYPES: 3 — INFLUENZA A, B, AND C.

(Practice experience: over 400 serologically proven cases or isolations; endemic cases were exceptional — Figs. 13 & 14)

This common disease has puzzled medical men for centuries. For many months no cases are encountered and then suddenly the doctor is called to a household in which several members have been stricken with an acute feverish bronchitis. One or 2 days later he is called to a different household in a similar predicament. This is the typical onset of an influenza epidemic.

An extensive epidemic of influenza is a nightmare experience for most family doctors. Work is suddenly doubled or trebled, many patients are very ill. Many others are frightened by the sensationalism of the popular press. Inevitably work is rushed. Throughout the epidemic three fears haunt the doctor:

1. Influenza can be a fatal disease, and although usually mild is capable of killing large numbers of any population.
2. The rush of work and consequent lowering of standards may cause him to overlook other cases of serious disease, meningitis, pneumonia, etc.
3. He may contract the disease himself and be forced to leave his patients and partners when they need him most.

EPIDEMIOLOGY

Influenza A virus (See Figs 13 and 14)

A family doctor over the years collects much epidemiological information about the common disease encountered. Influenza is a good example and is described in detail to illustrate the depth and continuity of observation available to any family doctor.

Between 1957 and 1972 routine paired sera were taken to check the diagnosis of 'flu' in as many suspected cases as possible. During this 15 year period over 1400 paired serology tests were performed and over 400 of these were positive.

Figures 13 and 14 summarise these findings on which the following account is based.

Originally I wanted answers to the following questions:

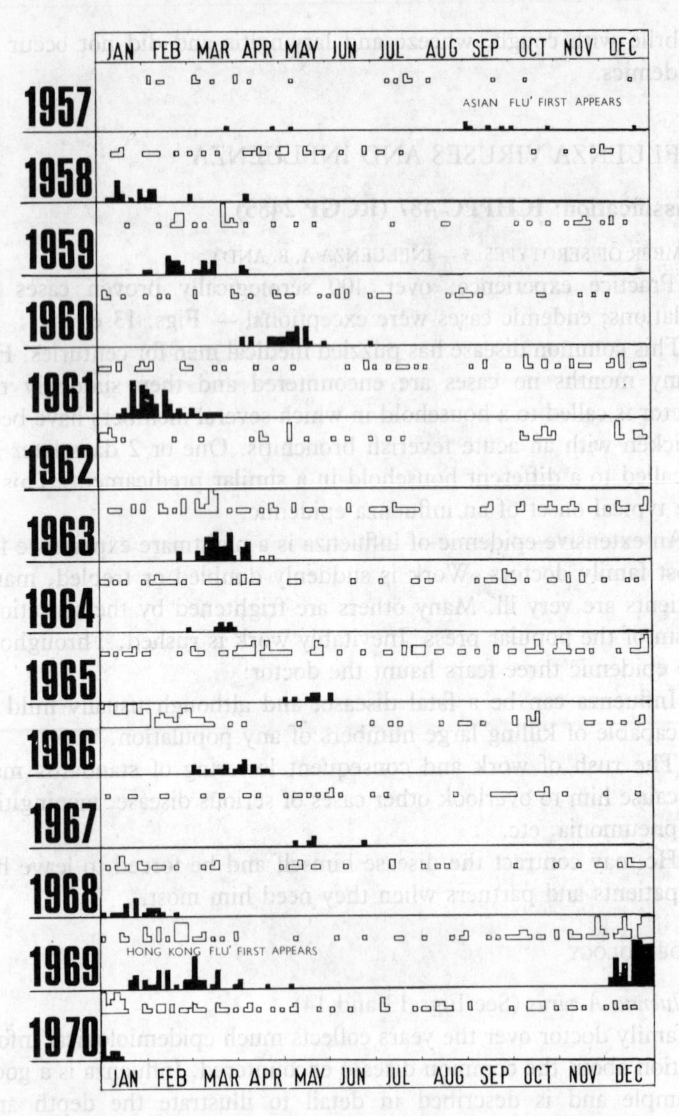

Fig. 13 Influenza A epidemics 1957–70. Each black square represents one proven case of influenza A. Serologically negative cases are outlined only, the scatter of these negative cases demonstrates the continuous search for positives. (For comments see text.)

1. Was it possible for an individual to have repeated attacks of influenza and for how many years did a clinical attack of 'flu' confer immunity?

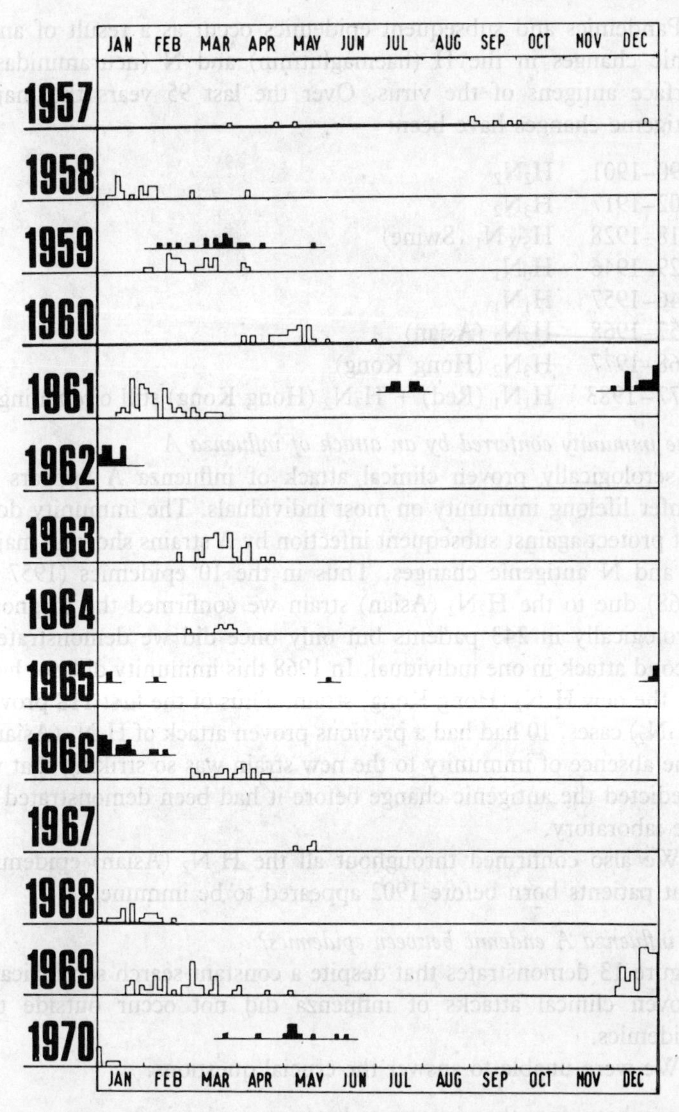

Fig. 14 Influenza B epidemics 1957–70. Each black square represents one proven case of influenza B. Proven cases of influenza A are outlined only. (For comments see text.)

2. Was 'flu' circulating in the community all the time between epidemics. If it was not where did it go to between epidemics and how did epidemics restart, i.e. where was the reservoir?

3. What causes an epidemic to stop?

Pandemics and subsequent epidemics occur as a result of antigenic changes in the H (haemaglutinin) and N (neuraminidase) surface antigens of the virus. Over the last 95 years the major antigenic changes have been:

1890–1901	H_2N_2
1902–1917	H_3N_2
1918–1928	$H_{SW}N_1$ (Swine)
1929–1946	H_0N_1
1946–1957	H_1N_1
1957–1968	H_2N_2 (Asian)
1968–1977	H_3N_2 (Hong Kong)
1977–1983	H_1N_1 (Red) + H_3N_2 (Hong Kong) still circulating

The immunity conferred by an attack of influenza A

A serologically proven clinical attack of influenza A appears to confer lifelong immunity on most individuals. The immunity does not protect against subsequent infection by A strains showing major H and N antigenic changes. Thus in the 10 epidemics (1957 to 1968) due to the H_2N_2 (Asian) strain we confirmed the diagnosis serologically in 243 patients but only once did we demonstrate a second attack in one individual. In 1968 this immunity did not hold for the new H_3N_2 (Hong Kong) strain. Thus of the first 118 proven (H_3N_2) cases, 10 had had a previous proven attack of H_2N_2 (Asian). The absence of immunity to the new strain was so striking that we predicted the antigenic change before it had been demonstrated in the laboratory.

We also confirmed throughout all the H_2N_2 (Asian) epidemics that patients born before 1902 appeared to be immune.

Is influenza A endemic between epidemics?

Figure 13 demonstrates that despite a constant search serologically proven clinical attacks of influenza did not occur outside the epidemics.

We were unable to answer the crucial questions:

- where does the virus go to between epidemics?
- where does the virus come from to start an epidemic?
- why when a new strain first circulated in 1957 and then in 1968 did it affect, clinically, only 18% of the almost un-immunised community (i.e. why does an epidemic stop?)
- where do the old strains disappear to when a new strain first appears? H_3N_2 (Hong Kong) and H_1N_1 (Red) are now both circulating in the community but this is unusual.

Perhaps the relationship is similar to that between the Herpes Zoster virus and outbreaks of Chicken Pox.

Hopefully such questions will encourage future family doctors to make the most of their epidemiological vantage point.

Influenza B virus (see Fig. 14)
Caused four epidemics (89 serologically proven cases) in the 14 years after 1957, *i.e.* 1959, 1961/62, 1965/66 and 1970. These epidemics were more erratic than influenza A. Two started in December and were preceded several months beforehand by a few isolated cases. The disease itself was clinically milder than influenza A and more likely to affect children. Epidemics of Influenza A & B often occur together in the same community. There is no cross immunity (Fig. 14).

Influenza C virus
Isolated from only three patients during the whole 15 year period.

DIAGNOSTIC RANGE (rates per 1000 population per year)
Personal: Suspected 18.2; Probable 5.0–10.0; *National* 6.0 All figures may be multiplied by a factor of up to 5 if there is a big epidemic.

AGE INCIDENCE
Patients of all ages are liable (Fig. 15).

INCUBATION PERIOD
One to 4 days.

CLINICAL POINTERS

1. High risk factors: (a) contacts; (b) immunity of the community to the circulating strain of virus (see p. 181 — epidemiology); (c) absence of previous infection (immunity) by current strain; (d) elderly and debilitated individuals; (e) nurses, doctors, ambulance drivers at special risk of infection.
2. High household attack rate. The possibility of an outbreak of influenza is raised whenever a G.P. is called to a household in which several members have been stricken by a sudden febrile respiratory illness. This is the most useful of all pointers.
3. Sudden onset is common but not invariable.
4. Cough (97%) is dry. After 2 to 4 days it becomes productive.
5. Retrosternal pain on coughing (49%) suggests a tracheitis and is characteristic.
6. Fever (78%) is frequently high and is probably always present in the early stages of the disease.

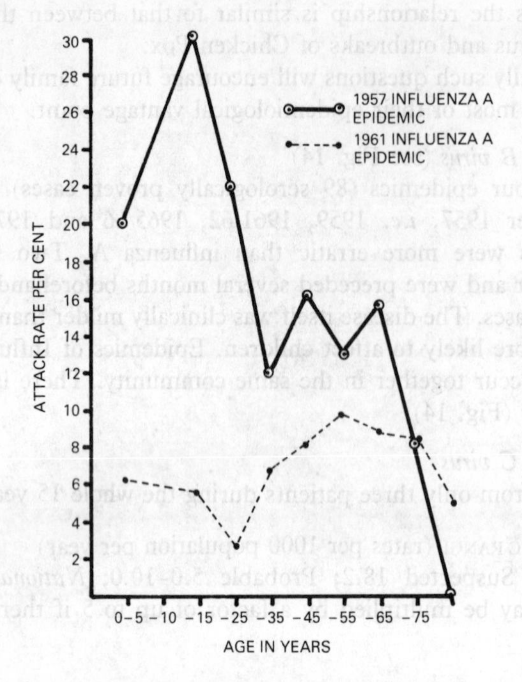

Fig. 15 Influenza A. Age incidence of 1957 epidemic (400 cases) and 1961 epidemic (300 cases). Note that the high attack rate in the 11–15 year olds in 1957 has created a low attack rate in this cohort 5 years later.

7. Backache and body aches (49%) are associated with any high fever.
8. Sore throat (44%).
9. Headache (33%).
10. Nosebleeds (6%), meningism (7%) and conjunctivitis (8%) tend to confuse rather than assist the diagnosis

NOTE. Meningism in influenza is transient and passes off in about 12 hours.

11. Attacks of diarrhoea are not caused by the influenza virus.

INVESTIGATION

Confirmation of the clinical diagnosis can be obtained in two ways: (1) isolation of virus from throat and nasal swabs in the first 3 to 4 days of the disease; (2) complement fixation tests on paired sera — serum is taken in the first 3 days and after the 12th day. Both tests are cumbersome and only give a result after the disease has subsided. Their chief use is at the onset of an epidemic when the G. P. wishes to know what type of virus he is to expect and if influenza is circulating in his community. A number of rapid methods of identifying viruses have now been developed but these are still very costly.

DURATION

The disease persists in an acute febrile form for 2 to 4 days. The fever then settles and the cough becomes productive and less painful. Convalescence is gradual from the 4th to 14th day. In the uncomplicated case recovery is complete after 14 days.

COMPLICATIONS

1. Pneumonitis (aspiration pneumonia)

(Practice experience: in one epidemic 7.8 per cent of patients developed a penumonitis with a positive chest X-ray; in another the rate was only 1.1 per cent.)

2. Lobar pneumonia

Tends to develop in patients who contract flu' and try to carry on. After 2 to 3 days the patient is forced to go to bed and the clinical picture is of a typical lobar pneumonia.

3. Fulminating (cyanotic or heliotrope) pneumonia

The incidence of this grim complication varies considerably in different epidemics. After 2 to 3 days of a comparatively mild illness the patient becomes desperately ill and cyanosed. Death may follow in 1 to 3 days. Empyema and lung abscess may develop. (Fortunately we have encountered very few of these cases.)

4. Mild degrees of depression

Common during convalescence.

MISLEADING FEATURES AND PITFALLS

1. Most of the mistakes made by the family doctor during a flu' epidemic arise directly from lack of time. Influenza presents in many ways and is always a potentially serious disease, but if care is taken mistakes are few.

2. Residual pneumonitis following flu' is easily overlooked. It may arise if the patient gets up before his temperature has returned to normal.

3. Serious disease such as acute infective polyneuritis, Guillain-Barré syndrome, poliomyelitis or encephalitis is overlooked because the patient's self-made diagnosis of flu' is accepted without corroboration.

4. Carelessness sometimes occurs because a doctor visits a house expecting to see one patient and finds that he has to see the whole household. Under these circumstances serious disease is easily overlooked in the extra patients. A mother who minimises her own condition because she wishes to 'carry on' is especially liable to suffer in this way.

5. In any influenza epidemic, instances of pseudoinfluenzal infection are observed. These patients report to the doctor saying that they have flu'. Examination reveals normal temperature and clinical findings. Paired sera fail to show evidence of influenza. These cases may be due to a coincidental cold; some are undoubtedly a result of mass suggestion.

DIFFERENTIAL DIAGNOSIS

Diseases that may be confused with influenza.

Common cold

Similar features: high household attack rate; fever; sore throat; cough.

Distinguishing features: fever rarely high; prostration absent; nasal symptoms predominate; confusion occurs only if patient is not seen until 3rd or 4th day.

Acute febrile tracheitis and bronchitis

Similar features: fever, cough with retrosternal pain.

Distinguishing features: preceding cold is common; fever in adults rarely high; prostration not marked; other members of household not affected.

Adenovirus infection

Similar features: high household attack rate; sudden onset; fever; cough with tracheitis; sore throat; body aches; conjunctivitis.

Distinguishing features: prostration slight; fever may be over 38°C but usually lower than flu'; differentiation serological not clinical; epidemics are rare and more localised.

Acute pharyngitis and exudative tonsillitis

Similar features; fever; sore throat.

Distinguishing features; cough is absent; exudate.

Encephalitis and meningitis

Similar features: fever; meningism.

Distinguishing features: back stiffness and neck stiffness is marked and not transient; the meningism of flu' passes off in a few hours.

MANAGEMENT OPTIONS

Prevention: Selective immunisation of high risk groups. Present vaccines give 90% protection for 1 year.

Established disease: (a) rest; (b) fluids; (c) symptomatic (BNF 4.7 and 3.9); (d) antivirals — BNF 5.3 (Ref. 0.1) — are occasionally needed; (e) antibacterials — BNF 5.1 — if special protection against secondary bacterial complications is needed; (f) follow up (often by phone) to ensure uncomplicated course.

VIRUS PNEUMONIAS

Several viral agents cause pneumonia. This statement depends on the definition of pneumonia, i.e. whether a radiological, clinical or histological definition is used.

[Practice experience suggests that in adults a number of viral agents cause an illness of medium severity that is characterised by: continued fever for 5 to 8 days; respiratory symptoms of cough; normal or slightly lowered white cell count; occasional chest X-ray changes suggesting consolidation (only a few of our cases showed this feature); almost complete absence of clinical signs in the chest (see also p. 411).

Mycoplasma pneumonia. Thirteen proven (endemic) cases.

Psittacosis. Six proven cases (three endemic and three in a single street that were reported in a period of 5 weeks). No ornithological or other vector was identified in any case.

Q Fever (*rickettsia burnetii or coxiella burnetii*). Six proven endemic cases.

In children respiratory syncytial, parainfluenza, adenovirus and influenza (A and B) viruses can all cause croup, tracheobronchitis bronchiolitis with evidence of pneumonia.]

AGE

All our proven cases were adults — perhaps a result of selection (blood tests on children are unpopular).

CLINICAL FEATURES

1. Prolonged fever was the most constant and striking feature. The general practitioner does not expect a fever to last longer than 4 or at most 5 days; when this occurs he should suspect virus pneumonia, infectious mononucleosis or serious disease such as brucella, typhoid, septicaemia, etc.
2. Cough was usually but not always present.
3. Few physical signs in chest.

4. Leucopenia.
5. Radiological evidence of consolidation.

EPIDEMIOLOGY
All our cases were endemic and no obvious vectors were discovered.

COMPLICATIONS
Rare.

MANAGEMENT OPTIONS
Prevention: Search for possible vectors (pets, birds, etc.) and contacts. Often negative.

Established Disease: (a) rest and home care; (b) follow until chest X-ray clear; (c) tetracyclines (BNF 5.1.3 Ref. 0.1) occasionally indicated in adults.

SEXUALLY TRANSMITTED (VENEREAL) DISEASES (STD)

Several widely different diseases come under this heading; each disease is therefore described separately. The primary care physician should remember the following general points:

1. Reported new cases have doubled in the last 10 years.
2. In Britain 500,000 new cases are treated at clinics each year; this suggests a mean rate of 10 fresh cases per 1000 patients per year.
3. Nothing like these rates are reported to family doctors.
4. Many sexual partners are infected without realising it.
5. Often more than one STD are present in the one individual.
6. Effective treatment is available for all these diseases (except Genital Herpes).
7. Many STDs are symptomless, or nearly so, at certain stages.
8. All these infections are spread mainly by casual sex and are avoidable.
9. Auto Immune Deficiency Syndrome (AIDS) — a rare but fatal disease — mainly affecting homosexuals, may become more prevalent.

Every family doctor should constantly search his practice for:
for:

- evidence of active Sexually Transmitted Diseases,
- symptomless cases and contacts,
- the possibility of more than one STD in a single patient.

To achieve this the doctor must develop a high index of suspicion and sensitivity to pointers in the following high risk groups:

- — Men and women aged 16 to 25 years.
- — The 'unattached' of both sexes.
- — Those on holiday or just returned from holiday.
- — Individuals (and their partners) whose job involves travel of any kind.
- — Individuals (and their partners) who have been treated previously for any STD.
- — Possible homosexuals.
- — Individuals with symptoms of cystitis, scabies, unexplained rashes, NSU (p. 194) and other complaints in which the possibility of sexual transmission may be overlooked.

The following Sexually Transmitted Diseases are described: (see below).

- — gonorrhoea (see below)
- — syphilis (p. 193)
- — genital Herpes (p. 163).
- — chlamydia (TRIC agent) infections. Non Specific Urethritis (NSU) (p. 194), Reiter's Syndrome (p. 194).
- — pubic lice (Crabs) (p. 200)
- — scabies (p. 201)

ACUTE GONORRHOEA

Classification: ICHPPC 098 (RCGP 0200)

AETIOLOGY

Neisseria gonorrhoea — a Gram negative intracellular diplococcus.

MODE OF SPREAD

By venereal contact. Direct infection occurs by urethra and endocervix. Occasionally direct infection occurs by anus, by conjuntiva (newborn) and pharynx. Homosexual groups are easily affected.

Since the advent of oral contraceptives, intrauterine devices and changing social mores, the incidence has greatly increased in the young adult population.

DIAGNOSTIC RANGE (rates per 1000 patients per year)

Personal: Suspected 8.0+, Probable 0.9, *National* 0.4 (Ref. 0.2). See Sexually Transmitted Diseases page 190. The true incidence is much higher because many patients report directly to hospital for treatment.

AGE INCIDENCE

Adults under 30, of which 25% are teenagers.

INCUBATION PERIOD

2 to 6 days, occasionally longer.

CLINICAL POINTERS

1. High risk factors: (a) contacts; (b) young adults, especially the unattached; (c) males on the move or with jobs that involve travel; (d) homosexual groups.

2. Half of all cases, male as well as female, are said to be symptomless and are potential carriers. Case finding by the general practitioner with a high index of suspicion is therefore essential.

3. Pointers in the male include:

— life style (see p. 191).
— urethral discharge;
— dysuria (often severe);
— frequent micturition;
— anal burning and discharge; anal infections are often asymptomatic;
— pharyngeal infections said to produce a follicular tonsillitis or asymptomatic infection.

4. Pointers in the female include:

— life style (see p. 191).
— increased vaginal discharge;
— dysuria;
— frequency;
— anorectal discharge.

5. Background knowledge, scabies, warts or pediculosis may all suggest possible venereal contact.

INVESTIGATIONS

1. Culture of all possible cases using special appropriate media. Culture after prostatic massage is sometimes used.
2. Serological tests are not very helpful.
3. Tests for concurrent syphilis infection.

COMPLICATIONS

Salpingitis, endometritis, bartholinitis, epididymitis, infertility and arthritis.

MISTAKES AND PITFALLS

1. Cystitis is common in women and the possibility of urethritis or veneral disease is not explored.

2. Urinary symptoms are treated without investigation and a carrier state induced.

MANAGEMENT OPTIONS

Prevention: (a) search for contacts (refer patients to special Clinic if necessary); (b) active case finding vital (see STD p. 190); (c) health education (Ref. 8.1) and avoid casual sex; (d) protective sheath (e) adequate follow up of treated cases.

Established cases: (a) referral; (b) appropriate antibacterials — BNF 5.1 (Ref. 0.1); (c) follow up.

SYPHILIS (EARLY PHASE)

Classification: ICHPPC 090 (RCGP 0195)

The early phase covers the first two years and includes the primary, secondary and early latent stage. This phase is significant because:

1. The patient should be regarded as potentially infectious.
2. Appropriate treatment prevents the late phase developing.
3. The high risk factors listed for STDs (p. 191) lead to the discovery of cases during this phase.

DIAGNOSTIC INCIDENCE

No cases encountered. Probably higher than this in many areas.

CLINICAL POINTERS

1. High risk factors as for other STDs

2. Any unexplained sore affecting genitalia, lips, breasts, hands or anal region.

3. Any unexplained rash especially associated with sore throat and fever in a teenager or young adult.

INVESTIGATIONS

1. Dark ground studies.
2. VDRL and other serology not always specific.

COMPLICATIONS

Late phase tertiary complications (see p. 203) should not arise with effective treatment.

MANAGEMENT OPTIONS

Prevention: (a) avoid casual sex; (b) health education (Ref. 8.1); (c) protective sheath; (d) active case finding (see p. 190).

Suspected and Established disease: Referral or close co-operation with specialist. Follow up, support and education are all crucial.

NON-SPECIFIC URETHRITIS (NSU)

Classification ICHPPC 0994 (RCGP 0205)

AETIOLOGY
This condition is venereal in most instances.
Viruses, Chlamydia (TRIC agent), mycoplasma, trichomonas, thrush and mixed bacteria have all been incriminated.

DIAGNOSTIC RANGE (rates per 1000 patients per year)
Personal: Suspected 1.0; Probable 0.5. As with other venereal diseases the incidence has increased in the past few years.

AGE INCIDENCE
15 to 30 years.

SEX INCIDENCE
Males are affected more than females (3:1)

CLINICAL POINTERS
1. High risk factors: (a) sexual contacts and partners; (b) young males especially those on the move or with travelling jobs.
2. Dysuria.
3. Frequency may occur.
4. Urethral discharge may be obvious or very slight. The discharge is purulent or clear and subsides fairly quickly.

INVESTIGATIONS
1. A urethral or prostatic smear excludes bacterial and gonococcal origins.
2. A check VDRL test after 2 months — not always specific.
3. Referral to a special (V.D.) clinic.

DURATION
The discharge subsides fairly quickly without treatment.

COMPLICATION
Conjunctivitis, fever and multiple arthritis (Reiter's Syndrome — 2 cases in 10 years) may be associated.

MISLEADING FEATURES AND PITFALLS
1. The discharge subsides quickly and it is easy to overlook the presence of other concurrent venereal disease.

2. Patients may fear 'V.D.' and create a traumatic discharge by continued milking of the penis in search of the feared discharge.

MANAGEMENT OPTIONS

Prevention as for gonorrhoea page 191.

Established disease: (a) Tetracyclines — BNF 5.1.3 (Ref. 0.1) or erythromycin — BNF 5.1.5 (during pregnancy), otherwise as for gonorrhoea.

Reiter's Syndrome: Anti-inflammatory non-steroidal drugs — BNF 10.1.1.2.

MONILIASIS (*CANDIDIASIS*)

Classification: ICHPPC 112 (RCGP 0225)

AETIOLOGY

Monilia — a fungus that infects mucous membranes. Common sites are: (1) the mouths of babies (especially bottlefed); (2) the vagina; (3) groins and genitalia; (4) axillae and under breasts; (5) napkin area in babies.

MODE OF SPREAD

Direct contact. Babies of mothers who had vaginal thrush during pregnancy are prone — possibly the vagina acts as a reservoir of infection. A similar reservoir that causes reinfection and spread to sexual partner is under the foreskin.

ORAL THRUSH

DIAGNOSTIC RANGE (rates per 1000 patients per year)

Personal: Probable 2.0+. Diagnosis rarely in doubt.

AGE INCIDENCE

Mainly the first year of life, usually in first 6 weeks.

CLINICAL POINTERS

1. High risk factors: (a) vaginal thrush in mother; (b) poor hygiene and bottle feeding; (c) previous attacks; (d) a course of antibiotics.

2. The characteristic white flecks on the inside of cheek or roof of mouth.

3. Refusal of feeds.

4. Restlessness and irritability.

INVESTIGATIONS
A therapeutic test with an application of gentian violet.

DURATION
Indefinite unless treated. Recurrences are common.

MANAGEMENT OPTIONS
Prevention: (a) Treat mother; (b) sterilise teats and bottles; (c) general hygiene.
Established disease: Apply Gentian Violet (1% aqueous solution) or other suitable anti fungals — BNF 12.3.2 (Ref. 0.1).

VAGINAL THRUSH

DIAGNOSTIC RANGE (rates per 1000 patients per year)
Personal: Probable 2.2+. Diagnosis rarely in doubt.

CLINICAL POINTERS
1. High risk factors: (a) women on the contraceptive 'pill'; (b) contacts; (c) pregnancy; (d) previous infections; (e) wearing tights (possibly); (f) a course of antibiotics; (h) immuno suppression.
2. Characteristic lesion may be profuse or sparse.
3. Irritation and soreness.
4. Vaginal discharge (white or brown).
5. Pregnancy is often associated.

INVESTIGATIONS
Vaginal swab or therapeutic test with antifungals.

DURATION
Indefinite unless treated. Recurrences are common and may follow use of constricting underwear or failure to treat male partner.

MANAGEMENT OPTIONS
Prevention: (a) treat both sexual partners; (b) avoid constricting tights etc.; (c) general hygiene.
Established disease: Antifungal pessaries — BNF 7.2.2 (Ref. 0.1).

MONILIA OF SKIN

Any enclosed sweaty area in adults is liable to develop a monilial skin rash.

Typical sites are: genitalia, groins, axillae or navel and under pendulant skin folds or breasts in obese individuals.

CLINICAL POINTERS

1. High risk factors: (a) obesity; (b) thrush elsewhere; (c) previous infections.

2. A red patch of skin looking like a ringworm with a clearly defined edge. The rash is distinguished from ringworm by: (a) small satellite lesions just beyond the edge; (b) the centre of the patch is not clear; (c) the rash is confined to the areas of skin contact.

3. Irritation: slight or absent.

4. Rash clears rapidly with antifungals — BNF 13.10.2 (Ref. 0.1).

DURATION

Persists indefinitely if not treated.

MANAGEMENT OPTIONS

Prevention: rarely practical.

Established rash: (a) frequent washing followed by a drying lotion; (b) topical antifungals — BNF 13.10.2 — these clear the rash in 2–3 days, but may have to be repeated every 2 to 3 months.

MONILIA OF NAPKIN AREA

(see p. 606, Napkin rash)

THREADWORMS (PINWORMS)

Classification: ICHPPC 127.4 (RCGP 0260)

AETIOLOGY

Enterobius vermicularis is a white thread-like worm 3 to 10 mm long. The worms develop in the small gut from swallowed ova and then inhabit the large bowel. The female migrates outside the anus to lay her eggs.

MODE OF SPREAD

The movements of the female worm in the perianal region cause irritation and the subsequent scratching distributes the eggs and reinfects the patient via the fingernails and mouth. Spread occurs in families and schools.

DIAGNOSTIC RANGE (rates per 1000 patients per year)

Personal: Probable 3.0+. *National*: 1.4 (Ref. 0.2). Diagnosis was rarely in doubt, but incidence may vary from year to year.

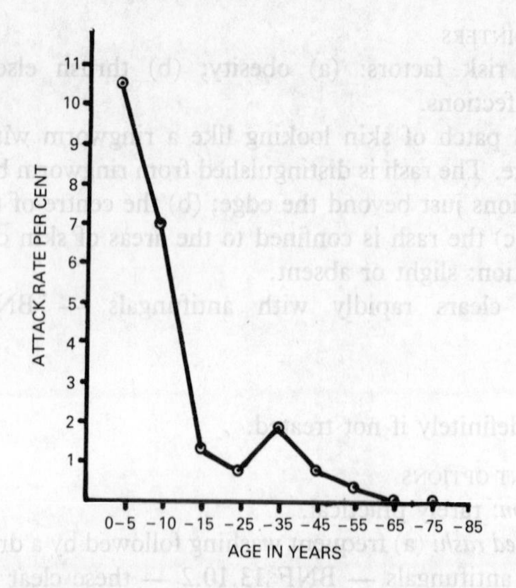

Fig. 16 Threadworms. Age incidence of 58 consecutive cases. Note the small peak at 25 to 35 years due to parental carriers.

AGE INCIDENCE

Toddlers are liable. Peaks occur at 5, 11 and 30 years (Fig. 16).

(Practice experience: analysis of family records revealed that the peak at 30 is entirely in parents of affected children; recurrent infections are common in the children from these families but were rare in other families; this suggests that the main reservoir of infection may be a few persistently infected adults.)

SEX INCIDENCE

Girls are affected more than boys (2:1). In women the worms are especially noticed during menstruation.

CLINICAL POINTERS

1. High risk factors: (a) family and school contacts; (b) families of infected adults; (c) poor toilet hygiene.

2. Irritation of the perianal region — worse at night. Nocturnal irritation causes (a) loss of sleep with irritability by day; (b) grinding of teeth during sleep; (c) puffiness or rings under the eyes.

3. Poor appetite.

4. Picking of nose.

5. Uncommon or misleading symptoms: (a) eating earth or similar perversions in toddlers; (b) anaemia, abdominal pain, enuresis and frequency of micturition.

INVESTIGATIONS

1. Inspection of a motion after an aperient usually confirms the diagnosis. Occasionally worms can be surprised outside the anus by separating the buttocks.
2. Examination of perianal area with selotape swab for ova.

DURATION

Indefinite unless treated.

MISLEADING FEATURES AND PITFALLS

Threadworms are occasionally found in the appendix and are said to cause appendicular pain.

MANAGEMENT OPTIONS

Prevention: (a) follow up to ensure cure of active cases; (b) adequate search for contacts; (c) general hygiene.

Established cases: (a) Antihelminthics — BNF 5.5.1 (Ref. 0.1); (b) treatment of suspected household contacts simultaneously; (c) follow up to establish cure.

PEDICULOSIS CAPITIS

Classification: ICHPPC 132 (RCGP 0270)

AETIOLOGY

Pediculus humanus capitis (head louse). The lice live in the scalp and attach their eggs (nits) to the base of the hairs. The nits hatch in about 12 days and are difficult to see until the growing hair has carried them away from the scalp.

MODE OF SPREAD

Direct contact.

DIAGNOSTIC RANGE (rates per 1000 patients per year)

Personal: Probable 1.0+, *National* 0.6 (Ref. 0.2) Cases are not discovered because they are not looked for. Many others are treated at home or by the school nurse.

AGE INCIDENCE

School age. Parents and siblings of school children are sometimes infected.

CLINICAL POINTERS

1. High risk groups: (a) school, family and occasionally sexual contacts; (b) overcrowded or disadvantaged homes and schools.

2. *Nits* are firmly attached to the hair and resemble small scales of scurf about 0.5 mm in diameter.
3. Irritation of the scalp.
4. Unexplained lymphadenitis of occipital or auricular nodes.
5. Impetigo of scalp.

MANAGEMENT OPTIONS

Prevention: (a) regular school and family inspection of scalp; (b) adequate follow up of active cases; (c) adequate search for contacts; (d) co-operation with school nurse and parents.

Established disease: (a) Parasiticidal applications BNF 13.10.4 (Ref. 0.1); (b) simultaneous treatment of all contacts; (c) follow up to establish cure.

PEDICULOSIS CORPORIS

Classification: ICHPPC 132 (RCGP 0270)

The lice, probably a variant of *Pediculus humanus capitis*, live on the body and clothes. (No cases in 10 years.)

PEDICULOSIS PUBIS

Classification: ICHPPC 132 (RCGP 0270)

The lice live on the pubic and other short hairs of the body, i.e. anal, axillary, chest or even eyebrows.

AETIOLOGY

Pediculus pubis (crab louse).

MODE OF SPREAD

Direct contact, usually sexually transmitted.

DIAGNOSTIC RANGE (rates per 1000 patients per year)

Personal: Probable 0.3+. Cases easily missed if not looked for.

AGE INCIDENCE

Adults.

CLINICAL POINTERS

1. High risk factors: as for Sexually Transmitted Diseases — Page 190.
2. *The lice* resemble minute dark-brown scabs, (1.0 mm across), and can be seen spreadeagled between two hairs.

3. Irritation.
4. Nits.

MANAGEMENT OPTIONS

Prevention: as for STDs — page 190.

Established disease: Parasiticidal applications — BNF 13.10.4 (Ref. 0.1).

SCABIES

Classification: ICHPPC 133 (RCGP 0275)

AETIOLOGY

Acarus scabiei.

MODE OF SPREAD

By prolonged direct skin contact or intermediate contact with infected bedding, etc. Many of the cases in young adults are sexually transmitted.

DIAGNOSTIC RANGE (rates per 1000 patients per year)

Personal: Probable 18.5+. *National*: 3.8 (Ref. 0.2). Confirmation by finding the acarus is time consuming and rarely necessary. In the last 10 years teenagers and young adults have reported many more infections.

AGE INCIDENCE

All ages.

CLINICAL POINTERS

1. High risk factors in children: (a) family and school contacts, (b) overcrowded and disadvantaged families, (c) inadequately treated households.

High risk factors in teenagers and young adults are STD — page 190.

2. Typical lesions: a burrow can sometimes be seen as a dirt-ingrained line running for a few millimetres through the superficial skin; it ends in a small vesicle. Often the vesicles are destroyed by scratching, leaving only the raw base. Burrows on loose skin cause induration.

3. Site of lesions is the best guide to diagnosis — interdigital clefts, genitals, umbilicus, breasts and buttocks. Facial lesions are rare.

4. Nocturnal irritation is intense.

5. Secondary infection.

INVESTIGATIONS

1. A therapeutic test.
2. The parasite can be 'winkled' out of its burrow with a needle.

DIFFERENTIAL DIAGNOSIS

Diseases that may be confused with scabies:

Papular Urticaria

Similar features: diffuse rash with nocturnal irritation and evidence of scratched vesicles.

Distinguishing features: early lesions occur in crops with well-marked urticarial weal; burrows absent; differentiation difficult.

Dermatitis Herpetiformis

Similar features: diffuse cropping rash; intense irritation; evidence of scratched vesicles; young adults affected.

Distinguishing features: lesions are general; genitals, umbilicus and interdigital clefts not especially affected; absence of burrows. Vesicles often large.

MISTAKES AND PITFALLS

1. The infection is kept at a minimal level by excessive washing.
2. The possibility of associated venereal disease is not considered.
3. The doctor fails to raise the question of infection and treatment of other household contacts.
4. The initial lesions of an atopic eczema in an infant mimic scabies.

MANAGEMENT OPTIONS

Prevention in children: (a) adequate search for contacts; (b) adequate follow up of active cases to ensure cure; (c) adequate treatment of whole household and bedding.

Prevention in teenagers and adults: (a) adequate search for household and possible sexual contacts; (b) test for possible concurrent STDs (see p. 190); (c) adequate treatment of whole household.

Established Disease in adults and children: (a) treat all household members simultaneously; (b) parasiticidal drugs — BNF 13.10.4 (Ref. 0.1); (c) clothes and bedclothes must be throughly washed at the same time. Materials need not be baked or boiled; (d) home nurse very helpful; (e) adequate follow up.

Table 8 Less common infective and parasitic diseases

Disease and distinguishing clinical pointers	Incidence per 1000 patients per year Suspected	Confirmed
Tuberculous meningitis Patients usually under 20; contacts; persistent headache, vomiting and fever; constipation; anorexia; neck stiffness; enlarged spleen. Tuberculin test.	1.0	1 in 10 years
Primary tuberculosis of bones and joints Patients aged 0 to 15; localised pain, e.g. limp or deformity; limitation of movement; low fever. Tuberculin test; ESR, X-ray changes.	0.1	2 in 10 years
Secondary tuberculosis of bones and joints Adults affected, tuberculosis elsewhere in body, localised pain, deformity and swelling, limited movement.	—	3 in 10 years
Lupus vulgaris Chronic scarring lesion with peripheral translucent greenish brown nodules on compression with a glass slide, face usually affected.	—	2 in 10 years
Tuberculosis of kidney and bladder Adults affected, tuberculosis elsewhere in body, chronic cystitis with haematuria. Sterile pyuria. ESR, X-ray changes.	—	2 in 10 years
Tuberculous endometritis and salpingitis Infertility, local lesion. Chest X-ray.	—	1 in 10 years
Miliary tuberculosis Similar to tuberculous meningitis.	—	1 in 10 years
Chancroid Rare STD. Indurated ulcer on genitalia. Early referral (See STD — p. 190)	—	0 in 10 years
Latent syphilis	0.1	0.1
Syphilitic aortitis Previous history, aortic incompetence and evidence of space-occupying mediastinal lesion — hoarseness. Serology and chest X-rays.	—	4 in 10 years
General paralysis of insane Progressive depression, delusions and mental deterioration. Serology, lumbar puncture.	0	0 in 10 years
Epidemics of vertigo, hiccup, stiff neck and laryngeal palsy Such epidemics are said to occur. Isolated cases may have occured but no epidemics were encountered in 10 years of practice.		
Hand, foot and mouth disease (see p. 179)	—	0 in 10 years
Malaria Patients from overseas, recurring febrile attacks with rigors. Blood smear at height of fever.	—	2 in 10 years
Leishmaniasis Patients from tropics, prolonged fever with splenomegaly. Blood smear.	0	0 in 10 years

Table 8 Cont'd

Disease and distinguishing clinical pointers	Incidence per 1000 patients per year Suspected	Confirmed
Schistosomiasis Patients from North Africa and Far East, chronic bowel or bladder symptoms.	—	1 in 10 years
Amoebic dysentery Chronic diarrhoea with abdominal pain, enlarged liver and raised dome of diaphragm. Examination of freshly passed stool for amoebae or cysts.	—	1 in 10 years
Toxoplasmosis Congenital infection — early fever, rash, jaundice, convulsions. Acquired infections in adults may resemble infectious mononucleosis or a virus pneumonia. Paired sera.	—	3 in 10 years
Tapeworms Passage of cylindrical white segments (1 to 2 cm long). Stool examination.	0.2	0.2
Roundworms Toddlers liable, passage of pale pink worm 10 to 30 cm long, few other symptoms. Stool examination for ova.	0.8	0.8
Sarcoidosis Doubtful aetiology; skin, lung and lymphoid lesions. Tuberculin negative. Often picked up on routine chest X-ray enlarged mediastinal nodes. Increasing incidence.	—	1 in 10 years
Roseola infantum Epidemics said to affect infants in first 2 years of life; rose-coloured macular rash with fever, tonsilitis and cervical lymphadenopathy.	0	0 in 10 years
Tabes dorsalis Neuralgic limb pains; loss of deep pain, proprioception and tendon reflexes; Argyll-Robertson pupils; legs affected most. Serological tests; lumbar puncture.	—	2 in 10 years
Gumma Localised, painless swelling at any site	0	0 in 10 years
Typhoid and paratyphoid fever Travel or contact 7 to 21 days previously; evidence of gradually progressing septicaemia, enlarged spleen, sparse or rubella-like rash. Leukopenia; blood culture and serology.	—	2 in 10 years
Brucellosis Possible source of infection, intermittent fever, malaise and body aches, enlarged spleen. Leukopenia, serology positive after a few weeks, blood culture (often negative).	0.3	0.1
Erysipelas Well-defined salmon-pink patch with raised edge that spreads slowly outwards, oedema in region of rash, face usually affected, fever and malaise, responds quickly to penicillin	0.3	—

Table 8 Cont'd

Disease and distinguishing clinical pointers	Incidence per 1000 patients per year Suspected	Confirmed
Diphtheria Possible contact 2 to 4 days previously, patient not immunised, membranous grey adherent exudate, cervical adenitis, toxaemia. Throat swab. (NOTE. Chronic nasal diphtheria may be present with local nasal symptoms only.)	0.3	0 in 10 years
Benign lymphocytic meningitis Contact cases, severe headache precedes other symptoms by 2 to 3 days, fever (often slight), back stiffness and meningism, vomiting; morbilliform rash occasionally, resembles viral encephalitis or early infective polyneuritis.	—	1 outbreak of 5 cases in 10 years
Adenovirus infection High household attack rate without epidemic elsewhere, painful cough, conjunctivitis (often absent), fever. Paired sera. see page 178.	—	2 outbreaks in 4 years
Epidemic winter vomiting High household attack rate without epidemic elsewhere, vomiting, 2 to 3 day interval between primary and secondary cases.	—	4 possible outbreaks in 4 years

9

Neoplasms

All neoplasms are arranged according to the system affected (see Index).

GENERAL COMMENTS ON THE EARLY DIAGNOSIS AND MANAGEMENT OF CANCER

Early diagnosis and clinical problems

As with other serious disease the family doctor must learn to develop a high index of suspicion for cancer. This involves a sensitivity to those factors which identify the high risk groups (given throughout Part II)

A check list of the most significant of such factors is:

1. General frequency and incidence rates of common cancers — (see Appendix VII, pp. 710–726)
2. Effects of age on the incidence rates of common cancers.
3. Effects of sex and parity on frequency (e.g. Uterine cancers).
4. Effects of race and climate (e.g. Sunlight, pigmentation for skin cancers).
5. Effects of occupation (e.g. Mining, chemicals, woodwork, etc.)
6. Factors in heredity and previous history (e.g. polyposis and cancer of colon).
7. Smoking and diet.

A similar check list of clinical factors which identify high risk groups is given below: (Note: Most patients are also aware of this list)

1. Coughing blood and persistent cough.
2. Blood in urine and stools.
3. Persistent changes in bowel habit — constipation, diarrhoea or mucus.

4. Unexplained bleeding, from vagina or during intercourse.
5. Unexplained lumps.
6. Ulcers and sores which fail to heal.
7. Any symptoms whose persistence and steady progression cannot be satisfactorily explained, e.g. of the headache of cerebral tumour.

These two lists may seem obvious but analysis shows that most failures to achieve early diagnosis of cancer, which occur with unfortunate regularity in even the best of practices, arise as a result of ignoring at least one of these factors.

The family doctor in training should make a habit of applying such clinical information by introducing it into his everyday diagnostic decision making.

It is occasionally argued that for some cancers early diagnosis makes little difference to survival time and may cause many months (or years) of worry instead of blissful ignorance. Several points against this argument should be emphasized:

1. The primary physician rarely knows the nature and survival rates of any cancer in its early stages.
2. The patient has usually considered the possibility of cancer before the doctor.
3. If a certain diagnosis of cancer is eventually made, patient or relatives (or both) may well feel that there has been needless delay.

EMOTIONAL PROBLEMS AND PITFALLS

Several points must be stressed:

1. 'Cancer' is correlated in most patients' minds with 'death'.
2. All of us accept our own death as being inevitable but as individuals we subconsciously insert a comforting interval of time between the present and the likely moment of our death.
3. A healthy 20-year-old will *accept* death in 30–50 years, a healthy 60-year-old will *accept* it in 14 years while a healthy 74-year-old may *accept* it in only 2 to 3 years. Any shortening of these subconscious, protective intervals is likely to be psychologically an extremely traumatic process. This may produce many different and unexpected reactions in:

— the patient
— the patient's loved ones, close relatives and friends
— the medical staff responsible.

For all of us unpleasant truths about ourselves are easiest to handle when we come to see them ourselves — not when they are pointed out by someone else.

4. Given time and the affection, love and *hope* of our friends, most individuals can come to terms with an unexpected shortening of their life span.

5. In most modern cultures any patient over 35 who is medically investigated is likely to have wondered — to a greater or lesser extent — if cancer (or a similar fatal disease) could be the cause.

6. The patient's questions are the doctor's best guide to the extent to which the patient has faced the reality of *early* death. If the patient has the courage to ask questions in which the words 'death', 'cancer', 'recurrence' are used — then the doctor can probably reply in the same courageous 'channel'. More commonly the patient's questions are diffidently concealed under a 'cover story'. The doctor is then left with the difficult and challenging task of bringing the patient to face the hidden reality of an early death.

PREVENTION OF CANCER

See chapter III and throughout Part II.

GENERAL MANAGEMENT OF EMOTIONAL PROBLEMS

A. THE PATIENT

The following points may be helpful:

- The individual solution for each patient, each doctor and each situation is different. There are no 'musts' and no 'nevers'. *How* things are done is often more important than *what* is done or said.
- Try to avoid deceiving patients (or relatives by implication). Remember that the family doctor is often sincerely able to be more hopeful than the specialist.
- The best time for the *doctor* to raise the possibility of cancer is often before a certain diagnosis is made i.e. *before* not *after* referral.
- A certain diagnosis of cancer may lead relatives, friends and doctors into an emotional no-man's-land of unspoken, subconscious isolation of the patient. This should be avoided.
- Friendship and affection leading to discussion, understanding and gradual realization are the best way of protecting the patient against the cruelty of isolation. Self-help groups and talking to other

patients may be a great help; appropriate addresses are given throughout Part II.

B. THE PATIENT'S CLOSE RELATIVES AND FRIENDS

- Try to involve close relatives as well as the patient in all decision making. Patient confidentiality is sometimes a problem here.
- Relatives often try to protect loved ones from realizing the truth. Encouraging shared activities (especially enjoyable ones) helps to discourage such isolating protection.
- Encourage relatives to share their fears with you — the doctor.

C. THE DOCTOR AND MEDICAL STAFF

- Combining hope with honesty may be difficult but is a constant aim.
- Try to avoid hiding your own 'hang ups' about death under jargon, scientific terms or rationalisations.
- Try to enjoy satisfying the *extra* demands of patients and relatives.
- Use and learn as much as you can from your local hospice.

10

Allergic, endocrine, metabolic and nutritional diseases

Please read the introduction for explanation of figures and analyses.

HYPERTHYROIDISM OR THYROTOXICOSIS

Classification: ICHPPC 242 (RCGP 0705)

Two types are encountered: *diffuse goitre* (or Graves' disease) patients are younger with marked eye and neurological signs; *nodular goitre* — affects older people, goitre often not obvious, eye signs may be absent and cardiac symptoms and signs predominate — very easily overlooked.

AETIOLOGY

Overproduction of thyroid hormones T_3 or T_3 and T_4. There is a negative feed back relationship with the Thyroid Stimulating Hormone (TSH). Thus TSH levels are usually reduced. An autoimmune origin is now thought likely. The causes of the exophthalmos are uncertain. Emotional shocks may influence onset.

DIAGNOSTIC RANGE (rates per 1000 patients per year)

Personal: Suspected 1.2. Probable 0.4. *National* 1.4 (Ref. 0.2).

SEX INCIDENCE

Women affected more than men [*Personal* 5: 1. *National* 8: 1]

AGE INCIDENCE

Adults.

CLINICAL POINTERS

1. Increasing nervousness.
2. Loss of weight, often marked.
3. Exophthalmos not related to severity and often absent in the elderly.
4. Thyroid enlargement may be diffuse or nodular and may be absent in the elderly.

5. Dislike of hot weather. Direct questions are usually needed to elicit this useful differentiating feature.

6. Irregularity of the menses.

7. Clinical features that can be confused with acute tension states: (a) palpitation; (b) sweating; (c) diarrhoea; (d) rapid collapsing pulse; a raised sleeping pulse is characteristic of hyperthyroidism; (e) a fine tremor of the extended hands. Sympathetic overactivity may be responsible for these five features.

8. Heart failure or auricular fibrillation in the elderly.

INVESTIGATIONS

1. Levels of thyroid hormone binding proteins (TBG) and thyroid hormones (T_3) are useful.

2. TSH levels after pituitary stimulation and radio assay, after referral.

3. Tests form a baseline for assessment of treatment.

DURATION

Mild cases occasionally recover after a few months without treatment. The results of treatment are good, but a few symptoms may persist.

COMPLICATIONS

Heart failure, auricular fibrillation and mental disturbances. (Hypothyroidism is not uncommon after treatment).

MISLEADING FEATURES AND PITFALLS

1. Thyrotoxicosis and acute tension states are confused.

2. Failure to recognise hyperthyroidism in the elderly. The two most obvious clinical signs (exophthalmos and thyroid enlargement) are sometimes absent in the older age-groups. Weight loss is accepted by the patient as a part of old age.

3. Diffuse physiological thyroid-enlargement may occur in girls of 15 to 25 years old.

4. In mild cases all laboratory tests may be marginal. The doctor should remember that several marginal test results may indicate a decreased, not increased, probability.

DIFFERENTIAL DIAGNOSIS

Diseases that may be confused with hyperthyroid disease:

Acute tension states

Similar features: nervousness; palpitation; sweating; rapid pulse; tremor of hands.

Distinguishing features: thyroid enlargement and exophthalmos absent; sleeping pulse normal; serum tests normal; hospital investigation may be indicated but should be avoided if possible.

Physiological goitre
Similar features: diffuse swelling of thyroid; young females affected; nervousness.

Distinguishing features: exophthalmos absent; palpitation, sweating, diarrhoea and weight loss absent; no preference for cold.

Exophthalmos associated with obesity
Similar feature: exophthalmos.

Distinguishing features: weight increases; menopausal women.

MANAGEMENT OPTIONS

Prevention: Nil.

Suspected disease: (a) referral for confirmation of diagnosis and choice of treatment; (b) antithyroid drugs — BNF 6.2.2 (Ref. 0.1); (c) radioactive iodine; (d) Surgery including orbital decompression.

MYXOEDEMA AND HYPOTHYROIDISM

Classification: ICHPPC 244 (RCGP 0710)

AETIOLOGY

Usually follows failure of thyroid gland — congenital, idiopathic, senile or following treatment for hyperthyroidism.

Rarer causes of thyroid failure: iodine deficiency, drugs and auto immune disease.

Failure of pituitary and hypothalamus may be responsible.

DIAGNOSTIC RANGE (rates per 1000 patients per year)

Personal: Suspected 4.0, Probable 2.4. *National* 2.1 (Ref. 0.2). Practices tend to collect patients under treatment.

SEX INCIDENCE

Women affected more than men (10+: 1).

AGE INCIDENCE

Over 45.

CLINICAL POINTERS

1. High risk factors (a) previous or treated hyperthyroidism; (b) middle aged women especially if anaemic; (c) menorrhagia.

2. Fatigue, weakness increasing 'slowness', usually ascribed by both doctor and patient to psychogenic causes.

3. Generalised aching and muscular cramps, usually ascribed by

both doctor and patient to psychogenic or osteoarthritic causes.

4. Dislike of cold weather. Direct questions are needed to elicit this useful pointer.

5. Hoarse voice. Perhaps the most useful sign because most sufferers are women and therefore the husky speech may alert the doctor at a time when other insidiously advancing symptoms remain unnoticed. The throat may be constantly cleared.

6. Loss of hair. This complaint should always alert the doctor.

7. Associated conditions that should alert the doctor to the possibility of myxoedema: refractory hypochromic anaemia; menorrhagia; treated thyrotoxicosis (especially operative treatment); carpal tunnel syndrome; ataxia and attacks of dizziness.

Refractory obesity, angina pectoris, constipation and loss of memory are all associated with myxoedema but are so easily explained by other more commonly occurring diseases that their significance is usually only realised after the diagnosis has been made. Acute psychiatric states may confuse.

8. Typical facies: (a) translucent bagginess of skin under (and around) the eyes — one of the signs that may alert the doctor early; (b) pallor and creamy skin with malar flush — a comparatively late sign; (c) loss of outer third of eyebrows — usually only noticed after the diagnosis has been made.

9. Other signs include slow pulse, low blood pressure, dry skin and characteristically sluggish reflexes.

INVESTIGATIONS

1. Radioactive iodine uptake and total serum T_4 (Serum T_3 levels unhelpful).

2. Thyroid stimulating hormone (TSH) levels are always raised if there is primary thyroid gland failure.

3. Hormone stimulation tests will distinguish central causes.

DURATION

Untreated cases may eventually prove fatal after a period of years.

MISLEADING FEATURES AND PITFALLS

1. Every experienced practitioner knows the dismay of discovering that for weeks, months or even years a 'classic case' or myxoedema has been developing under his 'unseeing eyes'. The only 'solution' is for the doctor to develop an unusually high index of suspicion for this serious but treatable disease.

2. Therapeutic tests with thyroid should be avoided — they may initiate needless but lifelong therapy if the patient shows a falsely-positive subjective response.

3. Apathy leads to uncomplaining acceptance of complaints.
4. Antidepressants may depress thyroid activity and cause harm and confusion.
5. Elderly patients, especially those living alone, are easily overlooked. A wrong diagnosis of senility anaemia, hypothermia or depression is easily made and delays correct diagnosis.

MANAGEMENT OPTIONS

Prevention: (a) continued follow up of treated hyperthyroid disease; (b) routine T_3 and T_4 estimates in middle aged and elderly women having blood tests for other reasons.

Established disease: (a) adequate Thyroxine BNF 6.2.1 (Ref. 0.1); (b) regular follow up.

DIABETES MELLITUS

Classification: ICHPPC 250 (RCGP 0720)

Defects of carbohydrate and fat metabolism lead to hyperglycaemia and glycosuria.

Two aetiologically distinct types of diabetes mellitus are recognised:

Type 1. the severer, juvenile onset or insulin dependent (IDD)
Type 2. the milder, maturity onset or non-insulin dependent (NIDD).

TYPE 2 MATURITY ONSET (NIDD)

AETIOLOGY

There is an insidious and genetically determined failure of the pancreatic islet B cells. The cause of the failure is uncertain but is related to both obesity and older age groups. These patients are insensitive to insulin and do not develop ketosis. Hyperglycaemia disappears as soon as obesity is reduced by diet. Heredity plays a part.

DIAGNOSTIC RANGE (rates per 100 patients per year)

Personal: Suspected 0.8. Probable 0.4. *National*: 2.3 (Ref. 0.2). An unknown number of patients remain under occasional dietary surveillance for this condition.

AGE INCIDENCE

Middle-aged and elderly patients (80% over 50).

SEX INCIDENCE

Women are affected more than men — probably because obesity is commoner in women.

CLINICAL POINTERS

1. High risk factors: (a) heredity; (b) age over 50; (c) obesity; (d) multiparity; (e) peripheral vascular disease.

2. Obesity is usual but may be absent in elderly patients.

3. A family history of diabetes is always suggestive.

4. Excessive thirst and frequency of micturition.

5. Recurrent infections of (a) skin, either staphyloccal or monilial, (b) urinary tract.

6. Perineal pruritus and an associated recurring balanitis are common.

7. Evidence of peripheral vascular disease including:
— gangrene or absent pulses in feet and claudication;
— retinitis and cataract;
— lesions in kidneys and CNS.

8. Nocturnal pains in legs may occur early.

9. Associated diseases which may mask or be masked by the diabetic process include:
— pulmonary tuberculosis;
— chronic alcoholism;
— monilia and intertrigo;
— recurring bacterial infections of skin and genito-urinary tract.

INVESTIGATIONS

As for type 1 see page 216.

DURATION

The disease may continue for many years if not recognised.

COMPLICATIONS

As for insulin-sensitive diabetes. Type 1 (IDD) is said to develop if the Type 2 (NIDD) is allowed to continue.

MISLEADING FEATURES AND PITFALLS

1. Practice experience: in five out of nine consecutive cases the history prior to diagnosis suggested that the disease may have been overlooked for periods of 1 to 5 years.

2. Renal thresholds may be raised in the elderly.

MANAGEMENT OPTIONS

Prevention and early diagnosis: Screening and case finding in high risk groups.

Established disease: (a) low calorie diet; (b) oral hypoglycaemics BNF 6.1.2 after trial of diet (Ref. 0.1) (c) patient education vital (Ref. 10.1); (d) regular follow up.

TYPE 1 JUVENILE ONSET (IDD)

AETIOLOGY

This is not certain. Virus damage and autoimmunity may both precipitate disease in individuals whose pancreatic islet B cells are genetically susceptible.

DIAGNOSTIC RANGE (rates per 1000 patients per year)

Personal: Suspected 0.9. Probable 0.5. Under surveillance 4.0.
National: 2.3 (Ref. 0.2).

AGE INCIDENCE

All ages.

CLINICAL POINTERS

1. High risk factors: (a) heredity; (b) post infection.
2. Onset is more sudden than in the obese type. In children ketosis may develop within 1 to 2 days. More commonly symptoms are present for several weeks before the doctor is consulted. An acute infection may precipitate the disease.
3. Thirst and frequency of micturition.
4. Loss of weight is marked although appetite may be excellent.
5. A family history of diabetes.
6. Pruritus and balanitis.
7. Incidents of skin sepsis.
8. Evidence of peripheral vascular disease in retina, kidneys, CNS and feet.
9. Ketosis and precoma. (a) The three D's — dyspnoea (air hunger) drowsiness and dehydration — in the absence of fever are characteristic of a rapidly developing diabetic ketosis. (b) Acetone in breath and urine. (c) Abdominal pain may confuse the diagnosis.
10. Diabetic coma is rare (no cases in 10 years).

INVESTIGATIONS

1. Glycosuria. Repeated tests 1 to 2 hours after meals.
2. Fasting and post-prandial blood sugar. Values of over 120 mg in a sample taken 2 hours after a normal breakfast indicate the need for a full investigation. Increasingly used to monitor surveillance.
3. Glucose tolerance test may be used by the family doctor.
4. Acetest of urine when ketosis is suspected.

DURATION

Indefinite.

COMPLICATIONS

The complications of diabetes are numerous. With the exception of diabetic coma, they mainly follow degenerative changes in the arterial tree: (a) eye — cataract and retinitis (with microaneurysms, haemorrhages and exudates); (b) kidney — nephropathy; (c) legs — gangrene; (d) neuropathy — neuritis, perforating ulcers of feet, and micro aneurysms of retinal arteries.

There is increasing evidence that maintaining normal blood sugar prevents more complications than maintaining a sugar-free urine.

MISLEADING FEATURES AND PITFALLS

1. Diabetes should be suspected in association with many common ailments (boils, moniliasis, cataract, loss of weight, etc.). It is easy for the busy doctor to omit the simple test for glycosuria.

2. A mild physiological glycosuria is often noted in pregnancy and true diabetes is easily overlooked.

3. In children a severe ketosis can develop very rapidly.

NOTE. Other causes of glycosuria. Non-pathological: (a) inadequate cleansing of the container; (b) lowered renal threshold; (c) pregnancy; (d) excessive ingestion of carbohydrate; (e) emotion, e.g. before a medical examination. Pathological: (a) raised intracranial pressure as in subarachnoid haemorrhage or cerebral tumour (two cases in 10 years of practice); (b) endocrine or chronic liver disorders (no cases in 10 years).

MANAGEMENT OPTIONS

Prevention: (a) Genetic counselling may be considered; (b) active case-finding in high risk groups.

Established disease: (a) diet — a balance between carbohydrate intake and total calories. Specialist advice usually required. (b) Insulin BNF 6.1.1 (Ref. 0.1). The correct balance between short, medium and the less often used long acting insulins usually requires specialist help.

Surveillance: (a) Patient education aimed at increasing patient independence and responsibility — a top priority (Refs. 10.1, 10.2, 10.3 and 10.4). (b) Blood tests *if feasible by patient) — aimed at maintaining normal* preprandial blood glucose levels. Urine tests: only when *blood* glucose levels not available. (c) Two injections of insulin per day may be better than one. (d) Patient awareness of indications for increasing (and decreasing) insulin dosage. (e) Close co-operation with family doctor. (f) Recently cheap electronic instruments for estimating blood sugar have encouraged better patient control.

DIABETIC AND HYPOGLYCAEMIC COMA

It is vital to differentiate between these two types of coma because the administration of insulin or sugar may be life saving.

HYPOGLYCAEMIC COMA

DIAGNOSTIC RANGE (rates per 1000 patients per year)
Personal: 0.3.

CLINICAL POINTERS

1. History. A known diabetic on treatment. No recent food.
2. Unconsiousness with evidence that a patient is a diabetic. A diabetic label or lumps of sugar may be found in the patient's pocket.
3. Sudden onset and absence of premonitory symptoms.
4. Drunken or abnormal behaviour commonly precedes unconsciousness for a few minutes.
5. Sweating is profuse and dehydration (with hypotension) absent.
6. Tremor, slurred speech and inco-ordinated actions.
7. Rapid recovery after the administration of sugar.

COMPLICATIONS

Permanent brain damage and death can occur if the condition is not treated quickly.

MANAGEMENT OPTIONS

Prevention: (a) patient understanding; (b) carrying sugar; (c) relatives and workmates able to give glucagon injection; (d) avoid unpunctual meals and unaccustomed exercise.

Established hypoglycaemia: (a) immediate treatment; (b) glucagon injection intramuscularly or intravenously. BNF 6.1.4 (Ref. 0.1). (c) 50 ml, 50% solution of glucose slowly intravenously.

DIABETIC COMA

Rare.
(No cases encountered in 10 years).

The clinical pointers are those of precoma and ketosis (see page 216).

MANAGEMENT OPTIONS

Immediate hospital referral.

GOUT

Classification: ICHPPC 274 (RCG 0770)

AETIOLOGY

Gout is caused by an excess of uric acid in the blood and tissue fluids. Symptoms of gout follow deposits of crystalline sodium urate in the joints, cartilage, subcutaneous tissues, etc. The body cannot metabolise uric acid which is a breakdown product of nucleoprotein; high serum uric acid levels arise from excessive ingestion of nucleoprotein or excessive breakdown of endogenous nucleoprotein as in leukaemia, polycythaemia or haemolytic anaemia. Renal disease or the use of diuretics may also raise serum uric acid by preventing excretion.

AGE INCIDENCE

Adults.

SEX INCIDENCE

Men most affected (6.1). Women more affected after menopause.

DIAGNOSTIC RANGE (rates per 1000 patients per year)

Personal: Suspected 2.2. Probable 1.1. *National*: 1.8 to 2.6 (Ref. 0.2). The incidence varies considerably in different communities.

CLINICAL POINTERS

1. High risk factors: (a) family history; (b) rich or excessive food; (c) excessive alcohol; (d) excessive fasting; (e) diuretics; (f) Down's syndrome; (g) renal disease.
2. Attacks of acute severe pain often in the early hours. Anyone joint may be affected but the big toe is common (70%). Ankle and knee also common.
3. Red, shiny swelling of overlying skin — looks like a cellulitis.
4. Deposits in subcutaneous tissues (tophi) — a late sign.

INVESTIGATIONS

1. Plasma uric acid is raised above 7.0 mg in men and 5.7 mg

per 100 ml in women (5.0 mg in women before the menopause).

2. Recovery of uric acid crystals from tophi or synovial fluid.

3. Radiology of hand. May show chronic punched out erosions.

DURATION

The tendency to suffer attacks of gout persists indefinitely.

COMPLICATIONS

1. Deformed joints.

2. Chronic renal disease — infections calculi, hypertension, etc., renal damage may then cause further rises in uric acid levels.

3. Diabetes mellitus.

MISLEADING FEATURES AND PITFALLS

1. A large joint is affected and the diagnosis is not considered.

2. A border-line or only slightly raised serum uric acid is given undue diagnostic weight.

DIFFERENTIAL DIAGNOSIS

Differential diagnosis is from cellulitis, inflamed bunion, infective arthritis and monoarticular rheumatoid or psoriatic arthritis. (Pseudo-gout is a similar condition involving calcium pyrophosphate instead of sodium urate crystals.)

MANAGEMENT OPTIONS

No real cure, only prevention of attacks.

Prevention of attacks: (a) modification of high risk and trigger factors — sometimes effective alone; (b) long acting and uricosuric drugs BNF 10.1.4 (Ref. 0.1).

Acute attacks: (a) rest; (b) simple analgesics; (c) anti-inflammatory non-steroidal drugs BNF 10.1.1.2 (Ref. 0.1).

OBESITY

Classification: ICHPPC 278 (RCGP 0785)

Obesity is often regarded as trivial, but is one of the greatest problems of Western civilisation.

AETIOLOGY

Eating more food than the body requires is the primary cause and it has been clearly shown that limiting daily calorie intake to 1000 to 1200 Kcal will lead to loss of weight in every adult. *In practice if weight loss is not achieved it is likely that patients are either consciously or more often subconsciously stretching their calorie intake to include 2000 or more Kcal.* The primary physician in a purely advisary position, has to deal with the many psychological and physical implications of this fact. Many of the solutions to obesity may thus resemble the solutions to excess alcohol intake.

Other aggravating factors are:

1. Patterns of modern life. These include boredom, advertising, lack of exercise and cheap, easily available high calorie foods.
2. Excessive alcohol and beer intake.
3. Heredity. Obesity tends to run in families.
4. Previous obesity. Fat storage cells once acquired may tend to be re-filled. This is one argument for not overfeeding babies.
5. Endocrine factors may explain the greater vulnerability of women especially in the puerperium and after the menopause.

(Obesity in childhood — see Behaviour problems in children).

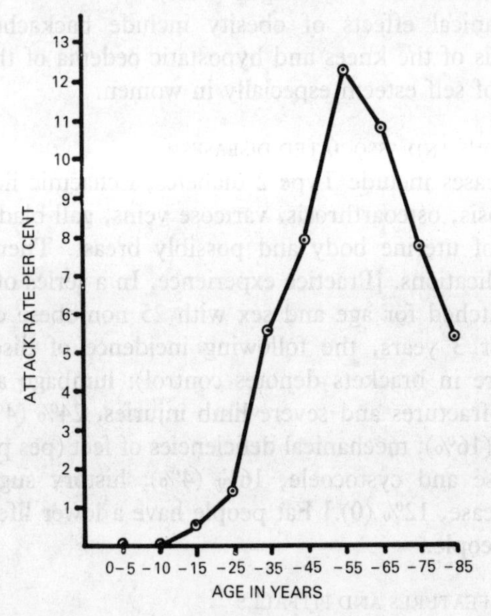

Fig. 17 Obesity. Age incidence curve of 122 consecutive female cases encountered in one year.

DIAGNOSTIC RANGE (rates per 1000 patients per year)

Personal: Suspected 30.7+. Marked 20.0+. *National*: 17.4+ (Ref. 0.2).

AGE INCIDENCE

The incidence steadily increases with age to reach a peak at the time of the menopause (Fig. 17). Old people tend to accept their obesity as part of old age and do not report it to the doctor.

SEX INCIDENCE

Women are affected more than men (6.1).

CLINICAL POINTERS

1. High risk factors: (a) pregnancy and menopause; (b) boredom; (c) cooking; (d) lack of exercise; (e) previous obesity; (f) alcohol; (g) heredity; (h) loss of confidence; (i) giving up smoking; (j) high carbohydrate/low fibre diets.

2. Fatness (100%). The patient often fails to relate her symptoms to the increase in weight.

3. Shortness of breath (40%).

4. Listlessness and easy fatigue (20%).

5. Mechanical effects of obesity include backache, flat feet, osteoarthritis of the knees and hypostatic oedema of the feet.

6. Loss of self esteem especially in women.

COMPLICATIONS AND ASSOCIATED DISEASES

Serious diseases include Type 2 diabetes, ischaemic heart disease, atherosclerosis, osteoarthrosis, varicose veins, gall-bladder disease, carcinoma of uterine body and possibly breast. There are many other complications. [Practice experience. In a series of 25 cases of obesity, matched for age and sex with 25 non-obese controls and followed for 3 years, the following incidence of disorders were noted (figure in brackets denotes control): lumbago and sciatica, 32% (8%); fractures and severe limb injuries, 24% (4%); varicose veins, 24% (16%); mechanical deficiencies of feet (pes planus), 16% (0); prolapse and cystocoele, 16% (4%); history suggesting gall bladder disease, 12% (0).] Fat people have a lower life expectancy than thin people.

MISLEADING FEATURES AND PITFALLS

1. An ovarian cyst is confused with obesity.

2. Obese patients easily acquire dependency on appetite suppressants.

MANAGEMENT OPTIONS

For both prevention and active weight reduction the problems of achieving adequate patient compliance are considerable and often time consuming.

Prevention: involves changing community attitudes. This is a major health education priority involving parents, schools, adults, media and eventually probably government.

Established obesity: (a) achieve patient co-operation by accurate explanation of problems and difficulties; (b) discuss modifications of high risk factors and set goals for limitation of calorie intake per day (Women 1000–1200 Kcals; Men 1000–1500 Kcals); (c) discuss long term methods of motivating patient using groups (Weight Watchers, etc.) and follow up; (d) avoid or limit use of appetite suppressants and short circuit operations; (e) obtain local information from dietician; (f) exercise programmes often acceptable.

MUSCLE CRAMPS AND RESTLESS LEGS

Classification: ICHPPC 7295, 355 (RCGP 1325)

Aetiology

Unknown. Relative deficiency of both Vitamin B complex and Vitamin E has been suggested.

DIAGNOSTIC RANGE (rates per 1000 patients per year)

Personal: Suspected 5.0+. Many cases never reported.

AGE INCIDENCE

Adolescents and adults.
Elderly patients are prone.

SEX INCIDENCE

Women are affected more than men (4 to 1).
Pregnant women are especially liable.

CLINICAL POINTERS

1. High risk factors: (a) pregnancy; (b) unaccustomed exercise; (c) certain chronic diseases i.e. venous insufficiency, demyelinating disease and diabetes; (d) possibly certain drugs, diuretics and the pill.

2. A constant desire to move the legs. Less commonly, actual cramp-like pains are felt.

3. The symptoms usually arise when the legs are rested after a period of activity.

MISLEADING FEATURES AND PITFALLS

1. Diabetes may be associated.
2. Confusion with intermittent claudication arises, if a careful history is not obtained.

MANAGEMENT OPTIONS

Established disease: (a) a variety of drugs are worth trying — vitamin B, Quinine (not in pregnancy), peripheral vasodilators — Parovan Cinnanzine-BNF 2.6.3 (Ref. 0.1) (b) self massage.

Table 9 Less common allergic, endocrine, metabolic and nutritional diseases

Disease and distinguishing clinical pointers	Incidence per 1000 patients per year	
	Suspected	Confirmed
Thyroid adenoma	0.6	0.6
Adults affected, hard round mass near larynx, mass moves on swallowing, possible evidence of retrosternal space occupying lesion, chest X–ray		
Physiological goitre		not uncommon
Diffuse rounded swelling of whole thyroid in teenage girls		
Thyroid carcinoma	—	1 in 10 years
Only early sign or symptom is a nodule that increases in size. Women over 45 most likely to be affected.		
Hashimoto's disease	—	1 in 10 years
Women under 50 with rubbery swelling of thyroid and evidence of myxoedema. Autoimmune.		
Cretinism	0.3	0.1
Typical facies, failure to develop, post-nasal obstruction, anaemia		
Simmond's (Sheehan's) syndrome	—	2 in 10 years
Incident of severe blood loss or shock, loss of pubic and axillary hair		
Pituitary infantilism	—	1 in 10 years
'Peter Pan' syndrome — failure to grow and mature		
Acromegaly	0	0
Enlargement of lower jaw and hands, bitemporal hemianopia		
Diabetes insipidus	0	0
Polyuria and polydipsia without glycosuria		
Cushing's syndrome	0	0
Adrenal virilism, hypertension, bitemporal hemianopia. Laboratory tests.		
Hyperparathyroidism	0	0
Polyuria, polydipsia, constipation, obscure bone pains, cystic changes in bones		
Adrenal cortex hyperfunction	0	0
Virilism, hypertension. Laboratory tests.		
Addison's disease	—	1 in 10 years
Listlessness, weakness, weight loss, pigmentation of skin and mucous membranes. Laboratory tests.		
Adrenal medulla tumour	0	0
Paroxysmal hypertension. Laboratory tests.		

Table 9 Cont'd

Disease and distinguishing clinical pointers	Incidence per 1000 patients per year	
	Suspected	Confirmed
Scurvy	0	0
Changes in gums; haemorrhages into skin, joints, etc.		
Rickets	0	0
Failure to thrive; bone deformities. Immigrant communities.		
Malnutrition	—	—
Occasionally encountered in old people, problem families, immigrants and indigents.		
Bronzed diabetes	—	2 in 10 years
Slow onset of dark silvery yellow pigmentation of skin (not mucous membranes), lassitude, occasional glycosuria, skin biopsy		
Exophthalmos with obesity	—	2 in 10 years
Persistent exophthalmos and obesity without evidence of thyroid overactivity		
Coeliac syndrome genetic inability to deal with gluten containing food.	—	1 in 10 years
Children affected, failure to gain weight, offensive bulky motions		
Cystic fibrosis	0	0
Failure to thrive. Steatorrhea, Anaemia, Chronic chest infection. Chest X–ray. Sweat test.		

11

Diseases of the blood and blood-forming organs

Please read the introduction for explanation of figures and analyses.

IRON DEFICIENCY (HYPOCHROMIC) ANAEMIA

Classification: ICHPPC 280 (RCGP 0900)

AETIOLOGY

The normal plasma iron level is 60 to 160 μ g per 100 ml. A daily intake of 5 to 10 mg. is probably adequate for most adults but should be two to three times this for babies, children, pregnant women and old people. A reduction of the mean corpuscular haemoglobin values (MCH) is the best indicator of an iron deficient anaemia

Possible causes should be considered under 5 main headings:

1. Blood loss — both obvious and hidden.
2. Deficient iron absorbtion.
3. Deficient iron intake and diet.
4. Deficient blood formation as in many chronic diseases and infections.
5. Increased destruction (haemolysis) of red cells.

Hypochromic anaemia is both common and often symptomless. Therefore, the family doctor must develop a high index of suspicion confirmed by blood tests. Successful identification of cases is most frequently triggered by the presence of one (or more) of the high risk factors mentioned below. [Practice experience: 60% (15 out of 25) consecutive patients with low haemoglobin levels had no symptoms of anaemia]

DIAGNOSTIC RANGE (rates per 1000 patients per year)

Personal: Suspected 30.0. Probable 11.0. *National*: 9.3 (Ref. 0.2). The number of patients treated depends on the thoroughness of the doctor's search and the MCH levels considered to be abnormal.

AGE INCIDENCE

Peaks of incidence occur in the twenties, forties and the seventies — due probably to child-bearing, menopausal menstrual irregularities and deficient diet, respectively (Fig. 18).

SEX INCIDENCE

Women are especially liable (7: 1).

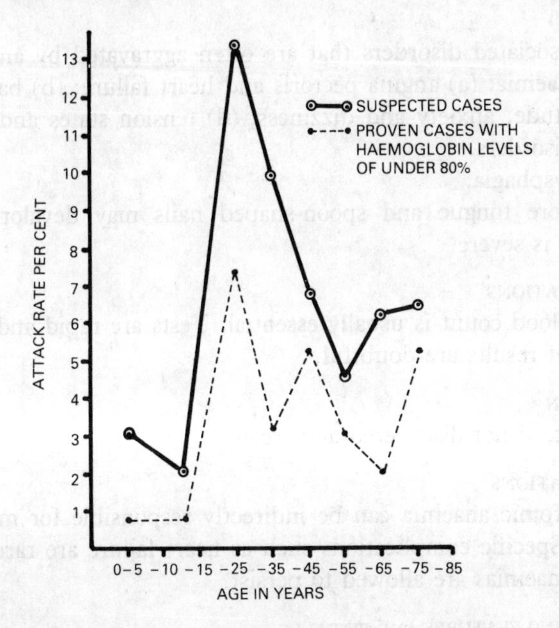

Fig. 18 Hypochromic anaemia. Age incidence of 111 consecutive cases encountered in one year.

CLINICAL POINTERS

1. High risk factors which justify a blood test in the absence of symptoms: (a) Blood loss— menorrhagia, child bearing, epistaxis, dental extractions, accidents and operations. Overt blood loss in diseases such as piles, peptic ulcer and cancer of gut, lung, bladder or kidneys. (b) Deficient iron intake — babies (especially premature), pregnancy, the disadvantaged, immigrant families and the elderly. (c) Chronic diseases (especially infections); also myxoedema and rheumatoid arthritis and chronic renal disease.
2. Onset is often insidious or symptomless.
3. Tiredness and easy fatigue.
4. Shortness of breath and palpitations.

5. In the elderly: confusion, dementia, giddiness and unexplained falls.

6. Pallor of skin and mucous membranes (44%) is difficult to assess: (a) face and cheeks; (b) lips (often masked by make-up); (c) conjunctivae; (d) palmar creases appear pink or orange instead of the normal red or purple.

7. Slight yellowness of the skin in severe cases. Not a true icterus.

8. Associated disorders that are often aggravated by an underlying anaemia: (a) angina pectoris and heart failure; (b) backache; (c) lassitude, anxiety and dizziness; (d) tension states and behavioural disorders.

9. Dysphagia.

10. Sore tongue and spoon-shaped nails may develop if the anaemia is severe.

INVESTIGATIONS

A full blood count is usually essential. Tests are rapid and cheap. Repeat if results are doubtful.

DURATION

Indefinite if not discovered and treated.

COMPLICATIONS

Hypochromic anaemia can be indirectly responsible for much ill-health. Specific complications such as heart failure are rare unless severe anaemias are allowed to persist.

MISLEADING FEATURES AND PITFALLS

1. Failure to realise that hypochromic anaemia is a common cause of ill-health.

2. Fear of doing too many *blood tests*. Most adults understand the need for accuracy although blood tests on children are avoided when possible.

3. Cosmetics and dark skins may conceal pallor.

4. Old people. Failure to realise that iron-deficiency anaemia is extremely common in the elderly. Symptoms are often absent or atypical.

5. Inaccurate clinical assessment of anaemia. [Practice experience: 121 consecutive cases were each assessed: (a) clinically, (b) by Tallqvist, (c) by laboratory. The variations in the clinical and Tallqvist assessments were large and led to treatment of 37 patients who were not anaemic and failure to diagnose 10 patients with

severe anaemia. The laboratory tests were consistently the most satisfactory.]

DIFFERENTIAL DIAGNOSIS

The family doctor should consider hypochromic anaemia as an additional not an alternative diagnosis.

MANAGEMENT OPTIONS

Prevention: (a) health education about causes and trigger factors; (b) effective early diagnosis by screening and case finding in high risk groups.

Established disease: (a) careful search for cause; (b) explanation to patient; (c) treat primary cause; (d) supplementary iron — BNF 9.1.1 (Ref. 0.1).

PERNICIOUS ANAEMIA

Classification: ICHPPC 281 (RCGP 0905)

AETIOLOGY

Failure by the stomach to produce an enzyme (intrinsic factor) that is needed for the absorption of vitamin B_{12} from the ileum causes this megaloblastic anaemia. One-third of cases have a family history. Similar anaemias are sometimes caused by gastrectomy, carcinoma or prolonged treatment with phenytoin (Epanutin). Achlorhydria is associated. Gastric cytoplasmic antibodies can be demonstrated in over 80% of patients. The disease is commoner in people of blood group A than blood group O.

DIAGNOSTIC RANGE (rates per 1000 patients per year).
Personal: Suspected 3.0. Probable 0.5. *National*: 1.6 (Ref. 0.2)

SEX INCIDENCE

Women are affected more than men [3: 1].

AGE INCIDENCE

Adults over 40; very rare under 30, most cases are 60 to 70.

CLINICAL POINTERS

Early clinical pointers

1. High risk factors: (a) elderly with unexplained symptoms; (b) previous gastrectomy, (c) certain drugs; (d) family history.

2. Insidious onset. Symptoms may be present for 9 to 18 months before the disease is recognised.

3. Sore tongue and patchy glossitis is commonly reported before clinical anaemia is apparent. Eventually the surface of the tongue becomes smooth and atrophic.

4. Listlessness and easy fatigue are usually reported before clinical anaemia is evident.

5. Attacks of diarrhoea are sometimes an early symptom.

6. A rapid pulse (over 100) is occasionally noticed as an unexplained finding before the diagnosis is made.

Late clinical pointers

1. When the haemoglobin has fallen below 65% the classical features appear: dyspnoea and palpitations; pallor and clinical anaemia; slight icterus and lemon yellow tinge of the skin (the conjunctivae and urine are normal colour); paraesthesia; ankle oedema; appetite is lost and weight falls.

2. A low-grade fever and a history of rigors may confuse the diagnosis.

3. Associated complaints: angina pectoris; dizziness.

INVESTIGATIONS

1. A full blood count reveals a large reduction of red cells with only a moderate reduction of cellular haemoglobin (MCH). The cells are macrocytic and the MCD and MCV values are therefore raised. Also, there is a neutropenia with an increase in the number of older cells.

2. A blood film shows variations in the shape, size and staining reactions of the red cells with immature nucleated red cells.

3. Serum level of vitamin B_{12} is reduced.

4. Schilling test, sternal marrow investigations, serum folate's and histamine test meal are best done in hospital.

DURATION

Indefinite if treated.

COMPLICATIONS

1. Subacute combined degeneration of the spinal cord. (No cases encountered in 10 years of practice.)

2. Heart failure and death may occur if the anaemia is allowed to persist.

3. Partial remissions. Patients sometimes manage for long periods without treatment.

4. Gastric carcinoma. [Practice experience suggests that other carcinomas may also be associated].

MISLEADING FEATURES AND PITFALLS

Confusion with hypochromic anaemia. Correct diagnosis may be delayed if iron treatment causes temporary improvement without the check of a full blood count.

DIFFERENTIAL DIAGNOSIS

Diseases that may be confused with pernicious anaemia:

Glossitis

Similar feature: persistent sore tongue. Distinguishing feature: a full blood count is the only certain way of excluding pernicious anaemia.

Hypochromic anaemias

Similar features: insidious onset; pallor; slight icterus; dyspnoea; palpitations; listlessness; dizziness; angina pectoris; sore tongue occurs in severe hypochromic anaemia.

Distinguishing features: cause of blood loss may be apparent; sore tongue uncommon and diarrhoea absent; full blood count.

Carcinoma of the gastrointestinal tract

Similar features: insidious onset; anorexia; loss of weight; clinical anaemia; megaloblastic blood picture said to occur; achlorhydria.

Distinguishing features: vomiting, pain or other evidence of gastrointestinal disease may differentiate; blood count may differentiate; hospital investigation indicated.

Septicaemia

Similar features: clinical anaemia; fever, tachycardia; enlarged spleen; rigors occasionally occur in pernicious anaemia.

Distinguishing features: onset sudden; high fever likely; rashes — purpura and other evidence of septic emboli common; blood picture (leucocytosis) and blood culture differentiate; hospital investigation indicated.

MANAGEMENT OPTIONS

Established disease: (a) Vitamin B_{12} injections — BNF 9.1.2 (Ref. 0.1); (b) careful regular follow up by doctor as well as nurse.

Table 10 Less common diseases of blood and blood-forming organs

Disease and distinguishing clinical pointers	Incidence per 1000 patients per year Suspected	Confirmed
Hodgkin's disease Persistently enlarged lymph nodes in young patient, fever, splenomegaly, raised ESR	—	1 in 10 years
Giant follicular lymphoma Progressive lymph node enlargement after middle age, biopsy	—	1 in 10 years
Multiple myelomatosis Progressive malaise, weight loss and bone pains, sternal tenderness, haemorrhages, greatly raised ESR, Bence-Jones proteinuria X–rays indicated.	—	2 in 10 years
Acute leukaemia Clinical picture resembles septicaemia, gum lesions, blood count	—	2 in 10 years
Chronic myeloid leukaemia Malaise, weight loss, haemorrhages, splenomegaly, blood and marrow investigation	—	1 in 10 years
Chronic lymphoid leukaemia Similar to chronic myeloid type but progression is slower and older patients are affected	—	1 in 10 years
Mycosis fungoides Areas of plum-coloured skin induration (fungating tumours form later)	—	1 in 10 years
Senile purpura A large purple patch is often noted on the limb of an elderly patient	—	Common
Purpura simplex A crop of purpuric spots may arise in an allergic reaction	—	—
Henoch-Schonlein purpura Intestinal haemorrhage or arthritis associated with purpura	—	2 in 10 years
Symptomatic purpura May arise in septicaemia	—	—
Sickle Cell Trait Any painful incident in a black child justifies investigation	—	—

12

Mental, psychoneurotic and personality disorders

Please read the introduction for explanation of figures and analyses.

CLASSIFICATION

A. Psychoses
  1. Organic dementias.
  2. Schizophrenia (including Paranoia).
  3. Manic-depressive syndrome (cyclothymia)

B. Psychoneuroses
  1. Simple anxiety
  2. Tension states (anxiety neurosis)
  3. Hysteria
  4. Obsessional neuroses (phobias and compulsions).
  5. Depression of psychoneurotic origin.

C. Psychosomatic disease
  Described under somatic headings.

D. Personality and behaviour problems

The psychoses bear no relation to normal behaviour. The patient lives in a world of his own and rapport is lost. Organic and biochemical changes are increasingly being shown to play a causative role.

By contrast, the psychoneuroses are extensions of normal behaviour; there is exaggeration of a normal trait. The basic normality of psychoneurotic disease explains many of the characteristics: (a) commonness; (b) the significance of upbringing and education in its development; (c) the irritations that psychoneurotic patients cause (no one likes to see his own faults mirrored and exaggerated in others); (d) the extreme difficulty of defining psychoneurosis and drawing the line between normality and abnormality.

In psychosomatic disorders, psychic influences are thought to cause organic disease. The patient's behaviour is normal, but personality is in some way linked to the development of somatic symptoms.

Psychoneurotic (better referred to as behavioural) disorders comprise a large section of primary care. In all such cases the physician's strategy for both questioning and management will vary greatly, depending on the many other influences affecting the patient's security. For example if a patient has no insight into the causation, referral to a psychiatrist may undermine self-confidence and aggravate insecurity. The significance of this fact is often not realized by either G.P.s or psychiatrists.

THE PSYCHOSES

THE ORGANIC DEMENTIAS

Classification: ICHPPC 290 (RCGP 1000)

The organic dementias often referred to as the chronic brain syndrome, are not uncommon and are of three types: (a) arterio-sclerotic or multi-infarct type (see p. 282); (b) senile or presenile dementia of Alzheimer's type (SDAT); (c) Secondary dementias due to other diseases e.g. fever, anaemia, cerebral tumour, etc.

DIAGNOSTIC RANGE (rates per 1000 patients per year)
Personal: Suspected 2.0+. *National*: 1.6 (Ref. 0.2). Many patients are able to cover up their early disorders of memory and disorientation. Agressive treatment at this stage may be counter productive if the primary cause is irreversible.

AGE INCIDENCE
Cases start appearing after 60. The majority are over 80.

CLINICAL POINTERS
1. High risk factors: (a) evidence of arterioselerosis elsewhere; (b) diabetes; (c) hypertension; (d) age; (e) living alone; (f) death of a spouse.
2. Increasing problems of orientation and recent memory.
3. Falls and giddiness.
4. Failures of self-care and toilet.
5. Increasing irritability, suspicion and social impairment.

MISLEADING FEATURES AND PITFALLS
A cerebral tumour, myxoedema, a fever, or severe anaemia can easily be mistaken for one of the less treatable organic dementias.

Pre-senile dementias of unknown aetiology usually affect patients in late middle age (one case in 10 years).

MANAGEMENT OPTIONS

Suspected disease: (a) treat treatable causes; (b) support patient and relatives at home as long as possible — this may involve home nursing services, home helps, regular visits to a day hospital or sheltered housing; (c) short stay hospital admission, holiday relief, etc; (d) psychogeriatric assessment; (e) institutional care as a last resort.

SCHIZOPHRENIA AND PARANOIA

Classification: ICHPPC 295 (RCGP 1020)

Schizophrenia is a serious mental disorder in which the patient lives in a world of his own and tends to believe that the outside world is threatening his dream world.

Paranoia is a form of schizophrenia that usually affects adults over 40 and in which fears of persecution are excessive.

AETIOLOGY

Uncertain — probably an underlying biochemical disturbance that interferes with the integration of the cerebral cortex and hypothalamus. The various high risk vulnerability factors are discussed below.

DIAGNOSTIC RANGE (rates per 1000 patients per year)

Schizophrenia. *Personal*: Suspected 1.7. Probable 1.1. *National*: 1.8 (Ref. 0.2). Many are in institutions not receiving primary care.
Paranoia. *Personal*: 0.4. *National*: 0.5 (Ref. 0.2).

AGE INCIDENCE

Schizophrenia: onset is between 15 and 30.
Paranoia: adults over 40.

CLINICAL POINTERS

1. High risk (vulnerability) factors: (a) positive family history; (b) major life events (pleasant and unpleasant); (c) relapses are fewer if patient lives alone or has low levels of emotional involvement with others; (d) over-concern or hostility from others; (e) attacks may be precipitated by organic disease; (f) upbringing, either strict or lax, is probably not a factor.

2. The patient is unaware of any abnormality. When relatives, not the patient, ask for the doctor's advice, schizophrenia or a psychotic depression is suspected. Relatives should be questioned about the patient's change of personality, attitude to work and family history.

3. The patient is less efficient — perhaps because his dream world becomes all-absorbing.

4. The patient gives the doctor a feeling of unreality. This feeling is difficult to describe but it often alerts the doctor. A patient will quite unaccountably not reply to a question or will suddenly make the most absurd or impossible remark. Unlike the hysteric, the remark is not underlined and the doctor may find himself like a comedian's stooge, suddenly asking the patient to repeat a curious remark. Many doctors when faced with the quiet certainty of an early schizophrenic must have wondered who is abnormal.

5. The so called 'first rank' early symptoms affecting the patient's perception: (a) auditory hallucinations i.e. voices talking or statements that their thoughts talk to them; (b) complex delusional beliefs about themselves in relation to others, i.e. that a newscaster is sticking needles into them; (c) that external forces are controlling their bodily functions or thoughts; (d) lack of insight about their beliefs, leading to odd or incongruous actions.

6. Negative symptoms: apathy, lack of drive, slowness of thought and movement, social withdrawal, depression, poverty of emotion and speech.

7. *Catatonic schizophrenia* causes the wild and bizarre posturing of obvious madness. Stupor may follow. Outlook in such cases may be good.

8. *Paranoia*. Trivial incidents are twisted to support the patient's rigid belief that he is being persecuted. The patient becomes so obsessed with these beliefs that normal life and relationships are increasingly interfered with.

INVESTIGATIONS

Early referral to a psychiatrist.

DURATION

Acute onset with well marked 'first rank' symptoms and few negative symptoms carries a good prognosis. Recurrences and prolonged illness are more likely if the onset is gradual and if negative symptoms predominate.

COMPLICATIONS

Suicide.

DIFFERENTIAL DIAGNOSIS

Distinction between an hysteric, an obsessional and a schizophrenic may be difficult and patients are referred to a psychiatrist.

MISLEADING FEATURES AND PITFALLS

1. Some trivial abnormality or remark raises the possibility of schizophrenia. Psychiatric investigation may upset an insecure personality or may be justified because early schizophrenia is suspected — a difficult decision which may be helped by discussion with the patient's relatives.

2. Schizophrenia is mistaken for neurosis. Schizophrenia causes inefficiency; the patient becomes depressed and develops an overlay which resembles hysteria or tension state.

The desire to impress the doctor and fear of being considered hypochondriac, so characteristic of the psychoneurotic is absent.

MANAGEMENT OPTIONS

Established disease: (a) referral for 'base line' assessment and anti-psychotic treatment — BNF 4.2 (Ref. 0.1); (b) regular follow up — the doctor should accept patients' delusions without disagreements which may raise 'emotional temperature'; (c) educate relatives to provide optimal contact and support; (d) group support of relatives to encourage sharing of problems and worries (Ref. 12.0).

MANIC-DEPRESSIVE SYNDROME

Classification: ICHPPC 296 (RCGP 1025)

This is a mental illness in which abnormal activity alternates with depression and lack of activity. The classic manic-depressive cycle is uncommon. Confusion arises because in practice the various definitions of depression overlap and merge to appear clinically as a continuum with severe (psychotic) depression at one end and mild psychoneurotic or reactive depression at the other.

AETIOLOGY

Uncertain.

DIAGNOSTIC RANGE (rates per 1000 patients per year)

Personal: Suspected 0.8. Probable 0.2. These figures refer only to patients considered to have the full manic-depressive cycle.

AGE INCIDENCE

Adults, especially in late middle age.

CLINICAL POINTERS IN THE DEPRESSIVE PHASE

(For comparison with reactive depression, see p. 256)

1. High risk vulnerability factors: (a) history of previous depressive or manic attacks; (b) genetic proximity to other depressives in

in the family; (c) puerperium; (d) menopause; (e) gynaecological operations; (f) major life events; (g) absence of family support; (h) lack of friends.

2. Onset gradual.

3. Persistence of depression. Sometimes the patient is especially depressed in the mornings but there is little change from day to day. This is the opposite of psychoneurotic depression in which the patient is worse when tired and the mood varies.

4. Slowing up of bodily functions. Anorexia, constipation and loss of libido.

5. Slowing up of intellectual powers. Loss of interest, confidence and drive.

6. Sleeping habits are disturbed. Early waking is characteristic of severe or psychotic depression.

> NOTE. This fact is now widely known amongst lay persons and is reported with increasing frequency in psychoneurotic depressions.

CLINICAL POINTERS IN THE MANIC PHASE

1. History of previous depressive incidents.

2. Sudden onset.

3. Abnormal increase in activity. Often the increased activity is not noticed until the patient gets up in the early hours to do some simple chore, e.g. decorating the bathroom. In acute cases the activity is so extreme that the patient may damage himself and others.

4. The patient has no insight. He is certain that any other 'intelligent' person would behave in the same way.

INVESTIGATIONS

Early psychiatric opinion.

DURATION

The depression may persist for long periods if not treated.

COMPLICATIONS

All depressives are potential suicides. Death from exhaustion can occur during acute mania.

MISLEADING FEATURES AND PITFALLS

1. A patient's judgement or activities are impaired by an endogenous depression. Consequent mistakes, e.g. business failure, are then wrongly considered by patient and doctor to be the cause of the depression. A severe psychotic depression may thus be wrongly treated as a simple reactive one.

2. A severe endogenous depression is mistakenly diagnosed as reactive and the patient is given of supply of drugs. The doctor unwittingly provides the means of suicide.

MANAGEMENT OPTIONS

Any mania or severe depression is best referred for psychiatric diagnosis and treatment (including ECT). Having done this the family physician should remember that his/her job has only just begun.

Once the patient is returned to the family doctor's care management is similar to that for milder (reactive depression (see p. 255).

THE PSYCHONEUROSES

The psychoneuroses are classified as:

1. Simple anxiety
2. Tension and anxiety states.
3. Hysteria
4. Obsessional neurosis and phobias.
5. Depression (reactive).

The fundamental feature of all psychoneurotic disorders is that they are extensions of normal behaviour.

Before discussing the different types of psychoneurosis several general points must be made.

Practical points relating to all psychoneurosis

1. Every normal individual (including the doctor) is capable of neurotic behaviour. If we as doctors are to understand and help sufferers we must first recognise such behaviour in ourselves. Every doctor's attitude should start with the humbling knowledge that 'there but for the grace of God go I'.

2. The best protection of every individual against psychoneurotic behaviour is a high level of security and self confidence.

3. Most individuals acquire and boost their self confidence from the following sources (see p. 110, Table 5):

— an affectionate caring childhood, especially in the first years.
— success in a role, i.e. in family, school, leisure or job. Even being a successful delinquent may give a teenager self confidence.
— supportive friendships with peers, family or parents. A single supportive confidant can play a powerful preventive role (Ref. 5.2).

— promotion or stable position in an organisational hierarchy e.g. school, profession, the armed services, many businesses or jobs.

4. Conversly the vulnerability of any individual is increased by those high risk factors that tend to lower self confidence:

— family insecurities
— feelings of failure — in a job, a marriage or community
— unemployment and boredom e.g. the 'empty nest'
— isolation from — peers, supportive friends or family
— role conflicts. Major life events such as death of a near relative, a change of job or domicile frequently precipitate such conflicts.
— ill health
— suggestions by friends (and doctors) that symptoms are 'imagined' i.e. manufactured.

5. Long term studies suggest that the majority of reported psychoneurotic behaviour is eventually self limiting. A poor prognosis is likely if: (a) symptoms are severe; (b) if there is no concurrent physical illness or; (c) if protective family and social networks are deficient.

6. Anxiolytic drugs BNF 4.1.2 (Ref. 0.1) are frequently prescribed and although initially helpful their long term benefits are uncertain. They can be counter productive for two important reasons. First, they can lead to dependence, second they can inhibit more effective but more demanding treatment because both patient and doctor consider that anxiolytics are sufficient.

7. Psychoneurotic disorders may be overlooked because family doctors are content to deal with a patient's trivial organic 'cover story' without exploring the underlying psychosocial causes.

Definitions and examples which help when discussing psychoneurosis with patients

1. SIMPLE ANXIETY

Definition: an exaggerated or unreasonable fear in a normal person.

EXAMPLE. When I was a medical student I read about hypothyroidism and because I felt tired and listless — probably a result of late nights worrying about success or failure in exams — I became convinced that I was myxoedematous. When I noticed that the outer third of my eyebrows was absent I became certain and consulted my family doctor. My symptoms disappeared after my exams.

In most cases of simple anxiety we find a similar sequence, i.e.

A conditioning experience

+

A physical complaint (often trivial)

↓

Unreasonable fear

↓

Further awareness and exaggeration of the symptom leading to further anxiety.

2. TENSION STATES

A collection of symptoms and signs that arise from faulty adaptation to the unresolved conflicts of life. We are unable to adapt because we are not fully aware of the cause.

EXAMPLE 1. Blushing. Insecurity is an internal conflict of roles between what we would like to be and what we actually are. An adolescent who is insecure in his relations with the opposite sex blushes — a typical tension symptom. It upsets the patient who is unable to control it. If some well-meaning doctor says 'It's up to you' or 'it's a question of will power', the symptoms are likely to get worse; the patient becomes increasingly aware of the symptom which in turn becomes more marked. The only cure will be when the patient resolves his conflict by acquiring social confidence.

EXAMPLE 2. The Monday morning feeling. Fatigue is a typical symptom of a mild tension state, e.g. 'I want a tonic, Doctor — I wake up tired'. The fatigue of Monday morning occurs because we fail to recognise the conflict between work and leisure. The malaise passes off as soon as we start work.

EXAMPLE 3. Thresholds. The headache or pain which disappears when we perform an interesting activity only to return when we are bored or when someone asks 'How is your headache'.

3. HYSTERIA

Definition: a collection of signs and symptoms are reproduced by a suggestible person for a motive of which he is unaware.

Hysteria is not a normal trait of most adults because they are not sufficiently suggestible. We can understand the problem by studying children who are able to overlook both logic and motive by suggestion. A child is able to believe that he is driving a car when he holds a toy steering-wheel attached to a chair. Similarly a child can develop an hysterical 8.30 a.m. sickness if he does not like school. A few adults — often those with immature personalities — retain this degree of suggestibility. They are potential hysterics, and may try to resolve some of their conflicts to their imagined advantage by hysterical self-deception.

4. OBSESSIONAL NEUROSES AND PHOBIAS

Definition: an unreasonable or exaggerated fear that cannot be overcome by reassurance or suggestion.

Unlike the schizophrenic, the obsessional admits that his fears are needless but still wants further reassurance.

> EXAMPLE. The householder who has to satisfy himself repeatedly that doors have been locked or gas turned off.

Obsessional disorders are classified as neuroses because these traits are present in all of us. A severe obsessional neurosis is so intractable and may upset a patient's life to such an extent that a psychosis is simulated.

5. DEPRESSION OF PSYCHONEUROTIC ORIGIN

Everyone knows the exogenous (reactive) depression which follows bad news or failing an examination — a direct conflict between what we want and what has happened. The depression of psychoneurotic origin is identical but the cause is not obvious to the patient. We all experience unaccountable moods of depression and know that in these moods something may happen that cheers us up; only then do we become aware of the cause of our depression.

The relationship between the frequent mild degrees of depression and the rarer severe psychotic depression is uncertain.

The work of Brown (Ref. 5.2) suggests that they are all part of a single spectrum.

The clinical descriptions of both extremes are given (p. 256) but most cases will probably fall somewhere between these end points.

Predisposing factors in psychoneurosis

The causes of insecurity, anxiety and depression in normal individuals have been discussed in Chapters 5 and 6, and the normal origins of so-called psychoneurotic behaviour have been stressed. Some of the more important factors in the production of such behaviour are described below.

HEREDITY

It is known that psychoneurotic tendencies run in families and the relative part played by inheritance or upbringing is difficult to assess. The practical point is that we cannot alter an individual's genes, but we may be able to influence his environment.

ENVIRONMENT AND UPBRINGING

Supportive family and social networks undoubtedly help to protect the individual against psychoneurotic behaviour.

Children (especially under 3 years) acquire their security and self confidence from the affection of their parents and loved ones. A number of family influences can interfere with this process:

1. The broken home. The parents are so concerned with their own affairs that they are unable to give affection to their children.

2. The excessively strict parents who are afraid of giving affection.

3. The excessively lax parents who are unable to understand that giving affection to children involves both discipline and integrity and does not mean saying 'yes' to every demand. School may help these children.

4. Parental interests outside the home become excessive and the members of the family cease to have emotional dependence on each other at an early age. Outward appearances are maintained but the children learn early on, to find affection as best they can in the outside world.

5. 'Sibling favouritism': a parent or grandparent may stress real or imagined inequalities. Lack of confidence and difficult behaviour arises in the unfavoured sibling. The favoured sibling may suffer later when he needs the support of peers not parents.

PARENTAL INSECURITY AND CONFIDENCE

A strong family network or a job appears to protect the parents of young families against psychoneurotic behaviour patterns. Single parents may be especially vulnerable.

The family doctor should never underestimate the way in which a young family can drain parental self confidence.

STRESS AND BOREDOM

Stress does not directly cause psychoneurosis. If increased responsibility leads to success then neurotic behaviour is unlikely. Loneliness, boredom and unemployment are potent sources of loss of self-confidence and may lead to neurotic behaviour.

SIMPLE ANXIETY

Classification: ICHPPC 3000 (RCGP 1040)

Simple anxiety can be defined as an exaggerated or unreasonable fear in a normal person whose thresholds of awareness have been lowered by insecurity or loss of confidence.

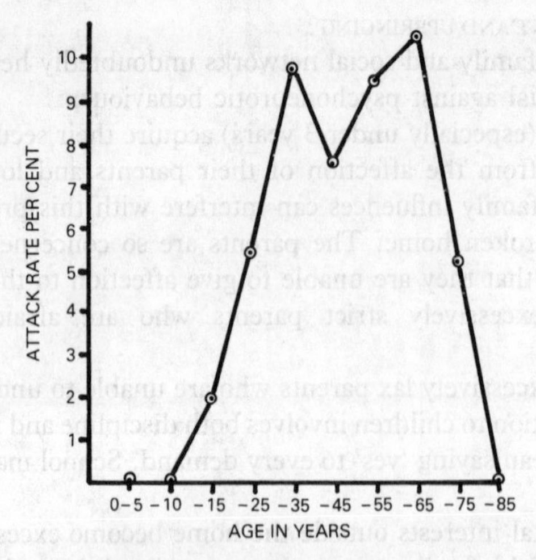

Fig. 19 Simple anxiety. Age incidence of 166 consecutive cases encountered in one year.

> EXAMPLE. A girl of 21 years was afraid that her headaches were due to blood pressure. During examination and reassurance it transpired that her aunt had died of subarachnoid haemorrhage 2 years previously.

A conditioning experience plus an organic symptom (often trivial) leads to an unreasonable fear; this in turn causes increased awareness and exaggeration of the original symptom. The impact of the conditioning experience, the suggestibility of the patient and the nature of the organic symptom affect the extent and persistence of the symptoms.

DIAGNOSTIC RANGE (rates per 1000 patients per year)

Personal: Suspected 120.1. Probable 56.0. *National*: 38.1 (Ref. 0.2). These figures also include all patients with tension states.

AGE INCIDENCE

Adults (Fig. 19).

SEX INCIDENCE

Women more than men (2.5 : 1).

CLINICAL POINTERS

1. High risk vulnerability factors: (a) genetic; (b) insecurity as a child especially under 3 years; (c) broken homes; (d) feelings of

failure at school or later in job or marriage; (e) isolation from supportive friends, family or peers; (f) role conflicts or role changes — these often follow major life events e.g. death of near relative, change of job, the 'empty nest', unemployment (see Table 5, p. 110).

2. Patients usually present their fears under a 'cover story'.

3. The presenting symptom. Often a small fibrositic pain is described in terms which indicate the patient's fear. Thus a woman who is afraid of heart disease complains of a pain over her heart, while if she fears cancer of the breast she describes the same pain as being in the breast.

4. Other symptoms of tension or fear include fatigue, listlessness, irritability, weeping, dizziness, sighing respiration, headache and depression.

5. Signs of fear or tension. The patient may be on the verge of tears, nervous or distraught.

6. The systematic questions and examination of the part complained of reveal no abnormality.

7. The symptoms clear within a few days of therapeutic examination and reassurance.

8. Common fears. Practice experience based on 90 consecutive cases — heart disease (20%); cancer (15.5%); tuberculosis (7.8%); fears of pregnancy (6.7%); sudden death (5.6%); madness (5.6%); diabetes (5.6%). Other fears include asthma, peptic ulcer, hole in the heart, gangrene, cerebral tumour, meningitis and appendicitis.

9. The conditioning experience may be known by the family doctor but is rarely volunteered by the patient until after full reassurance. It is of interest that conditioning experiences were usually related to diseases of friends and relatives and not to advertising, newspapers or television.

DURATION

Many patients are better within a year. A hard core remains as a chronic problem despite treatment. If symptoms persist the causes must be fully reconsidered and serious disease again excluded.

Persistent symptoms may be due to (1) serious organic disease; (2) trivial but persistent organic disease — listlessness or backache due to anaemia; (3) tension state, obsessional neurosis or psychoneurotic depression; (4) an early depression of psychotic origin.

MISLEADING FEATURES AND PITFALLS

1. A patient with serious organic disease is usually aware that something is wrong. Fear is predominant and anxiety may mask the true nature of the disease.

2. A depression is overlooked.

3. Lack of time (or interest) forces the doctor to prescribe a psychotropic drug and omit the important time-consuming steps of explanation, counselling and support. This mistake occurred frequently in the past with barbiturates and is easily repeated with modern tranquillisers.

MANAGEMENT OPTIONS

Prevention: Avoidance of high risk factors — often part of wider social problems. Unemployment, urban isolation, single parent families are all likely to cause increased prevalence. The family doctor may not be able to alter these factors in his/her surgery but can often have considerable influence as a concerned community member.

Established disease: (a) Exclude and initiate treatment for any organic disease; (b) Empathetic explanation — a top priority. Explanations should aim to *increase* the patient's self confidence. The doctor should stress that anxiety is a normal, often necessary, part of doing any job well; (c) explain that anxiety lowers thresholds of awareness and uncovers real and not 'imagined' symptoms; (d) Exploration of possible supportive family and social networks; (e) Strictly defined and limited use of anxiolytics BNF 4.1.2 (Ref. 0.1); (f) Supportive services, e.g. social worker often invaluable.

TENSION STATE (ANXIETY NEUROSIS, ETC.)

Classification: ICHPCC 3000 (RCGP 1040)

A tension state can be defined as a collection of symptoms that arise from faulty adaptation to the unresolved conflicts of a patient's life.

> EXAMPLE. An unmarried girl 16-year-old who is pregnant becomes listless, irritable and weepy because she does not want to face the conflicts created by her condition, but every day she is increasingly aware that this is impossible. As soon as she makes her decisions about the future, her symptoms subside. She will probably deal with the stresses of childbirth without a return of her former tension symptoms.

We all experience conflicts that we cannot resolve but we do not all develop tension states. The faulty adaptation which leads to tension is influenced by the following:

Insecurity — emotional, social or financial — is a characteristic of the patient who develops a tension state. Insecurity is felt when there is a conflict between what we would like to be and what we actually are.

Instability. An unstable individual has no fixed code of behaviour and few permanent standards. Such patients are prone to tension states because they are at the mercy of their uncertainties and have no proper yardstick to guide their decisions and resolve their conflicts. (See ch. 5.)

Self-confidence. Unresolved conflicts both internal and external usually undermine the patient's self-confidence. For this reason they affect the patient deeply and often involve one of the four areas from which most patients gain confidence, i.e. job or work, family relationships, marriage or sexual relationships, and social or group relationships.

DIAGNOSTIC RANGE

The dividing line between simple anxiety and an anxiety state is difficult or impossible to draw. The figures for simple anxiety include all tension states. In this practice about half of these would be labelled as having a tension state because of added tension symptoms.

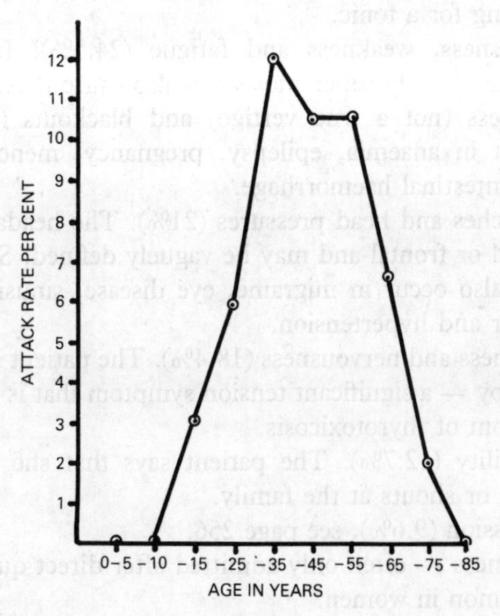

Fig. 20 Tension state. Age incidence of 167 consecutive cases encountered in one year.

AGE INCIDENCE

Adults (Fig. 20). Attack rates were high at all ages between 25 and 65 years.

SEX INCIDENCE

Women more than men (2.5 : 1).

CLINICAL POINTERS

A tension state may mask organic disease. The family doctor's first step must be to ascertain the extent of organic disease, by routine systematic enquiry and examination.

The following list of pointers and common symptoms is based on 224 consecutive patients in whom a diagnosis of tension state only was made.

1. High risk vulnerability factors, as for Simple Anxiety — page 243.

2. The patient's personality. Instability, insecurity and lack of self-confidence are often pointers.

3. Time relationships. The onset of symptoms and events precipitating the conflict correspond closely. Questions about these events should be discreet because patients may be reluctant to admit a cause and effect relationship at this early stage.

4. Symptoms of nervous origin. These patients often come to surgery asking for a tonic.

- Listlessness, weakness and fatigue (24.5%). In an adult, anaemia or early tuberculosis can also cause these symptoms.
- Dizziness (not a true vertigo) and blackouts (22.7%) also present in anaemia, epilepsy, pregnancy, menorrhagia and gastrointestinal haemorrhage.
- Headaches and head pressures (21%). The headache is often parietal or frontal and may be vaguely defined. Similar headaches also occur in migraine, eye disease, sinusitis, cerebral tumour and hypertension.
- Tenseness and nervousness (18.4%). The patient says that she is jumpy — a significant tension symptom that is also an early symptom of thyrotoxicosis.
- Irritability (12.7%). The patient says that she flies off the handle or shouts at the family.
- Depression (9.6%), see page 256.
- Weepiness — often only admitted after direct questioning — is common in women.
- Sighing respirations are typical tension symptoms and should always raise the possibility of added hyperventilation symptoms (p. 250).
- Other complaints include feelings of panic, palpitation, nausea and poor concentration.

- Insomnia is commonly associated. In tension states there may be difficulty in getting off to sleep — in psychotic disease there may be early waking.

5. The variability of symptoms is a characteristic of tension states. Symptoms vary from day to day. This is not always admitted by the patient but can be deduced by casual conversation. Thus a patient complains of listlessness and not wanting to do anything, but soon afterwards tells the doctor that he always enjoys certain TV programmes. The patient with depression of psychotic origin is consistently gloomy.

A psychotic depressive may give a history of diurnal variation of mood, but unlike the patient with a tension state, the depression is worst in the mornings.

6. Signs of nervous tension. The patient may be obviously apprehensive or tearful. A button is twisted or there is constant moistening of lips or swallowing. On examination there is tremor of hands and tendon reflexes are very brisk.

> NOTE. The extent of the examination varies. I like to examine the heart and lungs of patients with obvious tension states. This examination is usually therapeutic.

DURATION

Good prognostic features are absence of previous attacks, the presence of organic disease, a clear relationship to an acknowledged conflict, the presence of a strong family or social network. Patients from such backgrounds are often better within a year. Chronic sufferers are likely to show other evidence of long standing insecurity and lack of confidence.

All sufferers also tend to report more morbid disease than other patients. It is difficult to discover if physical ill-health has made them insecure or if they naturally have a lower threshold of complaint (see Ch. 5.)

[Practice experience. 33 consecutive patients with anxiety symptoms were matched for age and sex with 33 controls. The records of these matched pairs were analysed after 6 years (figure in brackets denotes control): number of incidents of psychoneurotic illness, 185 (92); number of incidents of organic illness, 576 (398).]

COMPLICATIONS

1. There are no serious complications, but patients with tension states may be extremely trying to deal with and may cause social complications in their families.

2. The patient is unaware of the origin of the symptoms and may be frightened by them. Fear in turn focuses the patient's attention on his symptoms. Explanation and understanding will reverse this vicious circle.

MISLEADING FEATURES AND PITFALLS

1. Tension states often mask organic disease.

2. Tension states are greatly aggravated by loss of self-confidence. Referral to a psychiatrist may aggravate the patient's loss of confidence and this action should be suggested tentatively.

3. Anxiolytic drugs are prescribed for long periods and the patient becomes dependent on these.

4. Anxiolytic drugs produce a short term benefit. Both patient (and doctor) are content with the temporary improvement and fail to attempt the more demanding and time consuming counselling procedures which may be of more permanent benefit.

MANAGEMENT OPTIONS

(As for Simple Anxiety — p. 246.)

HYPERVENTILATION SYNDROME

Classification: ICHPCC 3001 (RCGP 1150)

The syndrome is classified as a hysterical disorder. This is a mistake because it may lead to inappropriate treatment.

AETIOLOGY

In susceptible individuals hyperventilation produces an unusually prolonged fall in CO_2 blood levels and a rebreathing bag may be needed to stop the abnormal bout of hyperventilation. This unstable breathing response is cured by a course of breathing retraining combined with learned relaxation and *not* by tranquillisers. As with asthma, fear of an attack is more likely than anxiety by itself to act as a trigger.

DIAGNOSTIC RANGE

Uncertain. The majority of cases are identified at hospital level. Medical specialists and internists claim that 6 to 10% of all their referrals are due to the syndrome. Many cases are apparently overlooked at the primary level.

AGE INCIDENCE

All adults are liable. Onset is usually in younger (often male) adults.

SEX INCIDENCE

Uncertain.

CLINICAL POINTERS

1. High risk factors: (a) perfectionist, over conscientious individuals are said to be liable; (b) athletes, singers and those aware of their breathing may have a lowered threshold of susceptibility; (c) alcohol may also increase susceptibility.

2. Trigger factors: (a) Changes of mood or activity — laughter, worry or fear of an attack may all precede an attack; (b) alcohol.

3. Sighing respiration is always present but may need direct questioning to elicit. The patient is usually unaware of the relation of hyperventilation to the more spectacular symptoms which follow.

4. Palpitations, dizziness or feeling faint are common.

5. Listlessness and a feeling of exhaustion.

6. Chest pain often leads to referral.

7. Anxiety.

8. Absence of any evidence of physical disease.

INVESTIGATIONS

1. Asking the patient to hyperventilate will often replicate the symptoms.

2. Respirometry may demonstrate erratic or abnormal breathing patterns with wide variations in tidal volumes.

3. Referral and investigation in hospital.

DURATION

Most (70%) patients are cured by breathing re-education and learned relaxation. Untreated symptoms may persist for years.

COMPLICATIONS

There are no serious complications but symptoms may cause much anxiety and disruption of an individual's life.

DIFFERENTIAL DIAGNOSIS

The syndrome is difficult to differentiate from a tension state. Replication of symptoms by voluntary hyperventilation helps distinguish the two. The syndrome should be considered in anyone with tension symptoms (see p. 248) who admits to repeated attacks of sighing or air hunger.

MISLEADING FEATURES AND PITFALLS

1. Hyperventilation symptoms are regarded as due to tension and treated with tranquilisers.
2. A fear of heart disease is allowed to develop.

MANAGEMENT OPTIONS

Prevention: Early recognition.

Suspected cases: Early referral often helpful diagnostically and therapeutically.

Probable cases: (a) course of rebreathing education by physiotherapy department; (b) learned relaxation; (c) full optimistic explanation — the analogy of blushing or even asthma may be helpful. Implications that the condition is hysterical, neurotic or imagined are likely to aggravate, not reassure.

HYSTERIA

Classification ICHPPC 3001 (RCGP 1045)

AETIOLOGY

Hysteria and tension states both originate from a patient's inability to resolve a conflict. In hysteria, motive and suggestibility modify the picture.

Patients with hysteria are so suggestible that they are unaware of the origin of both their symptoms and their motive. Thus a young girl may develop a hysterical aphonia because she is afraid of her new job as a secretary. She protests that she is anxious to go to work but the aphonia persists. Suggestibility of this degree is normally found in children who in their play can believe that they are flying birds without being worried that they have no wings — logic has been overpowered by suggestion. It is not surprising that hysterics are usually immature personalities, and although the causes of hysteria are similar to those of tension states, the personality of the patient plays a larger part than family background or upbringing.

Hysterical symptoms can sometimes be cured by firm counter-suggestion — a sympathetic hearing, a therapeutic examination, perhaps an X-ray of chest and the tacit assumption that the patient's motives are beyond reproach.

DIAGNOSTIC RANGE (rates per 1000 patients per year)

Personal: Suspected 12.2 Probable 3.6. *National*: 1.9 (Ref. 0.2).

AGE INCIDENCE

All ages.

SEX INCIDENCE

Women more than men (3 : 1).

CLINICAL POINTERS

1. High risk vulnerability factors as for Simple Anxiety — page 244. Hysteria is most likely in immature individuals.

2. The patient's personality. Immaturity may be difficult to assess. Hysterics give a colourful history and yet seem unworried by their symptoms.

3. Previous attacks of hysteria.

4. Motive of which the patient is unaware, but which is usually obvious to the doctor.

5. Bizarre spectacular symptoms that do not fit a clinical picture are common but may simulate organic disease if the patient is knowledgeable. It is said that the only person capable of diagnosing hysteria in a neurologist would be a better neurologist. The symptoms vary from spectacular fits to trivial sensations which may be colourfully described as burning, excruciating, etc. Symptoms may be modified by the patient's idea of an illness and also by the ability of the symptoms to resolve the patient's conflict.

6. The patient does not appear to suffer because of his symptoms and seems almost pleased about them — la belle indifference.

DURATION

Minor degrees of hysteria may be cured by counter-suggestion. When there is a fixed motive, as in hypochondriasis or compensation cases, the duration may be indefinite.

COMPLICATIONS

Recurrences are common. Suicide may be attempted in a half-hearted way.

MISLEADING FEATURES AND PITFALLS

1. Failure to recognise organic disease in a patient whose symptoms have an hysterical overlay — a mistake that is easily made and may have disastrous consequences.

2. The doctor may react to difficult patients by wrongly labelling them hysterial. This is especially liable to occur with painful diseases that have no clinical signs, e.g. brachial neuralgia, migraine, etc.

DIFFERENTIAL DIAGNOSIS

Hysteria is only diagnosed after organic causes have been excluded. Many different and often serious diseases are easily confused with hysteria, e.g. disseminated sclerosis, cerebral tumour, epilepsy, prolapsed intervertebral disc, tuberculosis, sinusitis and even widespread carcinoma.

MANAGEMENT OPTIONS

Prevention: Encourage overprotective parents to give their children the challenges of responsibility.

Established disease: (a) exclude possibility of organic disease; (b) once a certain diagnosis is made — firm handling that tacitly assumes complete cure; (c) patients are often best not subjected to the threat of an open discussion of motives or exact diagnosis.

OBSESSIONAL NEUROSIS

Classification ICHPPC 3009 (RCGP 1055)

Simple anxiety is an unreasonable fear in a normal person — it is caused by suggestion and can be cured by further suggestion, i.e. careful reassurance. A phobia is an unreasonable fear which cannot be removed by reassurance although the patient may admit that the fear is needless. Grossly obsessional or phobic patients may resemble schizophrenic patients. Obsessional disorders are regarded as neurotic because most normal people experience obsessional tendencies, e.g. we may have to get out of bed three times to reassure ourselves that the front door is locked.

AETIOLOGY

Uncertain. The tendency runs in families, but the part played by heredity, rigid upbringing or the influence of obsessional parents is hard to define. The obsessional personality is said to be meticulous, rigid and stubborn.

DIAGNOSTIC RANGE (rates per 1000 patients per year)

Personal: Suspected 2.2. Probable 0.8. *National*: 2.1 (Ref. 0.2). The diagnosis was rarely in doubt.

AGE INCIDENCE

Adults.

SEX INCIDENCE

Females more than men (6 : 1).

CLINICAL POINTERS

1. High risk factors: as for other psychoneuroses. Background knowledge and past history may reveal obsessional traits, an immature or dependent personality.

2. Failure to respond to reassurance. A patient is worried and the doctor may spend 20 minutes taking a history, examining and reassuring her — only to be greeted with the identical fear that the patient presented at the start of the interview. It is as if the patient had not been listening. Often the patient admits that the phobia is absurd, but this is done with the resignation of someone who knows that the problem will not be overcome.

Some patients try to persuade their acquaintances that their fears have some substance and schizophrenia is simulated.

3. Persistence of the fears. In spite of reassurance and treatment a well-marked obsession is a most trying and intractable complaint.

4. Nature of fears: geographical — fear of going out, etc.; dirt and infection; sexual — fear of pregnancy, etc.; aggressive — fear of injuring others.

DURATION

The phobia may persist for many years.

COMPLICATIONS

The obsession usually affects the lives of the patient's family and may cause considerable social distress. Suicide is said to be unusual.

MANAGEMENT OPTIONS

Prevention: Uncertain probably similar to other psychoneuroses.

Established disease: (a) psychiatric referral if severe; (b) desensitisation combined with anxiolytics; (c) Support of patient and family at home; (d) treatment often unsatisfactory.

DEPRESSION

Classification: ICHPPC 3004 (RCGP 1060)

AETIOLOGY

Depression of mild or moderate degree is extremely common. The extent to which it is a part of normal behaviour and caused by environmental factors is uncertain. (The reader is referred to the section on depression in Chapter 5 page 91 and the section on the causes of individual insecurity in Chapter 6 page 110 and on manic depressive psychoses, p. 237.)

DIAGNOSTIC RANGE (rates per 1000 patients per year)
Personal: Suspected 20.0. *National*: 36.2 (Ref. 0.2). The diagnosis is rarely clear-cut.

CLINICAL POINTERS

1. High risk vulnerability factors (as For Simple Anxiety — p. 244) There are also a number of social factors which render the individual especially prone to depression.
   — Females, especially single parents and young mothers.
   — Several small children at home.
   — Low income group.
   — Absence of supportive family or social network.
   — Absence of supportive friends or confidant.
   — Absence of job or interest outside home.
   — Poor communication with husband or partner.
   — See also high risk factors for Severe Psychotic Depression — p. 237.

2. Differentiation between moderate and severe depression is necessary (Table 11) because early treatment may differ and suicides may be prevented.

Table 11 Differentiation between moderate and severe depression

Depression of psychoneurotic origin	Severe (psychotic) depression
Mood varies considerable from day to day	Mood variation slight
Depression worse when tired	Depression worse in mornings
Complaints vary	Complaints are unchanged and persistent
Reassurance helps	Reassurance ineffective
Behaviour and actions often belie statements	Behaviour and actions underline statements
Reactions not retarded	Retarded and slow
Depression causes little interference with life	Depression causes considerable interference with life, e.g. concentration poor, habits change
Sexual relations faulty — often a cause, not a result	Libido is lost
Suicidal in word not deed	Suicide likely (see below)
Difficulty in getting to sleep	Early waking

3. The distinction between the two extremes may be difficult. If there is no improvement in any depression after 3 to 5 weeks, a psychiatric opinion is obtained.

MISTAKES AND PITFALLS

1. Severity is underestimated and patient attempts suicide using antidepressant drugs.

2. Physician prescribes antidepressants but fails to provide either explanation or counselling which may be of great value in the many mild cases.

MANAGEMENT OPTIONS

Prevention: avoidance of high risk factors. As with the psychoneuroses this involves complex economic social and cultural changes which usually lie beyond the influence of the family physician.

Established disease: (a) antidepressants — BNF 4.3 (Ref. 0.1) very helpful; (b) explanations and support for the patient and family; (c) counselling once the patient is improving; (d) supportive services, especially social workers etc.

PSYCHOSOMATIC DISEASE

All psychosomatic disorders are described under somatic headings.

Note: In every psychosomatic complaint the doctor is in a dilemma. If he over-investigates or over treats the symptoms there is a danger of reinforcing and encouraging the patient's belief that serious disease is the cause. If the doctor under-investigates and under treats the symptoms, serious disease can be overlooked.

PERSONALITY AND BEHAVIOUR PROBLEMS

(See Chapters 5 and 6)

ATTEMPTED SUICIDE

Classification: ICHPPC 3009 (RCGP 5325, 5330)

Often referred to as self-poisoning or self-injury.

AETIOLOGY

Two types are recognised:

1. Attempted suicide following depression or psychotic illness (see previous section).
2. The 'cry for help' gesture in which the patient's main motive is a subconscious wish to gain recognition of his problems.

The practitioner's main problem is to diagnose and separate the two types. This is made more difficult because both overlap — the severely depressed patient can muddle their attempt and hunger for recognition while the patient who gives a 'cry for help' can be desperately unhappy and succeed in their attempt.

AGE INCIDENCE

All adult groups liable — especially those under 30 and the elderly.

SEX INCIDENCE

Attempts are twice as common in females.

SEASONAL INCIDENCE

Peaks are often noted in early spring and autumn.

DIAGNOSTIC RANGE

Personal: Probable 1.4. *National*: 1.7. (Ref. 0.2). Rates for unsuccessful attempts are increasing. Rates for successful attempts are static.

CLINICAL POINTERS

1. High risk factors. Sensitivity to the following high risk factors may be life saving:
   - Previous attempt (one in six).
   - Loneliness — under 30: when working or studying away from home; living alone.
     The elderly: after retiring to new community or after death of spouse.
   - Urban living, especially if unprotected by family or social network
   - Quarrel with sexual partner.
   - Unemployment and financial problems.
2. The patient is depressed
3. The patient admits to thoughts of suicide.
4. Sleep disturbances suggest depression.
5. Access to hypnotics or other drugs.

MISLEADING FEATURES AND PITFALLS

1. The majority of successful suicides have not previously seen a psychiatrist. A high index of both 'suspicion' and 'referral' is therefore essential.

2. In the elderly a common pattern is that of the couple who retire to new surroundings. One of the partners dies and the spouse later commits suicide. The doctor can often advise against such unwise retirement plans.

COMPLICATIONS

One attempt in six succeeds. Recurrences: One in six is liable to repeat the attempt.

MANAGEMENT OPTIONS

Prevention: Awareness of the vulnerability of patients in high risk groups can prevent the attempt. Flagging the record of patients who have made one attempt helps to alert the doctor and partners.

Established attempts: (a) emergency referral; (b) Counselling and support of patient after physical dangers have been dealt with. This is time consuming but should never be omitted. High risk factors can often be modified.

ALCOHOLISM AND ALCOHOL ADDICTION

Classification: ICHPPC 3031 (RCGP 1100)

Prosperity, increased availability and a less authoritarian society have led to a steady increase in alcoholism and related deaths in developed countries. Patterns of excessive drinking vary widely. Five types are recognised: Type 1(α) has a basic problem of insecurity and anxiety. Type 2(β) continued heavy drinking causes physical damage rather than dependence (publicans especially liable). Type 3(λ) continued 'bouts' of drinking with periods of abstention. Type 4(δ) is never quite drunk but always topping up. Type 5(ε) drinks till control is lost but may be sober between bouts.

AETIOLOGY

Behavioural causes are uncertain. Social inadequacy, poverty, boredom and insecurity play a part. Imitation is a powerful influence in teenagers. Role models may be traced to peers, parents and media sterotypes.

DIAGNOSTIC RANGE (rates per 1000 patients per year)

Personal: Known 3.0. Unknown to doctor, may be as many as 10–20 per 1000. These figures will vary according to culture, wealth and customs of community cared for.

AGE INCIDENCE

Adults. Rates for teenagers, including school children are increasing.

SEX INCIDENCE

Males more than females [3 : 1] Rates in women are increasing.

CLINICAL POINTERS

1. High risk factors: (Sensitivity to these factors is the family doctor's most potent early diagnostic aid.) (a) Occupation: especially those in the catering or drink trade or with jobs which involve travelling (sailors, fishermen, 'reps', lorrydrivers). Manual

workers with hot, dusty jobs. (b) The well off, retired or professional. (c) Those living alone. (d) The accident prone (especially motorists). (e) Attempted suicides. (f) The families of drinkers.

2. Smell of alcohol on the breath in clinic is always suggestive.
3. Unexplained falls and bruising especially in the elderly.
4. Morning discomfort, i.e. anorexia or tremor.
5. Marital disharmony; repeated absenteeism; repeated aggressive behaviour; repeated trouble with the police and unexplained debts.
6. Males who have evidence of depression.
7. Typical slightly 'bloated', red complexion of face.
8. Delirium with hallucinations (rare).
9. Cirrhosis of liver, a late sign.
10. Secret drinking — few obvious pointers except excessive use of deodorants, scent and sucking peppermints.

INVESTIGATIONS

1. The CAGE test — a mnemonic for:
   — Does drinker ever feel he should CUT down consumption?
   — Does drinker ever get ANNOYED by criticisms of consumption?
   — Does drinker ever feel GUILTY about consumption?
   — Does drinker ever have an EYE-OPENING drink to steady his nerves or for a hangover?

A 'yes' to all four, or even just the last, indicates there is a strong likelihood of alcoholism. A 'yes' to one (or more) of the first three questions indicates the need for care.

For further diagnostic questions see Ref. 0.3.

DURATION

Difficult to predict. Successful treatment is depressingly difficult to achieve but can be spectacular.

COMPLICATIONS

1. Progressive neuronal and hepatic cell loss leading to irreversible brain and liver damage. Damage is proportional to extent and duration of abuse. About 10% alcoholics show serious cell damage.
2. Delirium tremens, cirrhosis and Korsakoffs' syndrome are late pointers.
3. Pregnancy. The babies of heavy drinkers may show retarded growth, retarded mental state and more congenital abnormalities than normal.

4. Increases in respiratory and other common morbidity.
5. Increases in traumatic accidents.
6. Family and social complications. These are the most difficult and time consuming to deal with:
— Marital and family disharmony.
— Problems at work and with peers, or neighbours.
— Aggressive antisocial behaviour.
— Non-compliance.

MANAGEMENT OPTIONS

Prevention: (a) social rather than medical — family doctors can and should encourage local support groups such as A.A.; (b) early diagnosis and control of those with an 'alcohol dependency problem'.

Established alcoholism: (a) referral for advice about severity, possible drug therapy, desensitisation and group therapy; (b) assessment of patient motivation and compliance; (c) referral to A.A. group (Ref. 12.1) if compliance likely; (d) support family through Al-Anon and Al-teen organisations; family doctor will learn much that is helpful from these organisations (Ref. 12.2); (e) useful literature — Reader's Digest Family Medical Adviser (Ref. 0.3); also the Medical Council on Alcoholism (Ref. 12.3) — a voluntary body that informs doctors about the problems of alcoholism.

DRUG DEPENDENCE AND ADDICTION

Classification: ICHPPC 3048 (RCGP 1110)

There are two types of addiction:

1. Doctor-initiated (iatrogenic) — barbiturates, hypnotics and tranquillisers.
2. Patient-initiated — mainly alcohol, 'glue' sniffing amphetamines, LSD, cannabis and 'hard' drugs.

Iatrogenic addiction is common but reasonably controlled. Doctors are becoming increasingly aware of the problem — which often starts following a bereavement or a spell in hospital — and are avoiding hypnotics in these situations. Incidence is uncertain.

CLINICAL POINTERS IN IATROGENIC ADDICTION

1. Repeated requests for anxiolytic drugs, barbiturates, hypnotics, tranquillisers or analgesics.
2. Stories of prescriptions that have been lost or burnt.

3. Requests for such prescriptions that are on or just before the expiry date.
4. Reports from pharmacists or chemists.
5. Reports from near relatives.
6. Medical personnel.
7. Stories of unusually persistent or prolonged pain or other intractable symptoms.

Patient-initiated addiction is on the increase. Incidence is uncertain and early diagnosis may be difficult. Discovery may come as a surprise to doctor and parents. Rates vary for different communities. One survey suggested 6% of school children and 37% of university students.

CLINICAL POINTERS IN PATIENT-INTIATED ADDICTION

1. Young age, i.e. 16 to 26 years.
2. Uncertain way of life often with atypical or aggressive behaviour.
3. No regular employment.
4. Patient's clothing, hygiene and physical appearance may be neglected.
5. Skin puncture marks at injection sites.
6. Possibility of addiction may be denied.

COMPLICATION

Acute hepatitis A or B; malnutrition; death.

MANAGEMENT OPTIONS

Referral is usual.

COMMON SEXUAL PROBLEMS

Classification: ICHPPC 3027 (RCGP 1095)

Many of these problems are never reported although increasing numbers are seeking the help of doctors.

IMPOTENCE

There may be loss of interest (low libido), erectile failure (impotence) or ejaculatory problems (premature or delayed). Psychological trigger factors are common and should be investigated (see also male sterility p. 531).

AETIOLOGY

Usually emotional, occasionally due to organic neurological lesions, systemic disease, i.e. diabetes or drugs, alcohol, barbiturates, etc.

Male anxiety, once impotence has occurred, tends to aggravate the condition.

DIAGNOSTIC RANGE (rates per 1000 patients per year)

Personal: 0.8. *National*: 0.3 (Ref. 0.2). Many cases never reported.

AGE INCIDENCE

Peaks occur at 20 to 30 and 40 to 50 years of age.

CLINICAL POINTERS

1. High risk vulnerability factors: (a) 'performance anxiety' reflects, in an acute form, the effects of success and failure on confidence and performance, discussed on page 111; (b) ignorance, misunderstanding and communication failure; (c) feelings of guilt following adverse conditioning. Previous sexual trauma, parents, schools, and religion may contribute.

2. Nocturnal or early morning erections indicates that neurological pathways are intact and that causes are probably emotional.

3. Full history and therapeutic examination helps to rule out physical disease and pinpoint possible emotional problems, drugs, etc.

MISTAKES AND PITFALLS

1. The doctor shows uncertainty and lack of understanding. This aggravates patient anxiety.

2. The doctor for reasons of time or personal 'hang ups' does not wish to deal with such problems and patient anxieties are increased.

MANAGEMENT OPTIONS

See female sexual problems p. 265.

FEMALE SEXUAL PROBLEMS

AETIOLOGY

Most cases seen in general practice are emotional in origin. The 'pill' and other drugs may aggravate the condition. There may be (a) loss of interest (low libido); (b) general unresponsiveness (frigidity); (c) orgasmic difficulties; (d) vaginismus. Psychological vulnerability factors are common (see below).

DIAGNOSTIC RANGE (rates per 1000 patients per year)
Personal: 0.5+. *National*: 0.7+. (Ref. 0.2) Many cases not reported. One survey reports rates of 12% in sexually active women.

CLINICAL POINTERS

1. High risk vulnerability factors (a) women on the 'pill'; (b) fear of pregnancy; (c) fear of pain; (d) ignorance, misunderstandings and 'communication failures' with partner; (e) guilt following adverse conditioning by previous sexual trauma, parents, school and religion; (f) 'performance anxiety' is less likely in women than men; (g) marital problems (especially unresolved angers); (h) loss of self confidence and self esteem; (i) side effects of alcohol, drugs and disease.

2. Three main patterns are commonly reported:

• Simple immaturity. The girl reports early. Full discussion reveals relatively little in the way of previous psychological causes, examination is normal except perhaps for some vaginismus. Frank, unhurried discussion with husband and gentle deconditioning of the vaginismus frequently produce a cure.

• Hysterical causes. The girl, often attractively dressed and made up, usually reports late and gives a history of adverse childhood experiences or other possible hysterical aetiological factors. In discussion with her husband, fear of pregnancy, vaginismus and other marital difficulties may be reported. The patient is often reluctant to have any treatment. With a co-operative, sensitive husband the patient can often be encouraged to undergo what is, in effect, a course of behaviour modification.

• The 'normal' wife in whom fear of further pregnancy or other marital insecurities have led the patient to dread all sexual activity. Such cases are extremely difficult to treat because the complaint is long-standing and the primary cause is often intractable.

DURATION
Difficult to predict. Treatment is time consuming but justified by results.

MISTAKES AND PITFALLS
As for impotence (p. 263).

MANAGEMENT OPTIONS

Prevention: Long term modification of high risk vulnerability factors.

Established state: (a) correct assessment and modification of the relevant high risk vulnerability factors; (b) counselling to encourage the couple's understanding and communication; (c) greater concentration on mutually enjoyed love making and less striving after coital prowess; (d) nullifying guilt by open discussion and counter suggestion (Ref. 0.3); (e) short agreed periods of abstinence; (f) the specialised techniques of Masters and Johnson (squeeze procedures in male, etc.)

INSOMNIA

Classification: ICHPPC 3074 (RCGP 1175)

AETIOLOGY
Insomnia may be due to (a) external causes, i.e. shiftwork or a restless marital partner; (b) internal causes, i.e. tension state, depression, pregnancy or the discomforts of old age.

SEX INCIDENCE
Females are affected more than males [5 : 1].

DIAGNOSTIC RANGE (rates per 1000 patients per year)
Personal: Suspected 18.0. Probable 10.0. *National*: 9.6 (Ref. 0.2).

CLINICAL POINTERS

1. High risk vulnerability factors: (a) anxiety and responsibility; (b) a new baby or young family; (c) shift work or travel; (d) bereavement; (e) careless use of short term hypnotics by doctors or nurses especially in hospital.
2. Early waking is characteristic of possible early psychotic depression and is always a significant feature.
3. Difficulty in getting off to sleep is characteristic of a tension state.

DURATION
Often persistent. Habit prolongs the disorder.

MISLEADING FEATURES AND PITFALLS

1. Patients bring great pressure on doctors to prescribe hypnotics.
2. There is no evidence that long term sleeping habits are in any way improved by regular use of hypnotics.
3. There is evidence that hypnotics interfere with the normal sleep process.

4. The patient becomes dependent on hypnotics — *iatrogenic addiction* (p. 261).

MANAGEMENT OPTIONS

Prevention: Avoidance of hypnotics in high risk situations. *Established state*: (a) explanation vital, especially regarding high risk factors and the dangers and ultimate ineffectiveness of hypnotics; (b) encourage physical activity; (c) light reading and relaxation before or in bed; (d) short term hypnotics — BNF 4.1.1. (Ref. 0.1) as a last resort.

HYPOCHONDRIASIS AND COMPENSATION NEUROSIS

The motive is usually obvious to everyone but the patient. The complaints are often deeply entrenched making the condition highly resistant to treatment and extremely trying for those concerned.

DIAGNOSTIC RANGE (rates per 1000 patients per year)

Personal: Suspected 22.0. Probable rate: uncertain, but much lower than the suspected rate.

CLINICAL POINTERS

1. High risk factors: (a) motivation often involving escape from obligations to family or job; (b) investigation of possible serious disease; (c) the possibility or actuality of financial compensation; (d) removal of normal sources of confidence and security e.g. by unemployment, illness or hospital.

2. No particular symptom is characteristic.

MISLEADING FEATURES AND PITFALLS

1. Serious physical disease is overlooked — very easily done.

2. Every doctor's natural fear of overlooking serious disease leads to medical opinions and advice always being qualified. A healthy man with a minor cardiographic abnormality is at risk as long as diagnostic uncertainty remains.

MANAGEMENT OPTIONS

Prevention: Awareness and protection from the dangers of high risk situations.

Established state: (a) removal of source of motivation is rapidly effective but not always possible; (b) appropriate early tactful discussion may alert the patient to the dangers and disadvantages before the state becomes entrenched.

MATERNAL ANXIETY

The natural and understandable parental worries become exaggerated fears.

EXAMPLE. A parent put in an urgent call because her child was complaining of headache. The cause was tonsillitis — the maternal fear was of meningitis.

DIAGNOSTIC RANGE (rates per 1000 patients per year)

Personal: 12.6. Mild degrees of parental worry are shown by all parents.

Table 12 Other common behavioural problems in adults

	Incidence per 1000 patients per year suspected
Hysterical aphonia and functional laryngitis Many *normal* patients suffer from these disorders. Hoarseness or aphonia may last a few days to several weeks. Recurrences are common. Indirect laryngoscopy is a useful examination and reassures the patient. The vocal cords appear quite normal.	2.1
Separation, divorce and marriage problems Many such problems are either brought directly to the family doctor for advice or form a part of the 'hidden agenda' (motivations) that must be considered in the total management of a patient's problems. The number of these problems has steadily increased in the past 20 years. Today one child out of five during their formative first 15 years, will have parents who divorce or separate. For detailed discussion of these problems and management options see Chapter 6.	
Functional pharyngitis The throat is sore, especially when the patient is tired, but there is no evidence of inflammation	—
Functional gastritis There is no doubt that vomiting and indigestion of functional origin occur but many are probably mild cases of peptic ulcer (see p. 458)	10.8
Globus hystericus The motive is seldom obvious and the disorder is often part of a tension state. The patient feels a lump in the throat and is afraid of choking. Food does not stick and swallowing is normal — a distinguishing feature from organic oesophageal disease. Recurrences are common. One-third show a minor degree of gastric reflux.	1.6
Functional diarrhoea See page 499	—
Malingering The incidence probably varies according to the area, the patient's employment and the doctor's attitude. Definition: a complaint that is consciously invented or exaggerated for advantageous reasons. A fully recorded history and examination is the doctor's most useful weapon. Few patients can remember clearly and consistently what they told the doctor at the last interview.	3.0

BEHAVIOUR PROBLEMS IN CHILDREN

Most behaviour problems originate from a conflict — usually obvious to adults — in a child's mind between what he wants and what he has. Thus a spoilt child throws a tantrum when thwarted or a child of three with a new baby brother tries to regain the centre of attention by ceasing to eat.

Early diagnosis involves understanding the likely causes of the child's conflicts and insecurities. Management involves parents and doctor doing what they can to modify the conflicts and increase the child's security and confidence.

CLINICAL POINTERS

High risk vulnerability factors:

- Spoiling. The child is the centre of parental attention but parents cannot establish a routine of discipline.
- Parents are more concerned with their own problems than that of their children. Common in broken homes and socially deprived families. Insecurity in children follows.
- Family insecurities — sibling jealousy, parental favourites or a chronically ill sibling may all create insecurity in one or more member.
- School insecurities, bullying, fear of teachers, exams, etc.
- Sudden changes in a child's emotional environment, e.g. going into hospital, death of a parent (or grandparent), a parent taking a job, or a change of domicile.

MANAGEMENT OPTIONS

Prevention: Health education to modify or protect children in high risk situations. Not easy to do.

Established Problem: (a) counselling parents regarding ways of lessening high risk factors and giving child confidence; (b) supporting mother and family — relatives and social services are helpful; (c) referral occasionally indicated; (d) medication — use is usually limited or clearly defined.

Management aims to counter the conflict or insecurity: (1) negative therapeutic steps aim to ensure that abnormal behaviour does not achieve its end and is gently but persistently discouraged; (2) positive therapeutic steps aim to discover the origin of the conflict or insecurity and to persuade parents or school to compensate.

SLEEPING PROBLEMS IN CHILDREN

Classification: ICHPPC 3074 (RCGP 1175)

The common sleeping problem is that of the baby or toddler who will not go off to sleep — due to a bad habit that has developed through picking child up, often after illness or through fear of waking other members of the household. The sleeping habit can sometimes be re-established by kind but persistent firmness. This may take several weeks.

Night terrors
The child is very frightened and appears to be awake but does not recognise parents or recollect the experience.

Sleep walking
The child walks about, avoids obstacles and appears to be awake but is not. Both conditions settle in a few weeks.

DIAGNOSTIC RANGE (rates per 1000 patients per year)
Personal: 4.4.

MISTAKES AND PITFALLS

1. Hypnotics are used and deeper causes are not explored.
2. The child is cuddled on waking and subsequently stays awake to be cuddled.

MANAGEMENT OPTIONS
See Behaviour problems in children.

MENTAL DEFICIENCY AND BACKWARDNESS

Classification: ICHPPC 317 (RCGP 1220)

A paediatric opinion is advised before the child's diagnosis and subsequent management are discussed with the parents. Most primary physicians gain their practical knowledge in this area from those parents and institutions that are closely involved with the problems of mental handicap (Ref. 0.3 and 25.1) (see also Down's syndrome — p. 658)

DIAGNOSTIC RANGE (rates per 1000 patients per year)
Personal: 1.7.

BREATH-HOLDING ATTACKS

See page 293.

SPEECH PROBLEMS AND STAMMER

Classification: ICHPPC 316 (RCGP 1225)

DIAGNOSTIC RANGE (rates per 1000 patients per year)
Personal: 2.1.
A speech therapist's opinion is indicated.

DYSLEXIA **RCGP 1215**

Minor degrees of dyslexia are relatively common and easily overlooked. A child between 5 and 12 years is brought to the doctor because they are not doing well at school or are having difficulties with reading and writing but are otherwise bright. The condition is overlooked because the doctor fails to consider the possibility. If the condition is suspected by doctor or parents the child should be referred early to the appropriate educationalist or dyslexia association (Ref. 12.4).

EATING PROBLEMS IN CHILDREN

Classification: ICHPPC 312 (RCGP 1180)

The child, usually a toddler, is insecure — often from the presence of a younger sibling or from lack of parental affection. The greater fuss the more the child is likely to continue.

At a later stage bad feeding habits may follow poor parental example, e.g. fathers who are fussy about their food.

DIAGNOSTIC RANGE (rates per 1000 patients per year)
Personal: 2.9.

ENURESIS

Classification: ICHPPC 7883 (RCGP 1185)

AETIOLOGY

1. Delay in establishing control (seven out of 20 consecutive cases). The child has never been dry and is usually brought to the

doctor between 4 and 7 years of age. Upbringing may be responsible but often there is no obvious reason for the delay.

2. Psychological disturbances (ten out of twenty consecutive cases). There is a history of established control that has broken down. Insecurity may be caused by parental nagging when control is established late but usually the cause is obvious, i.e. a frightening schoolteacher or jealousy of a younger sibling. Most of these patients settle in a few weeks. A few (often those with unstable homes) continue to wet the bed until early adult life.

3. Chronic or recurrent urinary infection (three out of 20 consecutive cases). Both the infection and enuresis can become chronic. Pyuria may be intermittent. Congenital abnormalities may be associated.

DIAGNOSTIC RANGE (rates per 1000 patients per year)
Personal: 5.7. *National*: 2.5 (Ref. 0.2).

AGE INCIDENCE
Onset usually before 7 years; 0.6 per 1000 N.H.S. patients per year were over 20 years.

CLINICAL POINTERS

1. High risk vulnerability factors: (a) siblings with enuresis especially if sleeping in same bed; (b) authoritarian parental approach; (c) sibling jealousy and insecurity.
2. Wet beds.
3. Sleep. Some patients are heavy sleepers — they usually do well with treatment.

INVESTIGATIONS
Urine is checked for pus. Pyelogram and voiding cystogram.

DURATION
The majority of patients settle in a few months with reassurance, medication and regular self-charted progress reports. Patients with persistent enuresis are often cured when they gain confidence through a job or marriage.

MANAGEMENT OPTIONS

— As for all behaviour problems in children page 269
— Limit bedtime fluids (only occasionally effective)
— Star chart and encouragement (essential).
— Tricyclic antidepressants BNF 4.3.1 (Ref. 0.1).
— Bell and Pad (as a last resort).

ANOREXIA NERVOSA

Classification: ICHPPC 316 (RCGP 1170)

An individual usually an adolescent girl refuses food for fear of being obese.

AETIOLOGY

Uncertain. May be hormonal. A distorted self-image leads to a mistaken, largely subconscious, conviction of being over-weight.

DIAGNOSTIC RANGE

Personal: 3 in 10 years. *National*: Uncertain but increasing.

SEX INCIDENCE

Only one patient in 15 is male.

AGE INCIDENCE

15 to 30 years.

CLINICAL POINTERS

1. High risk factors: (a) female; (b) adolescence; (c) middle class; (d) strained family and emotional relationships (may be a result, not cause).
2. Failure to eat.
3. Loss of weight.
4. Vomiting usually self induced and concealed.
5. Amenorrhoea. Libido is lost in both sexes.
6. Reluctance to undress in front of others.

INVESTIGATIONS

Hospital admission may be needed to establish true facts.

DURATION

Several months to several years.

COMPLICATIONS

Severe loss of weight and anaemia. Death said to occur in 5% of cases.

MANAGEMENT OPTIONS

Established state: (a) obtain and maintain confidence of patient; (b) ensure that food is being retained; (c) agree with patient (not parents) on 'targets' for weight and regular visits to the doctor; (d) refer to a psychiatrist if patient agrees; (e) admit to hospital if regression occurs; (f) deal always directly with patient but support parents also.

Table 13 Table of common behaviour problems in children

Problem and common precipitating conflict or cause	Usual age of patient (years)	Diagnostic incidence per 1000 patients per year
Enuresis — page 271	4 to 16	9.5
Insecurity, infection, often some apparent		
Sleeping — page 270	1 to 5	4.4
Lack of parental routine		
Night terrors	5 to 8	—
Eating	1 to 5	2.9
Jealousy, lack of affection, poor parental example		
Tics	6 to 15	2.2
Often none apparent		
Tantrums	2 to 7	0.7
Lack of parental routine, spoiling, jealousy		
Sexual	12 onwards	0.7
Low I.Q., insecurity		
Jealousy	2 onwards	0.6
Insecurity, lack of affection		
Biting nails	5 onwards	0.5
Insecurity, anxious parents, often none apparent		
Vomiting	4 to 7	0.5
Fears, especially of school		
Continual crying	4 to 7	0.5
Fears, especially of school		
Frequency, incontinence of faeces and urine	4 to 8	0.4
Insecurity at school. Organic causes not uncommon. Often intractable		
Wandering	3 to 10	0.3
Insecurity at home		
Faecal soiling	5 to 10	0.2
1% children said to soil until 7 years. Sometimes resistant to treatment		
Stealing	7 onwards	0.3
Insecurity, poor parental example		
Thumb sucking	Normally should cease 3 to 7	0.2
No obvious reason for delay in stopping		
Rocking and head banging (*in sleep*)	1 onwards	0.2
Usually stops in adult life. Cause not known		

Management Options — see page 269

Table 14 Less common mental, psychoneurotic and personality disorders

Disease and distinguishing clinical pointers	Incidence per 1000 patients per years Suspected	Confirmed
Pseudo-cyesis Motive obvious, symptoms of early pregnancy including amenorrhoea	0.3	0.3
Disordered action of heart Motive, palpitation, chest pain, tachycardia	0	—
Homosexuality Childhood background often relevant, paternal rigidity noted, funnelling of anus or hypertrophy of labia, true incidence not known	0.3	—
Inadequate personality Patient always on move, unable to stick to one job, constantly in trouble or in need of support	0.9	—
Chronic (secret) alcoholism — page 259 Old ladies living alone, unexplained falls, irritability	0.8	—
Agoraphobia (Space phobia) — page 255 Fear of going out, mainly women, 20–35 years. Fear diminishes in company. No association with depression	—	3 in 10 years
Shoplifting in adults Middle aged women report for help as part of the 'empty nest' syndrome, motivation often not obvious and subconscious, previous behavioural problems common. Frequency increasing, teenagers and professionals rarely involve the family doctor	—	4 in 5 years

13

Diseases of the nervous system

Please read the introduction for explanation of figures and analyses.

CEREBRAL TUMOURS AND SPACE-OCCUPYING LESIONS OF SKULL

Classification: ICHPPC 199 (RCGP 0510)

1. Metastatic carcinoma — the commonest cerebral tumour.
2. The gliomas are primary cerebral tumours that are malignant and capable occasionally of forming metastases.
3. Meningiomas may grow slowly and calcify on the surface of the brain with few symptoms for many months or even years. They are usually operable.
4. Tumours arising from cranial nerves are slow to grow. An acoustic nerve neuroma may cause vague auditory symptoms which are ignored for 2 to 10 years.
5. Craniopharyngiomas, though rare, should be remembered as a possible cause of persistent headache and vomiting in children because they are treatable and more common than other cerebral tumours in the young.
6. Pituitary tumours produce characteristic defects in the temporal half of both visual fields. Hormonal changes may occur. (Cushing's syndrome, acromegaly and Simmond's disease.)

Other space-occupying lesions of skull

7. Cerebral abscess. Early diagnosis can prevent fatalities. The clinical picture is not typical of a space-occupying lesion (see p. 285).
8. Subdural and extradural haematomata (see pp. 670 and 671). (One case in 20 years.)
9. Cerebral aneurysm. (No cases in 10 years.)

DIAGNOSTIC RANGE (rates per 1000 patients per year)
Personal: Suspected 1.0. Proven 0.2. *National:* 0.1 (Ref. 0.2)

AGE INCIDENCE

All ages.

CLINICAL COURSE

A. The silent stage.

B. The focal stage of localising symptoms.

C. The stage of raised intracranial pressure.

D. Terminal stage — increased pressure leads to false localising signs and cone formation, i.e. the contents of the posterior cranial fossa are forced downwards into the conical foramen magnum.

CLINICAL POINTERS

A. During the silent stage.

Diagnosis is usually impossible. Frontal lobe tumours have a long silent phase.

B. During the focal or localising stage.

Diagnosis is difficult.

1. High risk factors: (a) symptom duration: more than 2 weeks and less than 6 months; (b) symptom progression: a suggestive symptom continues or is getting steadily worse; (c) the presence of other suggestive symptoms.

By the time most space occupying lesions are first reported one or more of the above three characteristics will apply to the presenting symptoms.

2. Epilepsy. A fit may be the first symptom, especially over the age of 30.

3. Steady progression of symptoms. Remissions may occur but only for 2 or 3 weeks.

4. Muscle weakness of organic origin is usually clearly defined and does not show the inconsistencies of an hysterical palsy. Diplopia may be an early symptom.

5. Muscular inco-ordination and unsteadiness may be difficult to assess but if associated with nystagmus or dysdiadokokinesis suggests a cerebellar lesion.

6. Sensory abnormalities may be of localising value. A defect of the optic fields can sometimes be shown by confrontation. Sensory abnormalities are difficult to assess because the family doctor gets so little practice.

7. Reflex abnormalities. Exaggerated tendon reflexes or abnormalities of the superficial reflexes may indicate a crossed cortical lesion. Unilateral sluggish tendon reflexes may suggest a cerebellar lesion on the same side.

8. Personality changes suggest a frontal lobe tumour.

C. During the stage of raised intracranial pressure.

1. Headache is often the first symptom in adults. It is made worse by coughing, straining and lowering the head. It may be intermittent and most marked in bed before getting up. Headache may be a late symptom in children.

2. Listlessness and lack of energy is often marked but is a feature of so many other diseases that it is rarely helpful.

3. Vomiting is a late symptom. It may be projectile; nausea is often absent.

4. Papilloedema is always present eventually. The disc is pink at first and the edge is blurred, later the disc becomes congested and haemorrhagic.

D. The terminal stage of coning and false localisation.

1. Paroxysmal headache — often very severe.
2. Drowsiness.
3. Mental irritability and dullness.
4. VIth cranial nerve palsy (external rectus).
5. Slow pulse.

INVESTIGATIONS

1. X-ray chest for primary bronchogenic carcinoma or bronchiectasis.

2. X-ray of skull may show: (a) calcification in a meningioma; (b) evidence of raised intracranial pressure, i.e. decalcification of the posterior clinoid processes and posterior part of pituitary fossa.

3. A raised ESR (see p. 681 Appendix 1B) suggests widespread carcinoma.

4. Diagnostic lumbar puncture should always be performed in a neurosurgical department.

5. CAT scans, EEG, air encephalography, cerebral angiography and ventriculography may be needed to complete the diagnosis.

DURATION AND COMPLICATIONS

The interval between the first symptom and death in a patient with untreated cerebral neoplasm varies from a few weeks to many years.

MISLEADING FEATURES AND PITFALLS

The first symptoms are easily labelled psychogenic.

The family doctor's dilemma is that if he refers every headache to a specialist, suggestible patients may suffer and an excessive burden is thrown on the hospital.

DIFFERENTIAL DIAGNOSIS

A. During focal stage

Diseases that may be confused with a space-occupying lesion:

Idiopathic epilepsy
Similar feature: fits.

Distinguishing features: starts between ages of 10 and 30 years; localising signs rare; hospital investigation indicated.

Hysterical paralyses
Similar features: evidence of motor paralyses; symptoms of inco-ordination; sensory disturbances.

Distinguishing features: repeated examination reveals inconsistencies; objective signs are absent; exaggeration of symptoms liable; hospital investigation should be avoided where possible.

Disseminated sclerosis
Similar features: evidence of motor paralyses; nystagmus; signs of inco-ordination; sensory disturbances (headache occasionally).

Distinguishing features: remission occurs and lasts for many weeks; further lesions elsewhere; hospital investigation indicated.

Cerebrovascular accidents
Similar feature: evidence of motor paralyses.

Distinguishing features: onset sudden; blood pressure sometimes raised; older age group usual; hospital investigation sometimes indicated; optic fundi show arteriosclerotic changes.

Migraine
Similar features: headache; disturbances of visual fields; occasionally migraine is associated with transient motor and sensory disturbances in face and limbs.

Distinguishing features: history of previous typical attacks; symptoms and signs are transient lasting a few hours only, and are followed by headache; hospital investigation rarely indicated.

B. During stage of raised intracranial pressure

Tension headaches
Similar features: headache; listlessness; anorexia and vomiting.

Distinguishing features: symptoms vary from day to day; localising features and papilloedema absent; hospital investigation should be avoided if possible.

Acute sinusitis
Similar feature: headaches — often severe, worse in mornings and after coughing or bending down.

Distinguishing features: local tenderness over affected sinus; history of cold and nasal discharge (often blood-stained); radiology; localising features and papilloedema absent; hospital investigation rarely indicated.

Migraine
Similar features: headaches associated with disturbances of vision; motor and sensory defects in the face and limbs sometimes occur.

Distinguishing features: history of previous attacks: symptoms and signs are transient lasting a few hours only; hospital investigation rarely indicated.

Malignant hypertension (and End Stage Renal Disease)
Similar features: headaches (often severe); papilloedema; CNS lesions present.

Distinguishing features: raised blood pressure; differentiation difficult; hospital investigation indicated immediately.

MANAGEMENT OPTIONS

Early referral: This should aim to be within 4 weeks of the patient first reporting. The doctor must avoid (by careful history-taking) referring large numbers of patients with symptoms eventually attributed to less serious causes.

Post hospital: (a) discussion; (b) medical and mental support; (c) family and group support (see p. 208).

CEREBROVASCULAR ACCIDENTS (CVA)

Classification: cerebrovascular disease ICHPPC 438 (RCGP 2105)

Known generally as strokes. These include any sudden disturbance of function of the CNS that follows interference with the cerebral blood supply.

Causes: (a) thrombosis (about 75%); (b) haemorrhage (about 20%; (c) emboli and spasm (about 5%) — hospital figures. Outside the hospital functional disturbance is often limited to a transient (less than 24 hours) ischaemic attack (TIA) (see p. 375), the cause of CVA is then difficult to identify.

AETIOLOGY

Arterial degeneration and vascular spasm are the immediate causes. Hypertension plays a clear but uncertain role.

DIAGNOSTIC RANGE (rates per 1000 patients per year)
Personal: Suspected 10.0. Probable 5.3. *National*: 5.9 (Ref. 0.2). Figures include both new and old cases and all TIAs. The rate over 10 years in our practice, for new cases with permanent damage, was 1.36.

AGE INCIDENCE
Over 60 years.

CLINICAL POINTERS
1. High risk factors: (a) age over 60 years; (b) previous underlying hypertension; (c) previous evidence of coronary artery disease; (d) previous attacks [44% (8 out of 18 consecutive cases)]; (e) previous possible TIA's are a common precursor of a major stroke.
2. Sudden onset. Thrombosis is said to start more slowly than haemorrhage.
3. Weakness or paralysis of the face or limbs is the common presenting symptom. The paralysis affects the side of the body opposite the lesion and may vary from a slight transient weakness to complete permanent hemiplegia.
4. Aphasia is usually associated with right sided hemiplegia.
5. Unconsciousness with stertorous breathing may be associated with a convulsion or generalised rigidity and is a bad prognostic sign.
6. Optic fundi may show evidence of arterial degeneration.
7. Evidence of upper motor neurone lesion on the paralysed side.
8. Dysphagia suggests a bulbar lesion.
9. Sudden acute vomiting with dizziness and cerebellar signs suggest a lesion of the cerebellar arteries. (Two cases in 10 years.)

DURATION
Transient attacks with little residual damage are common. [66% (12 out of 18) consecutive personal cases.]

COMPLICATIONS
Recurrences and death are common especially if there is permanent CNS deficit (28% of cases followed for 4 years had died and 17% had had recurrences).

MISLEADING FEATURES AND PITFALLS
Diabetes or a space-occupying lesion is overlooked.

MANAGEMENT OPTIONS
Prevention: (a) active case finding in all high risk groups is essential; (b) active appropriate safeguards against higher risk factors using

beta blockers or antihypertensives — BNF 2.4 and 2.5.; antiplatelets — BNF 2.9 and anti-coagulants — BNF 2.8 (Ref. 0.1).

Established cases with permanent deficits: (a) referral, about half can be treated at home; (b) early ambulation (foot-drop calliper, walking aids and instruction are essential; (c) full co-operation with Physio and Occupational therapy; (d) daily living assessments essential — followed by appropriate aids and adjustments to home; (e) support of patient and relatives by appropriate social services and allowances; (f) regular follow up and assessment; (g) sheltered housing, day-hospital, short stay (holiday) relief to support home care; (h) institutional care as last resort; (i) occupational therapy and physiotherapy at home if available; (j) useful information and addresses for any disabled patient are given in Reader's Digest — Family Medical Adviser (Ref. 0.3); (k) information about aids for the disabled (Ref. 13.1).

CEREBRAL ARTERIOSCLEROSIS (SENILITY)

Classification: ICHPCC 438 (RCGP 2105)

AETIOLOGY

Generalised degeneration of the cerebral arteries. See also the organic dementias (see p. 234).

DIAGNOSTIC RANGE (rates per 1000 patients per year)

Personal: Suspected 1.7+.

AGE INCIDENCE

Over 60 to 80 years.

CLINICAL POINTERS

1. High risk factors: (a) evidence of arteriosclerosis elsewhere; (b) diabetes; (c) hypertension; (d) age over 60; (e) living alone.
2. Gradual onset.
3. Falling about and dizziness (see also next entry.)
4. Mental changes: selfishness, obstinacy, loss of memory, lack of insight, euphoria, and emotional instability.
5. Evidence of other degenerative changes: cataract, retinitis, blindness, deafness, heart failure and osteoarthritis.
6. Incontinence.

DURATION

The disease is untreatable, slowly progressive, and may last for several years.

COMPLICATIONS

Cerebrovascular accidents and death. There may be a number of other associated clinical syndromes whose features depend on the site of the arteriosclerosis. The chief of these are: arteriosclerotic Parkinsonism (see p. 287); pseudo-bulbar palsy (Table 15, p. 303); carotid artery syndrome; vertebro-basilar artery syndrome (See below).

Pseudo-bulbar palsy

Characterised by slowly progressive difficulty in swallowing and speaking. The patient is in the arteriosclerotic age group and may show other evidence of cerebral arteriosclerosis. (Three cases in 10 years.)

Carotid artery syndrome

Usually arteriosclerotic; a carotid artery stenosis may affect younger patients. Attacks of transient dizziness, ipselateral blindness and contralateral paresis, paraesthesia and speech disturbance. Easily confused with migraine. (One case in 10 years.)

MANAGEMENT OPTIONS

See Organic dementias — page 235.

VERTEBRO-BASILAR ARTERY SYNDROME

AETIOLOGY

The cerebral blood supply is reduced as a result of temporary compression of the vertebral artery when moving the neck.

DIAGNOSTIC RANGE (rates per 1000 patients per year)

Personal: Suspected 2.5. Probable 0.9.

AGE INCIDENCE

Usually over 55 years.

CLINICAL POINTERS

1. High risk factors: (a) cervical osteoarthrosis; (b) evidence of arteriosclerosis; (c) unusual extension or twisting of neck.

2. A transient period of dizziness or unconsciousness follows either twisting or tilting the neck (often when decorating a ceiling, etc.)

3. Pallor, a fall in B.P. or even a small convulsion are occasionally noted.

MISTAKES AND PITFALLS

The condition is mistaken for a less easily treated CVA or TIA.

MANAGEMENT OPTIONS

Established disorder: (a) avoid precipitating movements; (b) cervical collar occasionally indicated; (c) explanation.

MULTIPLE OR DISSEMINATED SCLEROSIS

Classification: ICHPPC 340 (RCGP 1335)

AETIOLOGY

Uncertain. Possibly multifactorial. Heredity, diet, infection and immune processes have been varyingly incriminated.

DIAGNOSTIC RANGE (rates per 1000 patients per year)

Personal: Suspected 0.7. Probable 0.2. *National*: 0.9 (Ref. 0.2).

AGE INCIDENCE

The majority of patients start the disease between 15 and 35 years.

CLINICAL POINTERS

1. High risk factors: MS in first degree relative.
2. Disseminated onset. One transient lesion is followed months or years later by further lesions and remissions.
3. Disseminated lesions. A plaque of demyelinisation can produce a lesion anywhere in the central nervous system. Some commonly early pointers are: (a) transient weakness of a limb; (b) transient blurring of vision or blindness (retrobulbar neuritis); (c) transient diplopia; (d) lost abdominal reflexes and other evidence of upper motor neurone lesions; (e) poor co-ordination of limb movements — a limb feels stiff and clumsy; (f) nystagmus.

At first the lesions clear up in a few weeks; later, permanent lesions develop.

INVESTIGATIONS

Lumbar puncture and full hospital investigation.

DURATION

After a variable number of years the remitting character of the disease becomes buried in the permanent disabilities of paralysis and loss of sphincter control. The disease may progress steadily to death in a few years or may last for several decades.

COMPLICATIONS

Hypostatic pneumonia may cause death in the severely paralysed patient. Loss of sphincter control is a distressing and serious complication. Relapses: more likely during pregnancy and puerperium.

MISLEADING FEATURES AND PITFALLS

1. The early features of a cerebral space-occupying lesion may be confused with disseminated sclerosis.

2. Temporal pallor of the optic disc after a retrobulbar neuritis is difficult to assess because it is sometimes seen in normal discs.

3. Charcot's triad, i.e. nystagmus, intention tremor and scanning speech, is rare.

MANAGEMENT OPTIONS

Established disease: (a) a prolonged caring relationship essential; (b) each deterioration has to be countered with physiotherapy, home aids and modification of daily living that provide a maximum of hope; (c) drugs may be used to shorten acute attacks for muscle, spasm, tremor, pain, incontinence or depression; (d) main problems are when to inform patient of likely prognosis and; (e) support of patient and relatives at home — close co-operation between family doctor and hospital vital (Ref. 13.1); (f) patient information: M.S. Society of Great Britain (Ref. 13.2 and Ref. 0.3).

BACTERIAL MENINGITIS, CEREBRAL ABSCESS AND VIRUS ENCEPHALITIS

These three diseases of different aetiology are discussed together because they have certain features in common:

1. The consequence of a missed diagnosis is disastrous.
2. The combination of fever and signs of meningeal irritation may be the only indication of serious disease.
3. Immediate hospital investigation and lumbar puncture are usually indicated.

AETIOLOGY

Bacterial meningitis

Acute purulent inflammation of the meninges may be caused by the meningococcus, pneumococcus or *Haemophilus influenzae*. Now rarely seen.

Cerebral abscess

Follows chronic purulent lesions elsewhere in the body — otitis media, bronchiectasis or sinusitis. (Two cases in 10 years.) Rarely does an abscess form spontaneously.

Encephalitis

May complicate a number of virus infections: measles, mumps, vaccination, etc. Encephalitis is rare and occasionally causes death, permanent mental or Parkinsonian effects. Symptoms sometimes appear a week or so after the precipitating infection.

Aseptic meningitis (viral or benign lymphocytic meningitis etc.)
Not uncommon and may occur during the acute phase of mumps, Coxsackie, ECHO and other virus infections.

DIAGNOSTIC RANGE (rates per 1000 patients per year)
Personal: Suspected 1.8. Probable 0.8. A virus was usually responsible.

AGE INCIDENCE
All ages.

CLINICAL POINTERS
1. High risk factors: (a) low income group; (b) overcrowding; (c) contact sources of infection: mumps, polio, tuberculosis, virus and bacterial meningitis; (d) bodily source of infection: otitis media, bronchiectasis, mumps, other virus and T.B. infections.
2. Sudden onset. The patient becomes rapidly ill in 1 or 2 days. A more gradual onset may occur with tuberculous meningitis (2 to 3 weeks).
3. Headache is severe but may be absent in young children.
4. Fever. A convulsion may occur in children.
5. A purpuric rash or other evidence of septicaemia.
6. Signs of meningeal irritation. Sometimes slight but always persistent. Back stiffness, i.e. inability to kiss knees, is characteristic of a virus encephalitis and may be more marked than neck stiffness.
7. Vomiting, lethargy and irritability are common and may be marked in babies. A bulging fontanelle is always suggestive.
8. Localising signs. A cerebral abscess may show homonomous visual field defects and other evidence of a space-occupying lesion. Squints may occur in bacterial meningitis. Muscle weakness appears after a few days in poliomyelitis.

INVESTIGATIONS
Lumbar puncture and hospital investigation. Stools, nasopharyngeal swabs and 'paired sera' for virus studies.

COMPLICATIONS

Bacterial meningitis
Death, mental deficiency and epilepsy.

Cerebral abscess
Fatalities are common. Residual disability depends on the intracranial damage.

Encephalitis
Death, paralysis agitans or muscle paralysis when poliomyelitis is involved.

Aseptic or viral meningitis
Clears in 7 to 10 days and has few complications.

MISLEADING FEATURES AND PITFALLS

1. Antibiotics given in the early stages of a bacterial meningitis may mask or alter the development of the disease.
2. A transient meningismus is sometimes noted in the early stages of many febrile illnesses.

DIFFERENTIAL DIAGNOSIS

Diseases that may be confused with meningitis, abscess etc.:

Influenza
Similar features: fever; headache; body aches; signs of meningeal irritation.

Distinguishing features: contacts; cough and tracheitis; meningeal signs are transient; hospital investigation rarely indicated.

Acute exudative tonsillitis
Similar features: fever; headache; body aches and signs of meningeal irritation.

Distinguishing features: meningeal signs are transient; typical tonsillar exudate on 2nd or 3rd day; hospital investigation rarely indicated.

Subarachnoid haemorrhage
Similar features: fever; severe headache; signs of meningeal irritation.

Distinguishing features: onset of headache very sudden; fever rarely high, often absent; hospital investigation indicated.

PARALYSIS AGITANS OR PARKINSON'S DISEASE

Classification: ICHPCC 332 (RCGP 1315)

Two forms are described: the rare post-encephalitic Parkinsonism (onset usually under 40 with spasm of neck and eye muscles and associated with, or following, an attack of encephalitis); the much commoner arteriosclerotic Parkinsonism described below.

AETIOLOGY

Uncertain. The basal ganglia are usually affected.

DIAGNOSTIC RANGE (rates per 1000 patients per year)

Personal: Suspected 2.7. Probable 1.1. *National*: 1.2 (Ref. 0.2).

AGE INCIDENCE

Onset is usually in late middle age — after 55.

CLINICAL POINTERS

1. High risk factors: (a) previous strokes or encephalitis; (b) occasionally familial (20%); (c) Phenothiazines and other drugs — BNF 4.2.1 (Ref. 0.1).

2. Onset is slow over many months or years (90%). Vague aching or stiffness of limb muscles are often reported first.

3. Tremor (80%) affects hands, arms and legs. Tremor usually starts in one hand and spreads gradually to affect the whole of one and then both sides. The tremor may be inhibited by movement or sleep.

4. Characteristic facies (60%). Associated with tremor is rigidity of the affected voluntary muscles. This produces the characteristic fixed 'unblinking' expressionless facies that frequently alerts the doctor to the presence of the disease.

5. Slurred speech and the characteristic 'mincing' or festinating gait are usually late effects of the underlying muscle rigidity.

6. Weakness of the affected muscles (30%). Sometimes a very significant early complaint, whose significance is easily ignored.

DURATION

The disease is slowly and persistently progressive. A few cases may deteriorate comparatively rapidly in 2 or 3 years.

COMPLICATIONS

Mental powers may slowly disintegrate. There may be considerable emotional lability and a tendency to depression. Slow physical and mental deterioration can lead to confusion and dementia.

MISLEADING FEATURES AND PITFALLS

1. The patient complains of persistent weakness, the tell-tale tremor and unblinking facies have not yet developed; other signs of nervous disease are absent and the patient is labelled 'neurotic'. This adds to the patient's loss of confidence and depression, and

a vicious cycle is started that is only broken when the correct diagnosis is made.

2. The expressionless facies may lead to poor non-verbal communication and aggravate depression.

DIFFERENTIAL DIAGNOSIS

Differential diagnosis is from cerebral arteriosclerosis and psychogenic illness.

MANAGEMENT OPTIONS

Established disease: (a) Anti-parkinsonian drugs — BNF 4.9 (Ref. 0.1).

> NOTE: Anticholinergic drugs should not be used in Prostatism or Glaucoma while levodopa should not be started until there is clear difficulty with speech or limb movements.

(b) antidepressants (tricyclic) — BNF 4.3.1; (c) daily living assessment; (d) regular exercise and physiotherapy; (e) physical and housing aids; (f) sheltered housing; (g) support by relatives and social services; (h) regular follow up after establishing clear base lines for mental and physical capacity; (i) Parkinson's disease society hand books (Ref. 13.3).

EPILEPSY

Repeated transient disturbances of consciousness with few objective signs between episodes. Epilepsy may be difficult to differentiate from collapse, faints or blackouts. Major epilepsy is a disaster for the patient and the diagnosis is never made without full investigation.

The family doctor is in the best position to obtain an accurate description of the fit — he may actually witness it.

CLASSIFICATION

1. Minor epilepsy, or petit mal (see p. 304).
2. The para-epilepsies — narcolepsy and cataplexy (see p. 304).
3. Major epilepsy, or grand mal (see p. 290).
4. Symptomatic epilepsies:
   a. Breath-holding attack (see p. 293);
   b. Febrile convulsion (see p. 292);
   c. Convulsion following faint (see p. 291);
   d. Convulsion due to space-occupying lesion; (see p. 277);

e. Fit or sudden loss of consciousness due to cerebral arteriosclerosis (see p. 281);
f. Convulsion following cerebral damage (p. 671) or infection (p. 286).

MAJOR EPILEPSY (GRAND MAL)

Classification: ICHPCC 345 (RCGP 1370)

AETIOLOGY
Unknown. Heredity probably plays an important role. The onset is usually at puberty and in women attacks are often related to menstruation.

DIAGNOSTIC RANGE (rates per 1000 patients per year)
Personal: Suspected 5.7. Probable 2.8. *National*: 3.4 (Ref. 0.2).

AGE INCIDENCE
Onset 5 to 45 years, with peaks at puberty and between 2 and 5 years.

CLINICAL COURSE OF FIT
1. The aura lasts about 30 seconds; visual, olefactory or abdominal sensations may precede unconsciousness.
2. The tonic stage follows immediately and lasts about 30 to 60 seconds. Consciousness is lost and the patient stiffens becoming red or blue in the face and may utter a strange cry.
3. The clonic stage gradually supervenes and continues for 1 to 3 minutes. Generalised muscle twitching and tongue biting occurs.
4. A stage of flaccid coma develops as the twitching subsides. This may last 5 to 30 minutes.
5. Post-epileptic stage. As consciousness returns the patient remains drowsy and semi-automatic for about 1 to 2 hours. Odd behaviour may occur at this time. Headache may be marked.

CLINICAL POINTERS
1. High risk factors: (a) age i.e. peaks at 2–5 years and puberty; (b) family history; (c) menstruation; (d) possible previous petit mal or fits.
2. Nocturnal onset is common.
3. Convulsive movements. A history of twitching during a bout of unconsciousness helps to differentiate.
4. A history of tongue biting or personal injury during an attack strongly suggests epilepsy.
5. Stertorous or noisy breathing with frothing at the mouth during the tonic and clonic stage is common.

6. Drowsiness and odd behaviour after the attack.
7. Incontinence during attack.
8. Headache is of little differentiating value.

INVESTIGATIONS

An electroencephalogram.

DURATION

In the absence of treatment epilepsy persists.

COMPLICATIONS

Injury during an attack. Rarely, slow deterioration of character and intellect develops in uncontrolled cases. Status epilepticus — successive fits without return to consciousness.

MISLEADING FEATURES AND PITFALLS

1. Failure to obtain an adequate history may lead to confusion with migraine, febrile fits, petit mal, faints and Meniere's syndrome.
2. Casual diagnosis leads to needless suffering. Failure to give sufferers adequate information may lead to totally unnecessary suffering, stigmatisation and disbarring from crucial activities.
3. Occasionally a few convulsive squirming movements (not epileptic) occur during a faint.

DIFFERENTIAL DIAGNOSIS

Diseases that may be confused with epilepsy:

Faints and vasovagal attacks

Similar feature: episode of unconsciousness.

Distinguishing features: no aura; patient often standing; deathly white colour; sweating; shivering and vomiting often follow attack; convulsive movements usually absent.

Breath-holding attacks

Similar feature: episodes of unconsciousness.

Distinguishing features: attacks occur in children under three years; respiratory movements stop and unconsciousness occurs; convulsive movements rare; cyanosis marked; emotional tantrum or fright precedes attack.

Febrile convulsion

Similar features: unconsciousness with convulsive movements; deviation of eyes; followed by drowsiness; repeated attacks may occur.

Distinguishing features: attacks rare over age of seven; fever marked; cause of fever usually obvious.

Hysterical collapse
Similar feature: episodes of unconsciousness.

Distinguishing features: true hysterical convulsions are rare but hysterical collapse with a short period of apparent unconsciousness is common; emotional overlay apparent; audience present; injuries uncommon; incontinence absent; patient looks normal; closed eyelids flutter.

Stokes-Adams attacks
Similar feature: momentary episodes of unconsciousness sometimes associated with a generalised convulsion.

Distinguishing features: arteriosclerotic age groups usually affected (over 60); pallor during attack; pulse very slow (40); pulse may be absent for as long as one minute during attacks; face flushes with return of consciousness (see also drop attacks, page 375).

Cerebral tumours and space-occupying lesions of skull
Similar features: convulsions and headache.

Distinguishing features: age of onset is usually after 40 or before puberty; headache marked and progressive; fits are repeated; localising lesions in CNS.

MANAGEMENT OPTIONS

Prevention: genetic counselling if requested.

Established disease: (a) admission to hospital if diagnosis is in doubt; (b) control of seizures by antiepileptics — BNF 4.8 (Ref. 0.1); (c) full explanation — optimistic but objective — should be given to patient and relatives; (d) understandable parental over protectiveness must be countered; (e) full activities including sport, swimming and riding should be encouraged; (f) driving is allowed if free of fits for 3 years; (g) patient information: Epilepsy Explained (Ref. 13.4); British Epilepsy Association (Ref. 13.5); Fitness to Drive (Ref: 13.6).

Status Epilepticus: hospital admission after Slow intravenous diazepam BNF 4.8.2 (Ref. 0.1).

Pregnancy in a known epileptic: referral.

FEBRILE CONVULSIONS

AETIOLOGY

Fever. Recurrences are common. (Practice experience: acute tonsillitis, measles, mumps, chickenpox and influenza all precipitated fits.)

DIAGNOSTIC RANGE (rates per 1000 patients per year)
Personal: Probable 1.1. The diagnosis was rarely in doubt.

AGE INCIDENCE
1 to 7 years.

CLINICAL POINTERS
1. High risk factors: (a) previous attack; (b) fever.
2. The attack. The child goes vacant and stiff for a few seconds and then starts twitching. Cyanosis, frothing at the mouth, stertorous breathing and deviation of the eyes may occur. Drowsiness follows.
3. Fever is sometimes lowered temporarily after the attack.
4. The child is usually unconscious for a period of 0.5 to 5 minutes.

DURATION
Children grow out of the tendency.

COMPLICATIONS
Aspiration pneumonia sometimes occurs during the convulsion and is easily overlooked.

MANAGEMENT OPTIONS
Prevention (second attacks): (a) sedatives when child is febrile; (b) instruct parents about tepid sponging and positioning of unconscious child.
Established attack: (a) correct positioning of unconscious child; (b) rectal or intramuscular diazepam occasionally indicated — BNF 4.8.2 (Ref: 0.1); (c) hospital admission if prolonged or home care a problem.

BREATH-HOLDING ATTACKS

Classification: ICHPPC 312 (RCGP 4650)

Short episodes of unconsciousness which can be induced voluntarily by toddlers and young children.

AETIOLOGY
Emotional upsets or accidents precipitate an attack.

DIAGNOSTIC RANGE (rates per 1000 patients per year)
Personal: Probable 0.3. Confirmation of diagnosis depends on the mother's story. Many cases are probably not reported.

AGE INCIDENCE
Under 3 years.

CLINICAL POINTERS

1. High risk factors: (a) a thwarted or spoilt toddler; (b) known sibling jealousy; (c) parental audience.

2. The characteristic attack. The child holds his breath for a few seconds and then goes blue and limp for 30 to 60 seconds. Twitching sometimes occurs. Pallor may be marked on recovery.

3. The relationship to emotional upsets. The child may have been thwarted or frightened. An attack may follow an injury.

DIFFERENTIAL DIAGNOSIS
See major epilepsy, page 291.

MANAGEMENT OPTIONS

Prevention and established attacks: As for any toddler tantrum: (a) avoid making fuss; (b) reassure parents.

MIGRAINE

Classification: ICHPPC 346 (RCGP 1380)

AETIOLOGY
Uncertain. The aura of migraine is thought to be due to localised vasoconstriction in the cerebral cortex — on this theory the headache is caused by the reactionary vasodilatation. Heredity plays a part. Over-conscientious personalities are prone.

DIAGNOSTIC RANGE (rates per 1000 patients per year)
Personal: Suspected 16.0. Probable 4.8. *National*: 8.1 (Ref. 0.2). Many cases are not reported.

AGE INCIDENCE
The disease can start at any age between 5 and 45 years. Onset is common near to puberty.

SEX INCIDENCE
Women are affected more than men (4:1).

CLINICAL POINTERS

1. High risk factors: (a) family history; (b) diet — coffee, alcohol, nuts, cheese, chocolate, etc.; (c) puberty; (d) menstruation; (e) oral contraception; (f) hypoglycaemia, bright or flashing lights and fatigue may trigger attacks; (g) conscientious personality.

2. Repeated attacks (84%).

3. Transient aura (48%). Visual aura consist of blurring of vision, scotoma, flashes of light and fortification spectra. Less commonly abdominal pain or numbness of tongue, face or a limb occurs. Occasionally there may be a transient paralysis.

4. The headache (100%) is severe and starts as the aura subsides. It may be hemicranial and last for 2 to 24 hours. Occasionally it persists for several days. It is aggravated by quick movements or lowering the head.

5. Photophobia (20%).

6. Vomiting and nausea (54%) are associated with the headache.

7. A transient polyuria is often reported after the attack.

DURATION

The disease persists with remissions throughout middle life. It may subside after the age of 55 years.

COMPLICATIONS

None.

MISLEADING FEATURES AND PITFALLS

1. The early symptoms of cerebral tumours, disseminated sclerosis and hypertension may be labelled migraine.

2. The patient may awake with an attack of headache — the aura is then not noticed.

DIFFERENTIAL DIAGNOSIS

Diseases that may be confused with migraine:

Tension headache

Similar features: recurring episodes of headache; middle-age groups; emotional factors.

Distinguishing features: aura absent; headache central, vaguely described and not incapacitating; nausea uncommon; duration of headache variable.

NOTE: The two conditions may be present together.

Premenstrual headache

Similar feature: attacks of headache related to periods.

Distinguishing feature: may be a simple tension headache but often difficult to differentiate from migraine.

Refractive errors

Similar feature: headache in adolescents.

Distinguishing feature: definite relationship with use of eyes, reading, television, cinema, etc.

Acute sinusitis
Similar feature: · recurring episodes of headache, sometimes hemicranial.

Distinguishing features: history of cold or nasal discharge (often bloodstained); tenderness over affected sinus; dullness on transillumination; frontal sinus headache may start at a fixed time each day.

Disseminated sclerosis
Similar feature: transient attacks in young adults which suggest a CNS lesion; headache.

Distinguishing features: occasionally the early recurrences of MS (p. 284) may be ascribed to migraine; eye signs, muscle weakness, etc. last several days; headache is not marked; evidence of other CNS lesions common.

Hypertension
Similar feature: attacks of headache.

Distinguishing features: elderly patients; raised blood pressure; retinitis.

MANAGEMENT OPTIONS

Prevention of attack: Avoid high risk trigger factors where possible.

Established attacks: (a) analgesics — BNF 4.7.1; (b) antimigraine drugs — BNF 4.7.4. (Ref. 0.1) (Note: These may have to be stopped in pregnancy); (c) satisfactory treatment often difficult and patient education essential (Ref. 0.3) and Migraine Trust (Ref: 13.7).

ABDOMINAL MIGRAINE

Children sometimes give a history of repeated attacks of abdominal pain followed by sickness and headache. This diagnosis should be made by exclusion.

PERIODIC SYNDROME

A disease of doubtful aetiology. Toddlers and children said to be affected. Symptoms are said to be recurring attacks of abdominal pain associated with vomiting, pallor, headache and possibly fever. If the disease is a specific entity, there is difficulty in distinguishing it from mesenteric adenitis, recurrent pyelitis, appendicitis and abdominal migraine. Family doctors are wise to leave such technically difficult diagnosis to hospital doctors who can watch children closely enough to exclude more serious causes of pain. The diagnosis was not used in our practice.

BELL'S PALSY

Classification: ICHPPC 355 (RCGP 1395)

AETIOLOGY
Uncertain. Probably follows a virus infection (Coxsackie B was isolated from one of our cases).

DIAGNOSTIC RANGE (rate per 1000 patients per year)
Personal: Suspected 0.8. Probable 0.8. *National*: 0.3 (Ref. 0.2).

CLINICAL POINTERS
Sudden onset of one sided complete (lower motor neurone) facial paralysis. Diagnosis is usually obvious.

DURATION
80% recover in 2 to 8 weeks.

COMPLICATIONS
Recurrences. Permanent paralysis.

MANAGEMENT OPTIONS
Established disease: (a) early steroids — effect doubtful; (b) early referral for assessment of extent of muscle recovery followed by muscle stimulation and physiotherapy.

BRACHIAL NEURALGIA (NEURITIS)

Classification: ICHPPC 355 (RCGP 4010)

AETIOLOGY
1. Defects in the lower cervical spine. Osteoarthritis and prolapsed intervertebral disc.

2. Thoracic outlet syndrome. The brachial plexus may be put under tension.

3. Pressure from space-occupying lesions inside the chest or spinal cord — rare.

DIAGNOSTIC RANGE (rate per 1000 patients per year)
Personal: Suspected 5.0. Probable 4.6. *National*: 0.8 (Ref. 0.2). [Practice experience: in a series of 33 consecutive cases 33% (11)

X-rays suggested osteoarthritis of the cervical spine alone; 15% (5) X-rays suggested a cervical rib; 43% (14) the X-rays were normal or the history did not warrant an X-ray.]

AGE INCIDENCE

Over 30 (93%).

SEX INCIDENCE

Women more than men (2 : 1).

CLINICAL POINTERS

1. High risk factors: (a) middle age; (b) presence of cervical rib; (c) heavy arm loads e.g. shopping bags, typewriters, lifting baby out of cot, etc.
2. Repeated attacks of stiffness or pain in neck or shoulder (54%).
3. Pain, tingling or numbness of finger or hand (54%).
4. The effect of posture (66%). Certain positions aggravate the symptoms, e.g. pain is worse in bed.
5. Weakness of hand grip.
6. Evidence of muscle wasting, sensory loss and muscle fibrillation — late signs.
7. Local tenderness of lower cervical or upper dorsal region.

INVESTIGATIONS

X-ray of cervical spine and thoracic outlet.

DURATION

Self-limiting in most cases. [Practice experience in a series of 46 consecutive cases, 85% (41) were symptom-free after 1 to 4 weeks symptomatic treatment. The remainder cleared in 2 to 3 months with conservative treatment.]

COMPLICATIONS

Recurrences are common. (18% recurred within 2 years.) Gangrene of fingers with symptoms suggesting Raynaud's disease occasionally complicates a cervical rib.

MISLEADING FEATURES AND PITFALLS

A carcinoma at the lung apex occasionally causes a brachial neuralgia (Pancoast tumour).

DIFFERENTIAL DIAGNOSIS

Diseases that may be confused with brachial neuritis:

Rheumatoid arthritis
Similar features: stiffness and pain of hands associated with numbness of fingers; middle-aged women affected; remissions.

Distinguishing features: other joints affected; numbness does not follow any nerve distribution and is vaguely localised; little relationship with position; metacarpophalangeal joints are swollen; ESR raised; serological tests positive.

Carpal tunnel syndrome
Similar features: pain and numbness of hand; worse at night; wasting of thenar muscles; signs of median nerve compression; women commonly affected.

Distinguishing features: symptoms and signs localised to hand and wrists; tenderness between thenar and hypothenar regions.

Lesions in cerebral cortex
Similar feature: numbness and weakness of a hand.

Distinguishing features: pain is absent; other evidence of central nervous disease present.

Syringomyelia
Similar feature: numbness and wasting in hand.

Distinguishing features: very rare; temperature sense is lost; signs often bilateral.

MANAGEMENT OPTIONS

Prevention of attacks: (a) avoid high risk factors where possible; (b) cervical collar or surgery may be needed.

Established attack: (a) analgesics — BNF 4.7.1 (Ref. 0.1); (b) rest; (c) collar; (d) referral if intractable.

CARPAL TUNNEL SYNDROME

Classification: ICHPPC 355 (RCGP 1400)

AETIOLOGY

Compression of median nerve in carpal tunnel.

DIAGNOSTIC RANGE (rates per 1000 patients per year)

Personal: Suspected 0.9.

CLINICAL POINTERS

1. High risk factors: (a) rheumatoid arthritis; (b) myxoedema; (c) pregnancy; (d) rubella; (e) previous fractures; (f) obesity.

2. Tingling and pain of middle fingers — usually one hand only.

3. Symptoms worse at night. Pain never spreads above the wrist.
4. Muscle wasting (thenar); weakness of opposition and abduction of thumb are said to occur.

MISLEADING FEATURES AND PITFALLS

The carpal tunnel syndrome explains the patient's symptoms and for this reason an underlying myxoedema or arthritis is easily overlooked.

DIFFERENTIAL DIAGNOSIS

Differential diagnosis is from other causes of brachial neuralgia.

MANAGEMENT OPTIONS

Established disorder: (a) rest and splints; (b) analgesics — BNF 4.7.1 (Ref. 0.1); (c) diuretics — BNF 2.2; (d) local injection of steroids (Ref. 13.8) — BNF 10.1.2.2; (e) check for presence of high risk factors; (f) surgery — a last resort.

PROLAPSED INTERVERTEBRAL LUMBAR DISC

Classification: ICHPPC 7244 (RCGP 4005)

AETIOLOGY

Degeneration of the fibrous ring which surrounds the nucleus pulposus allows the disc to prolapse. The majority (70%) of patients relate the onset to trauma.

DIAGNOSTIC RANGE (rates per 1000 patients per year)

Personal: Suspected 36.4. Probable 17.7. *National*: 6.4. (Ref. 0.2).

AGE INCIDENCE

Adults liable.

SEX INCIDENCE

Males are said to be more affected than females. (In this practice the sexes were equally affected.)

CLINICAL POINTERS

1. High risk factors: (a) previous attacks; (b) manual work; (c) any unaccustomed bending or lifting (e.g. sport, garden or at work); (d) changes of lifestyle (or beds) as when travelling on holiday or moving house; (e) lifting or bending with back and not knees; (f) a sagging or soft mattress.
2. History of previous attack (55%). A definite diagnosis is often only possible when there has been more than one attack.
3. Relationship of onset to a specific incident of trauma or

bending (70%). The common story is that a patient bends down and is suddenly unable to straighten or move because of pain.

4. Back pain (85%). A severe shooting pain may immobilise the back in a certain position. Sometimes the pain remains as a dull ache.

5. Radiation of pain down leg (85%) is one of the most suggestive signs of a prolapsed disc. It is not always an early sign and may not develop until the second or third attack. The site of the disc protrusion will govern the distribution of the pain down the leg. An L5/S1 disc thus may cause radiation of pain to the ankle. Radiation of pain to buttocks or thigh suggests that the affected disc may be at a higher level.

6. Other characteristics of pain which suggest a disc lesion:

- The pain is eased in certain positions of rest and aggravated by bending movements (100%).
- The pain is aggravated by coughing (40%).
- The pain may be easier while the patient is sitting but is worse on getting up from this position (75%) — a common early feature that arises in few other diseases.
- The pain may be eased by walking about.

7. Straight leg raising test (65%). Passive raising of the straight leg in the prone position is limited to angles less than 60°. The test is not specific.

8. Compensatory scoliosis and flattening of the lumbosacral curve (35%) are late signs.

9. Signs and symptoms that suggest a nerve lesion and may develop after several attacks [55% (11 out of 20) patients followed for 5 years eventually developed evidence nerve lesion]. The site of the prolapse will govern the distribution of both pain and CNS signs.

- Tingling and numbness of feet or calf (15%).
- Area of anaesthesia over foot or calf (difficult to assess).
- Lost ankle or knee jerk (20%).
- Fibrillation of quadriceps or calf muscles.
- Wasting and weakness of quadriceps or calf muscles.

INVESTIGATIONS

X-ray of lumbar spine may show a decreased disc space at the site of the lesion.

DURATION

With rest and immobilisation most attacks settle within 1 to 6 weeks. Rapid relief can sometimes be achieved by manipulation.

COMPLICATIONS

Recurrences are common. [Practice experience: recurrences were noted in 75% (15 out of 20) suspected cases during a 5-year follow-up.]

MISLEADING FEATURES AND PITFALLS

1. A working man tells the doctor he has strained his back at work and wants a few days off. The absence of objective clinical evidence of an early disc lesion leads the doctor to the mistaken conclusion that the patient is malingering.

2. Secondary metastatic deposits in the lumbar spine may stimulate a disc lesion.

3. A spinal cord tumour may be overlooked.

DIFFERENTIAL DIAGNOSIS

Diseases that may be confused with prolapsed intervertebral lumbar disc:

Lumbar fibrositis

Similar feature: pain on movement in lumbar region.

Distinguishing features: previous attacks indefinite; pain does not radiate down leg; pain is not worse on coughing or on getting up after sitting; straight leg raising test usually negative; localised tenderness of lumbar muscles; CNS signs absent.

Tumour of spinal cord

Similar features: back pain with sciatic radiation; straight leg raising test positive; CNS signs of nerve lesion.

Distinguishing features: no previous attacks or trauma; symptoms gradually progressive; fibrillation, anaesthesia, muscle weakness and loss of reflexes appear early; wasting and CNS lesions are steadily progressive; lumbar puncture and myelography differentiates.

Collapsed lumbar vertebra

Similar features: back pain with sciatic radiation; straight leg raising test positive; CNS signs of nerve lesion.

Distinguishing features: elderly patient or previous history of cancer, tuberculosis or steroids may indicate diagnosis; local spinal tenderness marked; X-ray of spine differentiates.

MANAGEMENT OPTIONS

Prevention: (a) health education (especially those in high risk categories) regarding the right and wrong way to lift (Ref. 0.3); (b) hard (non-sag) bed; (c) regular exercise to strengthen and protect back.

Established attack: (a) rest; (b) analgesics — BNF 4.7.1 (Ref. 0.1); (c) manipulation; (d) splinting and lumbar jacket; (e) epidural and local injections; (f) surgery only as a last resort; (g) management often tedious and patient must be adequately prepared for this and appropriate preventive measures.

Table 15 Pointers that indicate some common lesions of the central nervous system

Lesion site	Pointers
Upper motor neurone lesion	Contralateral muscle weakness and sensory disturbance, clasp-knife muscle rigidity, tendon reflexes increased, clonus marked, skin reflexes absent, plantar response extensor, muscle wasting absent.
Lower motor neurone lesion	Muscle weakness, muscles flaccid, tendon reflexes absent or diminished, superficial reflexes unchanged (plantars flexor), muscle wasting marked
Frontal lobe	Personality changes, upper motor neurone lesion, speech defects
Parietal lobes	Upper motor neurone lesions, speech defects
Internal capsule	Hemiplegia
Temporal lobes	Optic radiations affected — quadrantic hemianopia, odd behaviour
Cerebellum	Signs are confined to side of lesion, hypotonia (i.e. tendon reflexes flattened), dysdiadokokinesia, poor muscle co-ordination, nystagmus on looking to side of lesion. Headaches from raised pressure arise early
Cerebellopontine angle tumour	Unilateral deafness and tinnitus for many years. Other localising signs arise late when operation may be impossible
Pituitary fossa	Bitemporal hemianopia, hormonal changes
Bulb and medulla	Difficulty with swallowing and speech

Table 16 Pointers that indicate abnormal neurological behaviour in neonates from brain damage

1. Apathy or poor movements
2. Floppiness
3. Hyperexcitability
4. Jitteriness or convulsions
5. Poor sucking
6. Shrill cry
7. Shallow, irregular respiration or apnoeic attacks

Table 17 Paralysis due to common peripheral nerve lesions

Peripheral nerve	Local lesion	Clinical pointers
Facial nerve	Bell's palsy	Unilateral weakness of all facial muscles
Radial nerve	Injury	Wrist drop, extensors of wrist and triceps weak or paralysed. Sensory loss radial side of hand
Median nerve	Carpal tunnel syndrome	Failure to oppose thumb or hold it in abducted position, lost sensation at tip of first and middle finger. (In above-elbow median nerve lesions hand grip may be weak)
Ulnar nerve	Brachial neuralgia; cervical rib syndrome; compression at elbow; injury	Failure to maintain adduction and abduction of fingers (from weakness of interossei). Sensory loss over ulnar side of hand
Sciatic nerve	Prolapsed lumbar disc at L5 S1 level	Lost ankle jerk, weak extension of ankle joint. Wasting of calf. Sensory loss of lower leg or foot variable

Table 18 Less common diseases of the nervous system

Disease and distinguishing clinical pointers	Suspected	Confirmed
Cerebral emboli (large) Left-sided heart disease and atrial fibrillation, sudden onset, hemiplegia, recurrences	0.2	—
Subarachnoid haemorrhage In young adults bleeding is from aneurysm, in older patients arteriosclerosis is responsible, sudden onset, severe headache, neck stiffness even when patient is unconscious, coma, lumbar puncture in hospital, (disorder must be distinguished from meningitis and diabetic coma)	0.3	0.1
Extradural and subdural haemorrhage See page 670 and 671	—	1 in 20 years
Hypertensive encephalopathy Late middle-aged patients, hypertension, retinitis, renal disease, cerebrovascular accidents, headaches	—	1 in 10 years
Symptomatic epilepsy History of injury, meningitis or space-occupying lesion; Jacksonian epilepsy	0.2	0.1
Petit mal Onset in childhood, repeated transient attacks of being vacant (child does not answer questions), odd behaviour after attacks. Grand mal often associated.	0.2	0.1
Narcolepsy Patient falls asleep or loses ability to move if upset or bored	—	2 in 10 years

Table 18 cont'd

Disease and distinguishing clinical pointers	Suspected	Confirmed
Carpo-pedal spasm Tingling and flexion of fingers at metacarpo-phalangeal joint occurs, tetany, excessive vomiting, uraemia or hysterical over-breathing are usually responsible (see hyperventilation p. 250)	—	3 in 10 years
Motor neurone disease Middle-aged patients, steady progression, muscle weakness and wasting, excessive muscle fasciculation, upper motor neurone lesions may develop Onset with bulbar lesions (dysarthria and dysphagia) has especially bad prognosis	—	2 in 10 years
Trigeminal neuralgia Middle-aged women liable, attacks of severe unilateral facial pain, trigger stimulus	0.5	0.1
Acute infective polyneuritis Symmetrical muscle weakness and paraesthesia that develops after an influenzal illness. CSF may show characteristic changes.	—	1 in 10 years
Pink disease Infants under 2 years, disease now never encountered since mercury has been removed from teething powders	—	2 in 20 years
Meralgia paraesthetica Lateral cutaneous nerve of thigh is pinched.	—	1 in 10 years
Myasthenia gravis May cause diplopia, dysarthria, dysphagia or difficulty in chewing and is therefore easily confused with cerebral tumour and other CNS diseases.	—	1 in 10 years

14

Diseases of the eye

Please read the introduction for explanation of figures and analyses.

All eye complaints that cannot be satisfactorily explained and treated are referred for a consultant ophthalmic opinion.

SIMPLE CONJUNCTIVITIS (PINK EYE)

Classification: ICHPPC 3720 (RCGP 1570)

AETIOLOGY
Bacterial.

MODE OF SPREAD
Close contact.

DIAGNOSTIC RANGE (rates per 1000 patients per year)
Personal: Suspected 32.0, Probable 21.3. *National*: 19.5 (Ref 0.2).

AGE INCIDENCE
All ages; babies and the elderly are especially prone (Fig. 21).

CLINICAL POINTERS (See Table 19)

1. High risk factors: (a) contacts; (b) schools and institutions.
2. Conjunctival injection (100%). Often unilateral.
3. Pain (100%). Irritation is followed by a painful gritty sensation.
4. Discharge is at first watery then purulent. The lids may stick together during sleep.
5. Associated disorders include chronic blepharitis, seborrhoea and acne rosacea.

DURATION
3 to 7 days. Local antibiotics usually clear the infection.

COMPLICATIONS
Recurrences. [Practice experience: 16% (4 out of 25) reported recurrences within 3 years.]

Table 19 Differential diagnosis of the pink or red eye

	Conjunctivitis	Iritis	Glaucoma	Keratitis (Foreign body, Corneal abrasion)
Discharge	Marked	None	None	Slight or none
Photophobia	None	Marked	Slight	Slight
Pain	Slight	Slight to marked	Marked	Marked
Visual acuity	Normal	Reduced	Reduced	Varies with the site of the lesion
Pupil	Normal	Smaller or same	Large, fixed	Same or smaller

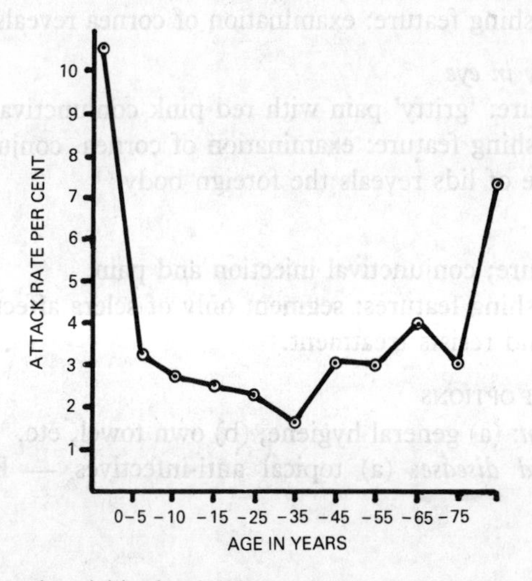

Fig. 21 Acute conjunctivitis. Age incidence of 262 consecutive cases in 3 years.

MISLEADING FEATURES AND PITFALLS

1. Failure to distinguish acute conjunctivitis from acute iritis, glaucoma, corneal ulceration and persistent foreign body.

2. Failure to realise that recurrent conjunctivitis may have an allergic origin.

DIFFERENTIAL DIAGNOSIS (See also Table 19)

Diseases that may be confused with acute conjunctivitis:

Allergic conjunctivitis

Similar feature: recurrent attacks of conjunctival injection.

Distinguishing features: other allergic complaints are commonly associated — asthma, allergic rhinitis and hay fever, response to antihistamines.

Acute iritis and acute glaucoma
Similar feature: conjunctival injection and pain in affected eye.

Distinguishing features: Acute iritis — pain is severe; conjunctival injection is maximal near iris; iris may be irregular and reacts sluggishly. Acute glaucoma — pain is severe; conjunctival injection maximal near iris; coloured haloes round light noted by patient; vision may be dimmed; pupil may be dilated or irregular with sluggish reaction; cupping of optic disc; increased tension in eyeball; immediate ophthalmic opinion indicated.

Corneal ulcer
Similar features: conjunctival injection; pain and discharge.

Distinguishing feature: examination of cornea reveals grey ulcer.

Foreign body in eye
Similar feature: 'gritty' pain with red pink conjunctiva.

Distinguishing feature: examination of cornea, conjunctivae and undersurface of lids reveals the foreign body.

Episcleritis
Similar feature; conjunctival injection and pain.

Distinguishing features: segment only of sclera affected; persists for weeks and resists treatment.

MANAGEMENT OPTIONS

Prevention: (a) general hygiene; (b) own towel, etc.

Established disease: (a) topical anti-infectives — BNF 11.3.1 (Ref. 0.1)

BLEPHARITIS

Classification: ICHPPC 3730 (RCGP 1580)

AETIOLOGY
The disease is probably a localised form of seborrhoea.

DIAGNOSTIC RANGE (rates per 1000 patients per year)
Personal: Suspected 10.6, Probable 4.9. *National*: 3.8 (Ref 0.2). Many cases are probably not reported to the doctor.

AGE INCIDENCE
All ages liable (Fig. 22).

CLINICAL POINTERS

1. High risk factors: (a) seborrhoea (acne, dandruff etc.); (b) previous attack.

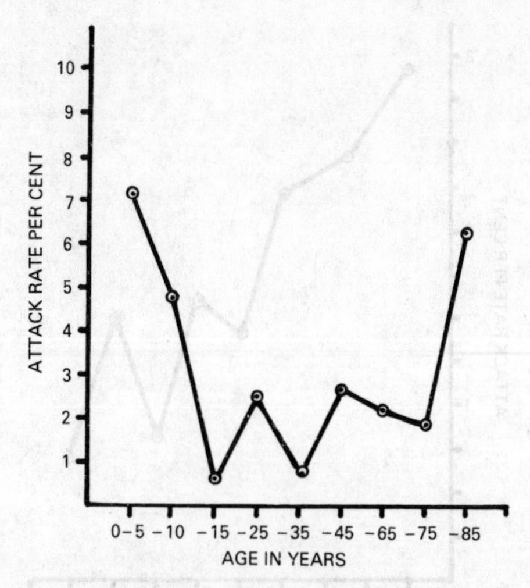

Fig. 22 Blepharitis. Age incidence of 106 consecutive cases in 1 year.

2. Redness of the eyelids (100%).
3. Desquamation. The scales, like those of seborrhoea, are removed by rubbing.
4. Irritation is common.

DURATION

Indefinite if not treated.

MANAGEMENT OPTIONS

Prevention: Treat high risk factors.

Established disease: (a) treat Seborrhoea and dandruff, (b) Topical anti-infective — BNF 11.3.1 (Ref 0.1).

STYES (HORDEOLUM)

Classification: ICHPPC 3730 (RCGP 1585)

AETIOLOGY

Staphylococcus pyogenes. Boils, seborrhoea and chronic blepharitis are often associated.

MODE OF SPREAD

1. From staphylococcal lesions in other parts of the body: axillae, fingernails, auditory meati, perineum, etc.
2. From the patient's nose.
3. From lesions in household contacts.

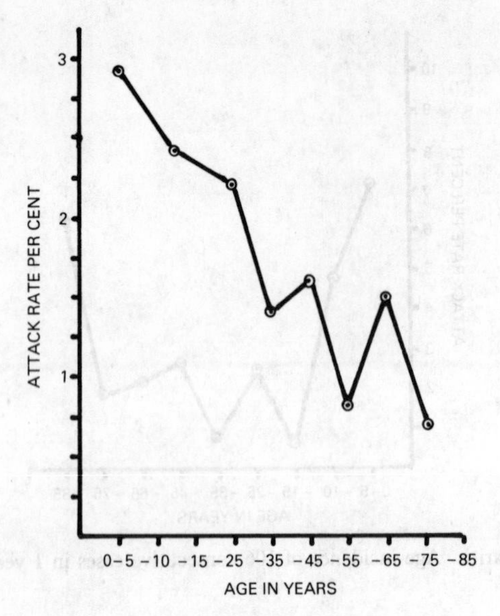

Fig. 23 Styes. Age incidence curve of 147 consecutive cases in 3 years.

DIAGNOSTIC RANGE (rates per 1000 patients per year)
Personal: Probable 18.8. *National*: 3.1 (Ref. 0.2). The diagnosis was rarely in doubt. Many cases are never reported.

AGE INCIDENCE
The incidence decreases steadily with age (Fig. 23).

CLINICAL POINTERS
1. High risk factors: (a) Other staphylococcal infections (b) Household contacts (c) Staphylococcal reservoirs in patient or others in household. Reservoirs are usually nasal but occasionally axillary or vaginal. (d) Recent stay in hospital ward.
2. Irritation of the lid. An early sign.
3. Redness, pain and swelling of the affected lid.
4. The boil.
5. Periorbital oedema.

DURATION
4 to 7 days.

COMPLICATIONS
Recurrences are common. Recurrent styes are occasionally associated with diabetes mellitus. Infection of others in household.

MISLEADING FEATURES AND PITFALLS
Periorbital oedema may appear early and obscure the local lesion.

MANAGEMENT OPTIONS
Prevention involves treating the whole household (see also Boils p. 592). This is difficult, tedious and rarely justified unless infections are annoying and entrenched: (a) nasal swabs are taken from all household members; (b) carriers treated with Naseptin — BNF 12.2.3 (Ref. 0.1); (c) all household members must comply with general hygenic measures.
Established disorder: (a) local bathing; (b) eye shade and dressing; (c) Naseptin — BNF 12.2.3, to prevent recurrences.

CORNEAL ULCERATION

Classification: ICHPPC 378 (RCGP 1560)

AETIOLOGY
Trauma or associated lesions in the surrounding skin. Contact lenses, especially plastic, predispose. Herpes Simplex Virus is often involved.

DIAGNOSTIC RANGE (rates per 1000 patients per year)
Personal: Suspected 1.1, Probable 0.4. *National*: 0.7 (Ref. 0.2).

CLINICAL POINTERS
1. High risk factors (as for Herpes Simplex, see p. 162): (a) unaccustomed, often reflected, sunlight from snow or sea; (b) trauma; (c) ophthalmic shingles; (d) Herpes Simplex infections elsewhere.
2. The ulcer appears as a pearly grey opacity on the cornea.
3. Associated conjunctivitis is common.
4. Pain is sometimes marked.
5. Associated lesions in surrounding skin, e.g. blepharitis, shingles, herpes simplex, acne rosacea, measles, etc.
6. A drop of fluorescein will outline a doubtful ulcer.
7. Photophobia.

DURATION
With treatment most corneal ulcers heal in a few days.

COMPLICATIONS
Scarring of the cornea is unlikely unless the ulcer is allowed to persist or the original damage to the cornea is so great that scarring is inevitable. Recurrences are common. Perforation can occur.

MISLEADING FEATURES AND PITFALLS

1. A corneal ulcer may be overlooked if the cornea of patients with acute conjunctivitis is not examined.

2. Eye drops containing steroids are used on a corneal ulcer of virus origin.

DIFFERENTIAL DIAGNOSIS

See Table 19

MANAGEMENT OPTIONS

Prevention: Goggles to protect from sun, chemicals, welding, flashes or power tools. Note: Protection at home is as important as at work.

Established ulcer: (a) rest eye with shade; (b) analgesics — BNF 4.7 (Ref. 0.1); (c) topical antivirals — BNF 11.3.1 (incl. acyclovir); (d) refer if no rapid improvement.

ACUTE IRITIS AND IRIDOCYCLITIS

Classification: ICHPPC 378 (RCGP 1530)

DIAGNOSTIC RANGE (rates per 1000 patients per year)

Personal: Suspected 0.4, Probable 0.3. *National* 0.5 (Ref. 0.2).

CLINICAL POINTERS

1. Severe pain in the affected eye.

2. Conjunctival injection maximal in the limbic area adjacent to the iris which appears pink and slightly swollen.

3. Irregular pupil with a sluggish reaction (not always present).

DIFFERENTIAL DIAGNOSIS

See Table 19.

MANAGEMENT OPTIONS

Refer if suspected.

REFRACTIVE ERRORS

Classification: ICHPPC 367 (RCGP 1545)

AETIOLOGY

The types and causes of refractive errors are numerous and most family doctors are content to leave elucidation and treatment to ophthalmologists and reliable opticians. The two refractive errors most commonly encountered are myopia (short sight) and presbyopia (inability to accommodate, that increases steadily with age).

DIAGNOSTIC RANGE (rates per 1000 patients per year)
Personal: Suspected 12.5, Proven 10.4. *National*: 6.9 (These figures represent the number of patients that a family doctor referred to ophthalmologists or opticians and does not indicate the number of people who wore glasses.)

AGE INCIDENCE
Refractive errors are usually not apparent until after the age of 4 years. The incidence then steadily increases until the age of 25. Myopia is common in the early decades. After 45 presbyopia becomes apparent.

CLINICAL POINTERS
1. High risk factors — family history of refractive errors.
2. Blurring of vision or difficulty with focusing.
3. Eye ache — often related to close work, watching the cinema or television.
4. Refractive errors can cause headache.
5. Inability to read small print suggests presbyopia.

CLINICAL POINTERS IN YOUNG CHILDREN
1. Holding books close to eyes.
2. Squints are often associated with refractive errors.

INVESTIGATIONS
1. Refraction.
2. Referral to a reliable optician for patients over 10 years.
3. Referral to ophthalmologist when there is doubt or for children under 10 years.

DURATION
Most refractive errors are permanent: some patients manage without glasses for long periods.

COMPLICATIONS
Detachment of retina may occur in short-sighted patients.

MISLEADING FEATURES AND PITFALLS
Overenthusiastic opticians occasionally overprescribe glasses

DIFFERENTIAL DIAGNOSIS.
Diseases that may be confused with refractive error:

Tension headache
Similar feature: headache related to close work.
Distinguishing features: differentiation often difficult; referral to reliable optician or ophthalmologist may be needed.

Migraine
Similar feature: headache associated with history of blurred vision.
Distinguishing features: time relationship of eye symptoms and headache; paroxysmal nature of attacks.

Acute glaucoma
Similar feature: eye ache and headache associated with visual disturbances.
Distinguishing features: headache is severe and pain is marked; haloes seen around objects; ocular tension raised; cupping of optic disc; immediate ophthalmic opinion indicated.

Chronic glaucoma
Similar features: deterioration of vision in the elderly; eye ache.
Distinguishing features: contracted visual fields; marked cupping of optic discs; ophthalmic opinion indicated.

MANAGEMENT OPTIONS
Referral.

SQUINT (STRABISMUS)

Classification: ICHPPC 378 (RCGP 1610)

AETIOLOGY
Weakness or paralysis of one or more of the external ocular muscles which may be congenital or hereditary or follow one of the infectious fevers such as measles. Refractive errors also play a part.

DIAGNOSTIC RANGE (rates per 1000 patients per year)
Personal: Suspected 4.3, Proven 1.5. *National*: 1.2 (Ref. 0.2).

AGE INCIDENCE
The majority (90%) of squints are reported between 1 and 7 years.

CLINICAL POINTERS
Divergence or convergence of the eyes may be obvious or may only occur when the child is tired or ill.

INVESTIGATIONS
An ophthalmic opinion is always indicated. Cover tests are helpful. Face to face: covering good eye leads to movement of squinting eye.

DURATION
Most squints can be cured if they are not severe and if treatment is instituted before the age of 7 years.

COMPLICATIONS

If the squint is inadequately treated, or if it is severe the image from the weak eye is suppressed (amblyopia). Monocular vision results.

MISLEADING FEATURES AND PITFALLS

1. Transient squints are observed in many normal infants in the first weeks of life before they have learned to accommodate.

2. Asymmetry of the nasal epicanthic fold may wrongly suggest a squint in a baby.

3. Occasionally a squint (or diplopia) follows an organic lesion of the central nervous system, space-occupying lesion or myasthenia gravis. Such lesions are easily overlooked.

MANAGEMENT OPTIONS

Referral for diagnosis and treatment (no child is too young if squint is suspected). Close co-operation between specialist, orthoptist, family doctor and parents for: (a) glasses or contact lenses; (b) exercises, plus occluding one eye to prevent ambliopia; (c) surgery.

CATARACT

Classification: ICHPPC 366 (RCGP 1540)

AETIOLOGY

Old age. Diabetes and injury may play a part.
Congenital cataract occurs.

DIAGNOSTIC RANGE (rates per 1000 patients per year)

Personal: Suspected 4.1, Probable 3.4. *National*: 1.2 (Ref. 0.2).

AGE INCIDENCE

The majority (75%) are over 70 years.

SEX INCIDENCE

Females affected more than males (3:1 — the result possibly of increased longevity in women)

CLINICAL POINTERS

1. High risk groups: (a) the elderly; (b) diabetics.

2. Failing vision (90%). The patient usually asks for fresh glasses.

3. Haziness of lens (100%). A hazy opacity can be seen when a light is focused on the lens. Characteristic radial opacities become more obvious if the pupil is dilated with homatropine.

4. The optic fundi may be obscured.

DURATION
Without treatment, the disease progresses steadily.

COMPLICATIONS
Blindness.

MISLEADING FEATURES AND PITFALLS

1. A cataract may mask other more serious diseases of optic fundus, e.g. retinitis or glaucoma.

2. Associated diabetes may be overlooked.

MANAGEMENT OPTIONS

Prevention: early diagnosis and management of high risk groups.

Established disease: referral for assessment and surgery if severe.

GLAUCOMA

Classification: ICHPPC 365 (RCGP 1535)

There is a profusion of terminology and the labels *primary* and *congestive* are best avoided. Raised intraocular pressure follows disturbances in the circulation of the aqueous fluid through the uveal tract. Acute or chronic forms of glaucoma may develop.

ACUTE (NARROW ANGLE) GLAUCOMA

Classification: ICHPPC 365 (RCGP 1535)

DIAGNOSTIC RANGE (rates per 1000 patients per year)
Personal: Suspected 0.9, Probable 0.3

AGE INCIDENCE
Adults are liable. Women of middle age are especially liable.

CLINICAL POINTERS

1. High risk factors: (a) premonitary attacks often in evening and passing off with sleep; (b) hypermetropic (short eyeball) eyes; (c) pupillary dilators.

2. Onset is moderately sudden, but two to three days may elapse before the patient seeks medical attention. A history of previous attacks is common. Angle closure may be precipitated by pupillary dilatation.

3. Pain is felt in the eye or as a severe headache over the eye and is often intense.

4. Coloured haloes are noticed around lights.

5. Conjunctivitis. Congestion may be noted around the pupil (limbus).

6. Vision is dimmed or obscured.

7. Vomiting is said to occur with acute attacks.

8. Fixed pupil may be dilated or irregular.

9. Signs which the family doctor may find difficult to assess, include:

- Increased intraocular tension.
- Cupping of the optic disc — the retinal vessels are seen rounding the rim of the enlarged cup, the rim is just inside the edge of the disc. Vessels are seen to be pulled away from macula area.
- Haziness of the cornea.

DURATION

Untreated, the disease occasionally remits. The prognosis with treatment is moderately good.

COMPLICATIONS

Blindness or gradual loss of vision.

MISLEADING FEATURES AND PITFALLS

1. Failure to distinguish between acute conjunctivitis and glaucoma.

2. Failure to distinguish between glaucoma and migraine.

3. Eye drops given to dilate the pupil aggravate the condition and must be avoided.

DIFFERENTIAL DIAGNOSIS (See also Table 19)

Diseases that may be confused with acute glaucoma:

Migraine

Similar features: severe hemicranial headache; vomiting; visual phenomenon.

Distinguishing features: visual phenomena precede headache; onset under 30; local eye signs absent. Pain improves with sleep.

Acute conjunctivitis

Similar features: pain in eye; conjunctival injection; visual disturbance.

Distinguishing features: pain rarely severe; local pupil changes absent; uniform injection; visual disturbance is from flecks of discharge.

Acute iritis and iridocyclitis
Similar features: severe pain in eye; local pupil changes; injection of conjunctiva around the pupil.

Distinguishing features: distinction may be difficult; immediate ophthalmic opinion indicated.

MANAGEMENT OPTIONS

Prevention: High index of suspicion in high risk cases.

Suspected disease: immediate referral. Avoid mydriatics, i.e. pupil dilators.

CHRONIC (SIMPLE) GLAUCOMA

Classification: ICHPPC 365 (RCGP 1535)

DIAGNOSTIC RANGE (rates per 1000 patients per year)
Personal: Probable 0.2. *National*: This type of glaucoma is said to occur in 2 per cent of all patients over 40.

AGE INCIDENCE
The elderly. It is thought that there is a symptomless period of 10 to 25 years while the disease is developing.

CLINICAL POINTERS

1. High risk factors: heredity; siblings and children on reaching 40 should be checked — reveals 10% of positives.

2. Onset insidious. Several members of a family are often affected.

3. Gradual failure of vision, especially of the peripheral visual fields.

4. Frequent requests for a change of glasses.

5. 'Cupping' of the optic nerve. The retinal vessels are seen to descend into the enlarged cup near the disc edge.

INVESTIGATIONS
Estimation of visual fields by confrontation. Diagnosis often very difficult.

Tests of tension are difficult to interpret unless the doctor has considerable practice.

DURATION
The disease is steadily progressive unless it is treated.

COMPLICATIONS
Blindness.

MANAGEMENT OPTIONS

Prevention: (a) routine case finding in patients with a positive family history; (b) routine case finding or screening of the elderly with tonometry and visual fields yields the occasional early case.

Established disease: referral for (a) drug therapy; (b) regular monitoring; (c) possible surgery.

RETINAL DETACHMENT

Classification: ICHPPC 378 (RCGP 1500)

DIAGNOSTIC RANGE (rates per 1000 patients per year)

Personal: Probable 0.2. The diagnosis was confirmed by a specialist in every case.

CLINICAL POINTERS

1. High risk factors: (a) myopia (especially high degrees); (b) trauma — often slight — to affected eye; (c) previous eye operations; (d) previous detachments.
2. The symptoms refer to one eye only.
3. Scotoma. A grey cloud, a black hair or spot is noticed over part of one visual field.
4. Visual outlines are blurred and may appear double or distorted.
5. Flashes of light may be noticed in the early stages.
6. Fundal examination reveals detachment. A portion of the retina looks grey or white. The retinal arteries on the surface appear black or grey. Areas of the fundus may be obscured by the detached portion. Folds of pale detached retina or even a torn hole may occasionally be seen.

DURATION

Progressive if treatment is not given.

COMPLICATIONS

Blindness.

MISLEADING FEATURES AND PITFALLS

1. The blurred visual outline may be described by the patient as double vision.
2. Both patient and doctor may fail to realise the urgency of the disorder because onset is painless and visual symptoms often slight.

MANAGEMENT OPTIONS

Prevention of serious effects: (a) high index of suspicion especially in high risk groups; (b) early referral of suspicious cases; (c) cryotherapy and lasers may prevent recurrent further separation.

Suspected detachments: (a) early referral for diagnostic confirmation and treatment to oppose separated layers — this includes rest, local pressure, surgery, lasers and cryotherapy; (b) careful follow up.

VITREOUS OPACITIES (FLOATERS)

Classification: ICHPPC 378 (RCGP 1620)

AETIOLOGY

Small haemorrhages into the vitreous are responsible in some cases. Often there is no obvious cause.

DIAGNOSTIC RANGE (rates per 1000 patients per year)

Personal: Probable 1.5. Many cases are never reported.

CLINICAL POINTERS

1. Floating visual opacities that are affected by posture.
2. A mobile shadow is sometimes seen with the ophthalmoscope.

INVESTIGATIONS

An ophthalmic opinion is occasionally indicated.

SUBCONJUNCTIVAL HAEMORRHAGE

Classification: ICHPPC 378 (RCGP 1575)

A wedge of the conjunctiva becomes bright red, either spontaneously or as a result of coughing or trauma. The haemorrhage is harmless and may spread over the whole conjunctiva. The area gradually goes brown and returns to normal in about 6 weeks. No treatment is indicated.

DIAGNOSTIC RANGE (rates per 1000 patients per year)

Personal: Probable 1.8. The diagnosis was rarely in doubt.

TARSAL AND MEIBOMIAN CYSTS

Classification: ICHPPC 3730 (RCGP 1585)

Small painless cysts that grow in the eyelids and form a chronic swelling that can be seen by everting the lid and treated if necessary by excision under local.

DIAGNOSTIC INCIDENCE (rates per 1000 patients per year)
Personal: Probable 1.5. Many cases are probably not reported because the cysts burst and cure themselves.

Table 20 Less common diseases of the eye

Disease and distinguishing clinical pointers	Incidence per 1000 patients per year Suspected	Confirmed
Chronic iridocyclitis Chronic progressive loss of vision, cause uncertain	—	1 in 10 years
Episcleritis Localised segment of conjunctivitis surrounds a small nodule (1 to 3 mm diam.) on sclera; lesion persists for several weeks, even months; recurrences occur.	0.4	—
Vascular accidents in the eye Sudden monocular loss of vision, emboli of central artery leave the fundus pale and bloodless, thrombosis of central vein causes gross venous congestion and haemorrhages	0.1	0.1
Subhyaloid and vitreous haemorrhages Occasionally cause blurring of vision in one eye which clears slowly according to the size. The fundal appearances are usually striking and may be out of proportion to the symptoms. The lesion is recognised because the retinal vessels, disc edges, etc. are obscured by it.	0	0
Blocked lacrymal ducts Constant tears (epiphora) cause periorbital excoriation.	0.3	0.3

15

Diseases of the ear and mastoid processes

Please read the introduction for explanation of figures and analyses.

OTITIS EXTERNA

Classification: ICHPPC 3801 (RCGP 1700)

An annoying but harmless superficial inflammation of the skin of the external auditory meatus.

AETIOLOGY

Uncertain. *Staphylococcus aureus* is common but *Streptococcus pyogenes*, *Proteus* and other organisms may be cultured.

AGE INCIDENCE

All ages. Babies are especially liable.

DIAGNOSTIC RANGE (rates per 1000 patients per year)

Personal: Suspected 18.4, Probable 12.3, *National* 8.8 (Ref. 0.2).

CLINICAL POINTERS

1. High risk factors: (a) seborrhoea; (b) chronic discharging otitis; (c) atopic eczema; (d) local irritants; (e) babies.
2. Debris or frank discharge (100%) — not always noted by the patient. Crusts of pale dry debris appear. Sometimes the debris is mixed with wax, giving the latter an unhealthy grey colour.
3. Irritation of the external auditory meatus (45%).
4. Deafness (35%) occurs when the debris blocks the meatus.
5. Pain (50%) is usually slight.

INVESTIGATIONS

Bacterial investigation is rarely necessary.

DURATION

The disease tends to recur or persists indefinitely. [Practice experience: 60% (12 out of 20 consecutive cases) recurred within 3 years.].

COMPLICATIONS

Boils in the external auditory meatus are a common and extremely painful complication.

MISLEADING FEATURES AND PITFALLS

Syringing the ears of patients with otitis externa may aggravate the symptoms or trigger off an underlying chronic otitis media.

DIFFERENTIAL DIAGNOSIS

Differentiation from chronic suppurative otitis media is occasionally difficult.

MANAGEMENT OPTIONS

Established disease: (a) deal with high risk trigger factors; (b) protective creams; (c) topical clioquinol with or without HCN — BNF 12.1.1 (Ref. 0.1). (d) astringents — aluminium acetate — BNF 12.1.1.

ACUTE OTITIS MEDIA

Classification: ICHPCC 3820 (RCGP 1710)

AETIOLOGY

1. Bacterial. *Streptococcus pyogenes* is the commonest infecting organism. It probably penetrates the middle ear from the throat via the Eustachian tube. [Practice experience: in a series of 91 consecutive cases of acute otitis media. *Strep. pyogenes* was cultured from the throat in 46% (42). This figure lies about half way between the normal throat carriage rates for *Strep. pyogenes* (5 to 15%) and the *Strep. pyogenes* carriage rate in acute exudative tonsillitis (72% in this practice). It would seem that other factors as well as the bacteria in the throat cause acute otitis media.]

2. Mechanical. Nose blowing and coughing probably help to drive the bacteria up the Eustachian tube from the throat. The following evidence bears this out:

- Acute otitis media complicates a wide variety of upper respiratory diseases, e.g. colds, coughs, measles and whooping-cough.
- Babies and children with their short Eustachian tubes are especially prone to acute otitis media (see age incidence chart).
- [Practice experience: in a series of 91 consecutive cases of acute otitis media 75% (69) had a nasal cold or cough prior to the otitis media.]

3. Age (Fig. 24). Acute otitis media is mainly a disease of the first 6 years of life.

4. Season. The prevalence of coughs and colds in the winter probably accounts for the increased incidence of otitis media at this time (Fig. 25). Summer infections are often associated with bathing and diving.

DIAGNOSTIC RANGE (rates per 1000 patients per year)
Personal: Suspected 66.2, Probable 43.8, *National*: 33.8 (Ref. 0.2).

AGE INCIDENCE
See Figure 24. There are peaks in the first and sixth years.

CLINICAL POINTERS
1. High risk factors: (a) previous attacks; (b) presence of a cough or cold; (c) mechanical pressure factors such as injury, blast, diving, flying.

2. Earache (90%). Babies may pull the affected ear. Occasionally a young child or toddler may develop an acute otitis without any complaint of earache.

3. Redness of the drum (70%) is probably always present, but the drum may be obscured by wax or discharge. At first the rim of the drum and handle of the malleus are red. Gradually the whole drum becomes acutely inflamed and may bulge outwards as fluid collects in the middle ear. If the drum perforates or pressure in the middle ear relaxes, the drum becomes dusky red, soggy and wrinkled with grey patches of desquamation.

4. Discharge (33%) appears after a few hours of pain. A history that the pain disappears with the onset of discharge is common. Patients occasionally present with a painless discharge; recurrences are more likely in such cases.

5. Fever is common and may rise rapidly to comparatively high levels (39.5°C). In young children the fever may be associated with vomiting.

6. Recurrent attacks. One attack predisposes a child to further attacks but this tendency disappears as the child grows and does not necessarily increase the likelihood of chronic suppurative otitis.

INVESTIGATIONS
When there is discharge a swab is cultured for organisms and sensitivity to antibiotics.

DURATION
The disease lasts for 1 to 4 days. If perforation occurs the discharge may persist. Treatment with antibiotics may reduced the duration and likelihood of perforation.

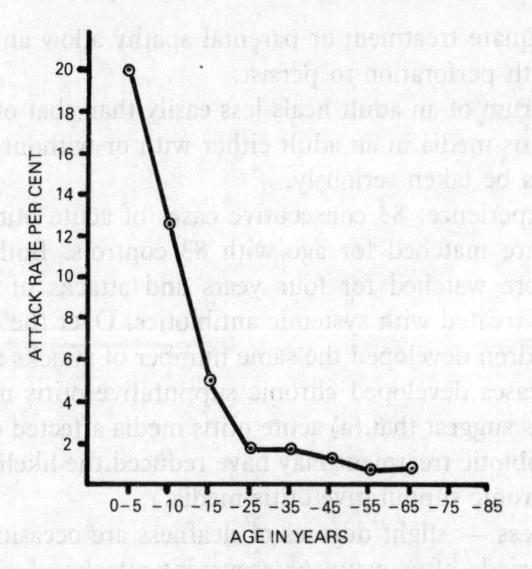

Fig. 24 Acute otitis media. Age incidence of 175 consecutive cases in 1 year.

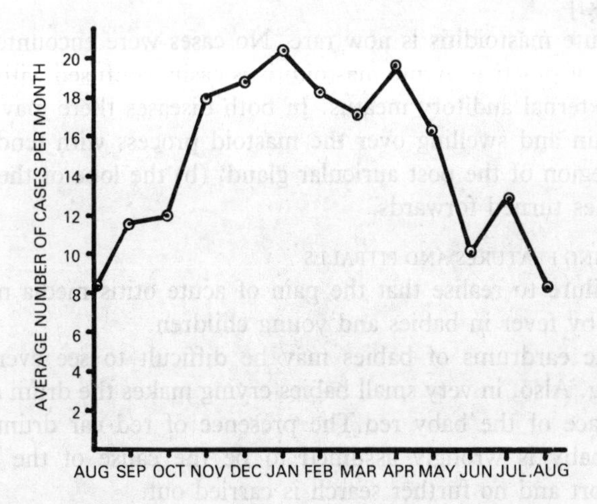

Fig. 25 Acute otitis media. Seasonal incidence of 731 consecutive cases reported over 4 years.

COMPLICATIONS

1. Chronic suppurative otitis media. The following factors are probably responsible for the development of this disease:

- Perforation of the drum allows a multitude of bacteria to replace the original infecting organism.

- Inadequate treatment or parental apathy allow an acute otitis media with perforation to persist.
- The drum of an adult heals less easily than that of a child.

Acute otitis media in an adult either with or without perforation must always be taken seriously.

(Practice experience: 83 consecutive cases of acute otitis media in children were matched for age with 83 controls. Both groups of children were watched for four years and attacks of acute otitis media were treated with systemic antibiotics. Over the 4 years, the control children developed the same number of attacks as the index cases. No cases developed chronic suppurative otitis media. These observations suggest that (a) acute otitis media affected every child, (b) that antibiotic treatment may have reduced the likelihood of developing chronic suppurative otitis media.)

2. Deafness — slight degrees of deafness are occasionally noted for long periods after acute or recurrent attacks of otitis media. [Practice experience: clinical deafness assessed by whisper tests was noted in 6% (5 out of 83 patients) who were tested 6 months after an attack.]

3. Acute mastoiditis is now rare. No cases were encountered in 20 years of practice. Acute mastoiditis is easily confused with a boil in the external auditory meatus. In both diseases there may be (a) acute pain and swelling over the mastoid process with tenderness in the region of the post auricular gland, (b) the lobe of the ear is sometimes turned forwards.

MISLEADING FEATURES AND PITFALLS

1. Failure to realise that the pain of acute otitis media may be masked by fever in babies and young children.

2. The eardrums of babies may be difficult to see even after cleansing. Also, in very small babies crying makes the drum as well as the face of the baby red. The presence of red ear drums in a crying baby is wrongly assumed to be the cause of the baby's discomfort and no further search is carried out.

DIFFERENTIAL DIAGNOSIS

Diseases that may be confused with acute otitis media:

Acute otitis externa

Similar feature: pain and discharge in ear.

Distinguishing features: adults mainly affected; history of previous irritation; external auditory meatus red and inflamed; drum is normal; systemic disturbance rare.

Boil in external auditory meatus
Similar feature: pain and discharge in ear of babies and children.

Distinguishing features: pain is acute; insertion of speculum into ear is painful; meatal boil with swelling, redness and discharge; drum normal; systemic disturbance rare.

Intussusception
Similar features: screaming attacks in an infant; vomiting; legs may be drawn up during pain.

Distinguishing features: attacks of pain are more definite; baby may go pale during an attack; abdominal mass; blood on rectal examination; eardrums normal; fever absent.

MANAGEMENT OPTIONS

Prevention: if children with cough can be kept quiet indoors the likelihood of secondary infection of lungs and ears may be reduced.

Established disease: (a) rest and warmth; (b) analgesics — BNF 4.7.1 (Ref. 0.1); (c) antibacterials — BNF 5.1 are usually given to prevent complications on the grounds that these are secondary bacterial infections; (d) follow up to check ears and hearing — essential.

SECRETORY OTITIS MEDIA (MUCOSEROUS CATARRH OF EAR)

Classification: ICHPPC 3811 (RCGP 1715)

A painless disorder in which fluid collects in the middle ear. The fluid often persists and may organise causing permanent deafness. The condition is therefore sometimes called *glue ear*.

AETIOLOGY

Uncertain. There may or may not be an obvious relationship with previous attacks of otitis media. The frequency appears to be increasing, a possible result of incomplete treatment and inadequate follow up.

DIAGNOSTIC RANGE (rates per 1000 patients per year)
Personal: Suspected 0.6, Probable 0.5.

AGE INCIDENCE

Children under 15 years.

CLINICAL POINTERS

1. High risk factors: (a) cleft palate; (b) enlarged adenoids

(doubtful); (c) inadequate compliance with antibacterials; (d) preceding acute otitis (not always present).

2. Deafness. The onset of deafness is gradual and pain is conspicuously absent.

3. The appearance of the drum may be normal. Sometimes fluid can be seen behind the drum. Redness and other evidence of inflammation is slight or absent. The lustre of the drum may be dulled.

DURATION

The fluid may remain in the middle ear for many weeks.

COMPLICATIONS

Deafness is sometimes permanent if treatment is inadequate and the fluid is allowed to remain.

MISLEADING FEATURES AND PITFALLS

1. The absence of pain and the insidious development of deafness may lead to inadequate treatment because the disorder is not considered serious.

2. The condition is missed because an acute otitis media is not adequately followed up.

DIFFERENTIAL DIAGNOSIS

Disease that may be confused with secretory otitis media:

Eustachian catarrh

Similar features: mild deafness; pain and redness of eardrum absent; light reflex dull.

Distinguishing features: adults usually affected; deafness follows cold and is slight, transient and non-progressive; eardrum is indrawn.

MANAGEMENT OPTIONS

Prevention: (a) ensure adequate parental compliance with antibiotics; (b) adequate follow up of all acute ear complaints.

Established disease: Early referral for diagnosis, management and base line hearing checks. Opinions on surgical treatment vary.

CHRONIC SUPPURATIVE OTITIS MEDIA

Classification: ICHPPC 388 (RCGP 1730)

AETIOLOGY

The key to the development of chronic otitis media lies with the eardrum. While the eardrum is perforated the middle ear is at risk and recurrent and then chronic infection may develop.

Under the age of 10 years the middle ear is most vulnerable and perforation and recurrent otitis media are common. Fortunately the drum at this age heals easily and with adequate treatment a perforated drum and chronic otitis media can be avoided.

In adults the drum heals less easily and although acute otitis media is less common there is a greater tendency for an acute infection to become chronic.

[Practice experience: 76 consecutive cases of acute otitis media in children were observed (and treated with antibiotics); 30 (40%) showed evidence of discharge or perforation. At follow-up 6 months later only one patient (aged 12) had a perforation. At a further follow-up 3 years later no cases of chronic suppurative otitis media or perforation were found.]

DIAGNOSTIC RANGE (rates per 1000 patients per year)

Personal: Suspected 2.8, Probable 2.2, *National*: 2.4 (Ref. 0.2). The number of cases appears to be falling in most practices.

AGE INCIDENCE

All ages are liable. (In practice the disease was confined to adults with a long history of otorrhoea.)

CLINICAL POINTERS

1. High risk factors: (a) inadequately treated acute otitis; (b) poor patient compliance; (c) disadvantaged socio economic groups.

2. Otorrhoea (100%) — may be continuous or intermittent. (Many patients can be kept free of discharge with regular full aural toilet.)

3. Perforation of the eardrum (100%). The so called 'safe' anterior perforation should be distinguished from the posterior, attic, perforation which is more likely to be associated over the years with all the serious complications.

4. Pain in the ear or over the mastoid is an unusual feature and may indicate an intracranial spread of infection.

5. Fever may indicate a spread of the infective process.

6. Cholesteatoma forms if there is much desquamating debris. It is sometimes associated with a spread of the infection to the surrounding bones.

INVESTIGATIONS

A swab of the discharge is useful if taken before treatment is started.

DURATION

The untreated case may continue indefinitely.

COMPLICATIONS

1. Deafness progresses slowly as long as active infection is present. [Practice experience: 44% (11 out of 25 consecutive cases) complained of varying degrees of deafness.]

2. Lateral sinus thrombosis and cerebral abscess. These two serious complications present with a swinging temperature, neck stiffness and pain in the affected ear. The patient is acutely ill and there may be paralysis of the 3rd, 4th, 6th or 7th cranial nerves. If the cerebral abscess is in the temporal lobe there may be homonomous defects of the visual fields. [Two cases encountered in 20 years of practice.]

3. Polyp formation is not uncommon.

MISLEADING FEATURES AND PITFALLS

1. Syringing an ear in which wax obscures a perforation may light up a latent chronic suppurative otitis media.

2. The significance of a posterior attic perforation is overlooked.

3. The spread of a chronic suppurative otitis media into the petrous bone and brain may be overlooked.

DIFFERENTIAL DIAGNOSIS

Diagnosis is rarely in doubt but cholesteatoma or otitis externa may occasionally confuse both diagnosis and assessment of progress.

MANAGEMENT OPTIONS

Prevention: (a) adequate follow up and treatment of acute otitis media, especially in adults or cases with discharge; (b) ear plugs or avoidance of swimming and diving as long as drum is perforated.

Established CSOM: (a) swab for bacteriology; (b) regular local toilet of meatus; (c) appropriate antibacterials, simultaneous, oral — BNF 5.1 (Ref. 0.1) and topical — BNF 12.1.1. Topical astringents — alum acetate — are used first, then topical anti-bacterials or steroids; (d) regular follow up; (e) referral often indicated.

WAX IN EARS

Classification: ICHPPC 3804 (RCGP 1705)

AETIOLOGY

Dusty atmospheres and syringing of the ears probably stimulate wax formation.

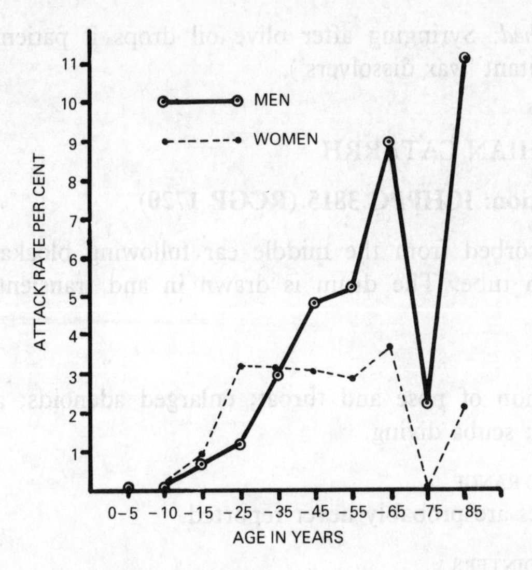

Fig. 26 Impacted wax in ears. Age incidence for men and women in 80 consecutive cases encountered in 1 year.

DIAGNOSTIC RANGE (rates per 1000 patients per year)

Personal: Proven 26.9, *National*: 20.1 (Ref. 0.2). Many cases are probably not reported.

AGE INCIDENCE

Adults become increasingly liable as they grow older (Fig. 26).

SEX INCIDENCE

Men are affected more than women (2:1)

CLINICAL POINTERS

1. Deafness.
2. The presence of wax (100%).
3. Earache is slight or absent.

MISLEADING FEATURES AND PITFALLS

1. The wax of babies is very soft and may run out of the external auditory meatus and be described by mothers as a 'running ear'.

2. The elderly may wrongly attribute increasing deafness to old age and fail to report (Fig. 26).

MANAGEMENT OPTIONS

Prevention: Wax production is normal. Needless cleansing of ears in the absence of symptoms should be discouraged.

Established: Syringing after olive oil drops if patient is deaf. (Avoid irritant 'wax dissolvers').

EUSTACHIAN CATARRH

Classification: ICHPPC 3815 (RCGP 1720)

Air is absorbed from the middle ear following blockage of the Eustachian tube. The drum is drawn in and transient deafness ensues.

AETIOLOGY

Inflammation of nose and throat; enlarged adenoids; air travel; swimming; scuba diving.

DIAGNOSTIC RANGE

Many cases are probably never reported.

CLINICAL POINTERS

1. High risk factors: (a) preceding respiratory infection; (b) mechanical pressure factors, e.g. diving, aviation, etc.
2. Deafness is slight and usually transient.
3. The indrawn drum is dull but not red.
4. Earache is occasionally present.

DURATION

The disorder rarely lasts for longer than a week.

MANAGEMENT OPTIONS

Prevention: Adequate precautions i.e. sucking sweets or ear plugs.

Established condition: (a) Encourage swallowing and Val Salva manoeuvre (b) waiting and watching (c) referral for insufflation.

DEAFNESS

Classification: ICHPPC 387 (RCGP 1780)

Deafness is a symptom, but the family doctor tends to regard it as an entity in itself because it is a specialist's problem (see Table 21).

DIAGNOSTIC RANGE

3.7 to 5.5 per 1000 patients per year. Many patients with mild deafness probably never report to the doctor.

MANAGEMENT OPTIONS

Early referral for diagnosis, management and establishment of base line hearing levels.

Table 21 Causes of permanent or progressive deafness

Cause of deafness	Age of onset	Clinical pointers
Congenital deafness	Birth	Backward speech and behaviour; possible prenatal causes — rubella, drugs etc.; other congenital defects.
Otitis media (chronic and serous)	5 to 20 years	Repeated infections and deformity of the middle ear. The drum may be normal in patients with secretory otitis media
Post infective nerve deafness.	0–20 years	Mumps, Measles, Meningitis
Otosclerosis	20 to 40 years	Familial; females especially liable; drum often normal; tinnitus
Industrial deafness (boilermakers')	Adults	Occupation; tinnitus; drum normal
Senile deafness	50 onwards	Tinnitus; drum normal

Table 22 Less common diseases of the ear

Disease and distinguishing clinical pointers	Incidence per 1000 patients per year Suspected	Confirmed
Acute mastoiditis Acute otitis media; earache, pain or fever that persists in spite of perforation and discharge; tenderness or oedema over mastoid; lobe of affected ear turned forward; meningeal irritation; the infection is easily confused with a boil in the external auditory meatus and a posterior auricular adenitis, both disorders can cause pain, tenderness and oedema over the mastoid. Refer early.	0.2	0
Meniere's disease Middle-aged and elderly patients, paroxysmal vertigo, nystagmus, nerve deafness and tinnitus often noticed before vertigo. Referral.	—	2 in 10 years

16

Diseases of the circulatory system

Please read the introduction for explanation of figures and analyses.

ACUTE AND SUBACUTE RHEUMATISM

Classification ICHPPC 390 (RCGP 1900)

AETIOLOGY

The basic pathological lesion — the Aschoff node — is said to arise at the site of inflammation in both cardiovascular and skeletal systems, but the aetiology is uncertain.

1. Streptococcal infections of throat, ears or wounds may precede the disease by 1 to 3 weeks (40%).
2. Hereditary and family influences. The incidence of rheumatic fever is high in some families.
3. One attack predisposes to others.
4. Allergic factors. The similarity between rheumatic fever and certain allergic reactions of joints and skin and the association with streptococcal infections has led to the suggestion that the disease is an abnormal immune or allergic reaction to a streptococcal infection.
5. Improved standards of living and increasing use of antibiotics appear to have contributed to its disappearance.

DIAGNOSTIC RANGE

Twenty years ago when this book was first written the range in this practice was 0.8 to 4.5 per 1000 patients. The disease is now mainly suspected in disadvantaged or immigrant families.

AGE INCIDENCE

Children between 5 and 15 years old are especially liable, but milder forms of the disease are not uncommon in adults under 35; onset over this age and in babies is rare.

THE PROBLEM OF ACUTE RHEUMATISM IN GENERAL PRACTICE

The classical clinical picture of rheumatic fever is of a child or young adult with fleeting joint pains, high fever and profuse sweats. The onset is a few days after tonsillitis and there may be evidence of early carditis. Diagnosis in such cases is not difficult and is confirmed by a raised erythrocyte sedimentation rate.

A study of the previous history of patients with known chronic rheumatic heart disease shows that an incapacitating valvular deformity can develop in the absence of the classical type of rheumatic fever. A period of ill-health or a vague history of occasional joint pains is often the only evidence of rheumatism.

CLINICAL POINTERS

1. High risk factors: (a) previous attacks, (b) previous streptococcal infection, (c) disadvantaged families.

2. Acute tonsillitis or other preceding streptococcal illness. Acute tonsillitis, pharyngitis, scarlet fever or otitis media may precede acute rheumatism by 2 to 21 days.

(Practice experience: this feature was present in 100% of confirmed cases and only 33% of unconfirmed.).

3. Joint pains (84%). Children between 5 and 10 years old may not complain of joint pains. The classical picture of fleeting joint pains, is often absent even in adults. Wrists, knees and elbows are most affected. A single joint may be affected.

4. Fever is variable and may be high. Patients who are examined in a surgery, especially in the mornings, may not show a rise of temperature, which only becomes evident at night.

5. A rapid pulse is common and levels over 120 may be noted. In children a high pulse rate does not necessarily indicate carditis.

6. A period of malaise. A history of listlessness, anorexia or fever that lasts for 10 days or more, after a possible streptococcal illness in a child, suggests active acute rheumatism. This feature may be difficult to assess because the ability of parents to observe their children objectively varies greatly.

7. Other pointers include (a) evidence of previous carditis, i.e. diastolic murmurs, etc., (b) large circinate rashes (erythema marginatum), and (c) rheumatic nodules, usually in the region of the olecranon (rare).

INVESTIGATIONS

ESR see page 681. Diagnosis is often dependent on this useful test, which is also a guide to the activity of the rheumatic process. The serum streptolysin level is a helpful pointer.

DURATION

Acute symptoms usually subside in 1 or 2 weeks. The rheumatic process as judged by the sedimentation rate may persist for several weeks.

COMPLICATIONS

1. Recurrences are common.

2. Carditis is the most serious complication and children are especially liable. It is suspected when the pulse rate remains raised or a systolic murmur develops at the apex or mitral region (this sign is not always significant). Mitral and aortic valves are commonly affected — the lesions develop slowly and may not become apparent clinically until months or years after an attck.

The frequency with which carditis complicates acute rheumatism is difficult to assess.

MISLEADING FEATURES AND PITFALLS

It is very easy to overlook the disease in a child, and even now this mistake is probably made more often than we realise.

DIFFERENTIAL DIAGNOSIS

Because of the cardiac complications the differential diagnosis has to be carefully considered in three types of case:

• GROUP I. The adult under 35 who complains of pain in one or more joints.

Rheumatoid arthritis

Similar features: pains in one or more joints; may be fleeting; fever, malaise and anorexia of over 7 days duration; raised ESR and response to salicylates.

Distinguishing features: differentiation difficult in young adults; preceding streptococcal illness absent; small joints of hands and feet commonly affected; serological tests said to be positive in 85% of established cases.

*Allergic arthritis (including serum sickness, erythema nodosum and erythema multiforme**)

Similar features: polyarthritis; fever; malaise; anorexia; raised ESR and response to salicylates.

Distinguishing features. Allergic arthritis — cause of allergy may be apparent; facial oedema and urticarial rashes usually present. Erythema nodosum — typical red lumps usually on front of shins.

*These diseases are probably closely related aetiologically to rheumatic fever.

Erythema multiforme — typical iris or 'flea bite' rash; lesions in mouth and occasionally in vagina.

Gout
Similar features: acute painful swelling of one joint; fever; raised ESR; response to salicylates.

Distinguishing features: rare under 40 years; small joints of hands and feet affected; tophi may be present; serum uric acid levels raised during an attack.

Septicaemic infections (brucella, meningococcus, staphylococcus, etc.)
Similar features: vague joint pains; fever, sweats and raised ESR.

Distinguishing features: rare; joint involvement usually indefinite; patient often acutely ill; rigors; spleen may be enlarged; embolic phenomenon; white-cell count or blood culture may differentiate; hospital investigation indicated.

• GROUP II. Children between 5 and 15 years who complain of pain in a single joint.

Acute hip syndrome
Similar features: one painful hip; slight fever.

Distinguishing features: settles in 3 to 10 days; constitutional disturbance slight; ESR only slightly raised or normal.

Acute septic arthritis
Similar features: acutely painful joint; marked constitutional disturbance.

Distinguishing features: rare; pain in joint is severe, progressive and continuous; joint is held in position of greatest comfort; source of infection elsewhere; hospital investigation indicated.

Acute osteomyelitis
Similar features: acute pain in region of joint; marked constitutional disturbance.

Distinguishing features: onset usually sudden; pain is severe, progressive and continuous; bone is tender to pressure in region of pain; focus of infection; immediate hospital investigation indicated.

• GROUP III. Children between 5 and 15 years old who complain of malaise and vague body aches.

Urinary tract infections
Similar features: malaise of over 7 days duration; low fever; anorexia; vague aches and pains; tachycardia.

Distinguishing features: nocturia and dysuria may be present in older children; preceding streptococcal illness absent; loins may be tender; facial pallor; urine contains pus cells.

Aspiration pneumonitis
Similar features: malaise over 7 days duration with low fever; anorexia; upper respiratory infection 7 to 14 days previously.
Distinguishing features: cough; localising signs in chest usual; slight cyanosis sometimes apparent; chest X-ray differentiates.

Behaviour problem
Similar features: apparent malaise and anorexia of over 7 days duration; vague aches and pains.
Distinguishing features: predisposing cause in school or family usually apparent; fever absent; ESR normal.

Infective and subclinical hepatitis
Similar features: malaise and anorexia of over 7 days duration; low fever; vague aches and pains.
Distinguishing features: icterus of sclerotics and skin after 4 to 7 days; pulse slow; vomiting and abdominal pain common; liver may be tender; motions light; urine very dark, stains clothing and contains bile.

Infectious mononucleosis
Similar features: malaise and anorexia of over 7 days duration; fever; muscle aches and pains; rashes may be present; illness may follow a sore throat.
Distinguishing features: spleen and glands palpable; serology and differential white-cell count usually distinguish; differentiation may be difficult.

MANAGEMENT OPTIONS
Prevention: (a) better living standards; (b) antibiotics — BNF 5.1.1 may be indicated in high risk groups.
Established disease: (a) rest; (b) anti-inflammatory analgesics — BNF 10.1.1 (Ref. 0.1) or steroids — BNF 6.3.2.; (c) specialist referral; (d) monitor progress (ESR etc.)

CHOREA

Classification: ICHPPC 390 (RCG 1900)

Aetiology

Chorea is thought to be related to acute rheumatism — a view that is based mainly on the clinical similarities of the two diseases.

DIAGNOSTIC RANGE (rates per 1000 patients per year)
Personal: Less than 0.3 per 1000.

AGE INCIDENCE
5 to 20 years.

CLINICAL POINTERS

1. High risk factors: (a) as for Acute Rheumatism, (b) Emotional upsets are said to precede the illness.
2. Involuntary purposeless movements of limbs and face may lead to clumsiness, 'dropping things' and grimacing. These are distinguished from nervous tics because they are not repetitive. The classical pendular knee jerk and other associated CNS signs are produced by these involuntary movements.
3. Fever may be present but is not high.
4. Chorea is said to be associated with pregnancy. This may be a true association, but many women give a history of increased clumsiness and 'dropping things' during an otherwise normal pregnancy.

INVESTIGATIONS
The ESR (see p. 681) is sometimes raised.

DURATION
The disease persists for several weeks — recurrences occur.

COMPLICATIONS
Chronic rheumatic endocarditis may follow chorea.

DIFFERENTIAL DIAGNOSIS
Disease that may be confused with chorea:

Tic
Similar features: similar age-groups affected; emotional upsets often precede the illness; grimacing common.

Distinguishing features: movements constantly repeated; clumsiness not apparent; ESR normal; no evidence of carditis; no fever.

MANAGEMENT OPTIONS
As for Rheumatic fever.

CHRONIC RHEUMATIC VALVULAR HEART DISEASE

Classification: ICHPPC 390 (RCGP 1905)

Chronic rheumatic endocarditis poses a diagnostic problem for the family doctor because early definite diagnosis is required for correct surgical and medical treatment. Unfortunately uncertainties of diagnosis may occasionally lead to needless cardiac investigation with subsequent development of cardiac neurosis.

AETIOLOGY

Many patients give a clear-cut history of rheumatic fever, but others can recollect no suggestive illness.

The rheumatic process may affect the myocardium and pericardium, but the endocardium is chiefly involved. The edges of the valves become adherent, the chordae tendineae shorten; valvular incompetence and stenosis follow. The aortic and mitral valves may be affected together or independently; disease of the tricuspid and pulmonary valves is rare.

DIAGNOSTIC RANGE (rates per 1000 patients per year)

Personal: Suspected 3.7, Probable 1.8, *National*: 1.4 (Ref. 0.2). This includes both fresh and established cases. In practice the number of fresh cases is steadily diminishing.

AGE INCIDENCE

From childhood onwards.

SEX INCIDENCE

Women are affected twice as often as men.

MITRAL INCOMPETENCE

Classification: ICHPPC 390 (RCGP 1905)

A well-marked apical systolic murmur is noted in a patient who gives a history of previous rheumatic fever. Cardiac compensation for the deficiency is usually good and symptoms may be few. Intensive cardiac investigations are avoided when possible. The disease is significant in the following circumstances:

1. If the patient is to undergo dental extractions — these are said to precipitate subacute bacterial endocarditis.
2. If the patient develops symptoms of cardiac failure.
3. If the patient is examined for life insurance.

MITRAL STENOSIS

Classification: ICHPPC 390 (RCGP 1905)

Mitral stenosis is the commonest form of chronic valvular disease and is the most amenable to surgical treatment.

CLINICAL POINTERS

1. High risk factors: (a) A definite history of rheumatic fever or chorea. A vague history of 'rheumatism', 'growing pains' or frequent sore throats may also be significant; such symptoms are so common that their causative role must be carefully assessed. (b) low socio-economic groups.

2. Symptoms and signs of pulmonary congestion:

- Dyspnoea — first apparent on exertion, sometimes nocturnal.
- Recurrent bronchitic cough is common.
- Haemoptysis, usually slight.
- Basal râles.

These symptoms are clinically significant because they indicate the necessity for an immediate full cardiological investigation.

3. Heart sounds:

- Diastolic murmurs — a soft diastolic blow or the more characteristic presystolic rumble; both murmurs may be heard after exertion at the apex or mitral areas.
- Accentuated pulmonary second sound indicates pulmonary hypertension. The opening snap is marked.

4. Evidence of cardiac enlargement.
5. Cyanosis is sometimes present.
6. Peripheral oedema is a late symptom.
7. Auricular fibrillation is a late sign.

INVESTIGATION

1. A straight chest X-ray is often extremely useful. It may show cardiac enlargement, pulmonary congestion, or dilatation of the pulmonary conus. Occasionally the outline of the right and left atria are seen along the right hand edge of the cardiac shadow.

2. Radiological screening enables the size of the left atrium to be assessed.

DURATION

In most cases the untreated disease progresses slowly but steadily and is accelerated by further attacks of acute rheumatism.

COMPLICATIONS

1. Recurrent attacks of bronchitis.
2. Auricular fibrillation.
3. Emboli originating in the heart may be trapped in any of the systemic capillary beds, e.g. brain, kidney or mesentery.
4. Myocardial failure, acute pulmonary oedema and death.
5. Subacute bacterial endocarditis. (Four cases encountered in

10 years of practice.) Incidence is increasing in patients with valve replacements.

MISLEADING FEATURES AND PITFALLS

1. The correct assessment of cardiac murmurs requires constant practice. Few family doctors are in a position to obtain this, but because surgical treatment at the right moment is so successful patients with doubtful heart sounds must be referred early for a second opinion.
2. In spite of a full cardiological examination which reveals no abnormality some patients remain fearful of heart disease and cardiac neurosis may follow.

DIFFERENTIAL DIAGNOSIS

In the early stages of the disease distinction between functional and organic murmurs is difficult. In the later stages the diagnosis is rarely in doubt.

MANAGEMENT OPTIONS

Prevention: Raised living standards,

Established disease: (a) early referral; (b) early cardiological assessment with specialist decisions on the surgical or medical alternatives; (c) antibiotic cover — BNF 5.1 (Ref. 0.1) if there is a risk of bacterial endocarditis.

AORTIC INCOMPETENCE

Classification: ICHPPC 390 and 424 (RCGP 1905, 1970)

Aortic incompetence is usually rheumatic but may be syphilitic. It is uncommon.

CLINICAL POINTERS

1. High risk factor. Previous attack of acute rheumatism.
2. Dyspnoea.
3. Aortic diastolic murmur.
4. Greatly enlarged left ventricle with displaced heaving apex beat.
5. Increased pulse pressure.

INVESTIGATIONS

1. Serological tests to exclude previous syphilis.
2. A straight chest-X-ray may show a 'boot-shaped' and enlarged left ventricle.
3. Radiological screening enables the size of the left ventricle to be assessed.

DURATION

Until the left ventricle ceases to compensate for the inefficient valve, symptoms are few. After heart failure has developed deterioration is often rapid.

COMPLICATIONS

1. Angina pectoris.
2. Heart failure and sudden death.
3. Subacute bacterial endocarditis.

MANAGEMENT OPTIONS

As for Mitral Stenosis.

AORTIC STENOSIS

Classification: ICHPPC 390 and 424 (RCGP 1905, 1970)

Aortic stenosis is rheumatic or arteriosclerotic in origin.

CLINICAL POINTERS

1. High risk factors: (a) previous attack of acute rheumatism; (b) evidence of arteriosclerosis.
2. Dyspnoea.
3. Aortic systolic thrill. An aortic diastolic murmur is also present.
4. Greatly enlarged left ventricle with heaving apex beat displaced to the left.
5. Pulse pressure is small.

INVESTIGATIONS

1. A straight chest X-ray shows greatly enlarged left ventricle and may reveal calcification of the aortic valve.
2. Radiological screening enables the size of the left ventricle to be assessed.

MANAGEMENT OPTIONS

As for Mitral Stenosis.

HYPERTENSIVE DISEASE

It is wise to regard hypertensives as a 'high risk group' who are vulnerable to certain diseases so long as their blood pressure remains high.

The chief known causes of hypertension are:

1. Physiological: emotion; exercise.

2. Pathological: chronic renal disease; endocrine disease (thyrotoxicosis, Cushing's syndrome, pheochromocytoma); coarctation of aorta; toxaemia of pregnancy.

In the majority of patients no reason can be found. This is Essential Hypertension.

Two crucial features make essential hypertension important: (a) it is reversible with drugs; (b) treatment decreases the likelihood of developing myocardial infarcts, heart failure and strokes. Under the age of 65 long term antihypertensive drugs reduce mortality rates by 17%. *Case finding of hypertensives is therefore an essential part of every family doctor's work* (Ref. 16.1).

The records of every patient aged 40 to 65, who are due for their 3- or 5-yearly blood pressure check are 'flagged'. A check is performed when next they attend. (See Chapter 3 — p. 57).

ESSENTIAL HYPERTENSION

Classification: ICHPPC 401 (RCGP 1910)

DEFINITION

Defining in any individual what is an abnormal blood pressure is difficult because we do not usually know the underlying cause.

The following diastolic levels are taken to warrant some form of treatment. *These levels are arbitrary and the therefore subject to 'change' as we learn more about hypertension.*

Men: 40 years or under — 100+ mmHg
40 to 64 years — 105+ mmHg
65 years and over — aggressive treatment of uncertain benefit

Women: 40 years or under — 110+ mmHg
40 to 64 years — 115+ mmHg
65 years and over — aggressive treatment of uncertain benefit

Establishing a 'true' level is usually done by arranging for the patient whose diastolic B. P. is over 95 to attend for two further checks. The mean of all three levels is then taken as the 'true' level.

DIAGNOSTIC RANGE (rates per 1000 patients per year)

Personal: Suspected 18.0, Probable 9.2, *National*: 22.4 (Ref. 0.2). Note these figures were collected before any active case finding policy. Today incidences two to three times greater might be expected.

AGE INCIDENCE

The majority of patients are over 60 but 'case finding' in younger age groups is a vital part of every doctor's work (see above and Fig. 27).

SEX INCIDENCE

Women are affected more than men. (Practice experience: 5:1; this difference is in part due to the greater longevity of women.) Hypertension in men is always more serious than in women.

CLINICAL POINTERS

Many patients with essential hypertension have no symptoms. This inevitably puts the responsibility of 'case finding' on the doctor.

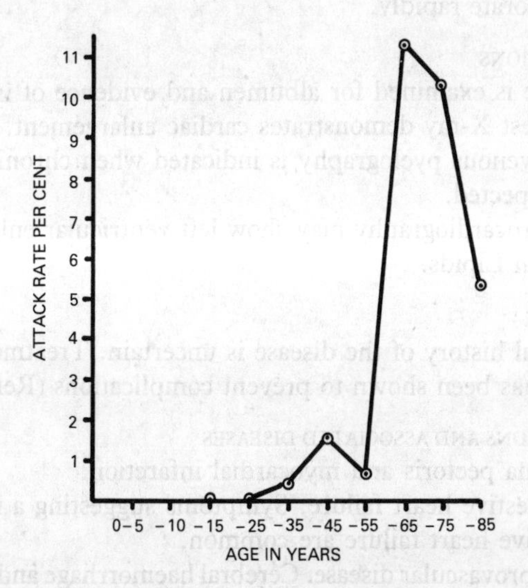

Fig. 27 Essential hypertension. Age incidence of 25 consecutive cases in one year.

1. High risk factors: (a) age; (b) family history; (c) high salt intake; (d) race (American negroes, Japanese, etc.); (e) high serum lipids.
2. Sphygmomanometer readings (as defined above). The reading should be confirmed on three separate mornings (100%).
3. Dizziness (45%).
4. Headaches (35%) — often difficult to assess.
5. Apex beat may be heaving and displaced to the left.

6. Retinal changes. In most cases hypertension leads to the discovery of retinal change rather than the reverse. The extent of the arterial disease can be judged by the retinal changes which are a better guide to prognosis than the level of the blood pressure:

Grade I Retinitis — silver wiring, narrowing and increased tortuosity is especially suggestive of arterial disease.
Grade II Retinitis — nicking of veins as they cross the arteries.
Grade III Retinitis — exudate and haemorrhages.
Grade IV Retinitis — papilloedema.

Patients with grade III and grade IV retinitis require immediate hospital investigation of possible malignant hypertension. Vision may deteriorate rapidly.

INVESTIGATIONS

1. Urine is examined for albumen and evidence of infection.
2. A chest X-ray demonstrates cardiac enlargement.
3. Intravenous pyelography is indicated when chronic renal disease is suspected.
4. Electrocardiography may show left ventricular enlargement.
5. Serum Lipids.

DURATION

The natural history of the disease is uncertain. Treatment of those under 65 has been shown to prevent complications (Ref. 16.1).

COMPLICATIONS AND ASSOCIATED DISEASES

1. Angina pectoris and myocardial infarction.
2. Congestive heart failure. Symptoms suggesting a mild degree of congestive heart failure are common.
3. Cerebrovascular disease. Cerebral haemorrhage and thrombosis may occur. Occasionally repeated small cerebrovascular accidents give a picture of hypertensive encephalopathy.
4. Obesity and hypertension are often associated.

MISLEADING FEATURES AND PITFALLS

1. The blood pressure of some individuals may vary considerably. (Practice experience: sphygmomanometer readings of one 53-year-old female, taken at monthly intervals for 8 years before the advent of modern antihypertensives, showed many random variations from 160/90 to 240/140. The patient was unaware of the variations and there were no apparent ill effects.)
2. The lay public regards a raised blood pressure as a serious disease; a diagnosis is not made lightly.

3. Surveys have shown that individuals (symptom free) found to have a raised blood pressure at routine screening have, after being treated, consistently lost more time off work than those not informed or treated.

'Marketplace case finding' and screening programmes of individuals not attending for other reasons has to be considered with caution (see Table 3, p. 56).

MANAGEMENT OPTIONS

Prevention: A case finding approach should be a routine for every family doctor. Diets low in saturated fat have not yet been shown to *prevent* hypertension.

Established hypertension: (a) exclude and treat primary causes and target organ damage; (b) use a step by step approach — first general measures; these include reducing weight, smoking, alcohol, saturated fat and salt intake; (c) drugs — thiazide diuretics — BNF 2.2.1 (Ref. 0.1); then Beta blockers — BNF 2.4 or calcium antagonists — BNF 2.6.1 (*Note*: these two should not be given together); finally other anti-hypertensives B.N.F. 2.5; (d) follow up, to monitor B. P. and compliance; (e) hypertension in pregnancy should be controlled — diuretics are best avoided; (f) treatment in the elderly (70 plus) is of doubtful benefit.

SIMPLE FAINTS (VASOVAGAL ATTACK)

Classification: ICHPPC 7802 (RCGP 4500)

A sudden fall in blood pressure leads to severe pallor and unconsciousness. Faints may follow internal haemorrhage or psychological causes. Faints are common in early pregnancy and in young girls. A short (non-epileptic) convulsion may occur during a faint.

DIAGNOSTIC RANGE (rates per 1000 patients per year)

Personal: Suspected 5.9, Probable 4.2. Many faints are not reported.

IDIOPATHIC (HYPOSTATIC) OEDEMA OF LEGS

Classification: ICHPPC 7823 (RCGP 4555)

Some otherwise normal adults (mainly women) appear to respond to periods of standing by a reduction of blood volume. Fluid intake is then increased and retained in the body. Heat, hormonal influences and long periods of standing aggravate the retention.

DIAGNOSTIC INCIDENCE (rates per 1000 patients per year)
Personal: Suspected 2.1. Probably many more unreported cases.

AGE INCIDENCE
Mainly middle aged housewives.

CLINICAL POINTERS
1. High risk factors: (a) housewives; (b) obesity; (c) hot weather; (d) menstrual and premenstrual days; (e) standing.
2. Oedema of feet and ankles as day progresses. Facial oedema often in mornings.

COMPLICATIONS
None.

MISTAKES AND PITFALLS
Myxoedema or other serious causes are overlooked.

MANAGEMENT OPTIONS
Established condition: (a) exclude serious causes; (b) modify high risk trigger factors; (c) extreme cases — monitor with twice daily weight chart, a 'no added salt' diet; (d) Spironolactone type diuretics if resistant — BNF 2.2.4 (Ref. 0.1).

ISCHAEMIC HEART DISEASE

Classification: ICHPPC 410–412 (RCGP 1945)

Occlusion of the coronary arteries (usually arteriosclerotic) may reduce the myocardial blood supply and cause the following diseases:

— angina pectoris
— myocardial infarction
— painless myocardial fibrosis
— congestive heart failure (see p. 357).

MYOCARDIAL INFARCTION (CORONARY THROMBOSIS)

Classification: ICHPPC 410 (RCGP 1940)

Recently a number of facts about the natural history of M. I. have emerged which have greatly changed our attitudes to management. These facts are:

— About 20% of proven M. I.s are 'silent' or with trivial unreported symptoms.

— In about 25% of the remainder death occurs in the first hour.
— In nearly 50% death occurs in the first 2 hours.
— In 63% death occurs before any medical attention is given.
— There is an average delay of 2 hours before calling the doctor and 45 minutes before the doctor arrives.
— Several well controlled studies have suggested that given these constraints good quality care at home may give slightly better overall outcomes than good quality care in hospital, which inevitably involves the added risk of transportation.

Three conclusions must be drawn:

1. Prevention must be every community's first aim. This must include anticipatory treatment for those in high risk groups. (See below).

2. Doctors and communities must co-operate to reduce the delay time between onset and doctor arrival.

3. Given the present variations in 'delay time', resources available and certainty of diagnosis, the family doctor must develop a flexible approach which enables the best combination of options to be chosen.

AETIOLOGY

Arteriosclerotic changes in the coronary arteries cause infarction.

Recently (Ref 16.1) there is clear evidence from the U.S.A., that in patients with very high serum cholesterol levels (top 5 per centile) a strict diet (with an increased ratio of unsaturated to saturated fats) will reduce: (a) serum cholesterol levels, (b) coronary atherosclerosis, (c) the risks of angina and MI.

DIAGNOSTIC RANGE (rates per 1000 patients per year)

Personal: Suspected 6.5. Probable 4.5. *National*: 3.8 (Ref. 0.2). In about three-quarters of these cases the diagnosis was clear. Most cases of sudden unexplained death in general practice are labelled 'coronary thrombosis'; some are probably due to pulmonary emboli or dissecting aneurysms of the aorta. Until 5 years ago the number of cases was steadily increasing. Recently the numbers appear to be decreasing. Incidence is also dependent on the social economic structure of the practice.

AGE INCIDENCE

Patients over 45 years are most commonly affected.

SEX INCIDENCE

Men are affected more than women.

CLINICAL POINTERS

1. High risk factors: (a) previous attacks; (b) angina, (c) hypertension, (d) diabetes, (e) claudication, (f) suggestive family history, (g) heavy smoking. The presence of more than one of these factors in a single patient of over 40 greatly increases the need for preventive action (h) diets high in saturated fats.

Other less certain high risk factors which may need modification are obesity, alcohol intake, sedentary life style and the contraceptive pill.

2. Pain is similar to that of angina (63% (nine out of 14)) i.e. a substernal or precordial tightness which radiates to arms throat or jaws. In most cases the pain is severe and continuous and even if there are confusing features (such as relationship to respiration or an unexpected radiation) the diagnosis is rarely in doubt. Less commonly the pain is mild and diagnosis difficult; in these cases, if the pain is felt in several places, is related to moving (or breathing) or has an atypical radiation, other causes must be considered.

3. Duration. The pain does not pass off with rest and may continue for some hours. [In 84% (13 out of 14) confirmed cases the pain lasted over an hour.] Occasionally the pain of an infarct is relieved by nitroglycerin.

4. Shock. The patient is sweating, grey and ill. They pulse may be shallow and rapid or irregular. When considering the problem of extensive transport the possibility of aggravating shock, breathlessness or bradycardia must be taken into account.

5. Fall in blood pressure is common and may remain low for long periods after the attack.

6. Auricular fibrillation or other arrhythmias may be precipitated by myocardial infarction. (Practice experience: in three out of 14 confirmed cases fibrillation was noted.)

7. Late signs and symptoms that may have prognostic significance because they tend to indicate a large infarct:

- Low fever on second day and after.
- Pericardial friction rub on third day and after.
- Slight icterus of face.

INVESTIGATIONS

1. Serum enzymes, (SGOT) are raised in a large proportion of patients with myocardial infarction. The increase begins within 24 hours and is present for 2 to 3 days. This test is extremely useful and a rising titre may enable a family doctor to diagnose a probable infarct with a doubtful cardiograph. The serum LDH is also useful because serum levels remain high for 4 to 7 days after an infarct.

2. Electrocardiography should be used to confirm an infarction.

3. ESR (see p. 681) and white-cell count may both be raised after 2 days. These rarely help diagnosis, but high readings, especially if associated with a fever or pericardial rub, indicate a bad prognosis.

4. Plasma cholesterol and low density lipoprotein (LDL) levels.

DURATION

As with most infarcts healing and fibrosis take place slowly and are said to be complete after 6 weeks.

COMPLICATIONS

1. Recurrences are common. A cardiographic record is very useful to the general practitioner for comparative purposes. Interpretation of any change is then a simple matter if recurrences are suspected.

2. Complete heart block with attacks of unconsciousness (Stokes-Adams attacks). Arrhythmias of all types are common.

3. Emboli from mural thrombi may fly off into the systemic or pulmonary circulation during the first few weeks.

4. Rupture of heart.

5. Death. [Practice experience: death occurred within 10 days of the onset in 63 per cent (nine out of 14) cases. These figures include cases of sudden death with a suggestive history and no cardiographic confirmation.]

MISLEADING FEATURES AND PITFALLS

1. Failure to realise that the chest pain of myocardial infarction is not always severe may lead to serious mistakes.

2. A paroxysm of atrial fibrillation may cause a continuous anginal pain that simulates a myocardial infarct.

3. Elderly patients may present with a history of collapse. Chest pain is entirely absent.

4. In the early stages, i.e., the first few hours, anxiety, new surroundings, an ambulance journey with sirens may all increase the dangers of fatal complications. Increasingly, practitioners are questioning the wisdom of admitting *all* suspected cases as a routine procedure. Six per cent of cases in one series died during transport.

5. A cardiac neurosis is created in a patient who has had inconclusive investigations.

DIFFERENTIAL DIAGNOSIS

Diseases that may be confused with myocardial infarction:

Angina pectoris
Similar features: character and distribution of pain; pain of infarction is sometimes partially relieved by nitroglycerin.

Distinguishing features: previous attacks common; pain related to exertion or heavy meal; rapid and complete relief with nitroglycerin; ECG and serum transaminase differentiate; hospital investigation may be indicated.

Atrial fibrillation
Similar features: a paroxysm of fibrillation may precipitate a latent angina and cause prolonged pain; a myocardial infarct may cause atrial fibrillation.

Distinguishing features: history of similar attacks; ECG and serum transaminase differentiate, hospital investigation may be indicated.

Pulmonary embolus
Similar features: sudden onset of severe continuous chest pain; shock.

Distinguishing features: source of embolus; pain aggravated by respiration; cough; dyspnoea marked; cyanosis; localising adventitious sounds; differentiation difficult; hospital investigation indicated; haemoptysis; pleural rub. Cardiograph and serum enzymes.

Reflux oesophagitis
Similar feature: character and distribution of pain.

Distinguishing features: pain related to posture; symptoms of indigestion; differentiation difficult; cardiograph, chest X-ray and serum enzymes; hospital investigation may be needed.

Perforated peptic ulcer
Similar features: sudden very severe substernal pain radiating to shoulder; shock.

Distinguishing features: history of indigestion; board-like abdominal rigidity; decreased liver dullness; pulse rate steadily increases; shoulder pain is on the right side. Cardiograph and enzymes.

Dissecting aneurysm
Similar feature: sudden continuous severe central chest pain that radiates to arm or chin.

Distinguishing features: shock slight; distribution of pain widespread, may extend gradually to both arms, abdomen or even legs; hospital investigation indicated. Chest and abdominal X-ray.

Spontaneous tension pneumothorax
Similar feature: sudden continuous severe chest pain.
Distinguishing features: dyspnoea; physical signs in chest.

MANAGEMENT OPTIONS

Prevention: (a) long term efforts to reduce high risk factors — hypertension, smoking, angina, diabetes, obesity and diets high in saturated fats (Ref. 16.1); (b) general health education regarding exercise, alcohol and diet; (c) practice and community action to prevent delays and fatal complications during the first 4 hours after onset — this involves creating practice protocols about urgent calls, training partners and staffs, use of radiopagers, appropriate emergency equipment and pressure on the local community for coronary care ambulances.

Established infarcts seen within 2 hours of onset: if transport distance is short — quick admission to hospital probably reduces fatality rates.

Established infarcts of longer than 2 hours duration: a selective approach to hospital admission may produce the best results provided the primary physician has discussed this beforehand with his local consultant: the major clinical considerations to be taken into account are:

— *Clinical*. Handling of arrhythmias and bradycardia. Handling of shock and effects of oxygen. Assessment of severity and handling of pain. The distances involved and the skills of the ambulance staff. The presence of acute pulmonary oedema.
— *Doctor*. Clinical confidence and time available.
— *Equipment and home facilities available*. Cardiograph, oxygen and appropriate drugs are essential.
— *Patient and relatives*. Their age, wishes, personality and socio-economic status.

Whatever decisions are made a brief but objective account of the doctor's underlying reasoning should be given to patient or relatives.

Subsequent management: (a) full explanation to patient and relatives; (b) agreed period of rest followed by graduated return to previous activity; (c) therapeutic attack on treatable high risk factors especially against smoking and by giving drugs including Beta blockers — BNF 2.4 (Ref. 0.1) and antihypertensives — BNF 2.5; (d) advice about exercise, diet and alcohol (e) regular follow up.

ANGINA PECTORIS

Classification: ICHPPC 412 (RCGP 1950)

AETIOLOGY

As for MI page 348. Arteriosclerotic changes in the coronary arteries narrow their lumen. Ischaemia is latent and is only unmasked by increased cardiac activity, anaemia or obesity. Occasionally syphilitic aortitis causes angina. Twenty-five per cent of cases follow a myocardial infarct.

In the last 10 years coronary bypass procedures (3% mortality) have become standard treatment. Symptomatic relief is excellent (80%) and life is prolonged in 13% if the obstruction is in the left main coronary artery. The rates of operation vary widely and may be high in countries where 'overservicing' may be a problem and probably too low in Britain where 'underservicing' is more likely (see Ch. 1 p 26).

The primary physician has a major role in guiding sufferers to the best decision.

DIAGNOSTIC RANGE (rates per 1000 patients per year)

Personal: Suspected 8.5. Probable 6.7. *National*: 4.5 (Ref. 0.2).

AGE INCIDENCE

Patients over 45 years are most commonly affected.

SEX INCIDENCE

Males to females: 2 to 1.

CLINICAL POINTERS

1. High risk factors: (a) previous myocardial infarct; (b) previous hypertension; (c) suggestive family history; (d) heavy smoking; (e) diabetes and claudication; (f) factors that increase the work required of the heart — anaemia, obesity, tachycardia; (g) diet (see MI p. 349); (h) high serum cholesterol levels.

2. Characteristic chest pain (100%) is a substernal tightness or feeling of constriction. Occasionally the pain is felt in the precordium or epigastrium. In most of the cases the pain was considered mild; in a third it was moderately severe and only rarely disabling.

3. Radiation of pain (50%). Pain radiates down one or both arms and occasionally to the throat or jaw. Sometimes patients complain of numbness in the arms of fingers rather than actual pain.

4. Relationship of pain to exertion (80%) is a characteristic feature of the pain. The pain may also follow a heavy meal or excitement.

5. Duration of pain. The pain passes in a few minutes if the patient rests. The possibility of myocardial infarction is raised when the pain continues and does not disappear with rest.

6. Relief of pain by anti-anginal vasodilators — BNF 2.6.1 (Ref. 0.1) is a helpful diagnostic feature.

7. Dyspnoea (65%).

8. Hypertension — i.e. as defined on page 344.

INVESTIGATIONS

1. Serum transaminase (SGOT) collected 24–36 hours after onset may differentiate between angina and myocardial infarction.

2. Haemoglobin estimation.

3. Serology for syphilis and serum lipid levels.

4. An electrocardiograph is often normal in angina pectoris but is indicated if myocardial infarction is suspected. A cardiographic record is always useful for comparison if further attacks suggest myocardial infarction.

5. An exercise cardiograph may be helpful but should be carried out with caution.

6. Coronary angiography should be considered in the 20% of severer cases who may have to be considered for bypass operation.

DURATION

Angina pectoris if untreated may continue for years without change or may be steadily progressive.

COMPLICATIONS

Myocardial infarction and death. Angina that is becoming more frequent or more severe is termed 'unstable' and may precede a full infarct.

MISLEADING FEATURES AND PITFALLS

1. Chest pain and anxiety may suggest a functional origin when in fact organic myocardial ischaemia is responsible.

2. A cardiac investigation or mention of a possible 'tired heart' may trigger off a cardiac neurosis in a patient with fibrositis of the chest wall and an entirely normal cardiovascular system.

3. The fear of being wrong leads the doctor to qualify his reassurances, e.g. 'Your heart is fine, but in a man of your age you never quite know.' This creates considerable needless doubt and increases the likelihood of a cardiac neurosis.

4. Bypass surgery may be chosen for inappropriate reasons — because changes in life style, e.g. smoking, diet, etc. appear too tedious.

DIFFERENTIAL DIAGNOSIS

Diseases that may be confused with angina pectoris:

Myocardial infarction

Similar features: nature and distribution of pain; pain sometimes relieved by nitroglycerin.

Distinguishing features: pain is not relieved by rest and continues for over 15 minutes; patient shocked; pulse rate may be raised; blood pressure falls and remains lower than previously in spite of recovery from shock; ECG changes present; serum transaminase raised; differentiation sometimes very difficult; second opinion indicated.

Reflux oesophagitis

Similar features: nature and distribution of pain; pain after meals.

Distinguishing features: not relieved by rest or nitroglycerin; pain related to posture not exertion; symptoms of indigestion — flatulence and water brash; differentiation may be difficult and require hospital investigation.

Chronic cholecystitis and peptic ulcer

Similar features: low substernal chest pain; after meals.

Distinguishing features: Chronic cholecystitis — pain radiates to back or right shoulder and is related to fatty foods; gall bladder is tender; cholecystitis and coronary disease sometimes arise in the same patient. Peptic ulcer — pain may radiate through to back and is relieved by food or alkalis; epigastric tenderness common.

Cardiac neurosis

Similar feature: pain in lower chest and precordium.

Distinguishing features: pain not clearly related to exertion; symptoms often disappear after careful questioning, examination and reassurance.

MANAGEMENT OPTIONS

Prevention: as for Myocardial infarction.

Established disease: (a) reduce high risk factors; (b) anti-anginal vasodilators — BNF 2.6.1; (c) coronary bypass surgery if symptoms are not easily controlled with drugs or there is evidence of disease in left main coronary artery — referral for an opinion about surgery should not be delayed too long; (d) diet, smoking, weight reduction etc. as for MI (page 353).

CARDIAC FAILURE

Cardiac failure may occur suddenly (acute cardiac failure) or slowly (congestive heart failure).

ACUTE CARDIAC FAILURE

May arise in myocardial infarction, ventricular fibrillation, cardiac tamponade or poisoning. The clinical picture is that of acute peripheral vascular collapse and shock. Death from failure of the cerebral circulation may follow.

CONGESTIVE HEART FAILURE

Classification: ICHPPC 428 (RCGP 2005)

A gradually progressive disorder in which impaired action of the heart slows up the circulation of the blood.

AETIOLOGY

The heart's action may be impeded by many factors which operate at a number of points in the circulation:

1. Arteriosclerosis and hypertension — the obstruction to the circulation is at the periphery.
2. Myocardial fibrosis and infarction — the flow of the circulation is impeded in one or both ventricles.
3. Auricular fibrillation — leads to inefficient filling and contraction of the ventricles. [Practice experience: 18% (six out of 33) patients with congestive heart failure had auricular fibrillation.]
4. Mitral stenosis and aortic valve lesions.
5. Diseases that produce an obstruction of the circulation within the lungs include emphysema, chronic bronchitis and asthma. [Practice experience: 9% (three out of 33) cases with congestive heart failure had gross pulmonary disease of this type.]
6. Excessive demands on the heart. In severe anaemias, thyrotoxicosis or obesity the demands on the heart may be so great that congestive heart failure occurs. Failure in these circumstances is sometimes called high output failure — an ambiguous term because cardiac output is always lowered when the heart fails. The term indicates that the cardiac output before the heart failed was higher than normal and that the excessive demands on the heart were a factor in producing the failure. Right- and left-sided failure — these convenient terms are used to describe the clinical pictures that follow obstruction to the circulation at different points.

Arteriosclerosis, hypertension and aortic valve lesions may lead to left-sided heart failure. Mitral valve lesions may lead to failure of the left atrium. As the left-sided failure progresses, pulmonary congestion and finally right-sided failure supervene.

Emphysema, chronic bronchitis and asthma may lead to right-sided heart failure *referred to as cor pulmonale.*

In many patients with congestive heart failure, the symptoms and signs of both right- and left-sided failure are present. It is difficult to say which predominates, because the heart acts as a whole unit and the two sides cannot function independently.

DIAGNOSTIC RANGE (rates per 1000 patients per year)
Personal: Suspected 11.1. Probable 8.8. *National*: 6.7 (Ref 0.2).

AGE INCIDENCE

The majority (90%) occur over the age of 60. Myocardial infarction, valvular disease, asthma or congenital heart disease may lead to congestive heart failure in younger patients.

I. CLINICAL POINTERS WHICH SUGGEST LEFT-SIDED HEART FAILURE

1. Dyspnoea (100%) is related to exertion, particularly going upstairs and as the disease progresses it becomes noticeable at rest (orthopnoea). Attacks of dyspnoea (often nocturnal) may occur — the patient wakes and finds that he is acutely short of breath — a bad prognostic sign. Such attacks of acute pulmonary oedema (see p. 443) indicate Acute Left Ventricular Failure and may follow any severe congestive failure or infarct.
2. Cough. A chronic cough is common.
3. Haemoptysis. Streaking of sputum with blood may occur with any pulmonary congestion, but is especially common in cases of mitral stenosis and infarct.
4. Cyanosis (central) is most obvious in lips, cheeks and hands.
5. Basal adventitious sounds (54%). Fine moist râles which persist after coughing are heard at both lung bases. A chest X-ray may show definite hilar congestion of both lungs when the bases are clinically clear.
6. Evidence of left ventricular enlargement. Clinical or radiological.
7. Accentuated pulmonary second sound. This sign is difficult to assess.

II. CLINICAL POINTERS WHICH SUGGEST RIGHT-SIDED HEART FAILURE

1. Evidence of left-sided heart failure. This is a frequent cause of right-sided heart failure.

2. History of chronic lung disease or emphysema. Asthma, chronic bronchitis and emphysema may cause right-sided heart failure. In these patients dyspnoea and cyanosis are often severe and are aggravated by the primary lung condition.

3. Peripheral oedema affects the dependent parts and is first noticed in one or both ankles at the day's end. The oedema appears over the sacrum, if the patient is in bed. Ascites or pleural effusion may develop if failure is prolonged or severe. [Practice experience: 42% (14 out of 33) patients with congestive heart failure had oedema.]

4. Anorexia and indigestion are thought to be due to venous congestion of the stomach.

5. Congestion of liver. An enlarged tender liver is often felt.

6. Distension of neck veins is a useful sign but may be difficult to assess.

7. Urine may contain albumen. Oliguria may be noted.

INVESTIGATIONS

1. Straight chest X-ray gives useful information about:

- Hilar and pulmonary congestion.
- Cardiac outlined and enlargement.
- Possible pulmonary lesions.

2. Radiological screening of the heart gives more accurate information about the cardiac enlargement.

3. Electrocardiograph may be helpful.

DURATION

A patient with congestive heart failure may live for years. Some patients default from treatment and appear to lead a contented life of reduced activity.

COMPLICATIONS

1. Lung infections are common and tend to be slow in both onset and recovery.

2. Death.

MISLEADING FEATURES AND PITFALLS

1. The slow sighing air hunger associated with a tension state is confused with the rapid panting dyspnoea of cardiac failure.

2. A patient with little or no evidence of congestive heart failure may develop a cardiac neurosis if a doctor hides his clinical doubts by using equivocal medical terms such as 'tired heart'.

3. Moderate degrees of cardiac enlargement, pulmonary congestion and peripheral oedema may be noted for some time before

there is much interference with the normal activities of the patient.

4. Confusing abdominal pain may be caused by digoxin or a congested liver.

DIFFERENTIAL DIAGNOSIS

Right- and left-sided failure may be associated and often mimic each other; differentiation may be difficult or impossible. Thus the pulmonary congestion of left-sided failure may produce a picture suggesting chronic bronchitis, while the pulmonary causes of right-sided failure are often associated with dyspnoea.

Diseases that may be confused with congestive heart failure:

Bronchogenic carcinoma

Similar features: dyspnoea; chronic cough; haemoptysis; basal râles.

Distinguishing features: younger patients affected; smoking; clinical differentiation may be difficult; chest X-ray differentiates.

Pulmonary TB in the elderly

Similar features: dyspnoea; chronic cough or history of bronchitis; older age-groups affected; haemoptysis.

Distinguishing features: contact cases; previous history; clinical differentiation difficult; chest X-ray differentiates.

Pneumonia in the elderly

Similar features: dyspnoea; cough; haemoptysis; basal râles; absence of fever.

Distinguishing features: these two diseases are surprisingly easily confused; chest X-ray differentiates.

Hypostatic oedema (*in the elderly or obese patient*)

Similar features: oedema of ankles; dyspnoea.

Distinguishing features: the patient may complain of dyspnoea from obesity; the absence of clinical or radiological evidence of cardiac disease differentiates.

MANAGEMENT OPTIONS

Prevention: case finding and early treatment of hypertensives and the many other diseases which may lead eventually to right or left heart failure.

Established CHF: (a) thiazide diuretics (+ potassium) — BNF 2.2.1 (Ref. 0.1) — progressing to (b) loop diuretics — BNF 2.2.2 and Cardiac Glycosides — BNF 2.1; (c) in intractable cases various peripheral vasodilator drugs may be used to reduce the peripheral load — BNF 2.5.1 and 2.6.2; (d) general: Re-organisation of life style and housing if required.

Acute LV Failure (a) morphine IV or IM — BNF 4.7.2; (b) frusemide IV or IM — BNF 2.2.2; (c) aminophylline (occasionally) — BNF 3.1.3 — (not if dysrhythmias are likely); (d) rest, in position of comfort; (e) then as for CHF above.

ATRIAL (AURICULAR) FIBRILLATION

Classification: ICHPPC 4273 (RCGP 1990)

AETIOLOGY

Rapid uncontrolled impulses in the atria stimulate irregular ventricular contractions. In the latter half of life, fibrillation may arise spontaneously.

DIAGNOSIS INCIDENCE (rates per 1000 patients per year)

Personal: Probable 4.3. The diagnosis was rarely in doubt.

CLINICAL POINTERS

In the elderly atrial fibrillation may be almost symptomless.

1. High risk factors: (a) age; (b) mitral stenosis; (c) hypertension and arteriosclerosis; (d) myocardial infarction; IHD; (e) thyrotoxicosis.
2. Palpitation.
3. Dyspnoea.
4. Pulse rate is irregular in both rate and volume. A 'pulse deficit' is often noted.
5. Congestive heart failure or angina pectoris may develop if cardiac efficiency falls.

INVESTIGATIONS

An electrocardiograph distinguishes atrial fibrillation from other arrhythmias.

DURATION

Atrial fibrillation may persist indefinitely with few symptoms. In other cases congestive failure and death gradually supervene. In a proportion [20%] of cases the fibrillation is paroxysmal.

COMPLICATIONS

1. Congestive heart failure.
2. Embolic phenomenon.

MISLEADING FEATURES AND PITFALLS

In the elderly patient with thyrotoxicosis, atrial fibrillation is such a striking finding and explains so many symptoms that the underlying thyrotoxicosis is easily overlooked.

DIFFERENTIAL DIAGNOSIS

Recurring runs of extrasystoles are most likely to be confused with atrial fibrillation. These can usually be distinguished by listening for the pause after the extrasystoles. Extrasystoles disappear with exertion. An electrocardiograph distinguishes.

MANAGEMENT OPTIONS

Prevention: (a) early treatment of high risk factors and rheumatic valve disease.

Established disease: (a) digoxin — BNF 2.1 (Ref. 0.1); (b) treat congestive heart failure (see p. 360).

PAROXYSMAL ATRIAL (SUPRAVENTRICULAR) TACHYCARDIA (PAT)

Classification: ICHPPC 4270 (RCGP 1990)

For short periods the heart beats regularly at two or three times its normal rate. The atrial origin may involve an ectopic focus or 're-entry'.

AETIOLOGY

Unknown. Healthy adults are commonly affected and it is only occasionally associated with serious heart disease.

DIAGNOSTIC INCIDENCE (rates per 1000 patients per year)

Personal: Probable 1.6. Diagnosis is easy once an attack is seen.

AGE INCIDENCE

Adults liable.

CLINICAL POINTERS

1. High risk trigger factors: (a) anxiety; (b) hypoglycaemia; (c) digestive upsets.
2. Sudden onset.
3. History of previous paroxysms.
4. Palpitations and awareness that the heart is racing.
5. Dyspnoea.
6. Regular rapid pulse — 120 to 240 beats per minute.
7. The attacks may settle with cautious pressure on one eye ball or carotid sinus. In my experience this is rarely effective.

INVESTIGATIONS

A cardiograph during an attack distinguishes; sometimes a second opinion is required to reassure the patient.

DURATION

Several minutes to a few days.

COMPLICATIONS

None.

MISLEADING FEATURES AND PITFALLS

Patients sometimes give a history that suggests a paroxysm of tachycardia. It is difficult to obtain clinical confirmation and these patients are mistakenly labelled neurotic.

DIFFERENTIAL DIAGNOSIS

Diseases that may be confused with paroxysmal tachycardia:

Tension states

Similar features: tachycardia and palpitations; rapid regular pulse.

Distinguishing features: pulse rarely over 120; onset and termination are not clear cut; symptoms and pulse rate are altered by exercise and sleep.

Thyrotoxicosis

Similar features: tachycardia and palpitations; rapid regular pulse.

Distinguishing features: exophthalmos and thyroid swelling; paroxysms absent; sweating; diarrhoea; loss of weight; patient prefers cold weather.

MANAGEMENT OPTIONS

Established disorder: (a) explanation and reassurance often sufficient; (b) sedatives — BNF 4.1. (Ref. 0.1) and anti-arrhythmics — BNF 2.3.1 — are occasionally needed if attacks are too frequent.

To stop attack: (a) prone position; (b) various manoeuvres — pressure on eyeballs or carotid sinus; sudden postural change or Valsalva — often not effective; (c) sedatives and reassurance — the attack often stops during sleep; (d) referral or intravenous verapamil — BNF 2.3.2 — occasionally needed.

PERIPHERAL ARTERIAL DISEASE

There are two main aetiological types.

1. Functional disease in which the symptoms are transient and are probably due to arterial spasm:
   - Congenital cold fingers and Raynaud's phenomenon.

- Chilblains.
- Erthrocyanosis, erythromelalgia and acrocyanosis (rare).

2. Organic disease in which the changes are irreversible and the symptoms are progressive:
   - Intermittent claudication.
   - Gangrene and arteriosclerotic changes.
   - A number of rare and obscure diseases, e.g. Buerger's disease and secondary Raynaud's phenomenon.

PRIMARY RAYNAUD'S PHENOMENON

Classification: ICHPPC 443 (RCGP 2210)

In cold weather, the fingers become dead and white — a result of arterial spasm. The disorder may last for minutes or hours and is followed by pain and flushing of the affected fingers when the circulation returns. The disorder sometimes called intermittent digital ischaemia or 'cold fingers' is present in about one-tenth of the population. In only a few is it reported or incapacitating.

DIAGNOSTIC RANGE (rates per 1000 patients per year)
Personal: Probable (reported) 5.0.

AGE INCIDENCE
Ages over 10 affected.

SEX INCIDENCE
Women are especially liable.

Secondary Raynaud's disease is a more serious condition in which gangrene of fingers may occur and may follow use of vibrating tools, severe anaemias, thoracic outlet syndrome, syringomyelia and some autoimmune disease (SLE, scleroderma and periarteritis nodosa).

MANAGEMENT OPTIONS
Established condition: (a) avoid cold; (b) gloves; (c) referral occasionally needed — especially secondary disease; (d) peripheral vasodilators not helpful.

CHILBLAINS

Classification: ICHPPC 994 (RCGP 5235)

AETIOLOGY
Cold weather, with modern central heating the incidence is declining.

DIAGNOSTIC RANGE (rates per 1000 patients per year)
Personal: Suspected 4.7. Probable 2.7. *National*: 1.0 (Ref. 0.2). Many cases are not reported.

AGE INCIDENCE
All ages. Teenagers are especially prone.

SEX INCIDENCE
Females report with chilblains more often than men (10:1)

CLINICAL POINTERS

1. High risk factors: (a) cold weather; (b) unheated bedrooms.
2. Characteristic appearance (90%) A blotchy purple area (2 to 8 cm diam.) develops on the fingers, toes, heel or just above the ankle.
3. Itching and pain. Pain, tenderness and secondary infection are common.
4. Swelling. Local oedema is sometimes marked, especially in babies' hands.

DURATION
The tendency persists throughout life.

DIFFERENTIAL DIAGNOSIS
The lesion of erythema nodosum resembles a chilblain but is usually found on the front of the upper shin — a rare site for chilblains.

MANAGEMENT OPTIONS
Prevention: (a) warm bedroom; (b) gloves; (c) peripheral vasodilators rarely helpful.

INTERMITTENT CLAUDICATION

Classification ICHPPC 443 (RCGP 2220)

AETIOLOGY
Arteriosclerosis. The disorder may arise in diabetics — a result of arterial degeneration.

DIAGNOSTIC RANGE (rates per 1000 patients per year)
Personal: Probable 2.0. Diagnosis rarely in doubt.

AGE INCIDENCE
Uncommon under 45.

CLINICAL POINTERS

1. High risk factors: (a) smoking; (b) diabetes; (c) hypertension; (d) evidence of arteriosclerosis elsewhere; (e) family history.

2. Characteristic history of pain. A severe cramp-like pain is felt in the calf muscles after exertion. The patient knows to a matter of yards how far he can walk before the pain forces him to stop. After resting a moment the pain goes. A pain that is present at rest or which starts with the first step is unlikely to be claudication.

3. Absence of arterial pulsation in legs. Pulsation in the dorsalis pedis or posterior tibial arteries may be absent. In severe cases popliteal or even femoral pulsation may be lost.

4. If associated 'rest pain' develops surgery should be considered. 'Rest pain' occurs in the foot at night, prevents sleep, is often severe and is relieved by hanging the foot out of bed.

INVESTIGATIONS

An X-ray of the leg may reveal arterial calcification.

Angiography if the condition deteriorates.

DURATION

The disease is slowly progressive.

(Improvement occurs spontaneously in 40%. A further 40% remain unchanged and only 20% come to operation.)

COMPLICATIONS

Gangrene of toes or feet.

DIFFERENTIAL DIAGNOSIS

This condition is occasionally simulated by *meralgia paraesthetica* in which the lateral cutaneous nerve of thigh is pinched during exertion. Sensory loss of the outer thigh confirms a diagnosis of the latter.

MISLEADING FEATURES AND PITFALLS

Diabetes mellitus is easily overlooked.

The likelihood of spontaneous improvement is not realised and a needless operation is performed.

MANAGEMENT OPTIONS

Prevention: Modifying the effects of smoking, diabetes and hypertension should be a part of every family physician's routine preventive practice.

Established disease: (a) graduated exercise to limit of pain; (b) stop smoking; (c) reduce weight; (d) peripheral vasodilators rarely effective; (e) surgery considered if symptoms are interfering with life style (or job), if there is 'rest pain' or if symptoms are steadily progressive.

THE ISCHAEMIC LEG AND ARTERIOSCLEROTIC GANGRENE

Classification: ICHPPC 443 (RCGP 2225)

DIAGNOSTIC RANGE (rates per 1000 patient per year)
Personal: 1.0. The diagnosis was rarely in doubt.

AGE INCIDENCE
Over 60 years.

CLINICAL POINTERS

1. High risk factors; (a) smoking; (b) diabetes; (c) hypertension; (d) evidence of arteriosclerosis elsewhere; (e) family history.
2. Sudden onset or any sudden change (over a few hours) in severity or progression of symptoms. This should raise the possibility of immediate embolectomy; then to be effective referral must be within 48 hours of onset.
3. The presence of 'rest pain' i.e. nocturnal pain, bad enough to keep the patient awake is always an indication for surgery.
4. Ulceration of the toes or foot. After a variable pregangrenous period, during which time the affected skin becomes shiny and purple, an indolent ulcer develops. Chiropody may start an ulcer.
5. Pain in the affected area varies according to the extent of infarction and the speed at which it occurs.
6. Circulation is very poor in the purple area which surrounds the ulcer. After gentle pressure the skin takes several seconds to return to its purple colour.
7. Absent arterial pulsation. Pulsation in dorsalis pedis, posterior tibial, popliteal or femoral arteries may be lost. Absence of femoral pulsation is always an indication for early surgical referral.

INVESTIGATIONS
X-rays may show arterial calcification. Urine test for sugar.

DURATION
The disease is slowly progressive and amputation may be necessary. Occasionally with treatment a gangrenous ulcer will heal.

COMPLICATIONS
Loss of a limb, foot or toe.

MISLEADING FEATURES AND PITFALLS
Diabetes mellitus is easily overlooked.

MANAGEMENT OPTIONS
Prevention: modifying the high risk factors involved should be a routine part of every family doctor's practice.
Established disease: early referral. For successful embolectomy referral within 48 hours is essential.

PULMONARY EMBOLISM AND INFARCTION

Classification: ICHPPC 415 (RCGP 1955)

AETIOLOGY
The possibility of an embolus should always raise questions about its source and trigger factors. Not infrequently the origin of an embolus is obscure.

DIAGNOSTIC RANGE (rates per 1000 patients per year)
Personal: Suspected 1.2. Probable 0.6. *National*: 0.3 (Ref. 0.2).

AGE INCIDENCE
The majority of patients are over 65. Operations and pregnancy may preciptate an embolus in younger patients.

SEX INCIDENCE
Women appear to be more affected than men (3 : 1).

CLINICAL POINTERS
1. High risk factors: (a) phlebitis especially legs, with or without varicose veins; (b) operations especially pelvic and after delivery; (c) heart disease especially valvular and MI; (d) bed rest; (e) the contraceptive pill.
2. Sudden death (20%) is caused by a large embolus.
3. Sudden onset (75%).
4. Chest pain (75%) is related to breathing and aggravated by coughing. A large embolus may cause severe central chest pain, associated with shock, dyspnoea and cyanosis.
5. Cough (60%) is dry and irritable.
6. Haemoptysis (50%) appears as a slight streaking or rustiness of the sputum and usually starts a few hours after the onset of pain. Occasionally loss is heavy.
7. Physical signs in the chest (25%). A few fine râles or pleural friction rub may be heard over the affected lung.

8. Fever. A moderate fever is not uncommon on the 2nd or 3rd day.
9. Tenderness of the calves suggesting phlebitis (30%).

NOTE. Pointers 4 to 8 are due to the pulmonary infarction that follows the pulmonary embolus.

INVESTIGATIONS
1. Chest X-ray may be helpful.
2. Electrocardiograph to explore the cardiac origins.
3. A leucocyte count.

In pneumonia, leucocytosis is high early — in infarcts it is moderate after 2 to 4 days.

DURATION
The lungs return to normal in two to four weeks.

COMPLICATIONS
Death. Heart failure is said to be precipitated by a large embolus.

MISLEADING FEATURES AND PITFALLS
Failure to realise that pulmonary infarction is common leads to it being overlooked.

DIFFERENTIAL DIAGNOSIS
Diseases that may be confused with pulmonary embolism:

Myocardial infarction
Similar features: sudden onset; severe chest pain and tightness; peripheral circulatory collapse; sudden death.

Distinguishing features: may be difficult to distinguish clinically from a large embolism; ECG may assist; hospital investigation.

Lobar pneumonia
Similar features: sudden onset; chest pain of respiratory type: rusty sputum; localised crepitations; pleural rub; fever.

Distinguishing features: distinction may be difficult; fever starts earlier, is higher and more prolonged; no obvious origin of embolus; chest X-ray, cardiograph and blood count may differentiate.

Spontaneous pneumothorax
Similar features: sudden onset; chest pain of respiratory type; respiratory distress.

Distinguishing features: chest X-ray differentiates; chest signs are characteristic; (a) Tension SP: breath sounds diminished or absent; percussion resonant; vocal resonance diminished; evidence of mediastinal shift; percussion is dull and tubular breath sounds are heard posteriorly where the lung is collapsed; (b) Non-tension SP: breath sounds are diminished or absent over affected area.

Bronchiectasis; pulmonary T.B.; neoplasm of lung; congestive heart (including mitral) diseases
Similar feature: haemoptysis.

Distinguishing feature: previous history and chest X-ray differentiate.

MANAGEMENT OPTIONS

Prevention: in all high risk groups, instructions to patients should aim for the middle course between 'activity' to prevent venous thrombi extending and 'rest' to prevent any formed thrombi breaking free.

Established emboli: (a) identify source; (b) small emboli — nil (c) larger emboli — refer or treat as lobar pneumonia (p. 415).

VARICOSE VEINS (LOWER LIMBS)

Classification: ICHPPC 454 (RCGP 2265)

AETIOLOGY

The valves of the superficial leg veins cease to function adequately — a result of: (1) pregnancy; (2) excessive standing as in shops or bench work; (3) a deep femoral vein thrombosis — the superficial veins take over the vital function of the deep veins.

DIAGNOSTIC RANGE (rates per 1000 patients per year)

Personal: Suspected 16.7. Probable 13.4. *National*: 9.6 (Ref. 0.2). Many cases not reported. Ten per cent of adult population said to be affected.

AGE INCIDENCE

Most patients first complain at child-bearing age, thereafter there is a steady increase in incidence (Fig. 28).

SEX INCIDENCE

Women are affected more than men (5 : 1).

CLINICAL POINTERS

1. High risk factors: (a) pregnancy and multiparity; (b) excessive standing; (c) positive family history; (d) constipation; (e) deep vein thrombosis; (f) low fibre diets.

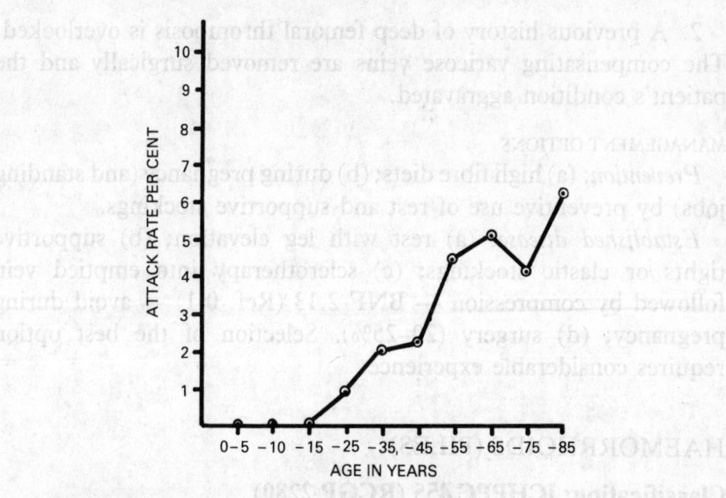

Fig. 28 Varicose veins. Age incidence of 115 consecutive cases in 2 years.

2. Distended tortuous superficial veins (95%).

3. Pain (60%) is worse after standing especially when the varicosities are small.

4. Discoloration or irritation of the skin precedes ulceration.

5. Swelling of the ankles is worse after standing.

6. A saphenous thrill (or impulse) can be felt — after a cough — over the saphenous opening when there is incompetence of the main valve — the Cough Test, Trendelenburgh test and Perthes test should be performed to identify the valves at fault and the state of the deep veins.

DURATION

The untreated disease tends to be slowly progressive.

COMPLICATIONS

1. Varicose eczema (10%). A brown irritant patch, often shiny and scaly, develops on the shin.

2. Varicose ulcer (20%). A slight abrasion frequently precipitates an ulcer that may take months to heal.

3. Thrombophlebitis. The vein is felt as a hard tender cord which may take several weeks to settle.

4. Pulmonary embolus. Uncommon.

MISLEADING FEATURES AND PITFALLS

1. The association between varicose phlebitis and pulmonary embolus is overlooked because it is uncommon.

2. A previous history of deep femoral thrombosis is overlooked. The compensating varicose veins are removed surgically and the patient's condition aggravated.

MANAGEMENT OPTIONS

Prevention: (a) high fibre diets; (b) during pregnancy (and standing jobs) by preventive use of rest and supportive stockings.

Established disease: (a) rest with leg elevation; (b) supportive tights or elastic stockings; (c) sclerotherapy into emptied vein followed by compression — BNF 2.13 (Ref. 0.1) — avoid during pregnancy; (d) surgery (20–25%). Selection of the best option requires considerable experience.

HAEMORRHOIDS (PILES)

Classification: ICHPPC 455 (RCGP 2280)

Internal piles (described below) are not true varicose veins but are due to abnormalities and prolapse of the special area above the sphincter.

External piles are external varicosities. The swelling is symptomless until thrombosis occurs. After a few days the thrombosed vein discharges a clot and heals.

AETIOLOGY

Like varicose veins, piles are probably the result of Man's upright stance and low fibre diet.

DIAGNOSTIC RANGE (rates per 1000 patients per year)

Personal: Suspected 14.5. Probable 9.0. *National*: 8.6 (Ref. 0.2). Many cases are not reported or only mentioned to the doctor incidentally.

AGE INCIDENCE

Adults liable. Peaks of incidence occur at the child-bearing age and just before retiring age (Fig. 29).

SEX INCIDENCE

Females are affected more commonly than males (3.2)

CLINICAL POINTERS

1. High risk factors: (a) pregnancy (66%) — Most women sufferers relate their piles to a pregnancy; (b) constipation and small or liquid stools; (c) positive family history; (d) low fibre diet.

2. Anal bleeding (50%) occurs at the end of defaecation.

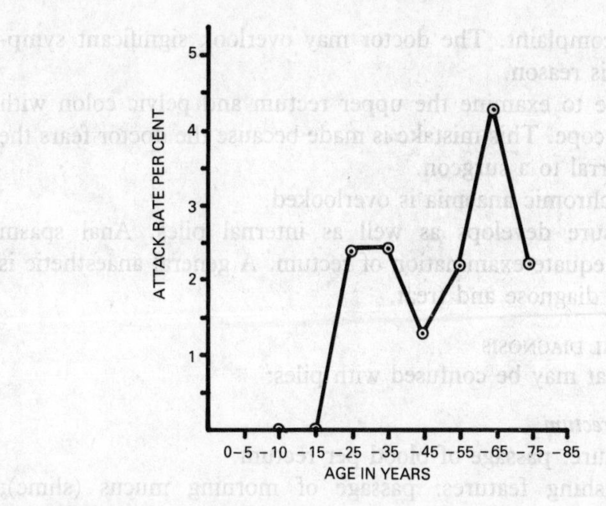

Fig. 29 Piles. Age incidence of 43 consecutive cases in 1 year. Note the peak at child-bearing age.

3. Rectal prolapse (60%). A sensation of something coming down is confirmed when the patient feels the tense tender rectal prolapse.

4. Irritation (10%) is an early symptom.

5. Pain (25%). Acute pain accompanies an irreducible prolapse.

6. Rectal examination is performed in every patient with suspected piles and helps the doctor to exclude cancer.

INVESTIGATIONS

1. Protoscopy is rarely of assistance.

2. Sigmoidoscopy may be the only way to exclude serious disease.

3. Barium enema is occasionally of assistance in outlining a carcinoma or colitis. It is not a substitute for sigmoidoscopy.

DURATION

Untreated piles usually improve spontaneously but tend to recur.

COMPLICATIONS

Hypochromic anaemia.

MISLEADING FEATURES AND PITFALLS

1. Failure to perform a rectal examination in an adult with symptoms of piles. If cancer is present, the omission is serious and will soon become apparent to both patient and relatives. Patients frequently report the symptoms of piles in an offhand way or as an

incidental complaint. The doctor may overlook significant symptoms for this reason.

2. Failure to examine the upper rectum and pelvic colon with a sigmoidoscope. This mistake is made because the doctor fears the fuss of referral to a surgeon.

3. Hypochromic anaemia is overlooked.

4. A fissure develops as well as internal piles. Anal spasm prevents adequate examination of rectum. A general anaesthetic is required to diagnose and treat.

DIFFERENTIAL DIAGNOSIS

Diseases that may be confused with piles:

Carcinoma rectum

Similar feature: passage of blood per rectum.

Distinguishing features: passage of morning mucus (slime); (rectal examination said to reveal growth in only 75% of rectal cancers); doubtful cases referred for sigmoidoscomy and Barium enema.

Carcinoma of colon (or pelvirectal junction)

Similar features: passage of blood per rectum; rectal examination negative.

Distinguishing features: change of bowel habit; passage of mucus may occur; blood intimately mixed with motion; surgical opinion indicated as well as radiology and sigmoidoscopy.

Ulcerative colitis and diverticulitis

Similar feature: passage of blood per rectum.

Distinguishing features: previous attacks common; diarrhoea and mucus; blood intimately mixed with motion. In colitis younger age-groups liable; sigmoidoscopy and proctoscopy may reveal typical granular inflammatory lesions and ulcerations. Barium enema.

MANAGEMENT OPTIONS (Internal piles)

Prevention: high fibre diets and active general exercise programmes especially during pregnancy.

Established piles: (a) high fibre diet; (b) active exercises for perineum; (c) suppositories to reduce swelling, pain and inflammation; (d) referral.

External piles cure themselves in 10–20 days.

Table 23 Less common diseases of the circulatory system

Disease and distinguishing clinical pointers	Incidence per 1000 patients per year Suspected	Confirmed
Dissecting aneurysm Young patients as well as elderly are occasionally affected; sudden onset; severe central pain in chest or abdomen with widespread radiation to jaw, arms or legs; secondary shock absent; CNS signs from vertebral artery obstruction	—	1 in 10 years
Extrasystoles Healthy adults affected; rapid or extra beats followed by a pause; atrial fibrillation simulated; coupled beats suggest digitalis overdosage; many cases are symptomless and never reported	0.9	0.9
Complete heart block Pulse regular at 45 or less; ECG	—	3 in 10 years
Stokes-Adams attacks Heart stops for up to 40 seconds; followed by unconsciousness and slow squirming convulsion — pulse reappears — a rosy flush spreads over the body as consciousness return. ECG.	—	2 in 10 years
Buerger's disease Onset before 40; intermittent claudication.	0	0 in 10 years
Periarteritis nodosa (see p. 626) Chronic progressive febrile illness; scattered muscle pains; hypertension; wasting; red cells in urine. Biopsy.	—	1 in 10 years
Temporal arteritis (see p. 635)		
Deep femoral vein thrombosis (*white leg*) Women (especially if anaemic) affected in the puerperium; pain tenderness and marked oedema of leg. If suspected immediate referral indicated.	—	2 in 10 years
Transient Ischaemic Attacks (TIA) Temporary loss of consciousness for a few seconds in the elderly. No residual symptoms or signs. Not uncommon. Attacks may precede a major stroke.	?	uncertain
Drop attacks Sudden fall without loss of consciousness in elderly patient. No residual symptoms or signs.	?	uncertain

17

Diseases of the respiratory system

Please read introduction for explanation of figures and analyses.

BRONCHOGENIC CARCINOMA

Classification ICHPP 162 (RCGP 0440)

AETIOLOGY

Uncertain. There is a proven link with cigarette smoking. The diagnosis should be questioned in any true non-smoker. The smoking link also makes nonsense of present health policies which spend so much on cure and so little on prevention.

DIAGNOSTIC RANGE (rates per 1000 patients per year)

Personal: Suspected 1.4. Probable 0.9. *National*: 1.0 (Ref. 0.2).

AGE INCIDENCE

Adults. 45 to 65 years.

SEX INCIDENCE

Men more than women.

CLINICAL POINTERS

1. High risk factors: (a) smoking; (b) asbestos and mining workers.
2. Duration of symptoms. 80% have had symptoms for less than 3 months when diagnosed.
3. Persistent cough of recent onset, in patients over 30 years, is suspect until proved otherwise. An early symptom.
4. Haemoptysis. Slight haemoptysis is an early symptom. Incidents may be single or repeated.
5. Dyspnoea is a distinctive early complaint.
6. Chest pain. A vague feeling of tightness or definite pleurisy. An early symptom. Occasionally severe pain is caused by invasion of the brachial plexus, or pathological fracture in rib or spine.

7. Weight loss is often an early symptom although appetite remains good until late in the disease.

8. Chest signs, cyanosis and clubbing of fingers are late signs. Pleurisy, pleural effusion or pulmonary collapse may occur in the final stages.

9. Fever indicates associated lung sepsis.

10. Supraclavicular glands are sometimes noted.

11. The latent pre-symptom period is thought to last many months.

INVESTIGATIONS

1. Chest X-ray may be normal in the early stages. Tomography or lateral views may be helpful. Radiological abnormalities include: (a) a dense irregular hilar expansion; (b) a dense well-defined peripheral opacity; (c) atelectasis or effusion.

2. Sputum cytology. Malignant cells may be seen.

3. Bronchoscopy. It is said that 80% of tumours can be visualised at an early stage by bronchoscopy.

4. Blood tests. Raised ESR (see p. 681).

5. A wide variety of tests and scans to assess the extent of spread.

DURATION

The patient usually dies within 15 months of the first symptom.

COMPLICATIONS

Blood-borne metastases may affect any of the great capillary beds, in the brain, bones or kidneys.

MISLEADING FEATURES AND PITFALLS

1. Pneumonia in the area of the growth often precedes other symptoms by a few months. Chest X-ray at this stage may reveal the pneumonia and then clear completely or leave minimal evidence of the underlying carcinoma.

2. Pneumoconiosis or pulmonary TB are confused. Persistent pain in such patients may indicate an added carcinoma.

3. Smoker's cough may mask the onset of cough from a carcinoma.

4. Failure to realise that surgery is rarely able to achieve complete removal (see Management).

DIFFERENTIAL DIAGNOSIS

Diseases that may be confused with bronchogenic carcinoma:

Bronchiectasis and chronic bronchitis
Similar features: haemoptysis; cough; dyspnoea.
Distinguishing features: long chest history; chest X-ray.

Asthma
Similar features: wheezing rhonchi; cough; dyspnoea; haemoptysis.
Distinguishing features: long chest history; generalised expiratory wheeze; symptoms relieved by ephedrine; the wheeze of an obstructing carcinoma is marked in inspiration and not relieved by decongestants; chest X-ray usually differentiates.

Pulmonary TB
Similar features: haemoptysis; cough; dyspnoea and loss of weight.
Distinguishing features: long chest history; low fever; history of contact; chest X-ray differentiates.

MANAGEMENT OPTIONS

Prevention: (a) avoid smoking; (b) use personal influence at national, local and patient levels to discourage smoking; (c) rigid control of asbestos working.

Established disease: referral for assessment and treatment using surgery, radiotherapy and/or chemotherapy.

Post hospital: (a) discussion; (b) medical and mental support; (c) family and group support (see pp. 207, 208).

ACUTE INFECTIOUS DISEASE OF THE RESPIRATORY TRACT IN PRIMARY CARE

This group of diseases includes about one-quarter of the general practitioner's work.

Aetiological classification of individual diseases is rarely possible. For example, in this practice for one year throat and nasal swabs were taken from the first four cases of respiratory disease encountered each week. The swabs were cultured for viruses and bacteria. Over the same period paired sera for virus studies were taken from every adult with fever and any evidence of respiratory disease.

This intensive search for the causes of respiratory disease in a single practice yielded disappointing results. Nearly 300 cases of respiratory disease affecting all ages were investigated. Positive evidence of the following aetiological agents was obtained:

Influenza A	9 cases
Influenza B	7 cases
Coxsackie B	4 cases

Parainfluenza I	1 case
Parainfluenza II	1 case
Parainfluenza III	1 case
Echo 9	1 case
Psittacosis	1 case

In six further cases the throat or nasal swab cultured bacteria that could have been responsible for an upper respiratory disease.

Acute respiratory disease illustrates very clearly the clinical problems that face the general practitioner today. He is expected to treat a large number of diseases about which our knowledge is limited. Faced with a crowded waiting-room and partners who know that the work must be done, even the most academically-minded practitioner is often forced to solve his problems by quick empirical methods.

There are two aspects of the subject: (1) the practical way in which the family doctor achieves his first objective of diagnosing and treating acute respiratory disease in all the patients for whom he is responsible; (2) the method by which a general practitioner attempts, with the limited time and crude facilities, to manage acute upper respiratory infection (AURI). When the new entrant to practice first accepts the challenge of dealing with this large mass of morbidity he discovers that: (a) his hospital training has not taught him much that is relevant; (b) diagnostic criteria are vague and ill-defined; (c) facilities for checking diagnosis are meagre and there is little encouragement to improve these; (d) the majority of patients get better regardless of treatment; (e) our knowledge of these diseases is surprisingly limited in spite of their common occurrence and the great opportunity for study provided by the National Health Service.

Like many practitioners I solve the problems of diagnosis, management and prevention in the following crude but practical ways:

A. DIAGNOSIS OF AURI

1. Acute respiratory disease is suspected when the patient's main complaint originates from the respiratory tract and is of short duration (less than a week).

2. A few quick questions then ascertain the point of maximal impact on the respiratory tree, their duration, severity and any suggestive associated pointers.

3. High risk factors of which I would expect to be already aware are: (a) relevant previous medical history e.g. previous attacks of

asthma, pneumonia or otitis media; (b) relevant features from family and social history e.g. asthma in father, poor compliance likely, lives 10 miles away but on the phone, etc.

4. A short list of the two to four likely diagnoses is considered and then checked if possible by a quick examination including temperature.

B. MANAGEMENT OPTIONS FOR ESTABLISHED AURI

The main aim is to prevent the complications of descending, secondary bacterial infections by the following steps:

1. The relative uncertainties of diagnosis and management are explained briefly to the patient (or parents).

2. Symptomatic treatment compatible with patient compliance is advised. This would include: (a) keeping the patient quiet in a warm room of uniform temperature; (b) advice about diet; (c) symptomatic treatment of pain, cough, etc.; (d) patients are asked to report back in 2 to 4 days or before, if they are worried.

3. Systemic antibiotics — BNF 5.1.1. (Ref. 0.1) — to protect against secondary descending bacterial infection, are considered in the following circumstances:

— the patient has an adverse previous history of infection, e.g. asthma, otitis media or pneumonia.
— parental or patient compliance is considered poor and likely to increase the risks of secondary infection.
— the patient is either very old or very young.

Further investigation and daily visiting are indicated if: (a) fever persists in spite of 4 to 5 days bed rest — virus pneumonia, or other serious infections warranting further investigation must therefore be considered; (b) haemoptysis suggests more serious disease; (c) there is pleuritic pain; (d) there is systemic evidence of serious pulmonary disease e.g. dyspnoea, rapid respiratory rate, cyanosis and in babies poor or grey colour, restlessness or subcostal recession.

If the patient is very old or very young daily visiting by doctor or nurse to monitor for such danger signs is usually *always* indicated.

Every practitioner will probably develop variations on this general scheme. If he has time he will attempt to be more accurate in diagnosis and more selective in treatment but his diagnosis will probably remain essentially anatomical; he will use antibiotics without really knowing if they are justified or not. If he is especially short of time, he will tend to prescribe more antibiotics because it is often better to safeguard his patients than to attempt a more selective diagnosis.

Teaching hospitals may be critical of these crude methods with their consequent rather liberal use of antibiotics. Several points should be remembered in this context:

1. Since the introduction of these methods, the incidence of many serious bacterial diseases has greatly decreased, e.g. meningococcal, streptococcal and staphylococcal infections.

2. The hospital physician is in a very different position to that of the primary doctor. Also laboratories could not deal with the massive work load if all such cases were swabbed.

3. When hospital physicians are faced with the primary situation in their own families they frequently resort to the same methods.

C. PREVENTION OF AURI

Further preventive measures e.g. immunisation etc, are unlikely to be possible until we have developed quicker simpler methods of identifying the many common viruses involved.

Tables 24 and 25 summarise the present overlapping anatomical and aetiological relationships.

For further information about the viruses that cause respiratory disease and their clinical and epidemiological characteristics see the end of Chapter 8 (p. 176 *et seq.*)

The family doctor will find that in practice all these virus diseases have a number of features in common.

1. Classification is predominantly clinical.

2. The relationship to the common cold. Many respiratory infections are triggered off by a cold.

3. A similar age distribution, regardless of the likelihood of viral or bacterial cause. See Figures 30 and 31.

4. The tendency of one acute respiratory disease to develop into another. Thus a cold may descend the respiratory tree causing a laryngitis, bronchitis and pneumonitis in turn. Observations in this practice suggest that physical activity aided by gravity promotes the downward spread of infection.

5. Relationship to season (see charts). The winter distribution of the common cold is followed.

6. Relationship to temperature and humidity. Observations in this and other practices suggest that sudden changes of temperature and possibly humidity play a part in the spread of acute respiratory illness between individuals.

Table 24 Probable primary acute infective respiratory diseases

Diseases	Suspected incidence per 1000 N.H.S. patients per year	Age incidence (years)	Seasonal incidence	Main symptoms	Main physical signs	Possible causative organisms
Acute exudative tonsillitis (p. 393)	86.8	All ages, mainly 2 to 10	All seasons	Sore throat (75%) Contact cases (25%) Nasal speech	Fever (85%) Exudate (100%) Offensive breath	Streptococcus Adenoviruses Coxsackie virus
Acute pharyngitis (p. 391)	75.9	All ages, mainly 0 to 10	Mainly winter	Sore throat (100%)	Fever (100%) Red fauces	As above. Also: Parainfluenza viruses Rhinoviruses
Colds (p. 384)	68.3	All ages, especially 0 to 10	Mainly winter	Sore throat Nasal catarrh (100%) Cough (40%) Contact cases	Fever, mainly in children	Rhinoviruses Parainfluenza viruses Adenoviruses Coxsackie virus Other viruses
Influenza (p. 181)	Epidemic (1957 A, pandemic affected one-fifth of all patients)	All ages	Usually winter	Sudden onset Cough (97%) Painful cough (49%) Body aches Contact cases Sore throat (44%)	Fever (78%) Red fauces Meningism (6%) Conjunctivitis (8%)	Influenza viruses A, B, C Adenoviruses Coxsackie virus Echo viruses
Lobar pneumonia (p. 413)	4.7	Adults		Sudden onset Dry cough Pleuritic pain Rusty sputum	High Fever Rapid breathing Cyanosis Crepitations	Bacteria: pneumococci, staphylococci, haemophilus, etc.
Virus pneumonia (p. 189)	?	Adults	Often with other virus epidemics	Sudden onset Cough (sometimes absent)	Fever (often for a week) Fine râles Positive chest X-ray	Eaton's Psittacosis Q fever Adenoviruses
Acute bronchiolitis (p. 404)	Epidemic	Infants		Contact cases Cough	Acutely ill Fever Cyanosis	Respiratory syncytial, Parainfluenza viruses

Table 25 Probable secondary acute infective respiratory diseases (mainly bacterial)

Disease	Suspected incidence per 1000 NHS patients per year	Age incidence (years)	Seasonal incidence	Main symptoms	Main physical signs
Acute bronchitis (p. 404)	119.1	Mainly 0 to 10, especially toddlers	Winter mainly	Cough (100%)	Fever (70%) Diffuse chest signs
Acute laryngitis, tracheitis and croup (p. 401)	33.4	All ages, especially 0 to 10	Winter mainly	Hoarse cough (90%) Hoarse voice (55%) Croup (10%) Pain on coughing (50%)	Fever (30%) (obstructive cases in babies — pallor grey colour, restlessness, cyanosis)
Benign aspiration pneumonia (p. 415)	28.1	All ages, especially 0 to 10	Winter mainly	Preceding respiratory illness (72%) Previous attacks (48%) Cough (96%)	Fever Localised chest signs (76%) Cyanosis Subcostal recession in babies
Acute otitis media (p. 323)	66.2	0 to 10	Winter mainly	Earache (90%) Recurrent attacks	Redness of drum (70%) Fever Discharge (33%)
Cough (without other features) (p. 441)	133.0	All ages, especially 0 to 10	Winter mainly	Cough (100%)	
Acute maxillary sinusitis (p. 387)	27.8	Adults mainly	Winter and spring	Preceding cold (75%) Headache (or face-ache) (60%)	Nasal discharge (100%) often bloodstained (25%) Tenderness over sinus Fever Dull transillumination
Acute frontal sinusitis (p. 390)	7.1	Adults mainly	Winter and spring	Preceding cold (50%) Frontal headache (100%) especially in mornings	Tender over sinus Bloody discharge (20%) Fever Dull transillumination

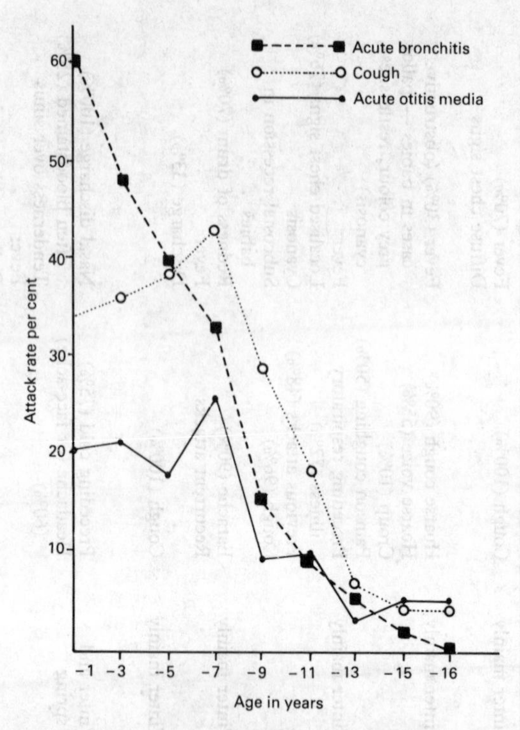

Fig. 30 Age incidence in 1 year for the three commonest secondary acute respiratory disease

7. The catarrhal child. Some children, between the ages of 2 and ten years, are especially prone to repeated attacks of all forms of infective respiratory disease. The cervical and other lymph nodes are often swollen concurrently. Fortunately most of these children grow out of the tendency.

NOTE. Families are specially likely to change their domicile when their children are between 2 and 10. The change is often blamed for the child's catarrhal troubles.

COMMON COLD

Classification: ICHPPC 460 (RCGP 2400)

AETIOLOGY

A large variety of viruses cause colds including rhinoviruses, adenoviruses, parainfluenza and Coxsackie viruses (see p. 176). Secondary bacterial infection is probably responsible for some of the later manifestations.

DIAGNOSTIC RANGE (rates per 1000 patients per year)
Personal: Suspected 120.1. Probable 68.3. *National*: 76.0 (Ref. 0.2). Most patients with colds do not report to the doctor.

AGE INCIDENCE
After a peak in the first years of life the incidence falls but increases again with age (Fig. 31).

SEASONAL INCIDENCE
Winter months (Fig. 32)

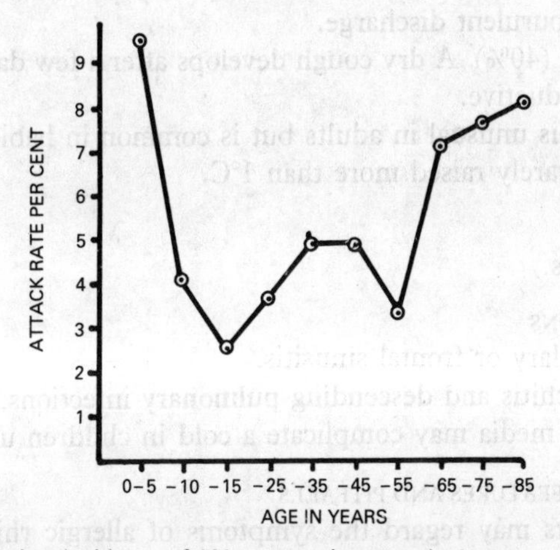

Fig. 31 Colds. Age incidence of 131 consecutive cases in 1 year.

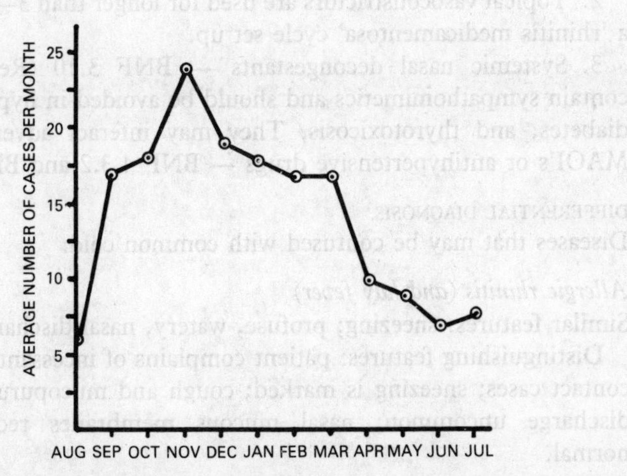

Fig. 32 Colds. Seasonal incidence of 675 consecutive cases reported over 4 years.

INCUBATION PERIOD

2 to 3 days.

CLINICAL POINTERS

1. High risk factors: (a) contacts — household attack rates are very high; (b) moving into a different community; (c) possibly changes in climatic conditions.

2. Sore throat is an early complaint. The pharynx sometimes looks red but is often normal.

3. Nasal catarrh (100%). A clear watery discharge is associated with a tendency to sneeze. After 1 or 2 days the nose is blocked by thick mucopurulent discharge.

4. Cough (40%). A dry cough develops after a few days and may become productive.

5. Fever is unusual in adults but is common in babies and children. It is rarely raised more than 1°C.

DURATION

4 to 14 days.

COMPLICATIONS

Acute maxillary or frontal sinusitis.
Acute bronchitis and descending pulmonary infections.
Acute otitis media may complicate a cold in children under 10.

MISLEADING FEATURES AND PITFALLS

1. Patients may regard the symptoms of allergic rhinitis, nasal polyp, recurrent sinusitis and influenza as being due to colds.

2. Topical vasoconstrictors are used for longer than 3–4 days and a 'rhinitis medicamentosa' cycle set up.

3. Systemic nasal decongestants — BNF 3.10 (Ref. 0.1) — contain sympathomimetics and should be avoided in hypertension, diabetes, and thyrotoxicosis. They may interact adversely with MAOI's or antihypertensive drugs — BNF 4.3.2 and BNF 2.5.

DIFFERENTIAL DIAGNOSIS

Diseases that may be confused with common cold:

Allergic rhinitis (and hay fever)

Similar features: sneezing; profuse, watery, nasal discharge.

Distinguishing features: patient complains of incessant colds; no contact cases; sneezing is marked; cough and mucopurulent nasal discharge uncommon; nasal mucous membranes redder than normal.

Nasal polyp
Similar feature: blocked nose with watery nasal discharge.

Distinguishing features: patient complains of frequent colds with blocked nose; examination with a nasal speculum reveals shiny, grey, translucent polyp.

Recurrent maxillary sinusitis
Similar features: blocked nose with mucopurulent nasal discharge.

Distinguishing features: recurring attacks of nasal discharge; headache; heavy sensation under eyes; sinus tenderness; nasal discharge — frequently bloodstained; transillumination or X-rays may confirm diagnosis.

MANAGEMENT OPTIONS (See p. 380)
If local or systemic decongestants are used for symptomatic treatment, the doctor should be fully aware of the adverse drug interactions involved.

There is no evidence that massive doses of Vitamin C prevent colds.

INFECTIONS OF THE ACCESSORY AIR SINUSES

There are four groups of accessory air sinuses:

1. Two frontal sinuses — situated above the orbit.
2. Two maxillary sinuses (antral) — situated below the orbit.
3. The ethmoidal air cells — situated medial to the orbit.
4. The sphenoidal air cells — situated above the posterior nasal space.

Infection may occur in any of these sinuses and may be acute, recurrent or chronic. Infections of the ethmoidal or sphenoidal sinuses are rare but may cause an acute illness with features of meningitis.

ACUTE MAXILLARY SINUSITIS

Classification: ICHPPC 461 (RCGP 2405)

The ostium through which the sinus drains into the nose is in the upper part of the antrum. The sinus, by virtue of man's upright position, is unable to drain by gravity and fills easily with mucus and pus after a cold. A secondary bacterial infection is usually held responsible.

DIAGNOSTIC RANGE (rates per 1000 patients per year)
Personal: Suspected 27.8. Probable 11.1. *National*: 13.5 (Ref. 0.2).

AGE INCIDENCE

Adults are liable (Fig. 33). The disease is infrequent in children and young adults and the age distribution is different from other respiratory diseases.

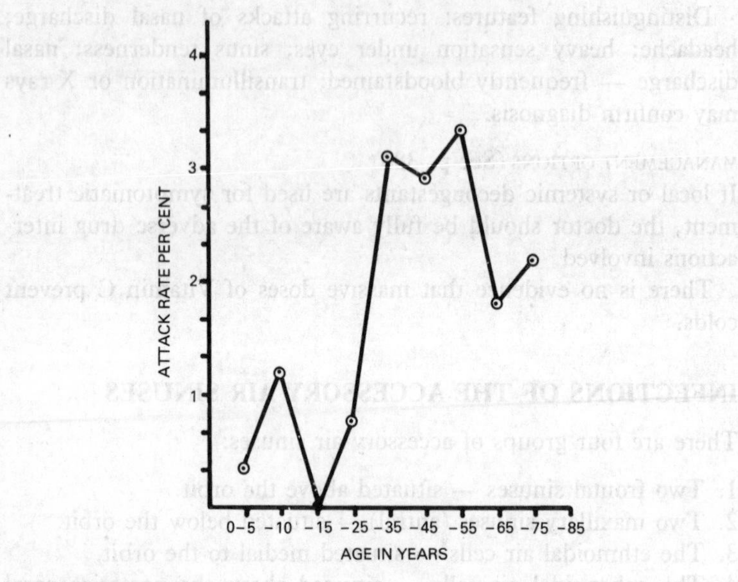

Fig. 33 Acute maxillary sinusitis. Age incidence curve of 54 consecutive cases encountered in one year.

SEASONAL INCIDENCE

A peak is reached in the spring.

CLINICAL POINTERS

1. High risk factors: (a) preceding nasal cold (75%) — usually 3 to 10 days previously; (b) an attack of allergic rhinitis; (c) previous attacks of sinusitis.

2. Headache or feeling of heaviness below the eyes (60%). A frontal headache is common. The pain is made worse by coughing, nose-blowing or lowering the head.

3. Nasal discharge (100%) is mucopurulent and varies considerably in consistency and quantity. In a proportion of cases (25%) the discharge is streaked with blood — a most useful confirmatory sign.

4. Tenderness to pressure over the affected sinus, i.e. at a point 1 cm lateral to the ala nasae. Slight swelling is occasionally noted.

5. Failure of the affected sinus to transilluminate.

6. Fever. A low-grade fever is sometimes present. Occasionally there is a high fever with oedema of the overlying cheek.

INVESTIGATIONS

X-rays of the maxillary sinuses confirm the clinical diagnosis — it may show fluid or thickened epithelial lining.

DURATION

Most attacks settle in 1 to 3 weeks.

COMPLICATIONS

Recurrences are common and may cause a chronic infection of the antrum. [Practice experience: 25% (5 out of 20) consecutive cases recurred within 3 years.]

DIFFERENTIAL DIAGNOSIS

Diseases that may be confused with acute maxillary sinusitis.

Tension headache and acute tension states

Similar feature: frontal headache.

Distinguishing features: mucopurulent or bloodstained discharge absent; fever absent; other features of tension present — sighing respiration, irritability, etc.; headache unaffected by posture.

Refractive error

Similar feature: frontal headache.

Distinguishing features: headache is related to ocular activities; nasal catarrh absent.

Migraine

Similar feature: frontal headache, aggravated by lowering head.

Distinguishing features: history of aura with nausea, vomiting and photophobia; local tenderness and nasal catarrh absent.

Space-occupying lesions of skull

Similar feature: recurring headache aggravated by coughing, nose-blowing or lowering head.

Distinguishing features: progressive evidence of raised intracranial pressure, i.e. listlessness, nausea and papilloedema; localising signs in the CNS; local tenderness and nasal catarrh absent.

Dental abscess (upper jaw)

Similar features: face-ache; oedema of cheek; fever; acute local tenderness.

Distinguishing features: affected tooth tender to touch; gum beside tooth red and swollen; sinuses transilluminate normally; history of cold absent.

MANAGEMENT OPTIONS (see p. 380)

Established disease where symptoms are severe, systemic antibiotics — BNF 5.1.1. (Ref. 0.1) — combined with decongestants (either systemic — BNF 3.10 or local — BNF 12.2.2) may be indicated.

RECURRENT AND CHRONIC MAXILLARY SINUSITIS

Classification: ICHPPC 461 (RCGP 2405)

Apart from the chronicity, the clinical picture of acute and chronic maxillary sinusitis is similar.

COMPLICATIONS

Bronchiectasis complicates chronic sinusitis surprisingly often.

MISLEADING FEATURES AND PITFALLS

Chest complications are easily overlooked.

MANAGEMENT OPTIONS

As for acute maxillary sinusitis. Referral to ENT Surgeon often needed.

ACUTE FRONTAL SINUSITIS

Classification: ICHPPC 461 (RCGP 2405)

AETIOLOGY

The headache of frontal sinus is thought to arise in two different ways.

1. The vacuum headache

The ostium becomes blocked by a mild catarrhal inflammation and the air from the main body of the sinus is absorbed. The headache is produced by the negative pressure inside the sinus.

2. The positive pressure headache

When the sinus fills with pus and the ostium becomes blocked free drainage cannot occur, the pressure inside the sinus rises and headache follows.

DIAGNOSTIC RANGE (rates per 1000 patients per year)

Personal: Suspected 7.1, Probable 4.5.

AGE AND SEASONAL INCIDENCE
The same as acute maxillary sinusitis.

CLINICAL POINTERS
1. High risk factors: (a) preceding nasal cold (50%); (b) previous attacks.
2. Characteristic headache (100%) is severe, is over the affected sinus and tends to start at a fixed time each morning.
3. Tenderness over the affected sinus.
4. A bloodstained nasal discharge (20%).
5. Fever. Occasionally there is an acute systemic reaction to an acute frontal sinusitis. Fever may be over 38°C and may persist for 3 to 4 days. Oedema over the sinus may then be marked and pain with local tenderness is severe.
6. Transillumination of frontal sinuses is rarely helpful because it is impossible to decide if a frontal sinus is dull or absent.

INVESTIGATIONS
An X-ray of the frontal sinuses.

DIFFERENTIAL DIAGNOSIS
As for maxillary sinusitis.

MANAGEMENT OPTIONS (see p. 380)
Established disease: where symptoms are severe systemic antibiotics — BNF 5.1.1 (Ref. 0.1) may occasionally be indicated. Local decongestants — BNF 12.2.2 assisted by gravity may relieve pain rapidly.

ACUTE PHARYNGITIS

Classification: ICHPPC 460 (RCGP 2400)

The clinical picture of acute pharyngitis is ill-defined because:
1. Redness or injection of the fauces is an unreliable sign — many healthy throats are red.
2. A sore throat is a common complaint in patients who are mentally tired or depressed. Such functional pharyngitis is often referred to by patients as a 'relaxed' throat.
3. A sore throat is a very convenient pseudo-complaint for a child who wishes to avoid school or an adult who wants a few days off work.
4. A sore and inflamed throat without exudate is sometimes present for 2 to 3 days in the early stages of acute exudative tonsillitis.

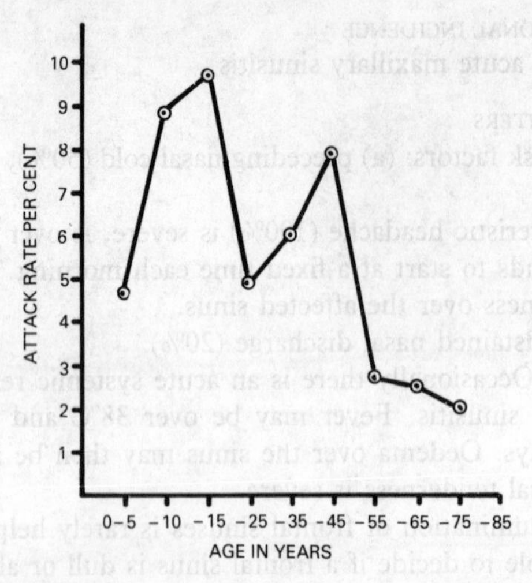

Fig. 34 Acute pharyngitis and sore throat. Age incidence curve of 197 consecutive cases encountered in 1 year.

AETIOLOGY

1. Bacterial — *Streptococcus pyogenes*.
2. Virus — rhinoviruses, parainfluenza and influenza viruses can all cause pharyngitis (see p. 176). Responsible for most acute infections.

DIAGNOSTIC RANGE (rates per 1000 patients per year)
Personal: Suspected 75.9. Probable 44.5. *National*: 91.3 (Ref. 0.2).

AGE INCIDENCE

A peak is reached in the first year at school, thereafter there is a steady decline (Fig. 34).

CLINICAL POINTERS

1. Sore throat (100%). The back of the pharynx is painful on swallowing. A sore throat which starts in the evening suggests a functional origin.
2. Fever (30%).
3. Redness of the fauces.

DURATION

3 to 10 days.

COMPLICATIONS

Scarlet fever, acute rheumatism and acute nephritis occasionally follow streptococcal pharyngitis.

MISLEADING FEATURES AND PITFALLS

Infective and functional pharyngitis may be confused.

DIFFERENTIAL DIAGNOSIS

Diseases that may be confused with acute pharyngitis:

Common cold

Similar features: sore, red throat; low fever.

Distinguishing features: streaming nasal discharge; sneezing.

Acute exudative tonsillitis

Similar features: sore, red throat with fever; pain on swallowing.

Distinguishing features: fever high; onset sudden; exudate appears after 1 to 3 days.

Acute exudative adenoiditis

Similar features: sore, red throat with fever and pain on swallowing.

Distinguishing features: fever high; onset sudden; nasal speech; inspection of the adenoids on 2nd or 3rd day with pharyngoscope reveals adenoidal exudate.

Functional pharyngitis

Similar feature: (relaxed throat) sore, red throat.

Distinguishing features: usually occurs in the evening; fever absent; persists for one or more weeks; psychological causes.

MANAGEMENT OPTIONS (see p. 380)

ACUTE EXUDATIVE TONSILLITIS

Classification: ICHPPC 463 (RCGP 2410)

AETIOLOGY

Streptococcus pyogenes can be cultured from the exudate in many patients (73% of 100 consecutive cases. Most of these cases were children. The streptococcal carriage rate for healthy school children is 25–35%). Viral infections probably account for about half the cases with exudate.

MODE OF SPREAD

Said to be by droplet; but dummies and feeding utensils may also be responsible. The interval between household contact cases may vary from 3 days to several weeks.

DIAGNOSTIC RANGE

Personal: Suspected 86.8. Probable 75.5.

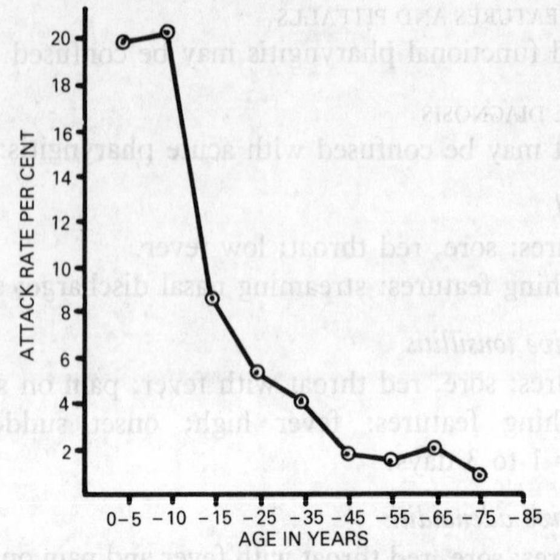

Fig. 35 Acute exudative tonsillitis. Age incidence curve of 254 consecutive cases encountered in 1 year.

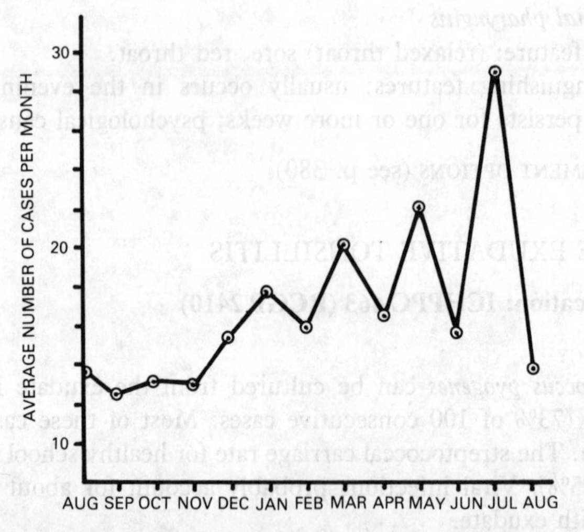

Fig. 36. Acute exudative tonsillitis. Seasonal incidence of 860 consecutive cases reported over 4 years.

AGE INCIDENCE

The condition is uncommon during the first year of life. The incidence rises steeply until the first year of school, when over a third of all children may be affected; the incidence falls thereafter (Fig. 35).

SEASONAL INCIDENCE

The disease is common at all times of the year, especially summer (Fig. 36).

CLINICAL POINTERS

1. High risk factors: (a) contact cases (25%) — The exact source of infection is often difficult to trace; (b) previous attacks.

2. Onset is usually sudden.

3. Sore throat (75%) is the significant presenting symptom. It may be absent in children under 10 years.

4. Fever (85%) is usually high and occurs early in the disease. It is associated with body aches, headaches, malaise, dizziness, feeling hot and cold and shivering. Occasionally a rigor occurs.

5. Pharyngeal exudate (100% by definition). In most cases several follicles are filled with an obvious purulent exudate. In others the exudate is reticular, orange-brown and more evenly spread over the tonsil.' This type is often streptococcal. Sometimes the whole tonsil is covered with a continuous yellowish-white membrane which on swabbing may show a surprising absence of bacterial pathogens. In adults (and possibly children also) this type is suggestive of an EBV (glandular fever) infection. The exudate usually becomes apparent on the first day of the disease, but in some patients, especially children, it may not appear until the second or third day.

6. Redness of the fauces is invariable unless the inflammation is settling.

7. Nasal speech is common and suggests adenoidal involvement.

8. Offensive breath and coated tongue are common after the exudate has appeared.

INVESTIGATIONS

Throat swab is essential if the tonsillar exudate is membranous or in any way suggestive of diphtheria. Occasionally a throat swab is indicated if a type 12 haemolytic streptococcal infection is suspected. Blood tests for mononucleosis are indicated if the fever or exudate persist or are excessive.

DURATION

2 to 4 days. The patient is liable to feel listless and sweaty for a further 4 to 5 days.

COMPLICATIONS

1. Acute cervical lymphadenitis is common in children. The tonsillar glands of one or both sides are swollen and tender.

2. Scarlet fever. A typical fine pinpoint scarlet rash may develop during the first 3 days.

3. Acute otitis media may arise at any time during the acute phase.

4. Acute rheumatic fever may develop up to 3 weeks after an attack.

5. Acute glomerulonephritis (see p. 511), although rare, is becoming more common. It arises within 3 weeks of the throat infection and may be associated with a type 12 haemolytic streptococcus.

MISLEADING FEATURES AND PITFALLS

Most mistakes occur in children under 10 years because at this age the disease has a number of atypical features:

1. Late development of the exudate. The child is feverish for 2 to 3 days before the typical exudate appears.

2. Absence of sore throat.

3. Associated abdominal pain. A high proportion of children complain of abdominal pain during the early stages of the illness. In most cases the pain clearly precedes vomiting, but in a few it is continuous and associated with central or localised abdominal tenderness. Differentiation from appendicitis and pyelonephritis may be difficult.

4. Neck or back stiffness is transient and is associated with the high fever at the onset of the disease. Differentiation from meningitis or virus encephalitis may be difficult if the patient is seen before the appearance of exudate.

5. Enlargement of spleen is a rare feature and may cause confusion. A blood count and tests for infectious mononucleosis are indicated.

6. Non-pathogenic exudate on the tonsils. In the tonsillar crypts of some children, pus is visible for long periods. The absence of local redness of the fauces and tonsils helps to distinguish these cases from acute exudative tonsillitis.

In the early stages of the illness when exudate is absent, children with abdominal pain or persistent meningism may occasionally have to be observed in hospital.

DIFFERENTIAL DIAGNOSIS

Diseases that may be confused with acute exudative tonsillitis:

Influenza

Similar features: sudden onset; high fever; body aches; headaches; red throat.

Distinguishing features: cough is invariable; the absence of tonsillar exudate after the 3rd day usually differentiates.

Acute upper respiratory infections
Similar feature: sudden high fever.

Distinguishing features: cough and adventitious sounds in the lungs differentiate.

Infectious mononucleosis (glandular fever)
The possibility should be considered in every adult case. Many cases of EBV infection in children are mild and probably remain undiagnosed because blood tests are avoided.

Acute appendicitis
Similar features: fever; rapid pulse; abdominal pain and tenderness.

Distinguishing features: high fever is unusual; in the absence of exudate, observation in hospital is occasionally indicated.

Meningitis and virus encephalitis
Similar features: fever; backache; meningism.

Distinguishing features: sore throat absent; meningism persists; differentiation may be difficult during first 3 days and observation in hospital is occasionally indicated.

Acute rheumatism
Similar features: high fever; sore throat; body aches and headache.

Distinguishing features: previous history of rheumatism; joint pains and evidence of carditis may differentiate; fever persists for more than 4 days; ESR is markedly raised; the two diseases are sometimes associated.

Vincent's angina, diphtheria, and certain virus infections
All may cause tonsillar exudate with enlarged cervical glands and fever (Ch. 8).

MANAGEMENT OPTIONS (see p. 380)
Many doctors give simple antibiotics routinely to all patients with tonsillar exudate on the grounds that exudate indicates a bacterial origin. This assumption is probably not justified.

ACUTE EXUDATIVE ADENOIDITIS

Occasionally the family doctor encounters patients with high fever, sore throat, nasal speech and offensive breath. The picture suggests acute exudative tonsillitis, but the fauces appear normal. If the adenoids are inspected with an indirect laryngoscope (reversed) they are inflamed and covered with typical follicular exudate. The lymphoid tissue beside the root of the tongue may be affected in the same way. *Management*: see acute tonsillitis (p. 380 and 397).

ACUTE CERVICAL ADENITIS

Classification: ICHPPC 683 (RCGP 3620)

AETIOLOGY

Acute cervical adenitis is probably always secondary to infections elsewhere.

Tonsillectomy is occasionally followed by attacks of acute cervical adenitis.

DIAGNOSTIC RANGE (rates per 1000 patients per year).

Personal: Suspected 17.5. Enlarged cervical glands are often noted in children, and it may be impossible to say if they are causing symptoms.

AGE INCIDENCE

Patients of all ages are liable. Most cases (70%) occur in children under 10.

CLINICAL POINTERS

1. High risk trigger factors. The site of the swollen gland often suggests the original trigger: (a) throat and tonsil infections — the glands below the jaw are swollen; (b) local skin sepsis of face and neck — glands affected depend on site; (c) scalp infections and pediculosis — auricular or occipital glands; (d) Herpes Simplex (type 1) virus infections — glands affected depend on site. Sometimes no obvious trigger factors are present and a wider differential diagnosis (see below) must be considered.
2. Tender swelling in the cervical lymph gland chain [100%].
3. Sore throat or tonsillitis (55%) precedes the adenitis by one to 20 days.
4. Fever (50%) often persists for several days.

INVESTIGATIONS

1. Throat swab is rarely necessary unless diphtheria is suspected.
2. Tuberculin test if tuberculous origin is considered.

DURATION

Fever may persist for over a week.

The glandular enlargement may be noted for months after active inflammation has settled.

COMPLICATIONS

1. Suppuration may occasionally occur.

2. Recurrences are common. [25% (5 out of 20) patients had more than one attack in a period of 4 years.] Tonsillectomy does not always prevent recurrences.

MISLEADING FEATURES AND PITFALLS

1. Pseudomeningism. The tender swollen glands may prevent flexion of the head and neck stiffness is simulated. The adenitis is distinguished by local pain and tenderness over the affected glands.

2. Occasionally spasm of the sternomastoid muscle over the inflamed glands causes a torticollis.

DIFFERENTIAL DIAGNOSIS

Diseases that may be confused with acute cervical adenitis.

Mumps

Similar feature: tender swelling in the region of jaw.

Distinguishing features: contact cases; absence of preceding local infection; ramus of the mandible not palpable; pain on eating; redness of salivary duct orifices.

Rubella (before rash)

Similar feature: tender swelling in the region of jaw.

Distinguishing features: contact cases; typical rash after 2 days; auricular and occipital glands only affected; absence of preceding local infection; glands rarely big.

Infectious mononucleosis

Similar features: preceding sore throat with exudate; fever; enlarged cervical glands.

Distinguishing features: enlarged glands elsewhere; enlarged spleen; fever persists for more than five days; blood smear and Paul-Bunnell test (or monospot) differentiate.

Diphtheria

Similar features: sore throat with membranous exudate; local cervical adenitis.

Distinguishing features: exudate is continuous and adherent to tonsil; patient usually toxic; all cervical glands are swollen (bull neck); immediate throat swab indicated for all doubtful cases.

Tuberculous cervical adenitis

Similar feature: unilateral cervical adenitis.

Distinguishing features: onset gradual; swelling persists for weeks and may suppurate; absence of preceding tonsillar or local infection.

Reticuloses and leukaemias
Similar feature: cervical adenitis and fever.

Distinguishing features: onset usually gradual; enlargement of glands elsewhere; enlargement of spleen; presence of haemorrhagic phenomenon; blood count, ESR and referral indicated.

MANAGEMENT OPTIONS

Prevention: Appropriate treatment of trigger factors.

Established disease: simple systemic antibiotics — BNF 5.1.1 (Ref. 0.1)

ACUTE MESENTERIC ADENITIS

Classification: ICHPPC 2891 (RCGP 0935)

AETIOLOGY

Closely related to acute exudative tonsillitis. It is probable that the abdominal pain which sometimes occurs in tonsillitis is due to an associated mesenteric adenitis.

DIAGNOSTIC RANGE (rates per 1000 patients per year)

Personal: Suspected 2.4+. It was rarely possible to confirm the diagnosis.

AGE INCIDENCE

Children are chiefly affected.

CLINICAL POINTERS

1. High risk factors: (a) children of 'tonsillitis' age; (b) previous similar attacks although a part of this syndrome are also characteristic of acute appendicitis.
2. Abdominal pain.
3. Abdominal tenderness may be central or in either flank.
4. High fever helps differentiate mesenteric adenitis from appendicitis. It is not always high.
5. Sore throat is sometimes present.

MISLEADING FEATURES AND PITFALLS

Acute mesenteric adenitis and acute appendicitis are easily confused. Doubtful cases must be handled as cases of appendicitis.

MANAGEMENT OPTIONS

Suspected Disease: (a) acute appendicitis is suspect until proven otherwise; (b) admission to hospital for observation may be needed.

ACUTE TRACHEITIS, ACUTE LARYNGITIS AND CROUP

Classification: ICHPPC 464 (RCGP 2415)

AETIOLOGY

Acute inflammation of the larynx interferes with the laryngeal function and causes the symptoms.

DIAGNOSTIC RANGE (rates per 1000 patients per year)

Personal: Suspected 30.2, Probable 10.0. *National*: 19.7 (Ref. 0.2).

AGE INCIDENCE

There is the usual peak during the first years of life, after which the incidence falls and remains steady throughout adult life (Fig. 37).

SEASONAL INCIDENCE

October to April as for other respiratory diseases (Fig. 38).

CLINICAL POINTERS

1. High risk factors: (a) contacts; (b) heavy smoking habits.
2. Hoarse cough (90%) is characteristic and easily recognised.
3. Hoarse voice (55%) suggests an acute laryngitis. The voice may be altered or completely lost.
4. Croup (10%) is common in children under 5 years — a result of their small larynx.
5. Cough associated with retrosternal pain (50%) suggests tracheitis.
6. Fever (30%) is absent or slight in adults. In children — temperatures of over 38°C are common.

INVESTIGATIONS

1. Laryngoscopy usually reveals a normal larynx and excludes more serious disease.
2. Chest X-ray if symptoms persist for longer than 21 days.
3. The opinion of an ENT consultant is obtained if laryngeal symptoms persist for longer than 28 days.

DURATION

Seldom longer than a week. Recurrences are common. [Practice experience: 30% (six out of 20) consecutive patients reported more than one attack over a 3 year period.]

COMPLICATIONS

1. Basal pneumonitis (aspiration pneumonia)
2. Laryngeal obstruction

In babies the possibility of this complication may be raised. The

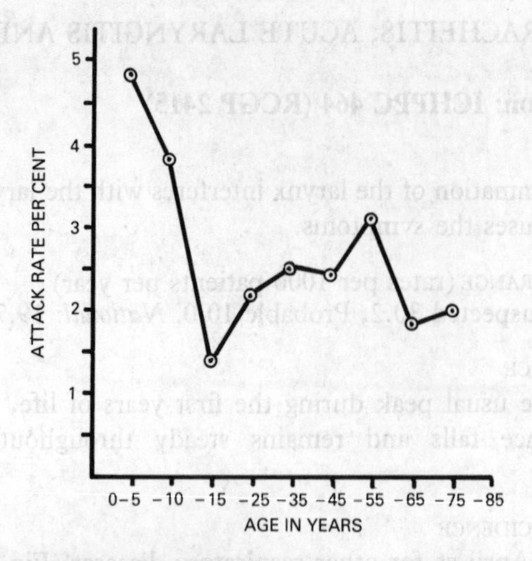

Fig. 37 Acute tracheitis, acute laryngitis and croup. Age incidence curve of 94 consecutive cases encountered in 1 year.

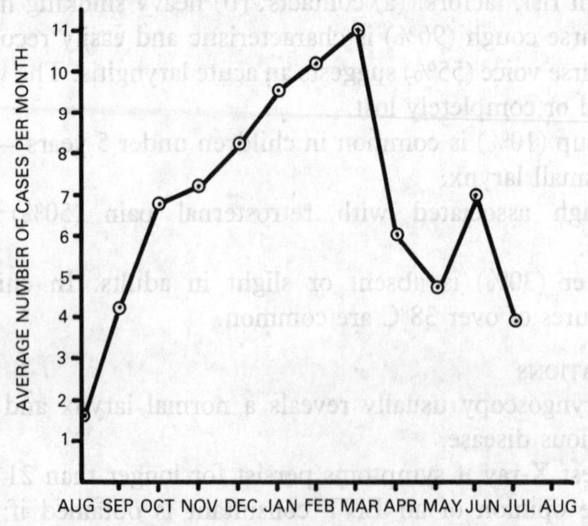

Fig. 38 Acute laryngitis and tracheitis. Seasonal incidence of 322 consecutive cases reported over 4 years.

doctor gets a call late at night to a baby with marked croup and fever. Hospital admission may be indicated.

The situation can deteriorate rapidly in babies and children (see below).

MISLEADING FEATURES AND PITFALLS

1. Heavy smokers may develop a recurring laryngitis.

2. Parents may confuse the hoarse bark of tracheitis or laryngitis with the inspiratory stridor which follows the coughing spasm of pertussis.

DIFFERENTIAL DIAGNOSIS

Diseases that may be confused with acute laryngitis and tracheitis:

Influenza and other respiratory virus infections

Similar features: fever; painful cough; croup or wheeze.

Distinguishing features: contact cases; high household attack rates; fever over 38°C.

Functional laryngitis

Similar feature: hoarse voice.

Distinguishing features: cough or fever absent; recurrences likely; duration over 7 days.

Space-occupying lesion of upper mediastinum

Similar feature: hoarseness and barking cough.

Distinguishing features: slowly progressive; laryngoscopy may differentiate; chest-X-ray and second opinion indicated.

MANAGEMENT OPTIONS (see p. 380)

Established disease: If the doctor is satisfied that there is no likelihood of airway obstruction (see below) humidification with a steam kettle is helpful.

ACUTE UPPER RESPIRATORY INFECTIONS WITH OBSTRUCTED AIRWAY

This situation may arise in babies or young children and although relatively uncommon should be remembered because early admission to hospital may be needed.

In the first 2 years of life hospital admission should be considered if a diagnosis of either croup or bronchiolitis is suspected and there is:

— subcostal recession
— restlessness
— grey, toxic or cyanotic appearance.

From 2 to 15 years epiglottitis, though rare, can cause sudden death from closure of larynx. The condition should be suspected if the child, usually 3 to 10 years, is febrile, clearly very ill and is sitting up in bed or drooling. A brassy cough is said to occur. *If epiglottitis is suspected the throat should not be inspected as depression of the tongue can cause a sudden complete closure of the larynx.* A lateral X-ray of the throat frequently reveals both the epiglottic oedema and the narrowed airway.

BRONCHIOLITIS

Classification: ICHPPC 466 (RCGP 2420)

Usually caused by respiratory syncytial virus in babies and young children. A cold is followed rapidly by an incessant wheezy cough. The infant is grey and extremely ill with evidence of hyperventilation. Mainly a winter disease; epidemics can occur. Respiratory failure and death sometimes occur. Hospital admission is usual.

[Practice Experience: 0.3 cases per 1000 patients per year].

ACUTE BRONCHITIS

Classification: ICHPPC 466 (RCGP 2420)

All patients with cough of short duration, fever or adventitious sounds in the chest, and no other respiratory disease have been labelled acute bronchitis. This definition is arbitrary and it may be possible in the future to split this group into more clearly defined entities.

AETIOLOGY

The disease frequently follows a cold.

DIAGNOSTIC RANGE (rates per 1000 patients per year)

Personal: Suspected 50.4. Probable 39.8. *National*: 70.3 (Ref. 0.2).

AGE INCIDENCE

There is a peak in the first 3 years of life (Fig. 39).

SEASONAL INCIDENCE

A peak of incidence occurs in the winter months (Fig. 40).

CLINICAL POINTERS

1. High risk factors: (a) previous cold; (b) previous attacks; (c) heavy smokers.
2. Cough (100% by definition). The cough is loose and slightly productive. It has usually persisted for 3 to 7 days before the patient reports to the doctor.
3. Adventitious sounds in the chest (70%). Coarse rhonchi are

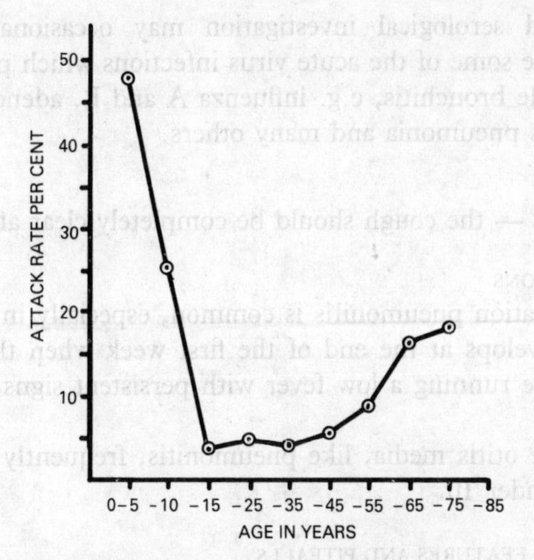

Fig. 39 Acute bronchitis. Age incidence curve of 269 consecutive cases encountered in 1 year.

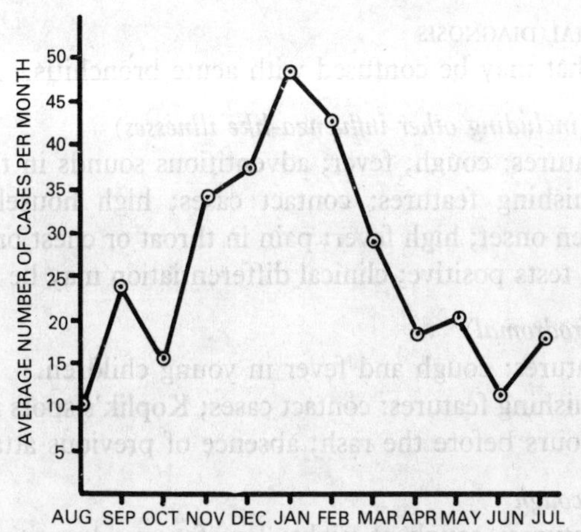

Fig. 40 Acute bronchitis. Seasonal incidence of 1239 consecutive cases reported over 4 years.

common in adults, but in small children they may be fine or absent.

4. Fever (45%). In babies and children, fever may be high, i.e. over 39°C, but in adults it is rarely over 38°C.

INVESTIGATIONS

1. Chest X-ray is occasionally helpful if lung damage is suspected.

2. Paired serological investigation may occasionally help to differentiate some of the acute virus infections which present as an acute febrile bronchitis, e.g. influenza A and B, adenovirus infections, virus pneumonia and many others.

DURATION

A few days — the cough should be completely clear after 14 days.

COMPLICATIONS

1. Aspiration pneumonitis is common, especially in children. It usually develops at the end of the first week when the patient is found to be running a low fever with persistent signs at one lung base.

2. Acute otitis media, like pneumonitis, frequently develops in children under 10.

MISLEADING FEATURES AND PITFALLS

A complicating pneumonitis is easily overlooked, especially if an acute bronchitis is inadequately followed up.

DIFFERENTIAL DIAGNOSIS

Diseases that may be confused with acute bronchitis.

Influenza (*including other influenza-like illnesses*)

Similar features: cough; fever; adventitious sounds in the chest.

Distinguishing features: contact cases; high household attack rate; sudden onset; high fever; pain in throat or chest on coughing; serological tests positive; clinical differentiation may be impossible.

Measles (*prodromal*)

Similar features: cough and fever in young children.

Distinguishing features: contact cases; Koplik's spots may appear 12 to 36 hours before the rash; absence of previous attack.

Whooping cough

Similar features: cough at night; low fever; adventitious sounds; children affected.

Distinguishing features: contact cases; spasmodic nocturnal cough; typical cough spasm followed by vomit or whoop; differentiation in first 10 days may be difficult.

Pneumonitis (*aspiration pneumonia*)

Similar feature: cough with low fever and adventitious sounds in the chest.

Distinguishing features: a complication of other respiratory diseases; fever and localised adventitious sounds persist after primary disease has settled.

Acute lobar pneumonia
Similar features: cough; fever; adventitious sounds in chest.

Distinguishing features: onset frequently acute; fever high; cough sometimes absent in early stages; patient ill; respiration rapid; subcostal recession in children; cyanosis; pleuritic pain; chest X-ray may differentiate.

Virus pneumonia (*Bronchiolitis*)
Similar features: cough; fever.

Distinguishing features: onset like influenza with cough and high fever; after 2 to 3 days a few adventitious sounds may develop; clinical examination frequently negative; chest X-rays and serological tests help to differentiate. Fever persists for 4 to 8 days. *Bronchiolitis* is suggested if a baby or toddler is acutely ill with incessant wheezy cough.

MANAGEMENT OPTIONS (see p. 380)

CHRONIC BRONCHITIS

Classification: ICHPPC 491 (RCGP 2490)

Classically chronic bronchitis is defined as a chronic productive cough which recurs at intervals in response to irritation of the bronchial mucous membrane by respiratory infections, smoke, fog, dust, fumes, etc.

The syndrome is clear enough in theory, but in practice it is often impossible to distinguish between chronic bronchitis and such diseases as smoker's cough, asthma, congestive heart failure, emphysema and bronchiectasis.

[Practice experience: 20 consecutive patients of over 40 years old who were diagnosed as chronic bronchitics, i.e. repeated attacks of productive cough over several years (without any clinical evidence of asthma, heart failure or bronchiectases), were followed for 4 years: seven did not report recurrences in the subsequent 4 years; six were later considered to have bronchiectasis following a radiologist's report on a straight chest X-ray; three followed the classic picture of chronic bronchitis and reported repeated attacks of productive winter cough; two later developed an associated asthma; one was found to be suffering from pulmonary tuberculosis and not chronic bronchitis; one left the district.]

AETIOLOGY

Chronic bronchitis appears to be a stage in a slowly progressive morbid process following repeated irritation and lung infections which in turn lead to loss of pulmonary elasticity, generalised emphysema (p. 418) and chronic asthmatic bronchitis (chronic obstructive lung disease) (p. 423). The overlap between these three diseases is considerable.

DIAGNOSTIC RANGE (rate per 1000 patients per year)

Personal: Suspected 10.9. Probable 9.0. *National*: 14.2 (Ref. 0.2). Possibly two or three times this number of patients have some degree of chronic bronchitis or obstruction but never report.

AGE INCIDENCE

Most patients (85%) are over 50.

SEX INCIDENCE

Men are affected more than women.

SEASONAL INCIDENCE

Most attacks (70%) occur in the winter months.

CLINICAL POINTERS

1. High risk factors: (a) smoking; (b) urban smoke pollution and 'smog'; (c) industrial dusty working conditions (mining, etc.); (d) previous lung infections.
2. Chronic productive cough (100%). Attacks follow a cold; eventually the cough becomes continuous.
3. Scattered rhonchi.
4. Dyspnoea and increasing emphysema are late features.

INVESTIGATIONS

1. A straight chest X-ray is obtained for all patients whose cough has persisted for more than 4 weeks.
2. Bacteriological examination of sputum is occasionally performed if pulmonary tuberculosis is suspected.
3. Peak flow pulmonary function tests (See p. 681).

DURATION

The disease progresses slowly and its course is extremely variable.

COMPLICATIONS

1. Emphysema is common.
2. Asthma. A symptomatic asthma often develops in the later stages of the disease (See chronic asthmatic bronchitis, p. 423).
3. Bronchiectasis.
4. Right-sided heart failure is a late complication.

MISLEADING FEATURES AND PITFALLS

The patient accepts his chronic cough and makes his own diagnosis of bronchitis. It is very easy for the G.P. to accept the patient's evaluation and serious disease may be overlooked.

(Practice experience: out of 76 consecutive patients with chronic cough, pulmonary tuberculosis was overlooked in three patients for varying periods up to 6 months.)

Pulmonary neoplasms and early heart failure can be overlooked in the same way.

DIFFERENTIAL DIAGNOSIS

Diseases that may be confused with chronic bronchitis:

Bronchiectasis

Similar features: productive chronic cough; aggravated by upper respiratory infections; dyspnoea; emphysema and asthma.

Distinguishing features: sputum and coughing worse on getting up in mornings; haemoptysis; febrile incidents; localised rhonchi; chest X-rays help to differentiate; bronchography.

Smoker's cough

Similar feature: chronic cough.

Distinguishing features: history of heavy smoking; cough not productive; physical signs in chest absent; chest X-ray negative.

Pulmonary tuberculosis

Similar features: chronic cough in adults over 50; productive sputum; dyspnoea.

Distinguishing features: history of contact; immigrant; history of preceding cough shorter than in chronic bronchitis; evening fever; loss of weight and appetite; incidents of indigestion, nausea and haemoptysis; physical signs in chest often absent; chest X-ray differentiates; sputum may contain acid-fast bacilli.

Bronchogenic neoplasm

Similar features: chronic cough in adults over 40; dyspnoea; smoking.

Distinguishing features: preceding cough of short duration (smoker's cough may confuse); dyspnoea appears early; fever and haemoptysis common; systemic disturbance slight at first; pneumonic illness may precede other symptoms; chest X-ray may differentiate; bronchoscopy usually differentiates; sputum cytology.

Congestive heart failure

Similar features: chronic cough in adults over 60; dyspnoea; basal râles.

Distinguishing features: history of heart disease; peripheral oedema; distended neck veins; enlarged liver; response to diuretics; chest X-ray shows hilar congestion.

MANAGEMENT OPTIONS

(see Chronic Asthmatic Bronchitis p. 424)

Prevention: (a) avoid smoking; (b) avoid atmospheric pollution; (c) use of protective masks at work; (d) prompt antibiotic treatment of infections; (e) prolonged antibiotics and vaccines (except for influenza) inadvisable.

Established disease: (a) early antibiotics with full bacteriological control — BNF 5.1 (Ref. 0.1); (b) symptomatic — BNF 3.1, 3.7 and 3.9; (d) warm bedroom and humidified atmosphere; (e) hospital admission especially if in ventilatory failure.

COT DEATHS OR SUDDEN INFANT DEATH SYNDROME (SIDS)

Classification: ICHPPC 7889 (RCGP 4905)

A baby usually between 4 weeks and 14 months old is put to bed apparently well or with a slight cold. The mother (or sometimes a nurse) is horrified to find the child dead in the early hours of the next morning. At post mortem no obvious cause of death can be found. These catastrophies at first were attributed to accident, inhalation of vomit, inadvertent asphyxia, overlaying by the mother, etc. Much needless suffering and guilt were created in mothers as a result.

Recent work suggests cyclic attacks of hypoxia-apnoea lead to deepening hypoxia and then cardiac arrest. This vicious cycle being triggered off in babies by a minor respiratory infection.

DIAGNOSTIC RANGE (rates per 1000 patients per year)

Personal: Probable 0.2. *National*: 1 for every 500 live births.

AGE

Babies of 2 weeks to 8 months are susceptible.

CLINICAL POINTERS

1. High risk factors: (a) any baby noted to have prolonged apnoea cycles while in hospital; (b) suggestive family sibling history; (c) the presence of a minor infection. Such infections are so common (and SIDS is so rare) that it is unjustifiable and unkind to warn parents of this remote danger. The doctor should however

remember the possibility when dealing with parents of babies suffering from minor infections.

2. There are no specific pointers. A number of retrospective surveys have isolated many non-specific symptoms.

COMPLICATIONS

1. Guilt reactions are common in the parents (sometimes also in the doctor if he has been treating the baby).

2. Subsequent increased reporting of any ill-health in siblings. This may be noticed for several years after and must be sympathetically handled by the doctor.

3. A baby is seen in a busy clinic with a minor infection. The doctor's hurried reassurances or abrupt manner makes the mother feel she is bothering the doctor needlessly. The baby is found dead in the cot next morning and not unnaturally the doctor is blamed by the parents.

(The Sheffield survey revealed a distressingly large number of such complaints.)

MANAGEMENT OPTIONS

Prevention: (a) 'apnoea alarms' — very occasionally indicated if apnoea attacks are noted in hospital; (b) the family doctor must often consider cot death as a remote possibility without raising his fears with parents. The difficulties of prevention remain.

If SIDS occurs: (a) support both parents with immediate careful explanations aimed to reduce their inevitable feelings of guilt; (b) provide continued 'running' support during bereavement period (p. 94) by giving information and literature — Family Medical Adviser — Reader's Digest (Ref. 0.3) — use of health visitor; referring to other parents who have previously had a SIDS; Foundation of Sudden Infant Deaths (Ref. 17.1); (c) guide parents through legal requirements; (d) counter all suggestions of suffocation etc., as a cause; (e) use specialists if necessary to reinforce your support; (f) avoid explanations which *decrease* your feelings of guilt but *increase* those of the parents.

PNEUMONIA

Classification: ICHPPC 486 (RCGP 2475)

A. VIRUS PNEUMONIAS — Classification: ICHPPC 486

(See p. 189)

1. Psittacosis.

2. Mycoplasma pneumoniae (syn. Eaton's agent, primary atypical or cold agglutinin pneumonia).
3. Q fever.
4. Adenovirus infections occasionally.

B. BACTERIAL PNEUMONIAS — Classification: ICHPPC 486

1. Pneumococcal pneumonia (syn. acute lobar pneumonia).
2. Staphylococcal pneumonia.
3. Haemophilus pneumonia.
4. Tuberculous pneumonia.

C. ASPIRATION PNEUMONIAS — Classification: ICHPPC 519

1. Aspiration pneumonias following infection elsewhere in the respiratory tract:
- Benign aspiration pneumonia (localised aspiration).
- Acute bronchopneumonia (generalised aspiration).

2. Breakdown of the normal defence mechanism of the lung as in unconsciousness, laryngeal paralysis and hypostatic pneumonias of the elderly or post-operative patient.

3. Inadequate drainage of a portion of lung following bronchial damage, e.g. bronchiectasis or carcinoma of bronchus.

This classification is useful as a guide, but in general practice many cases cannot be labelled with certainty. Few diseases illustrate so clearly the general practitioner's dilemma of reconciling accurate with early diagnosis. If on the one hand pneumonia is suspected, the family doctor cannot afford to delay treatment until the picture becomes definite, while on the other a full hospital investigation is rarely justified at the start of the disease.

MANAGEMENT OPTIONS

Suspected disease: 1. Decide on clinical grounds whether the infection is a bacterial or an aspiration pneumonia — a preceding illness or underlying reason for aspiration helps to make this decision.

2. Give a simple antibacterial — BNF 5.1 (Ref. 0.1).

3. After 3 to 4 days of antibiotic the position is reviewed. Patients who are responding are kept under observation at home. Patients who are suspected of having a bacterial pneumonia but who are not responding are admitted for investigation in hospital. No antibiotics other than penicillin are given by the family doctor.

Patients suspected of having aspiration pneumonitis but who are not responding to treatment are kept at home, provided their general condition is not deteriorating. One of the broad-spectrum antibiotics is then given. An X-ray of chest is obtained for all patients as soon as they are well enough.

ACUTE LOBAR PNEUMONIA (PNEUMOCOCCAL PNEUMONIA)

Classification: ICHPPC 486 (RCGP 2475)

The classical picture of fully developed lobar pneumonia is now rarely encountered in general practice.

AETIOLOGY

The pneumococcus (*Strep. pneumoniae*).

DIAGNOSTIC RANGE (rates per 1000 patients per year)

Personal: Probable 4.7. *National*: 3.4 (Ref. 0.2). (It is seldom possible to confirm the diagnosis because treatment modifies the disease.)

AGE INCIDENCE

All ages are liable. Young adults are especially prone.

CLINICAL POINTERS

1. High risk factors: (a) the elderly and debilitated; (b) diabetes; (c) congestive heart failure; (d) postoperative; (e) previous attack.
2. Sudden onset. Sometimes a rigor occurs.
3. Cough is dry, short and frequent.
4. Pleuritic pain localised to one part of the chest or shoulders, is aggravated by respiration or coughing.
5. Rusty sputum is suggestive. Sometimes sputum is frankly bloodstained.
6. Fever is high (over 39°C).
7. Respiratory rate is raised in most cases. In young patients the respiratory rate is greater than in older patients — grunting respiration occurs.
8. Physical signs in the chest: (a) fine adventitious sounds (crepitations) may be heard persistently over the affected lung; (b) a pleural friction rub may be heard if the overlying pleura is involved.

The physical signs of consolidation or pleural effusion may appear on the third to fifth day of the illness, if treatment has not been effective.

9. Cyanosis is unusual and appears late. Prognosis is bad if it is present during the first 3 days.

10. Subcostal recession suggests pneumonia in babies.

INVESTIGATIONS

1. White blood-cell count is useful in doubtful cases. Counts of over 14 000 per mm^3 are common in pneumonia.

2. Chest X-ray confirms the diagnosis, but if the patient is being treated at home it may not be feasible.

DURATION

The classical course of the disease with resolution by crisis after 7 to 10 days is rarely observed — a result of modern antibiotic treatment. In the treated case the fever should show signs of settling after 2 to 3 days.

COMPLICATIONS

1. Herpes labialis frequently develops on the second or third day.

2. Pleural effusion occasionally appears after a few days. Admission to hospital is indicated because an empyema may develop.

3. Pneumococcal meningitis is rare. (One case in 10 years.)

MISLEADING FEATURES AND PITFALLS

1. The absence of cough. Occasionally patients are seen in whom the absence of cough fails to alert the doctor to the respiratory origin of the disease.

2. Meningism — a transient neck stiffness is sometimes observed at the onset.

3. Splenomegaly occasionally arises in patients with pneumonia.

DIFFERENTIAL DIAGNOSIS

Disease that may be confused with acute lobar pneumonia:

Pulmonary infarct

Similar features: sudden onset; cough; pleuritic pain; rusty or bloodstained sputum; fever; cyanosis; rapid respirations; localised crepitations; pleural rub; signs of consolidation.

Distinguishing features: fever is absent or low in first few days; origin of embolus may be apparent; distinction may be extremely difficult.

Pulmonary tuberculosis

Similar features: cough; fever; rapid respiration; pleuritic pain; bloodstained sputum; cyanosis.

Distinguishing features: onset less sudden; history and contacts may be suggestive; fever fails to settle with antibiotics; chest X-rays and sputum examination differentiate.

Bornholm disease (*epidemic myalgia*)
Similar feature: sudden onset of acute pleuritic pain and fever.

Distinguishing features: contact cases; pain severe; physical signs in chest absent.

Acute cholecystitis, perforated duodenal ulcer and acute appendix
Similar feature: pleuritic pain.

Distinguishing features: previous history is suggestive; fever is slight or absent; physical findings point to abdomen not chest.

MANAGEMENT OPTIONS

Prevention: antibiotic cover of high risk groups.

Established disease: (a) rest; (b) fluids; (c) antibacterials — BNF 5.1 (Ref. 0.1) — bacteriological control may be indicated; (d) careful follow up.

BENIGN ASPIRATION PNEUMONIA

Classification: ICHPPC 519 (RCGP 2475)

(For convenience this term is often shortened to 'pneumonitis'.)

This mild disease is the commonest of the pneumonias. Children are especially liable.

AETIOLOGY

The common precipitating infections are colds, acute bronchitis, influenza viruses, measles and whooping cough. A descending respiratory infection is often precipitated by physical activity in a child that is allowed to get up and go out before the primary illness has settled. A bronchus becomes blocked with mucus and the portion of lung which it supplies becomes collapsed and infected.

DIAGNOSTIC RANGE (rates per 1000 patients per year)

Personal: suspected 28.1. Probable 16.3. In 16.3 per 1000 patients per year the diagnosis was confirmed by chest X-ray.

AGE INCIDENCE

All ages are liable but most (66%) cases are in children under 10 (Fig. 41).

SEASONAL INCIDENCE

A peak is reached between December and April (Fig. 42).

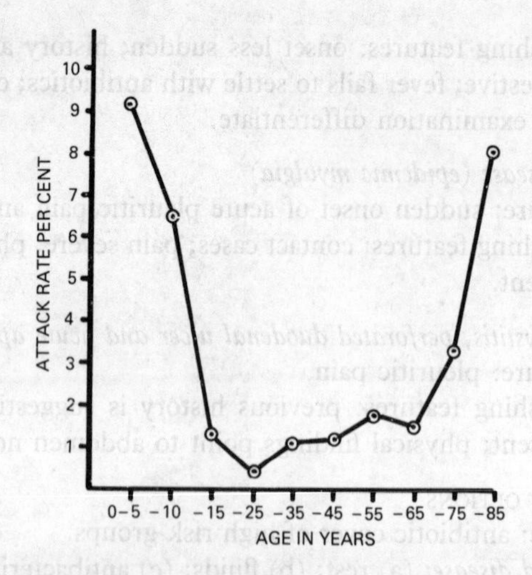

Fig. 41 Aspiration pneumonitis. Age incidence of 118 consecutive cases in 1 year.

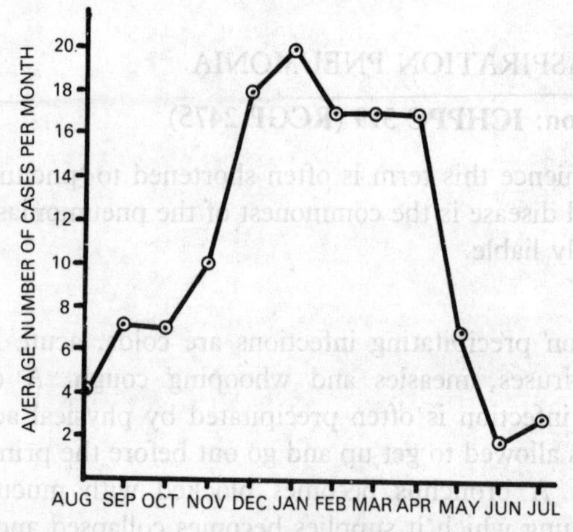

Fig. 42 Aspiration pneumonia. Seasonal incidence of 118 consecutive cases reported in 1 year.

CLINICAL POINTERS

1. High risk factors: (a) preceding upper respiratory infection (72%); (b) previous history of lung infections; (c) excessive physical activity while under treatment for any upper respiratory infection.

2. Onset: In children the disease may present in two ways: (a) pneumonitis follows the primary illness immediately — the cough, malaise and fever merely prolong the preceding illness; (b) the child

improves from the primary illness and tries to get back to normal, 7 to 14 days after the onset of the original illness he is brought back to the doctor because he is not right and still coughing. In adults the precipitating illness is usually a chronic bronchitis or bronchiectasis.

3. History of previous similar attacks.
4. Persistent cough (96%) may be productive or irritant.
5. Fever and malaise. Fever is frequently only slightly raised and rarely over 39°C.
6. Persistence of localised adventitious sounds in the chest (76%). Fine râles or crepitations are common. Persistent rhonchi are also heard. Signs of pneumonic consolidation are usually absent.
7. Increased respiratory rate (21%); any high fever may increase a child's respiratory rate.
8. Subcostal recession may occur in babies and toddlers.
9. Cyanosis (12%). Slight degrees of cyanosis are sometimes noted in the cheeks or lips of children. Occasionally this sign draws the attention of the doctor to the pneumonitis of a convalescent child.

INVESTIGATIONS

Chest X-ray. The radiological changes are often minimal and there may be difficulty in assessing the extent of the disease process.

DURATION

The condition clears up with treatment in 1 to 2 weeks.

COMPLICATIONS

1. Recurrences are common in children under 10 years [32% (eight out of 25) recurred within 4 years]. In adults recurrences are associated with bronchial damage or chronic sinusitis.
2. Bronchiectasis. Clinical and radiological evidence suggests this complication is not uncommon.

MISLEADING FEATURES AND PITFALLS

An aspiration pneumonitis is frequently overlooked. Mistakes occur for three reasons: (1) failure to ensure that fever has subsided before a patient with febrile respiratory illness is allowed to get up; (2) failure to examine the chest of a patient who has recovered from a respiratory illness but who still complains of cough and not feeling right; (3) failure in an adult presenting with a pneumonitis, to investigate the possibility of an underlying carcinoma of lung.

DIFFERENTIAL DIAGNOSIS

Diseases that may be confused with aspiration pneumonitis:

Other forms of pneumonia
Similar feature: clinically it is often impossible to distinguish between the different types of pneumonia.

Distinguishing features: sudden onset and absence of primary illness; early development of signs of consolidation suggests a possible bacterial origin; sputum cultures occasionally assist diagnosis.

Whooping cough
Similar features: delayed onset of fever; progressively increasing spasmodic cough — worse at night; children especially liable.

Distinguishing features: contacts; cough is spasmodic not irritant; child goes red in the face; vomiting and whoop follow the coughing spasm; cough persists for 4 to 10 weeks; differentiation may be difficult before the whoop appears.

Pulmonary tuberculosis
Similar features: the two diseases may be confused in adults; cough; gradual onset; bloodstained sputum; minimal chest signs.

Distinguishing features: contacts or preceding TB history; gastric symptoms often present; localised physical signs at apex (usually a late finding); chest X-ray and sputum examinations differentiate.

Urinary tract infection
Similar features: children affected; listlessness; prolonged fever, anorexia.

Distinguishing features: urinary symptoms (often absent in children); pyuria; cough absent.

MANAGEMENT OPTIONS

Prevention: early antibacterials — BNF 5.1 (Ref. 0.1) — in high risk groups.

Established disease: (a) rest; (b) antibacterials — BNF 5.1; (c) follow up with chest X-ray.

GENERALISED CHRONIC EMPHYSEMA

Classification: ICHPPC 492 (RCGP 2495)

Localised or compensatory emphysema arises in healthy lung tissue which is adjacent to collapsed lung. Generalised (chronic) emphysema affects all the lung tissue and is usually associated with chronic bronchitis. A picture of chronic obstructive lung/airways disease (COLD) then arises (see Chronic Asthmatic Bronchitis, p. 423).

AETIOLOGY

Generalised emphysema is thought to follow — loss of pulmonary elasticity, partial bronchial obstruction and chronic overdistension of the lungs. Recent work suggests that smoking and infection may cause emphysema by upsetting lung enzymes as well as causing loss of elasticity.

DIAGNOSTIC RANGE (rates per 1000 patients per year)

Personal: Suspected 2.8. Probable 0.7. *National*: 1.1 (Ref. 0.2). Many cases are diagnosed as chronic bronchitis.

AGE INCIDENCE

Patients over 40 are liable. (Reversible generalised emphysema occurs during an asthmatic attack, at any age.)

CLINICAL POINTERS

1. High risk factors: (a) smoking; (b) chronic or recurrent lung infections (especially asthma); (c) pneumoconioses and air pollution.
2. Dyspnoea (100%).
3. Barrel-shaped chest. The chest becomes gradually held in a position of overdistension. Full expiration becomes impossible and the vital capacity is correspondingly reduced.
4. Physical signs in the chest. Resonance is increased and breath sounds are diminished.
5. Associated diseases. Bronchiectasis, chronic bronchitis and asthma. Loss of weight is commonly associated.

INVESTIGATIONS

1. Straight chest X-ray confirms the diagnosis.
2. Peak flow pulmonary function test (see p. 681).
3. Vitalograph.

DURATION

The disease, once it has become irreversible, is slowly progressive.

COMPLICATIONS

Right-sided heart failure and death.

MISLEADING FEATURES AND PITFALLS

The physical signs of emphysema are easily confused with those of a small spontaneous pneumothorax.

MANAGEMENT OPTIONS

Prevention: (a) avoid smoking; (b) early treatment of chronic lung infections (See Chronic Bronchitis, p. 407).

Established disease: (a) stop smoking; (b) bronchodilators — BNF 3.1 (Ref. 0.1); mainly Adrenoceptor stimulants (BNF 3.1.1) and anticholinergics (BNF 3.1.2) graduated fitness and exercise programmes are often crucial; (d) supplementary oxygen; (e) referral (see also Chronic Bronchitis); (f) peak flow rate monitoring of all therapy; (g) regular follow up.

ASTHMA

Classification: ICHPPC 493 (RCGP 2500)

Any illness in which bronchospasm causes an expiratory wheeze can be classified as asthma. Within this loose clinical definition a number of aetiological types emerge:

1. Acute wheezy bronchitis (bronchospasm in children).
2. Simple asthma (allergic asthma).
3. Chronic bronchitis with asthma (chronic asthmatic bronchitis).
4. Cardiac asthma (see pp. 358 and 443).

Although these four types of asthma overlap, the prognosis varies for each and the doctor should try to classify every case. (For a list of distinguishing features see p. 425).

ACUTE WHEEZY BRONCHITIS (BRONCHOSPASM IN CHILDREN)

This disorder is chiefly encountered in babies and young children. The baby develops a bronchitis and scattered expiratory rhonchi are heard over the chest. Wheezing may occur every time a baby has a respiratory infection; some babies wheeze for weeks without apparent discomfort.

AETIOLOGY

1. Mechanical. An asthmatic wheeze is produced in the small bronchi when they are narrowed by inflammation and expiration.

2. Allergic. Clinical similarity apart, there is little to suggest that wheezy bronchitis in babies is related to true allergic asthma.

DIAGNOSTIC RANGE (rates per 1000 patients per year)
Personal: Suspected 8.6+. Many cases are probably not reported. One in five children under 5 are said to wheeze at some time.

AGE INCIDENCE
The majority (67%) are aged 3 years or under.

CLINICAL POINTERS

1. An expiratory wheeze (100%) is heard when the baby has a respiratory infection.
2. Fever is sometimes present.

INVESTIGATIONS

1. Chest X-rays are normal.
2. Pulmonary function tests sometimes indicated (See p. 681).

DURATION

The attack of wheezing may last several weeks. The child usually grows out of the tendency before school age.

COMPLICATIONS

None.

MISLEADING FEATURES AND PITFALLS

Much unnecessary worry is caused if the term asthma is used to parents before a certain diagnosis has been made.

MANAGEMENT OPTIONS

As for any minor respiratory infection (see p. 380).

SIMPLE ALLERGIC ASTHMA

Classification: ICHPPC 493 (RCGP 2500)

Sometimes defined as 'reversible airways obstruction'.

AETIOLOGY

1. Heredity. A family history of asthma or hay fever is common.

2. Allergy is thought to play a big part and a history of other allergic diseases is usual. In a few patients sensitivity to a specific substance, e.g. feathers, pollen, etc., can be demonstrated, but antihistamines and attempts at desensitisation rarely give much relief.

3. Psychological factors are said to play a part. It is often difficult to separate the fear that precipitates an attack from the fear of the attack itself. Excessive parental domination is often noted.

DIAGNOSTIC RANGE (rates per 1000 patients per year)

Personal: Suspected 10.3. Probable 8.3. *National*: 13.4 (Ref. 0.2). The diagnosis was rarely in doubt after school age.

AGE INCIDENCE

Simple asthma usually starts in early childhood. In a few patients (20%) the onset is later, i.e. in adolescence or early youth.

SEASONAL INCIDENCE

Attacks may occur in the pollen season, i.e. June to September.

CLINICAL POINTERS

1. High risk factors: (a) presence of allergic stigmata (70%), these include: family history of asthma or hay fever, a previous history of atopic eczema, hay fever or allergy; (b) possible attacks of 'wheezing' previously.

2. Attacks of difficult breathing associated with cough and tightness of chest (100%). In young children, frequent attacks of febrile bronchitis are sometimes the first sign of the disease.

3. Scattered expiratory wheeze associated with difficult expiration (100%). During an attack the chest is held almost fully expanded and may with repeated attacks become permanently barrel shaped and emphysematous.

4. A low-grade fever may be present.

INVESTIGATION

1. X-rays of the chest are normal or show hyperinflation.
2. Blood count. Eosinophilia may occur during an attack.
3. Peak flow rates (PFR) — see page 681.
4. Vitalograph and other pulmonary function tests.

DURATION OF THE ATTACK

The height of the attack is reached in a few hours. It then gradually recedes in the next 1 to 2 days. In severe cases the attacks may become continuous (status asthmaticus).

DURATION OF THE ILLNESS

When the onset is in early childhood, the majority (80%) grow out of the tendency as puberty is reached. If the onset is after puberty, attacks are more severe and more persistent.

COMPLICATIONS

1. Chest deformities and emphysema.

2. Liability to attacks of pneumonia.

3. Status asthmaticus suggests a bad prognosis, but is not common.

4. A chronic asthmatic bronchitis may develop after years of repeated lung infections and simple asthmatic attacks.

5. Death may occur in very severe attacks.

6. A vicious circle sometimes starts in which great relief is obtained from a single measure, e.g. admission to hospital, use of an inhaler, steroids or injection. The patient is then frightened in future attacks if this measure is not used again; dependency follows.

DIFFERENTIAL DIAGNOSIS (see p. 425)

MANAGEMENT OPTIONS

Prevention: (a) occasionally a specific allergen can be identified — Avoidance or desensitisation may then prevent attacks; (b) anti-asthmatic drugs (cromoglycate etc.) — BNF 3.3. (Ref. 0.1); (c) encourage normal activities; (d) avoid dust and smoking.

Established attacks: (a) bronchodilators — BNF 3.1; (b) short course of steroids — BNF 3.2; (c) referral occasionally needed; (d) peak flow monitoring of all therapy; (e) regular follow up — Antibiotics rarely indicated; (f) self help groups and physiotherapy; (g) full normal activities.

CHRONIC ASTHMATIC BRONCHITIS OR CHRONIC OBSTRUCTIVE LUNG DISEASE (COLD)

Classification: ICHPPC 492 (RCGP 2490)

Other names for this late stage of chronic bronchitis (see p. 407) are chronic airways obstruction and irreversible airways obstruction.

Chronic asthmatic bronchitis usually develops in the latter half of life and is associated with varying degrees of emphysema (see p. 418).

AETIOLOGY

Smoking, chronic bronchitis and recurring lung infections, precipitate the disease. It is not certain whether the infection produces the asthma by an allergic mechanism or by damaging the lungs.

DIAGNOSTIC RANGE (rates per 1000 patients per year)

Personal: Suspected 6.7+. The diagnosis was sometimes difficult to confirm.

AGE INCIDENCE

The age of onset depends upon the nature and severity of the precipitating lung infection. It is uncommon before the age of 35 years.

SEASONAL INCIDENCE

Like many respiratory diseases, attacks are more frequent in the winter months.

CLINICAL POINTERS

1. High risk factors: (a) smoking; (b) chronic or recurring chest infection or irritation (70%); (c) cold winter climates and cold bedrooms.

2. Attacks of difficult breathing, tightness of the chest and cough (100%).

3. Scattered expiratory wheeze associated with difficult expiration (100%).

4. Fever is common.

5. Breathlessness is a useful guide to the progress of the disease in its irreversible form.

The following four progressive stages are useful markers:

- Able to walk with people of similar age but is unable to keep up on hills and stairs.
- Unable to keep up with others on the level but can walk long distances at own pace.
- Unable to walk more than 100 yards on the level without being short of breath.
- Breathless on washing, dressing, walking a few steps or on talking.

Each of these steps will correlate with decreases in PFR (The division of patients into 'pink puffers' and 'blue bloaters' is essentially a late stage hospital classification.)

INVESTIGATIONS

1. X-rays of chest and sinuses may reveal the presence of chronic infection, emphysema and over-inflation.

2. Peak flow rates are used to monitor the effectiveness of treatment and the progress of the disease.

DURATION

The tendency to wheeze may persist for long periods. The disease is steadily progressive.

COMPLICATIONS

1. Emphysema and barrel-shaped chest deformity are common.
2. Right-sided heart failure (cor pulmonale).
3. Status asthmaticus (i.e. severe continuous asthma).
4. Death may be sudden in an attack or from complications (rare).

MISLEADING FEATURES AND PITFALLS

Occasionally wheezing is inspiratory as well as expiratory and then asthma simulates a space-occupying lesion of the mediastinum.

MANAGEMENT OPTIONS

Prevention: (a) smoking avoidance; (b) early antibacterials for chronic bronchitis and recurrent lung infections; (c) winter 'flu' immunisation

Established disease: (a) stop smoking; (b) bronchodilators — BNF 3.1.1 and 3.1.2 (Ref. 0.1); (c) graduated exercise programmes; (d) warm bedrooms; (e) peak flow rate monitoring of all therapy; (f) regular follow up; (g) referral, antibacterials and oxygen may all be indicated in severe cases. Beta blockers — BNF 2.4 — should be avoided.

Differential diagnosis of different types of asthma

Acute wheezy bronchitis
Distinguishing features: Affects children mainly under 3 years old. Child grows out of tendency to wheeze in a year or two, is not associated with allergic stigmata. Clinical differentiation from simple allergic asthma may be impossible in babies and young children.

Simple allergic asthma
Distinguishing features: Onset usually between 2 and 25 years old; other allergic stigmata are present; onset after 15 years old associated with severe attacks.

Chronic asthmatic bronchitis
Distinguishing features: Onset usually from 35 years onwards; precipitating pulmonary illness (pneumonia, bronchitis, bronchiectasis, etc); attacks last longer, are frequently febrile and become progressively more severe.

Cardiac asthma and congestive heart failure
Distinguishing features: Onset usually after 50; precipitating heart lesion usually obvious; attacks are often nocturnal and of short duration; peripheral oedema may be present; chest X-ray reveals evidence of heart enlargement and hilar congestion. Acute pulmonary oedema is the immediate cause.

ENLARGEMENT OF TONSILS AND ADENOIDS

Classification: ICHPPC 474 (RCGP 2450)

AETIOLOGY
Hypertrophy of the tonsils and adenoids is normal in children and is part of the generalised lymphoid hypertrophy that starts in infancy and progresses steadily for the first 8 to 10 years of life. After this the tonsils and adenoids regress. Excessive hypertrophy may cause:

1. An obstructed nasal airway with snoring, mouth breathing nasal speech and possibly 'glue ear'.
2. Chronic infection with recurrent tonsillitis and otitis media.

DIAGNOSTIC RANGE (rates per 1000 patients per year)
Personal: Suspected 10.7. Probable 3.8. *National*: 1.7 (Ref. 0.2). There are wide differences amongst doctors (and patients) about what is an 'acceptable' enlargement.

AGE INCIDENCE
The majority of patients (79%) are 3 to 8 years old.

CLINICAL POINTERS
1. Mouth breathing and snoring (80%).
2. Nasal speech.
3. Previous attacks of tonsillitis and otitis media (70%).

INVESTIGATIONS
The adenoids can be inspected by means of an indirect laryngoscope (reversed).

DURATION
The enlargement persists until the child is 10. If chronic infection is then present, recurring tonsillitis may continue into adult life.

COMPLICATIONS
Recurrent infection of the tonsil and middle ear are common. [Practice experience: 70% (14 out of 20) consecutive cases had an associated infection.] Chronic infection of the nasal sinuses is occasionally associated.

MISLEADING FEATURES AND PITFALLS
Tonsillectomy is easily regarded by both parents and doctor as a cure for all respiratory ailments of childhood. It is not without risk (one death in 10 years of practice) and is only performed for certain definite indications.

MANAGEMENT OPTIONS
The following criteria are considered as indications for referral for possible surgical removal:

- Repeated attacks (i.e. more than three in any year) of acute tonsillitis or adenoiditis.
- Progressive obstruction as judged by mouth breathing, snoring and nasal speech.
- The child should be over 5.

Some doctors consider that removal prevents recurrences of acute otitis media and 'glue ear'.

COMPLICATIONS OF TONSILLECTOMY

1. Secondary haemorrhage from operation site [10% (two out of 20) consecutive cases] may occur within 5 days of operation.
2. Aspiration pneumonia.
3. Acute otitis media.
4. Acute cervical adenitis.
5. Death.

TONSILLAR DEBRIS

Classification: ICHPPC 474 (RCGP 2450)

DIAGNOSTIC RANGE (rates per 1000 patients per year)
Personal: Suspected 1.2. Many cases are not reported to the doctor.

AGE INCIDENCE
Adults are liable.

CLINICAL POINTERS

1. High risk factors: Tonsils which have not atrophied during the 'teens'.
2. Offensive breath.
3. Chronic sore throat. Occasional.
4. Yellow debris lies in a crypt or hidden above the tonsil behind the fauces. Two spatulae are need both to visualise and dislodge the debris. The debris may collect again after an interval.

MISLEADING FEATURES AND PITFALLS
The condition is easily overlooked.

MANAGEMENT OPTIONS
Regular removal of debris. Surgery rarely indicated.

QUINSY (PERITONSILLAR ABSCESS)

Classification: ICHPPC 463 (RCGP 2455)

DIAGNOSTIC RANGE (rates per 1000 patients per year)
Personal: Suspected 1.3. The diagnosis was often in doubt because many abscesses subside without incision.

AGE INCIDENCE
Adults are mainly affected. Rare under 10 years.

CLINICAL POINTERS

1. Sore throat and inflammation of the tonsil. Breath is offensive when tonsillar exudate is present.
2. Nasal speech; often with trismus.
3. Unilateral swelling of the fauces. The tonsil and soft palate may be displaced.
4 Fever and malaise. Prostration is often marked.

DURATION

The untreated abscess points and discharges within 4 to 10 days.

COMPLICATIONS

Recurrences are likely.

MANAGEMENT OPTIONS

Established abscess: Antibacterials rarely effective. If the abscess has not drained spontaneously in 2–4 days referral for surgery indicated.

NASAL CATARRH

Classification: ICHPPC 519 (RCGP 2440)

Nasal catarrh is often regarded as a disease, but it is in fact a symptom that results from many different irritant processes.

Acute nasal catarrrh

This follows irritation of the nasal mucous membrane, e.g. colds, inhalation of irritants, decongestives or a foreign body.

Recurrent or chronic nasal catarrh

This may occur in the following disorders:

1. Allergic rhinitis (vascomotor rhinorrhoea). The discharge is watery and sneezing frequent. The nasal mucous membrane is red and oedematous.
2. Recurrent or chronic sinusitis. The discharge is mucopurulent and profuse. The nasal catarrh which persists after a cold is probably a result of an infection in the maxillary antra.
3. Nasal drip or snuffles. A mucopurulent discharge of toddlers and small babies due to a low-grade infection which may remain for weeks because the nasal passages are small and the patient unable to blow the nose. Congenital syphilitic snuffles is a rare nasal periostitis affecting the new-born.
4. Atrophic rhinitis (ozaena) is rare (two cases in 10 years). It is characterised not so much by catarrh as by a chronic crusting. Nasal

obstruction is slight but an offensive smell may cause great distress.

5. Iatrogenic rhinitis may be induced by prolonged use of decongestive solutions, some antihypertensives (BNF 2.5.2 and 2.5.3) and occasionally the 'pill'.

CLINICAL POINTERS

Nasal discharge and obstruction (100%) are the main complaints. Snoring and mouth-breathing may be associated.

MISLEADING FEATURES AND PITFALLS

Patients frequently diagnose and treat themselves for what they term *nasal catarrh*. This may be an allergic rhinitis which has been aggravated by the use of decongestives. If the doctor accepts the patient's evaluation, he may aggravate the symptoms by prescribing further decongestives.

DIFFERENTIAL DIAGNOSIS

Obstruction of the nasal passages may be produced by mechanical defects such as deviated nasal septum, broken nose, foreign body or nasal polyp. Thorough examination with a nasal speculum differentiates.

MANAGEMENT OPTIONS

These depend on the underlying cause.

NASAL POLYPI

Classification: ICHPPC 519 (RCGP 2435)

AETIOLOGY

Nasal polypi follow either prolonged allergic rhinitis or chronic sinusitis.

They may arise in response to a specific allergen and are said to occur in fibrocystic disease. Why some individuals should suffer from such a localised oedema of the nasal mucosa is unclear.

DIAGNOSTIC RANGE (rates per 1000 patients per year)
Personal: Suspected 3.0. Probable 2.3.

AGE INCIDENCE

Adults are affected.

CLINICAL POINTERS

1. High risk factors: (a) other allergic stigmata; (b) chronic nasal or sinus infection.

2. Chronic nasal obstruction with mouth-breathing and snoring.

3. The polyp is a round shiny grey opalescent obstruction which may fill the nasal passage. It is easily seen with a nasal speculum.

DURATION
Prolonged if not treated.

COMPLICATIONS
Nasal polypi are liable to recur after surgical removal. Extensive intra-nasal surgery is sometimes required to prevent recurrence.

MANAGEMENT OPTIONS
Referral usually indicated because local treatment is ineffective.

HAY FEVER

Classification: ICHPPC 477 (RCGP 2460)

AETIOLOGY
The pollens of grasses and other plants are commonly incriminated. Allergens cause degeneration of sensitized mast cells. This releases histamine which causes the localised symptoms.

DIAGNOSTIC RANGE (rates per 1000 patients per year)
Personal: Suspected 3.1. *National*: 11.3 (Ref. 0.2). Many cases not reported.

AGE INCIDENCE
Onset 5 to 25 years in most (80%) cases.

SEASONAL INCIDENCE
This is influenced by the plant life of the area. (June and July in the U.K.).

CLINICAL POINTERS
1. High risk factors: (a) allergic stigmata; (b) other known sensitivities.
2. Seasonal recurrences (80%) in spring and summer.
3. Irritation of mucous membrane of nose and eyes (100%). Streaming nose and eyes with sneezing and injection of the nasal mucous membranes and conjunctivae.
4. Mild asthma attacks or tightness of the chest are associated.

INVESTIGATIONS
Skin tests for sensitivites.

DURATION
Many years. Older patients are less inconvenienced.

MANAGEMENT OPTIONS

Prevention: (a) course of specific desensitisation (not without danger) — BNF 3.4.2; (b) anti-allergics — BNF 3.4.1 and 12.2.1 (topical) (Ref. 0.1) used prophylactically; (c) allergen avoidance.

Established attacks: (a) anti-allergics — BNF 3.4.1 and 12.2.1 (topical).

ALLERGIC CONJUNCTIVITIS

Classification: ICHPPC 372 (RCGP 1570)

This disorder is part of the hay fever complex. The nasal symptoms are minimal. Allergic and infective conjunctivitis are easily confused.

MISTAKES AND PITFALLS

Other more serious diseases occasionally present as a chronic conjunctivitis.

MANAGEMENT OPTIONS

As for Hay fever — local anti-allergics for eye — BNF 11.4 (Ref. 0.1).

Referral indicated if treatment is ineffective.

ALLERGIC RHINITIS

Classification: ICHPPC 477 (RCGP 2465)

AETIOLOGY

Specific allergens are incriminated less commonly than in hay fever. Iatrogenic causes — see Nasal catarrh (p. 429).

DIAGNOSTIC RANGE (rates per 1000 patients per year)

Personal: Suspected 9.4+. Certain diagnosis often difficult.

AGE INCIDENCE

Over 10 years.

SEASONAL INCIDENCE

Apart from a slight peak in the summer, there are no clear seasonal variations.

CLINICAL POINTERS

1. Recurrent rhinorrhoea or frequent so-called colds (100%). The discharge is not purulent although crusting of the mucous membrane may occur.
2. Polyp formation is commonly associated.

INVESTIGATIONS
Skin tests may suggest sensitivity to a specific allergen.

DURATION
Many years.

COMPLICATIONS
Severe crusting (atrophic rhinitis) with offensive smell (ozaena). Nasal polyps.

MANAGEMENT OPTIONS
As for hay fever (p. 431). Referral indicated if treatment is ineffective.

PLEURISY AND PLEURAL EFFUSION

Inflammation or irritation of the pleura may produce either sticky dry fibrin (dry pleurisy) or fluid (pleural effusion). It is wise to assume that both types of pleurisy indicate underlying lung disease. A dry pleurisy may develop into a pleural effusion, but the dry form is usually associated with acute and often slight lung disease; an effusion suggests serious pulmonary disease.

DRY (FIBRINOUS) PLEURISY

Classification: ICHPPC 5110 (RCGP 2520)

A fibrin exudate forms on the two surfaces of the pleura. Occasionally the exudate organises with subsequent adherence and calcification of the two layers.

AETIOLOGY

1. Trivial disease. [Practice experience. In 65% (13 out of 20) cases no underlying lung disease could be demonstrated by clinical or radiological means.]

2. Lung disease. Dry pleurisy may be caused by the following types of lung disease:

(a) Any pneumonic process, e.g. lobar pneumonia, bronchiectasis with pneumonitis.

(b) Pulmonary infarction (p. 368).

(c) Pulmonary tuberculosis (p. 147).

(d) Carcinoma, i.e. pleural metastases (p. 377).

3. Trauma. Pleuritic pain and friction rub occasionally follow trauma to the chest wall. Pain may start after an interval of 1 or 2 days.

DIAGNOSTIC RANGE (rates per 1000 patients per year)
Personal: Suspected 3.1. Probable 2.3. *National*: 1.1 (Ref. 0.2).

AGE INCIDENCE
The majority [90%] of patients are adults.

CLINICAL POINTERS

1. High risk factors: (a) smoking; (b) underlying lung disease; (c) injury to chest wall, (d) possible source of embolus or metastases.
2. Sudden onset.
3. Pleuritic pain (95%) is well localised and aggravated by coughing, deep breathing or moving. Occasionally the pain of a myocardial infarct is aggravated by respiration.
4. Cough (80%) is dry. Pain and spasm of the respiratory muscles give it a staccato character.
5. Fever (40%) is high when there is underlying pneumonia but more commonly it is only slightly raised or absent.
6. Friction rub (30%).

INVESTIGATIONS

1. A chest X-ray is always indicated.
2. Patients with persistent or recurrent pleurisy are referred to a chest physician.

DURATION
When underlying lung disease cannot be demonstrated, the pleuritic pain and friction rub should disappear in 1 to 5 days.

COMPLICATIONS
Depend on the nature of the underlying pathology. Recurrences occur: [Practice experience: 15% (three out of 20; recurred in 3 years].

MISLEADING FEATURES AND PITFALLS
Pneumonia, pulmonary tuberculosis and carcinoma are easily overlooked if patients with pleurisy are not X-rayed.

DIFFERENTIAL DIAGNOSIS
Diseases that may be confused with dry pleurisy:

Myocardial infarct
Similar features: pain in chest; low fever on second or third day.

Distinguishing features: pain is continuous and not related to coughing or deep breathing; radiates down an arm; BP depressed; cardiograph differentiates.

Spontaneous pneumothorax (non-tension)
Similar features: sudden onset of pleuritic pain; fever absent.

Distinguishing features: tension symptoms are absent when the leak of air into the pleura is slight; breath sounds and vocal resonance diminished; friction rub absent; chest X-ray differentiates.

Bornholm disease (epidemic myalgia)
Similar features: sudden onset of pleuritic pain; fever.

Distinguishing features: contact cases; fever often over 38°C pain severe; friction rub absent.

Fibrositis of chest
Similar features: pain in chest aggravated by movement and coughing; fever absent.

Distinguishing features: history of exertion or muscle strain common; localised muscle tenderness; cough and friction rub absent.

Shingles
Similar features: pain in chest; low fever.

Distinguishing features: rash appears 2 to 3 days after onset of pain; friction rub absent.

Acute upper abdominal disease
Similar feature: pain in chest of pleuritic type.

Distinguishing features: peptic ulcer and cholecystitis are rarely confused with pleurisy if a careful description of pain is obtained.

MANAGEMENT OPTIONS

Depend on the underlying causes.

PLEURAL EFFUSION

Classification: ICHPPC 5119 (RCGP 2525)

AETIOLOGY

The main causes are:

1. Lung infection:
   - acute pneumonia, pneumonitis or pulmonary infarction;
   - Primary or secondary tuberculous lung infection.
2. Pulmonary neoplasm:
   - Bronchogenic carcinoma;
   - Metastatic carcinoma.

   The effusion is often bloodstained.
3. Congestive heart failure and renal disease may lead to a collection of transudate.

DIAGNOSTIC RANGE (rates per 1000 patients per year)
Personal: Suspected 0.8. Probable 0.4. *National*: 0.2 (Ref. 0.2).

AGE INCIDENCE
A pleural effusion may arise at any age. In teenagers and young adults an effusion suggests primary tuberculosis. After 40 an effusion suggests neoplasm, tuberculosis or congestive heart failure.

CLINICAL POINTERS
1. High risk factors: (a) smoking; (b) asbestos worker; (c) underlying lung disease (infective or neoplastic); (d) cardiac or renal failure.
2. Preceding dry pleurisy. The pain and friction rub of a dry pleurisy disappear and are replaced, when the effusion develops, by a vague feeling of discomfort.
3. Cough is common.
4. Dyspnoea is marked when the effusion or lung disease are extensive.
5. Malaise and fever.
6. Classical signs of pleural effusion. Stony dullness to percussion, poor breath sounds, diminished vocal resonance and aegophony just above the fluid.

INVESTIGATIONS
1. Chest X-ray.
2. A white blood-cell count and ESR (see p. 681)
3. Diagnostic paracentesis for cytology, etc.
4. Full hospital investigation is usually indicated.

DURATION
Depends on the underlying disease and treatment.

COMPLICATIONS
Empyema, i.e. purulent effusion, occasionally develops in a post-pneumonic pleural effusion. (Two cases in 10 years of practice.)

MISLEADING FEATURES AND PITFALLS
1. Effusions may be missed if the lung bases of patients with serious pulmonary or cardiac disease are not examined regularly
2. Effusions may be overlooked when a dry pleurisy is replaced by a less painful effusion — the chest is not examined because the patient says the pain is better.

DIFFERENTIAL DIAGNOSIS
The thickened pleura which arises after repeated lung infections may be confused with an effusion.

MANAGEMENT OPTIONS
Depend on the underlying cause.

SPONTANEOUS PNEUMOTHORAX

Three types are described: (1) closed, (2) open, (3) valvular or tension.

CLOSED SPONTANEOUS PNEUMOTHORAX

Classification: ICHPPC 519 (RCGP 2530)

It is thought that an emphysematous bulla ruptures and air leaks into the pleural cavity. This event may complicate asthma.

AETIOLOGY
Trauma and coughing. Usually there is no obvious underlying cause.

DIAGNOSTIC RANGE (rates per 1000 patients per year)
Personal: Suspected 1.3. Proven 0.3. *National*: 0.2 (Ref. 0.2).

AGE INCIDENCE
Young adults are especially liable.

CLINICAL POINTERS
1. Sudden onset.
2. Dry cough is usually but not always present.
3. Pleuritic pain in the region of the affected lung.
4. Diminished breath sounds over the affected lung.

INVESTIGATIONS
Chest X-ray confirms the diagnosis.

DURATION
The lung takes 2 to 10 weeks to re-expand, depending on the degree of collapse.

COMPLICATIONS
1. There is always a slight risk that the closed type will develop into the more serious valvular type.
2. Recurrences affecting the same lung are not unusual.
3. Surgical emphysema at the base of the neck may occur.
4. Asthma may obscure the picture.

MISLEADING FEATURES AND PITFALLS
A ferbile respiratory illness may be wrongly diagnosed.

DIFFERENTIAL DIAGNOSIS

Pleurisy, Bornholm disease and fibrositis of chest may be confused with a pneumothorax. A chest X-ray differentiates.

MANAGEMENT OPTIONS

Established disease: (a) full explanation (risks, etc.); (b) limited activity until reabsorption confirmed; (c) follow up with chest X-rays.

OPEN PNEUMOTHORAX

Air flows freely between the lung passages and the pleural cavity. A bronchopleural fistula of this kind is rarely encountered outside hospital and is associated with serious pulmonary disease.

VALVULAR OR TENSION PNEUMOTHORAX

The communication between the lungs and the pleural cavity allows the passage of air into, but not out of the pleural cavity. Instead of ceasing as the lung collapses, the valve action persists even after considerable tension has been built up inside the pleural cavity. This leads rapidly to dyspnoea, cyanosis and occasionally death. (One case — not fatal — encountered in 10 years of practice.

CLINICAL POINTERS

1. High risk factors: (a) presence of non-tension pneumothorax; (b) other serious lung disease.
2. Sudden onset.
3. Severe chest pain worse on breathing.
4. Severe dyspnoea.
5. Cyanosis (not always present).
6. Increased resonance on one side of chest.
7. Evidence of mediastinal shift away from affected side.
8. Absent or diminished breath sounds on affected side.

INVESTIGATIONS

In an emergency the following quick test is useful. A sterile 5 mm syringe is filled with sterile water. A serum needle with the syringe attached is then introduced into the pleural cavity via a suitable intercostal space. The barrel of the syringe is then held vertically and the plunger withdrawn. Air will escape through the water seal if a tension pneumothorax is present.

MANAGEMENT OPTIONS

Immediate referral — doctor should accompany patient.

BRONCHIECTASIS

Classification: ICHPPC 491 (RCGP 2505)

Repeated bronchial infection leads to abnormal dilation of the bronchi. The disease may be reversible in children but rarely in adults.

AETIOLOGY

1. Atelectasis and aspiration pneumonitis. The onset of bronchiectasis is often associated with lung collapse. When a portion of lung collapses following an aspiration pneumonitis, the space is filled in two ways: (a) emphysema of the healthy surrounding lung; (b) dilatation of the affected bronchi which are at the same time crowded together. Chronic or recurrent infection prevents re-expansion of the collapsed lung.

2. Nasal sinus infections. (Practice experience: evidence of chronic sinus infection in 50% of the children and 20% of adults.)

3. Fibro-cystic disease. (One case in 10 years of practice.)

DIAGNOSTIC RANGE (rates per 1000 patients per year)

Personal: Suspected 2.8. Probable 1.3. *National*: 0.8 (Ref. 0.2).

AGE INCIDENCE

Experience in this practice suggests that there are two groups of approximately equal size:

1. Children — onset between 3 and 6 years. The disease follows repeated incidents of basal pneumonitis with lung collapse.

2. Adults — onset after the age of 30. The disease follows many years of repeated chest infection and is usually irreversible.

CLINICAL POINTERS

1. High risk factors: (a) previous recurrent or chronic basal lung infection or collapse; (b) chronic sinusitis; (c) asthma — it may be difficult to decide which is the primary disease. (Practice experience: asthma was noted in 70% of adult bronchiectatics.)

2. Repeated attacks of cough (100%). The cough is loose or productive and may persist indefinitely; it is often affected by posture, i.e. worse on getting out of bed.

3. Sputum. Adults — the sputum is profuse, frothy and mucopurulent. Children — the sputum is less obvious, either because it is swallowed or because the quantity is smaller.

4. Fever. Children — fever is present in half the cases and is often high. It may indicate a concurrent aspiration pneumonitis. Adults — fever is low or absent.

5. Haemoptysis (adults 40%; children — rare). Staining of the sputum occurs. Frank haemorrhage is less common.

6. Chest signs (70%). Persistent moist sounds are heard over one or both bases, at the same place with each attack. Dullness to percussion at one or both bases is common and may result from thickened pleura or chronic lung damage. The classical signs of pulmonary collapse or consolidation are rarely found.

7. Dyspnoea, asthma and clubbing of the fingers are late signs. Other late signs include loss of weight and right-sided heart failure.

INVESTIGATIONS

1. Chest X-ray may not show conclusively that a patient has bronchiectasis, but it often provides strong indirect evidence, e.g. heavy basal markings, lung collapse or crowding of the basal bronchi.

2. X-ray of accessory air sinuses.

3. Bronchography is rarely justified unless lobectomy is contemplated.

4. Bacteriological examination of the sputum is indicated if there is any possibility of pulmonary tuberculosis.

5. Referral to a chest physician.

DURATION

Rigorous treatment in childhood may prevent recurrence and gradual progression of the disease in adult life; once fully developed in adults, the disease is slowly progressive unless the affected lung is excised. Most adult patients report to the doctor for help one to three times each year.

COMPLICATIONS

1. Asthma.
2. Right-sided heart failure — rare.
3. Cerebral abscess is said to occur. (No cases encountered.)

MISLEADING FEATURES AND PITFALLS

1. Parents and patients resign themselves to the chronic cough. It is easy for the doctor to accept the patient's evaluation.

2. Failure to X-ray the accessory air sinuses. A potent source of reinfection may thus be overlooked.

DIFFERENTIAL DIAGNOSIS

Diseases that may be confused with bronchiectasis:

Chronic bronchitis
Similar features: recurring productive cough with febrile incidents and a tendency to asthma.

Distinguishing features: adults affected; cough and production of sputum unaffected by posture; both lungs are equally involved; haemoptysis absent; chest X-ray (and bronchography) fail to show localised lesions.

Pulmonary tuberculosis
Similar features: chronic productive cough with febrile incidents.

Distinguishing features: contacts; patient's condition is liable to deteriorate; history often short; lung bases are clear; chest X-ray differentiates.

MANAGEMENT OPTIONS

Prevention: (a) adequate follow up and rigorous treatment of childhood respiratory infections; (b) early, full anti-bacterial treatment — BNF 5.1 (Ref. 0.1) — of all descending secondary infections of the respiratory tract; (c) early postural drainage to prevent irreversible changes.

Established disease: (a) postural drainage; (b) graduated exercises; (c) appropriate antibacterials after bacteriology — BNF 5.1; (d) referral usually indicated; (e) surgery.

EPISTAXIS

Classification: ICHPPC 7847 (RCGP 4595)

Usually follows local trauma e.g. a knock, over vigorous blowing or picking of nose. Sometimes bleeding is spontaneous or during a fever such as influenza. Rarely it may be associated with hypertension, anticoagulant therapy, diseases of the blood or uraemia. Often no cause is apparent.

DIAGNOSTIC RANGE (rates per 1000 patients per year)
Personal: 5.8. Many cases are never reported.

MANAGEMENT OPTIONS

Established bleed: (a) exclude serious causes; (b) exclude possible anaemia from blood loss; (c) identify site of bleed if possible — many are from anterior septal (Little's) area where bleeding is controlled by firm nasal compression or cautery; (d) reassurance and rest; (e) nasal pack or even referral to hospital are sometimes needed if above measures fail.

HAEMOPTYSIS

Classification: ICHPPC 7863 (RCGP 4635)

In many cases there is no obvious cause but underlying lung disease should be suspected and a chest X-ray or referral arranged.

DIAGNOSTIC INCIDENCE
Cases without obvious cause — 1.4 per 1000 patients per year.

COUGH (WITHOUT OTHER CLINICAL FEATURES)

Classification: ICHPPC 7862 (RCGP 4630)

Cough is usually one manifestation of the ubiquitous common cold. In practice, however, the single complaint of cough without any other evidence of disease is so common that it is managed as a separate clinical entity. The following description refers solely to those patients who complain of cough of short duration without fever or other evidence of disease.

DIAGNOSTIC RANGE (rates per 1000 patients per year)
Personal: Suspected 133+. Most coughs are never reported to the doctor.

AGE INCIDENCE
A peak is reached in the first year of school (Fig. 43).

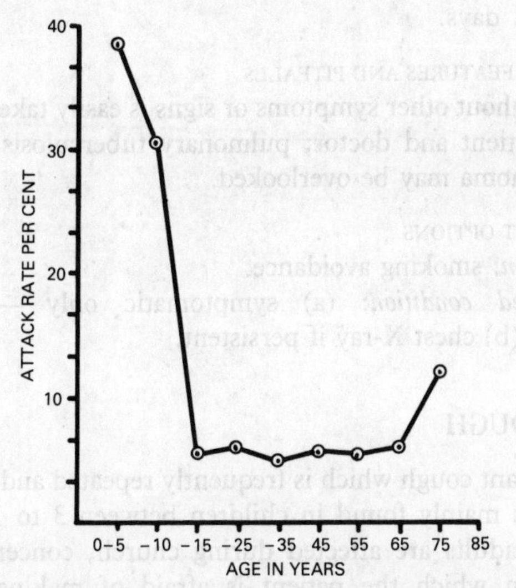

Fig. 43 Cough. Age incidence curve of 345 consecutive cases encountered in 1 year.

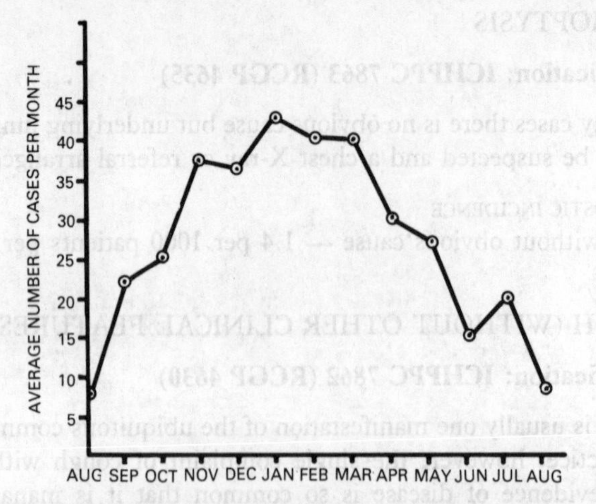

Fig. 44 Cough. Seasonal incidence of 1374 consecutive cases reported over 4 years.

SEASONAL INCIDENCE

The highest incidence is in the winter months (Fig. 44).

CLINICAL POINTERS

1. High risk factor: smoking.
2. Cough without other evidence of disease [100%].

DURATION

Three to 21 days.

MISLEADING FEATURES AND PITFALLS

A cough without other symptoms or signs is easily taken for granted by both patient and doctor; pulmonary tuberculosis or bronchogenic carcinoma may be overlooked.

MANAGEMENT OPTIONS

Prevention: smoking avoidance.

Established condition: (a) symptomatic only — BNF 3.9 (Ref. 0.1); (b) chest X-ray if persistent.

HABIT COUGH

A mild irritant cough which is frequently repeated and is of nervous origin. It is mainly found in children between 3 to 10 years, but sometimes adults are affected during church, concerts or similar functions in which the patient is afraid of making a noise. It disappears during sleep or when the patient's attention is fixed.

DIAGNOSTIC RANGE

1.1 per 1000 patients per year.

SMOKER'S COUGH

This common complaint is directly related to excessive smoking. The diagnosis can only be made after serious pulmonary disease has been excluded. *Management*: Smoking avoidance.

Table 26 Less common diseases of the respiratory system

Disease and distinguishing clinical pointers	Incidence per 1000 patients per year Suspected	Confirmed
Carcinoma of tonsil	—	1 in 10 years
Staphylococcal and haemophilus pneumonia Influenza epidemic (sporadic cases occur when influenza is not epidemic), evidence of early consolidation, cyanosis, chest X-ray	—	3 in 10 years
Tuberculous pneumonia Contact and prevous history, clinical pneumonia that fails to settle with antibiotics, chest X-ray	—	1 in 10 years
Acute bronchopneumonia Babies and elderly patients liable, clinical picture ill-defined	—	—
Virus pneumonia (including psittacosis) Influenzal illness (with cough, high fever and tracheitis), chest signs — a few basal râles on 4th to 7th day, illness lasts 7 to 14 days, rarely severe, white blood-cell count normal (or low), paired sera prove the infection, radiological findings show consolidation or congestion, (See p. 189)	1.0	0.5
Q fever (see p. 189) Sudden onset; high fever that persists for 5 to 9 days; cough, chest pain and body aches are slight; occasional râles in chest; white blood-cell count is normal; chest X-ray may show congestion Reservoir may be in sheep and goats.	—	6 in 10 years
Deviated nasal septum Nasal obstruction, septal deviation	0.8	0.8
Foreign body in nose Nasal obstruction, unilateral bloodstained nasal discharge. Mainly children.	0.6	0.6
Empyema Post-pneumonic pleural effusion with fever, paracentesis	—	2 in 10 years
Acute pulmonary oedema (cardiac asthma) Heart disease, sudden onset, acute dyspnoea (often nocturnal), cyanosis, numerous scattered adventitious sounds, (see pp. 358, 361).	0.4	0.4

18

Diseases of the digestive system

Please read the introduction for explanation of figures and analyses.

IMPACTED WISDOM TOOTH

Classification: ICHPPC 520 (RCGP 2600)

During early adult life the wisdom teeth erupt and sometimes crowd the other teeth. This may cause pain or infection of the wisdom tooth socket. Facial neuralgia is common. Extraction is usual.

TEETHING SYNDROME

Classification: ICHPPC 520 (RCGP 2600)

Opinions differ about the extent and nature of the symptoms produced by the eruption of the milk teeth. In babies many minor ailments are ascribed to teething when in fact other diseases are responsible. Undoubtedly an erupting tooth makes a baby restless, but there is no evidence that fever, respiratory illness or systemic disturbances are caused by teething. The diagnosis of teething should therefore be made by exclusion.

DIAGNOSTIC RANGE (rates per 1000 patients per year)
Personal: Suspected 5.6. The diagnosis is difficult to confirm.

AGE INCIDENCE
Three to 18 months (95%).

CLINICAL POINTERS
1. Restlessness, crying and general irritability (60%).
2. Pulling the ears and excessive chewing of hands, etc.
3. Evidence that a tooth is erupting.
4. Other diseases absent, e.g. absence of cough, fever, enteritis, nappy rash, otitis media, etc.

DURATION

Intermittent; each bout of restlessness rarely lasts longer than 1 or 2 days.

MISLEADING FEATURES AND PITFALLS

These are avoided if the diagnosis is made by exclusion.

MANAGEMENT OPTIONS

(a) Exclude other causes of restlessness; (b) 150 mg soluble aspirin.

DENTAL CARIES

Classification: ICHPPC 520 (RCGP 2600)

AETIOLOGY

Western low fibre/high sugar diets, sweets and fluoride content of water all play a part.

DIAGNOSTIC RANGE (rates per 1000 patients per year)

Personal: Suspected 11.7+. Many cases not reported.

MANAGEMENT OPTIONS

Prevention: (a) fluoridation; (b) dental hygiene; (c) diet.
Established state: dental referral.

DENTAL ABSCESS

Classification: ICHPPC 520 (RCGP 2600)

In children the abscess points on the outer side of the gum as a gumboil.

DIAGNOSTIC RANGE (rates per 1000 patients per year)

Personal: Suspected 6.7+. Many cases not reported. The diagnosis was rarely in doubt.

AGE INCIDENCE

All ages liable.

CLINICAL POINTERS

1. Persistent pain in the jaw. This is the rule except in children.
2. Tenderness in the affected tooth when tapped.
3. Swelling and redness of surrounding gums (not always present).

INVESTIGATIONS

X-ray of jaw if local signs are absent.

MANAGEMENT OPTIONS
Dental referral.

DENTAL EXTRACTIONS

DIAGNOSTIC RANGE (rates per 1000 patients per year)
Personal: 6.0. Many cases are not reported.

COMPLICATIONS
1. Persistent socket infection.
2. Haemorrhage is often referred to the G.P.

NOTE. Persistent haemorrhage is occasionally an early sign of a reticulosis

CHRONIC GINGIVITIS AND PYORRHOEA

Classification: ICHPPC 520 (RCGP 2605)

These two conditions of the gums may occur together. Pyorrhoea is a simple infection of the gums in which a small quantity of pus can be expressed from the space between tooth and gum.

Gingivitis causes a red spongy painful swelling of the gum which bleeds easily from friction. Gingivitis may follow simple infection such as pyorrhoea. Occasionally it indicates the presence of serious systemic disease:

- Reticulosis. The spongy gums are haemorrhagic and proliferate after extraction. (Two cases in 10 years.)
- Metal poisoning: lead, bismuth, etc. A black line forms along the gum edge. (One case in 10 years.)
- Scurvy. (No cases in 10 years of practice.)

DIAGNOSTIC RANGE (rates per 1000 patients per year)
Personal: Suspected 2.5. Many cases are never reported.

MANAGEMENT OPTIONS
Established condition: (a) exclude serious disease; (b) dental referral.

APHTHOUS ULCERS OF THE MOUTH

Classification: ICHPPC 528 (RCGP 2635)

AETIOLOGY
Uncertain. The ulcers resemble those of herpetic stomatitis and

may be a manifestation of chronic *herpes simplex virus* infection (see p. 161).

DIAGNOSTIC RANGE (rates per 1000 patients per year)
Personal: Suspected 10.5+. Many cases are probably never reported. The diagnosis was rarely in doubt.

AGE INCIDENCE
All ages are affected; children are especially liable.

CLINICAL POINTERS

1. High risk factors: (a) previous similar ulcers or primary HSV stomatitis; (b) parental HSV infections; (c) poor oral hygiene.
2. Sore painful spot inside mouth (100%).
3. The presence of an ulcer (100%). Shallow ulcers, 2 to 10 mm diameter, on the tongue, floor of the mouth and inside of cheeks.
4. Offensive breath.
5. Recurrences are characteristic.

DURATION
Each ulcer takes about 4 to 10 days to heal. The tendency to develop these ulcers persists for many years.

MANAGEMENT OPTIONS

Prevention: Good oral hygiene.

Established ulcer: (a) analgesics; (b) topical (protective, steroid etc.) — BNF 12.3.1.(Ref. 0.1).

ANGULAR CHEILOSIS

Classification: ICHPPC 528 (RCGP 2640)

A chronic condition characterised by red painful excoriation at the angles of the mouth and cheek.

AETIOLOGY
Deficiency of riboflavin is said to be the cause, but treatment is disappointing. The disorder is said to be associated with hypochromic anemia — not confirmed in this practice. Sometimes there is an associated monilia infection.

DIAGNOSTIC RANGE (rates per 1000 patients per year)
Personal: Suspected 1.3+. Many cases not reported.

AGE INCIDENCE
All ages. In young babies a severe form of the condition is said to arise in congenital syphilis.

MANAGEMENT OPTIONS

Established disease: Local protectives especially at night — BNF 12.3.1 (Ref. 0.1).

GLOSSITIS

Classification: ICHPPC 528 (RCGP 2650)

This is a convenient term which is used to cover a number of clinical conditions of the tongue. The aetiology of many of them is uncertain.

In practice the clinical types of glossitis are as follows:

1. Simple glossitis
Aetiology unknown. Soreness is associated with redness of the papillae, most marked at the edges of the tongue. The condition is very persistent and difficult to treat.

2. Atrophic glossitis
Associated with pernicious anaemia. At first a sore patchy redness of the tongue appears. Later, as the condition progresses, all the papillae are lost and the smooth pink atrophic tongue of Addisonian anaemia appears.

3. Brown (or black) hairy tongue
Said to be due to a fungus infection and may follow the use of antibiotics. The middle and posterior part of the tongue becomes coated with a thick brown (or black) hairy fur that is harmless.

4. Geographical tongue
Aetiology unknown. The superficial epithelium desquamates in patches, giving the tongue a harmless map-like appearance.

Note: Leukoplakia, gumma and deficiency diseases that affect the tongue are rare. (No cases seen in 10 years of practice.)

DIAGNOSTIC RANGE (all types) (rates per 1000 patients per year)
Personal: Suspected 2.5+. Many cases are never reported.

MISLEADING FEATURES AND PITFALLS

1. The sore tongue of pernicious anaemia may appear several months before the other symptoms of this disease.

2. A sore tongue may develop with severe hypochromic anaemia.

3. A considerable amount of thick white fur on the tongue is normal for some patients, and the doctor may be consulted about this fancied sign of ill health.

DISEASES OF THE OESOPHAGUS, STOMACH AND DUODENUM

The diseases that occur in these three organs can be classified into a number of distinct pathological entities. The family physician's main difficulty is to separate these disorders by clinical means. The problem is made more difficult because (a) the clinical features of each entity are often similar; (b) the diagnostic tests at the disposal of both G. P. and specialist are not infallible.

CLASSIFICATION OF COMMON DISORDERS

A. Oesophagus

1. Oesophageal carcinoma.
2. Achalasia and cardiospasm.
3. Globus hystericus and functional dysphagia.
4. Reflux oesophagitis.
5. Hiatus hernia.
6. Plummer-Vinson syndrome.

B. Stomach and duodenum

1. Gastric carcinoma.
2. Peptic ulcer syndrome, including: ulcer-type dyspepsia; gastric ulcer; duodenal ulcer; anastomotic ulcer.
3. Acute gastritis.
4. Functional gastritis (nervous dyspepsia).

> NOTE. Chronic gastritis may exist as a separate pathological entity, but for practical purposes it can be regarded as part of the peptic ulcer syndrome.

[A survey of all patients reporting with indigestion was carried out in this practice and in three other practices covering a total NHS practice population of 19 619 patients (Ref. 2.1). Three hundred and fifty-one patients were investigated, of whom 251 were all subjected to the following investigations — barium meal, blood group and secretor status assessments, and serum pepsinogen investigation. The clinical descriptions of the following diseases in this section are based largely upon this material: duodenal ulcer, 136 cases; gastric ulcer, 13 cases; reflux oesophagitis with hiatus hernia, 29 cases; cholecystitis, 16 cases; ulcer-type dyspepsia, 67 cases.]

CARCINOMA OF OESOPHAGUS

Classification ICHPPC 151 (RCGP 0405)

A form of carcinoma in which there is probably a long period of silent growth before symptoms appear. The prognosis is therefore poor. The lower half of the oesophagus is most commonly affected.

DIAGNOSTIC RANGE (rates per 1000 patients per year)
Personal: Suspected 0.3, Probable 0.1, *National*: 0.1 (Ref. 0.2).

AGE INCIDENCE
Adults over 50.

SEX INCIDENCE
Men are affected more than women.

CLINICAL POINTERS

1. Dysphagia. Food is felt to stick behind the sternum at a point corresponding to the level of the growth. Any adult who says that food 'sticks after swallowing' requires an immediate full investigation of the oesophagus.
2. Loss of weight occurs early.
3. Substernal pain associated with swallowing food is common.
4. Regurgitation of food or mucus stained with blood sometimes occurs.

INVESTIGATIONS

1. Barium swallow sometimes fails to outline the growth.
2. Oesophagoscopy is the only certain method of excluding carcinoma. It is not without risk.

DURATION
Few cases are operable and in the untreated patient death usually occurs within 2 years of onset. Only 7% operated cases live 5 years.

MISLEADING FEATURES AND PITFALLS
Failure to take an adequate history may lead to confusion between the true dysphagia of carcinoma and the more vague sensations of globus hystericus.

DIFFERENTIAL DIAGNOSIS
Diseases that may be confused with oesophageal carcinoma:

Oesophagitis (reflux)
Similar features: dysphagia; substernal pain.

Distinguishing features: pain is marked; weight loss is slight; hospital investigation indicated.

Achalasia
Similar features: dysphagia; regurgitation of food.

Distinguishing features: young adults affected; pain and weight loss slight at first; hospital investigation indicated.

Functional dysphagia (globus hystericus)
Similar features: feeling of lump in throat or behind sternum.

Distinguishing features: no true dysphagia; sensation is not related to food or swallowing; weight loss absent; response to reassurance; hospital investigation rarely indicated.

MANAGEMENT OPTIONS

Suspected disease: early referral.

Post-hospital: (a) discussion; (b) medical and mental support; (c) group support (see p. 207 *et seq*).

REFLUX OESOPHAGITIS AND HIATUS HERNIA

Classification ICHPPC 530 (RCGP 2660) and ICHPPC 551 (RCGP 2730)

These two conditions are closely linked aetiologically. Many cases of hiatus (diaphragmatic) hernia are symptomless and are discovered incidentally during radiological examinations for other reasons. When symptoms arise from hiatus herniation they are said to follow, not the hernia, but the associated reflex oesophagitis and possible high gastric acidity.

AETIOLOGY

1. Reflux oesophagitis
The cardiac sphincter fails to prevent stomach contents from entering the oesophagus when the patient lies down.

2. Hiatus hernia
Congenital short oesophagus, para-oesophageal and oesophago-gastric hernia are described. With the exception of congenital short oesophagus, the aetiological factors are as for other hernias.

DIAGNOSTIC RANGE (rates per 1000 patients per year)
Personal: Suspected 3.3, *National*: 1.5 (Ref. 0.2).

AGE INCIDENCE
Adults over 40.

SEX INCIDENCE
Women are more affected than men (2:1). Those who are fat, short or pregnant seem especially prone.

CLINICAL POINTERS
These are those of reflux oesophagitis.

1. High risk factors: (a) excessive bending or lying; (b) previous

attacks; (c) high gastric acidity; (d) known hiatus hernia.

2. Onset. Symptoms increase slowly and intermittently over many years.

3. Pain felt behind the lower sternum or in the epigastrium. Sometimes there is radiation to the neck or arms with simulation of myocardial ischaemia. Pain at night is very common (65%). Pain that occurs daily over long periods is very suggestive of reflux (40%). Sometimes the pain shows marked periodicity with relief by alkalis and a peptic ulcer is closely simulated. The pain usually starts within an hour of food (50%).

4. The pain is affected by posture and is aggravated by lying down and bending (50%). Sitting up may relieve the pain.

5. Heartburn is frequent (60%). Waterbrash may be reported. Both these symptoms occur in duodenal ulceration.

6. Other symptoms of little differentiating value:

- The relation of the pain to food or alkalis.
- Vomiting.
- Increased resonance over the left lower chest, also noted in many normal individuals.
- Haematemesis.

INVESTIGATIONS

1. Straight X-ray of chest occasionally reveals evidence of the disorder.

2. Barium meal X-ray. Hiatus herniation or gastric reflux may be difficult to outline. The Trendelenburg position and a sip of cold water may be needed before herniation can be demonstrated.

DURATION

The condition persists indefinitely unless it is corrected by operation.

COMPLICATIONS

Oesophageal stricture and fibrosis are said to occur. Some authorities claim that the so-called congenital short oesophagus is due to an acquired fibrosis following oesophagitis and is not a congenital defect.

MISLEADING FEATURES AND PITFALLS

Peptic ulcer and myocardial infarction are common conditions. Reflux oesophagitis can mimic both diseases.

DIFFERENTIAL DIAGNOSIS

Diseases that may be confused with reflux oesophagitis.

Peptic ulcer
Similar features: epigastric or low substernal pain related to food; waterbrash and heartburn; similar age distribution; haematemesis.

Distinguishing features: pain affected by posture but usually relieved by lying down, not sitting up; pain relieved by alkalis; periodicity marked; radiation of pain to jaw, neck, or arms absent; epigastric tenderness present; clinical distinction often difficult; barium meal differentiates.

Myocardial ischaemia and infarction
Similar feature: substernal pain lasting several hours and radiating to jaw, neck or arms.

Distinguishing features: history of effort angina common; pain is not relieved by changes in posture; waterbrash and heart burn absent; patient may be shocked and blood pressure lowered; cardiograph and serum transaminase differentiate.

Carcinoma of oesophagus
Similar features: food felt to stick behind lower sternum; retrosternal pain; barium swallow may be similar; haematemesis.

Distinguishing features: dysphagia is progressive; pain is often slight and unaffected by posture; weight loss marked; investigation in hospital indicated; oesophagoscopy or laparotomy may be only certain method of differentiating.

> NOTE. Cholecystitis (and angina pectoris) may occur concurrently and the history may be difficult to differentiate from that of reflux oesophagitis.

MANAGEMENT OPTIONS

As for Peptic Ulcer Syndrome p. 464. Referral for surgery if intractable and due to hernia.

CARCINOMA OF STOMACH

Classification: ICHPPC 151 (RCGP 0410)

A common form of cancer with a poor prognosis which is aggravated by delays in diagnosis because:

1. The symptoms and signs vary according to the site of the carcinoma:

- Prepyloric growths present a clinical picture of pyloric obstruction. Two-thirds of stomach cancer are said to originate here.

• Growths in body of the stomach cause few symptoms until late in the disease.

• Growths at the fundus produce signs of oesophageal obstruction.

2. There is probably a silent period before onset of symptoms.

3. A prior history of many years indigestion due to a known or suspected ulcer is not uncommon. This may cause delays in diagnosis.

AETIOLOGY

Uncertain. Heredity, race and diet may play a part.

DIAGNOSTIC RANGE (rates per 1000 patients per year)

Personal: Suspected 0.9, Probable 0.7, *National* 0.4 (Ref. 0.2).

AGE INCIDENCE

Adults — a peak is reached at 50 to 60 years.

SEX INCIDENCE

Men are said to be affected three times more than women.

CLINICAL POINTERS

1. High risk factors: (a) positive family history; (b) pernicious anaemia; (c) race i.e. Japanese.

2. Symptoms of indigestion that appear for the first time in middle-aged patients. Gastric and dyspeptic symptoms due to other causes are common.

3. Failure of indigestion to remit with treatment. Patients with gastric carcinoma may improve for two to three weeks on an ulcer régime. After this, progressive deterioration with daily pain is apparent.

4. Loss of weight is a constant and significant early symptom.

5. Vomiting is a feature of all types of gastric carcinoma. In prepyloric growths it is profuse. Vomitus contains food eaten long before. Loss of weight and vomiting are often the only early symptoms. Haematemesis (and melaena) may occur.

6. Anorexia is a surprisingly late symptom.

7. Anaemia is usually a late sign.

8. Abdominal mass or supraclavicular lymph node enlargement are late signs which indicate extensive spread.

9. Pernicious anaemia. Gastric carcinoma is a common complication of this disease. (In 10 years, out of nine patients with pernicious anaemia four died of a gastric carcinoma.)

INVESTIGATIONS

Negative results do not exclude cancer and reliance should only be placed on positive findings.

1. ESR (see p. 681) is unfortunately not always raised in the early stages of gastric carcinoma.

2. Haemoglobin estimation may be normal.

3. Occult blood in faeces warrants a full and immediate gastrointestinal investigation. Unfortunately occult blood cannot be detected in all cases of gastric carcinoma.

4. Barium meal. Radiology fails to reveal the growth in 25%.

5. Fractional test meals and gastroscopy are helpful.

DURATION

Without treatment, death usually occurs within 2 to 12 months of onset of symptoms.

COMPLICATIONS

Carcinomatosis and death.

MISLEADING FEATURES AND PITFALLS

1. Patients who have a gastric carcinoma are acutely aware that they are organically ill, although the symptoms may be vague. It is easy to confuse this genuine apprehension with the mild anxiety so often encountered in gastric patients.

2. The family doctor is lulled into a sense of false security by the negative results from X-rays and other tests.

3. The family doctor forgets that gastric carcinoma is a cause of simple hypochromic anaemia.

4. The association between pernicious anaemia and gastric carcinoma is forgotten.

DIFFERENTIAL DIAGNOSIS

The separation of cases of gastric carcinoma from the many patients complaining of dyspeptic symptoms may be extremely difficult.

Diseases that may be confused with gastric carcinoma:

Peptic ulcer and ulcer dyspepsia

Similar features: upper abdominal discomfort related to food; loss of weight; vomiting; anorexia; temporary relief of symptoms by alkalis.

Distinguishing features: most peptic ulcers start before the age of 40; most gastric carcinomas start after this; vomiting and loss of weight are late signs; hospital investigation indicated.

Hiatus hernia and reflux oesophagitis
Similar features: daily pain; onset after age of 40; discomfort related to food; vomiting; temporary relief by alkalis.

Distinguishing features: steady progression of all symptoms is absent; weight loss and occult blood in stools unusual.

MANAGEMENT OPTIONS

Suspected disease: early referral for possible surgery, often palliative.

Post hospital: (a) discussion; (b) medical 'whole person' support; (c) group support (see pp. 207–208); (d) diet.

ACUTE GASTRITIS

Classification: ICHPPC 536 (RCGP 2700)

AETIOLOGY

Any gastric irritant may produce repeated vomiting, but in practice there appear to be three main causes: (a) fever — a common cause in children under 10 years; (b) excessive alcohol intake; (c) unsuitable food.

DIAGNOSTIC RANGE (rates per 1000 patients per year)

Personal: Suspected 19.6+. Many cases not reported. Diagnosis difficult.

AGE INCIDENCE

Many cases (38%) are in children under 15 years.

CLINICAL POINTERS

1. High risk factors: (a) unsuitable food; (b) fever; (c) alcohol.
2. Repeated vomiting starts suddenly and lasts 1 to 2 days.

DURATION

1 or 2 days.

COMPLICATIONS

If vomiting is severe, dehydration or even tetany (1 case in 10 years) may occur.

MISLEADING FEATURES

Young children sometimes complain of upper abdominal pain just before vomiting or when they are feeling sick.

DIFFERENTIAL DIAGNOSIS

Other more serious causes must be excluded.

MANAGEMENT OPTIONS

Established attack: (a) rest; (b) fluids.

NERVOUS DYSPEPSIA (FUNCTIONAL GASTRITIS)

(see also p. 268).

Classification: ICHPPC 536 (RCGP 2700)

Vomiting is the main symptom. Psychological causes are apparent. In children the sickness may occur every morning before going to school. Occasionally a child may be sick to get its own way.

In adults the condition develops in a tension state or if a patient is convinced that he has serious organic disease.

DIAGNOSTIC RANGE (rates per 1000 patients per year)

Personal: Suspected 10.8+. It was rarely possible to confirm the diagnosis.

CLINICAL POINTERS

1. High risk factors (a) possible psychological triggers; (b) previous attacks.
2. Vomiting. The quantity of vomit is small and questioning reveals that there is much retching or that vomiting is self-induced.
3. The absence of other clinical pointers.

DURATION

The condition rarely lasts longer than 2 days.

COMPLICATIONS

Vomiting of psychological origin occasionally upsets the body biochemistry sufficiently to perpetuate the tendency to vomit. This vicious circle vomiting settles rapidly with removal to hospital.

MISLEADING FEATURES AND PITFALLS

As with other diseases of psychological origin, the common pitfall is to diagnose functional gastritis in an anxious patient whose vomiting has an organic basis. Vomiting of pregnancy may be overlooked.

MANAGEMENT OPTIONS

Prevention: Learn to accept or avoid trigger factors.

Established attack: (a) encourage normal activities; (b) minimum of symptomatic treatment — antacids BNF 1.1 (Ref. 0.1).

PEPTIC ULCER SYNDROME

This syndrome is conveniently divided into three groups:

1. Gastric ulcer (ICHPPC 533 (RCGP 2675)
2. Duodenal ulcer (ICHPPC 532 (RCGP 2685);
3. Ulcer-type dyspepsia (ICHPPC 533 or 536 (RCGP 2695) — a useful term which covers any condition with the clinical features of an ulcer but in which the diagnosis has not been confirmed.

[Practice experience. Barium studies of 144 such patients revealed that half the men (46 out of 95) and only 16% of the women (eight out of 49) had a demonstrable duodenal ulcer.]

AETIOLOGY

The production of gastric acid and pepsin in the stomach when food is seen or ingested is an initial step in normal digestion. We know the thought of food and its presence in the stomach normally stimulate it to produce acid and pepsin through neural and chemical mechanisms. Thus *gastrin*, *histamine* and other chemotransmitters stimulate acid/pepsin levels while *secretin* and other hormones inhibit their secretion. We also know that ulceration does not occur in the absence of gastric acid and pepsin. We do *not* know how healthy gastric and duodenal mucosa is protected from ulceration in individuals without ulcers.

From a practical management point of view it is therefore helpful to know:

- — those factors which probably enhance the natural mucosal protection
- — those factors which interfere with the protection
- — those factors which either decrease or neutralise acid and pepsin in the stomach and duodenum.

Factors which protect the gastric duodenal mucosa

1. Heredity factors. Peptic ulcers occur three times more often in patients with blood group O and in patients who fail to secrete blood group antigens in their saliva. Certain bodily antigens thus play a protective role.

2. Sex factors. Women appear to be protected against duodenal ulceration until the menopause. The ulcer rates for men and women then approximate.

3. Small frequent meals, certain foods and the presence of fat in the duodenum may all have a protective effect.

4. Ulcer healing drugs e.g. cimetidine — BNF 1.3 (Ref. 0.1).

Factors which may interfere with the natural protection of the gastric and duodenal mucosa

1. Abnormally high levels of acid and pepsin in stomach and duodenum.
2. Dietary factors: Irregular or hurried meals; long periods between meals; certain foods especially fried and spicy foods.
3. Smoking. Smoking delays ulcer healing.
4. Gastric irritants: Alcohol — especially spirits; certain drugs e.g. aspirin, phenylbutazone, anti-inflammatory drugs and steroids — BNF 10.1 (Ref. 0.1).
5. Stasis and reflux of duodenal and stomach contents. Rapid emptying of stomach acid may aggravate a duodenal ulcer.
6. Psychological factors such as anxiety or tension may possibly play a part by affecting neurological control.

Factors which either neutralise or reduce the effect of gastric acid and pepsin

1. Further food or milk. These may also cause rebound acid increases.
2. Antacids — BNF 1.1. (Ref. 0.1). Different antacids cause varying degrees of rebound.
3. Antispasmodics (including anticholinergics) — BNF 1.2.
4. Stomach histamine (H_2 receptor) blockers and ulcer healing drugs cimetidine, etc. — BNF 1.3.

DIAGNOSTIC RANGE (rates per 1000 patients per year)
Personal: Ulcer Type Dyspepsia: Suspected 29.3. Probable 6.6.
Gastric ulcer: Proven 1.7. *National*: 0.8 (Ref. 0.2)
Duodenal ulcer: Proven 6.5. *National*: 4.0 (Ref. 0.2).

AGE INCIDENCE
Most cases begin before 35 years (Fig. 45).

SEX INCIDENCE
Men are liable to develop duodenal ulcers (4 : 1). Young males are especially prone to duodenal ulcers.

SEASONAL INCIDENCE
Peaks of incidence occur in late autumn and late spring (Fig. 46).

CLINICAL POINTERS

1. High risk factors: (a) previous history; (b) positive family history; (c) job involving irregular meals — driving, night work,

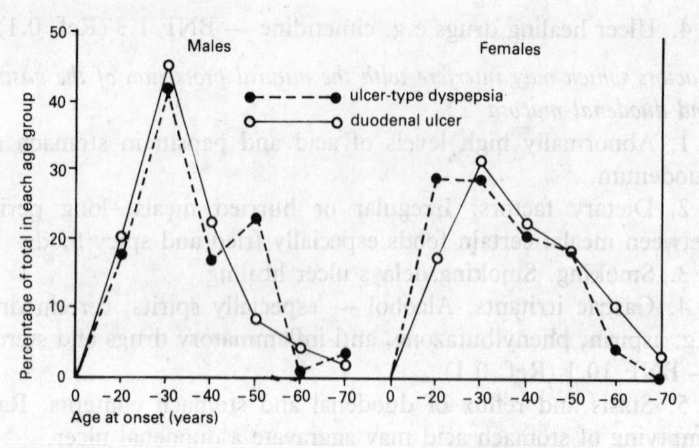

Fig. 45 Distribution curves for onset of duodenal ulcer (136 cases) and ulcer-type dyspepsia (67 cases).

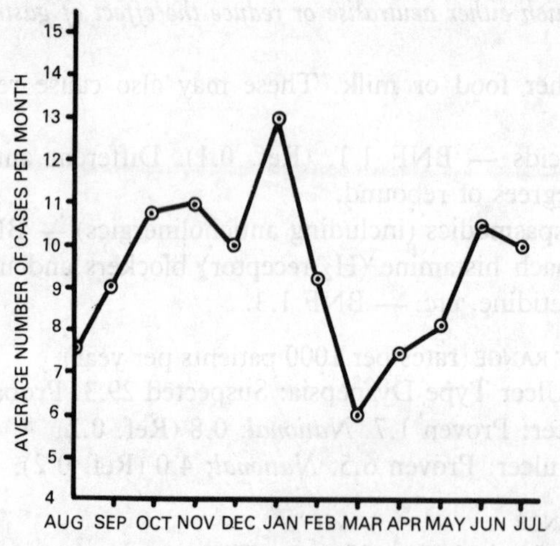

Fig. 46 Ulcer dyspepsia. Seasonal incidence of 406 consecutive cases (including recurrences) encountered in 4 years.

etc.; (d) diet — fried spicy food; (e) smoking; (f) gastric irritants — drugs, alcohol.

2. Periodicity (90%). A history of previous attacks with symptom-free periods is given.

3. Abdominal pain (90%) is epigastric in most cases (75%). The pain is felt in the right hypochondrium by some patients with duodenal ulcer; in others it may radiate through to the back. This latter feature suggests severe ulceration.

4. Pain or other symptoms are relieved by taking further food or alkalis (85%).

5. The onset of the pain is related to food intake (80%). In gastric ulcers the pain tends to arise soon after a meal. In duodenal ulcers the pain may not start for 1 to 2 hours; it is often worse at night and may wake the patient in the early hours. In such cases the patient may connect the pain with hunger and not the preceding meal.

6. Epigastric tenderness (80%) may be difficult to evaluate.

7. Other common symptoms of less differentiating value:

• Heartburn — a burning sensation that is felt behind the sternum after meals, a common symptom in oesophagitis.

• Waterbrash — a collection of clear salty fluid at the back of the throat. It should be distinguished from vomitus and suggests duodenal ulceration.

• Belching of wind and feeling of abdominal distension.

8. Features that arise in the peptic ulcer syndrome, but which also suggest a gastric carcinoma:

• Vomiting is common in gastric ulcers and frequently relieves the pain. If the vomiting is excessive or contains food that has been ingested long before, carcinoma should be suspected.

• Daily pain or other symptom.

• Anorexia is not common in peptic ulcers and is very suggestive of carcinoma. Some patients with gastric ulcers are afraid to eat and this tendency should not be confused with true anorexia.

• Loss of weight may occur when a patient with a gastric ulcer is afraid to eat, but it is a common early symptom of carcinoma.

• The presence of haematemesis, melaena or hypochromic anaemia.

INVESTIGATIONS

1. Barium meal is useful but in the early stages it may be falsely negative in both maligant and benign ulceration. Clinical rather than radiological features are the best guide to diagnosis. Barium meal should only be used if there is real doubt about a more serious diagnosis.

2. Occult blood in the stools. The benzidine test is useful. A positive test may indicate simple or malignant ulceration. A negative test is of no diagnostic value.

3. Haemoglobin estimation. Hypochromic anaemia can occur with a simple ulceration but always suggests carcinoma.

4. ESR (see p. 681). Sometimes helps to differentiate simple from malignant ulcers.

5. Gastroscopy and fractional test meals. Hospital admission for these tests may be indicated.

DURATION

The tendency to form peptic ulcers is lifelong, and is only partly modified by treatment. As a result there is a steady cumulative rise in the numbers of cases in the older age groups. Some patients after years of suffering may suddenly become symptom free for much longer intervals.

COMPLICATIONS

1. Perforation.

2. Haematemesis. Frank blood or coffee-ground vomit may occur. (Practice experience: a 4-year study revealed that 30% of proven cases bled at some time.) Recurrent haematemeses occur in older patients. Careful questioning may be needed to distinguish between a haematemesis and haemoptysis.

3. Melaena occurs less often than haematemesis and is easily overlooked because the patient does not realise its significance. It should be remembered as a cause of unexplained faints and anaemia.

4. Pyloric stenosis may follow chronic duodenal or prepyloric ulceration and is suggested by excessive vomiting, evidence of gastric dilatation, i.e. a gastric splash, or visible gastric peristalsis.

5. Hypochromic anaemia.

6. Carcinoma of stomach. It is not certain that peptic ulceration predisposes to gastric carcinoma. Both conditions are, however, relatively common and may therefore occur in the same patient.

MISLEADING FEATURES AND PITFALLS

Most mistakes arise from two difficulties: (a) obtaining proof of a peptic ulcer; (b) distinguishing between peptic ulceration and carcinoma of stomach.

1. A family history of ulcer is common. Unfortunately a G.P. may become mistakenly prejudiced against the diagnosis if the patient appears to know all the answers as a result of this family experience.

2. A patient with an ulcer is often worried and anxious. In the absence of conclusive evidence of an ulcer, the busy G. P. tends to assume that the symptoms are solely functional when in fact they are organic as well.

3. The G.P., because of his own uncertainties, avoids frank discussion and uses equivocal terms such as gastritis, dyspepsia,

etc. The patient then discusses his symptoms with a relative or workmate who has a proven ulcer, and reaches the conclusion that he too has an ulcer and that a mistake has been made.

4. The symptoms of gastric carcinoma may improve temporarily on a diet of rest and alkalis. A peptic ulcer is thus simulated.

5. A high gastric ulcer can occasionally produce a substernal pain that suggests coronary artery disease.

DIFFERENTIAL DIAGNOSIS

Diseases that may be confused with the peptic ulcer syndrome:

Cholecystitis

Similar features: attacks of epigastric pain radiating through to back and related to meals; tenderness in right hypochondrium; belching sensation of abdominal distension after meals.

Distinguishing features: fat women especially liable; indigestion related to fatty foods; jaundice may occur; periodicity and attacks of pain are less frequent than with an ulcer; pain radiates to the shoulder; fever sometimes present; Murphy's sign positive; abdominal X-rays and cholecystogram distinguish; gall stones and peptic ulcer may present in the same individual; the ulcer is only discovered after the removal of the gall bladder.

Reflux oesophagitis and hiatus hernia

Similar features: epigastric or low substernal pain which is related to meals; heartburn and waterbrash; haematemesis.

Distinguishing features: pain usually substernal, comes on daily during a meal; it is aggravated by lying down and relieved by getting up; a barium meal in the Trendelenburg position differentiates.

Gastric carcinoma

Similar features: epigastric pain and vomiting after meals; loss of weight; absence of previous indigestion; haematemesis; melaena; anaemia.

Distinguishing features: onset out of blue usually over 40; steady progression of symptoms; pain sometimes absent; daily symptoms; vomiting and evidence of pyloric obstruction common; anorexia and loss of weight; early differentiation difficult and usually requires gastroscopy and full hospital investigation.

Acute appendicitis

Similar feature: attacks of epigastric pain.

Distinguishing features: occasionally attacks start with pain in epigastrium and differentiation is difficult; pain not related to meals and not relieved by food or alkalis; low fever and right-flank tenderness suggest appendicitis.

MANAGEMENT OPTIONS

Prevention: Advice about modifying high risk factors especially smoking, diet and way of life.

Established disease: (a) advice on frequency and nature of meals; (b) rest if severe; (c) antacids — BNF 1.1 (Ref. 0.1); (d) antispasmodics — BNF 1.2; (e) ulcerhealing drugs (cimetidine etc.) — BNF 1.3; (f) referral if refractory.

PERFORATED PEPTIC ULCER (RCGP 2680, 2690)

DIAGNOSTIC RANGE (rates per 1000 patients per year)
Personal: Suspected 0.6. Proven 0.4.

AGE INCIDENCE

Adults liable; there is a peak of incidence in the forties and fifties.

SEX INCIDENCE

Men are said to be affected 20 times more often than women. (Practice experience confirms this.)

CLINICAL POINTERS

1. High risk factors — (as for Peptic Ulcer) — history of previous dyspepsia (100%). Apart from a history of previous attacks, perforation is usually preceded by a few days of dyspepsia.

2. Sudden onset of pain (66%) is usual, but sometimes the onset of perforation is blurred by the presence of previous pain from the ulcer.

3. Abdominal pain (100%) is usually upper abdominal or epigastric. Occasionally it starts in the right flank. As the stomach contents become widespread, the pain becomes diffuse and may be felt in the shoulders, back or flanks. The pain is very severe and the doctor is usually called within 3 hours of onset.

4. Abdominal rigidity (100%). The abdomen is held rigid, feels board-like. The patient's whole body is held tense and abdominal respiratory movements are absent because movement aggravates the pain. Occasionally, in the early stages, the rigidity and tenderness are confined to the upper abdomen. Board-like rigidity is not easy to assess because apprehension plays such a large part in its production.

Less constant or late pointers

5. Absence of excessive vomiting. A patient who perforates rarely vomits more than once.

6. Shock develops 3 to 4 hours after perforation and is often absent when the general practitioner first sees the patient.

7. Diminution of liver dullness is due to the presence of gas under the diaphragm. It is sometimes helpful but is a difficult sign to assess.

8. The absence of peristaltic sounds. Ileus develops after the peritonitis has been present for a few hours.

9. Low fever appears after a few hours and follows the development of peritonitis.

INVESTIGATIONS

Straight X-ray of abdomen may reveal gas under the diaphragm, or at a later stage, the fluid levels of paralytic ileus.

DURATION

The untreated patient deteriorates rapidly after the first few hours. Paralytic ileus develops and the patient may die within 24 to 48 hours.

COMPLICATIONS

1. Localised abscess formation, i.e. subphrenic or pelvic.
2. Peritoneal adhesions with subsequent obstruction.
3. Paralytic ileus and death.

MISLEADING FEATURES AND PITFALLS

1. The stage of reaction. After 3 to 4 hours, the peritoneum reacts to the chemical peritonitis by producing fluid. The patient may say that he is better because the pain eases. The doctor may wrongly leave such a patient overnight.

2. The absence of pain. Occasionally an elderly patient may perforate with very little pain. Such a case may present as an acute obstruction from paralytic ileus.

3. Perforation with steroids. Patients who are on steroid treatment are said to perforate without pain.

DIFFERENTIAL DIAGNOSIS

Diseases that may be confused with a perforated peptic ulcer:

Acute exacerbation of a peptic ulcer

Similar feature: severe epigastric pain with a board-like rigidity of upper abdomen, in a case of known peptic ulcer.

Distinguishing features: onset is more gradual; the pain is not so severe and has usually persisted for a few hours before doctor is sent for; shoulder pain absent; liver dullness unchanged; admission to hospital may be indicated.

Acute cholecystitis and gallstone colic
Similar features: previous indigestion; sudden onset of severe upper abdominal pain radiating to shoulder; rigidity and tenderness of upper abdomen.

Distinguishing features: pain is intermittent; low fever common; Murphy's sign positive; flatulent dyspepsia associated with fatty foods.

Acute pancreatitis
Similar feature: sudden onset of severe upper abdominal pain with board like rigidity and shock.

Distinguishing features: it is usually impossible for the G. P. to distinguish these two conditions; immediate hospital admission.

Acute appendicitis
Similar feature: sudden onset of upper abdominal pain.

Distinguishing features: in the first few hours it may be impossible to distinguish the two conditions; immediate hospital admission.

Myocardial infarction
Similar features: sudden onset of severe pain in epigastrium; pain may radiate to shoulder; shock.

Distinguishing features: previous angina; absence of previous indigestion; pain radiates to arm or jaw; abdominal rigidity and tenderness usually absent. Hospital admission often indicated.

MANAGEMENT OPTIONS
Early diagnosis with immediate admission.

CONGENITAL PYLORIC STENOSIS

Classification: ICHPPC 758 (RCGP 4235)

AETIOLOGY
Unknown.

DIAGNOSTIC RANGE (rates per 1000 patients per year)
Personal: Suspected 0.4. Probable 0.05. The condition appears to be decreasing.

AGE INCIDENCE

The first 3 months of life. Most patients are under 5 weeks.

SEX INCIDENCE

Male babies are especially prone.

CLINICAL POINTERS

1. High risk factors: (a) male; (b) first born; (c) positive family history.

2. Projectile or forcible vomiting. The vomit spouts out of the baby's mouth and covers a wide area of bedding or floor. Most of the previous feed is brought up. Vomiting occurs up to 4 hours after a feed, but in most cases it arises within an hour. The characteristic vomit is at first occasional, but later all feeds are affected. Vomitus — curdled and sour.

3. Visible gastric peristalsis can be seen if the baby is placed in an oblique light. The waves of peristalsis are seen to move across the left upper quadrant of the abdomen towards the midline.

4. Constipation may be partial or complete and starts as soon as the vomiting becomes excessive. It is usually present.

5. Palpable pyloric tumour is felt in proven cases, but repeated and painstaking examinations may be required. The baby must be examined while feeding, with the source of light to its right side and the examiner seated on its left. Every member of the trio must be comfortable. The right upper quadrant of the baby's abdomen is palpated with the tip of the examiner's left middle finger. A small mass, which feels like a lymph node about ½ inch (15 mm) long, is felt in the right upper quadrant of the abdomen on the posterior abdominal wall under the liver; it may be hardened by a wave of peristalsis.

6. Dehydration, loss of weight and wasting depends on the severity of the vomiting.

INVESTIGATIONS

A stomach wash-out (performed with a Ryles' tube) is helpful in doubtful cases after admission to hospital. Characteristically the contents are profuse, sour and curdled.

DURATION

If untreated, the baby's condition may deteriorate and death occurs from dehydration. In some mild cases the baby outgrows the disease after a variable period of vomiting.

COMPLICATIONS

Dehydration, wasting, intercurrent infection and death.

MISLEADING FEATURES AND PITFALLS

Early recognition of the disorder depends largely on the mother's account of the vomiting. It is easy to underestimate the significance of such hearsay accounts. The baby looks well between each feed, the doctor is tempted to diagnose maternal anxiety.

DIFFERENTIAL DIAGNOSIS

Disease that may be confused with congenital pyloric stenosis:

Feeding problem

Similar features: persistent vomiting after feeds; babies affected in first 12 weeks of life; maternal anxiety.

Distinguishing features: vomiting rarely forcible and does not affect whole feed; dehydration, visible gastric peristalsis and palpable pyloric mass are absent; differentiation difficult; hospital investigation or second opinion may be indicated.

MANAGEMENT OPTIONS

If the diagnosis is suspected admission of mother and baby, for observation and decision regarding: (a) antispasmodics; (b) surgery.

ACUTE APPENDICITIS

Classification: ICHPPC 540 (RCGP 2715)

AETIOLOGY

Uncertain.

DIAGNOSTIC RANGE (rates per 1000 patients per year)

Personal: Suspected 10.4. Probable 4.8. *National*: 2.0 (Ref. 0.1). [Practice experience: the problem of acute appendicitis in general practice is well shown by the following analysis of 134 consecutive cases of suspected appendicitis: 73 (54%) were watched at home — of these patients four had to be admitted to hospital after observation at home of 24 hours or less and operation revealed an acute appendicitis in all four; 61 (45.5%) were admitted straight to hospital — of these over half (33) were operated on and in 26 the diagnosis of acute appendicitis was confirmed, 36 were managed conservatively in hospital. Thus in only 30 (22.2%) was the diagnosis confirmed conclusively by operation. Similar figures have been reported from many other practices.]

The consequences of a mistaken diagnosis are serious and the family doctor must be prepared to overdiagnose acute appendicitis.

AGE INCIDENCE

Patients of all ages are affected. Rare in babies and toddlers.

CLINICAL COURSE

The clinical course is variable and it is not surprising that the diagnosis of acute appendicitis gives the family doctor some very difficult problems. Two factors are mainly responsible for the great variation in the clinical picture:

1. The patient's age. Mistakes in diagnosis occur most frequently at the extremes of age. In children the picture may be confused by unusually marked reflex and systemic reactions, thus, vomiting is sometimes profuse and the temperature is occasionally surprisingly high. In elderly patients the reverse tends to occur and the early signs and symptoms may be slight.

2. The position of the appendix. The inflamed appendix may irritate a variety of structures and cause different clinical features:

Structure	*Sign or symptom*
Bladder	Frequency and dysuria
Large bowel	Diarrhoea
Anterior abdominal wall	Rigidity, guarding and absent movement on respiration
Psoas muscle	Psoas spasm

In other cases these signs and symptoms may be masked because the inflamed appendix is buried in a roll of protective omentum or in the pelvis.

In view of the varied symptomatology it is a mistake for the family doctor to think of acute appendicitis in terms of rigid clinical patterns. He must develop the ability to consider this diagnosis in a very wide range of circumstances, then to use his clinical experience to decide if the patient should be admitted to hospital for observation or operation.

CLINICAL POINTERS

There are two clinical features of acute appendicitis that are rarely absent. These are abdominal pain and tenderness on the right side of the abdomen (or rectum).

1. Abdominal pain (100%). All complaints of abdominal pain raise the possibility of acute appendicitis. The following characteristics of the pain are particularly suggestive:

• A central abdominal or right flank pain — the classical picture of a central abdominal pain which shifts in a few hours to the right iliac fossa is uncommon.

• The pain is continuous.
• Previous attacks of a similar pain.
• A pain that wakes the patient at night.
• A pain of less than 24 hours duration. [Practice experience: the doctor is called to most cases of proven acute appendicitis within the first 10 to 24 hours of the onset.]
• A continuous abdominal pain that suddenly stops for one to 2 hours and then starts again should suggest the possibility of perforation.

2. Right-sided tenderness of the abdomen. (Practice experience: right-sided abdominal tenderness was noted in 80% of proven and 58% of non-proven cases.) If this sign is found in association with abdominal pain, the patient should be treated as a case of acute appendicitis until there is proof to the contrary. Operation may be the only way to obtain such proof. Guarding or rigidity of the muscles of the anterior abdominal wall overlying the right iliac fossa may be associated with the tenderness. This finding suggests acute appendicitis but is often absent, especially in early cases. Generalised guarding or rigidity suggests the presence of general peritonitis but is often difficult to assess. Sometimes rectal tenderness on deep pressure of the right side of the rectum is noted when there is no tenderness on the right side of the abdomen.

Other signs and symptoms should only influence the diagnosis, if either of these two main clinical pointers is equivocal, e.g. if the pain has stopped before the arrival of the doctor, or if the patient is too young to give reliable replies about tenderness.

3. History of previous attacks of pain. (Practice experience: a previous history of attacks was reported in 50% of proven and 30% of non-proven cases.)

4. Temperature. A low fever — 37° to 38°C (98.6° to 100°F) is suggestive. Occasionally higher fevers occur in children. (Practice experience: temperatures 37° to 38°C were noted in 50% of proven cases and in 33% of non-proven cases.)

5. Pulse rate is often unaffected in the early stages, but a pulse of over 100 in the absence of a corresponding rise in temperature may suggest a rapidly progressing attack of appendicitis. (Practice experience: a pulse of over 100 was noted in 40% of proven cases and 5% of non-proven cases.)

6. Coated tongue and foetid breath. A faecal taint of the breath

is especially suggestive of acute appendicitis. (Practice experience: a coated tongue was noted in 33% of proven cases and 25% of non-proven cases.)

7. Vomiting is an early sign and is often the first indication of the possible seriousness of the symptoms. Occasionally it occurs before the onset of pain. One or two isolated vomits are more suggestive of appendicitis than repeated vomiting. (Practice experience: vomiting was noted in 40% of proven cases and in 25% of non-proven cases.)

NOTE. Young children often complain of abdominal pain before they are sick from any cause.

8. Diarrhoea is a particularly misleading symptom because it is often associated with colic. Abdominal pain in the presence of diarrhoea should only be diagnosed as due to gastroenteritis after appendicitis has been carefully excluded. (Practice experience: diarrhoea was noted in 9% of proven cases and 20% of non-proven cases.)

9. Dysuria and frequency. These two symptoms occur surprisingly often in proven cases of appendicitis and they can therefore be misleading. It is dangerous to assume that the combination of abdominal pain and urinary symptoms indicate a urinary infection. Such a diagnosis is justified only after microscopic examination of the urine has revealed pus. (Practice experience: dysuria and frequent micturition were noted in 33% of proven cases and 14% of non-proven cases.)

10. Psoas spasm. The right leg is flexed at the hip or pain may be felt if the right hip is hyperextended — an uncommon sign.

11. Absence of abdominal respiratory movement is associated with guarding or rigidity of the anterior abdominal wall. It is usually a late sign and difficult to evaluate.

12. Rovsing's type tenderness is an uncommon and unreliable sign i.e. pain on the Right with pressure on the Left side.

13. Release or rebound abdominal tenderness suggests an acute appendicitis but is uncommon in the early stages. (Practice experience: rebound tenderness was noted in 23% of proven and only 4% of non-proven cases.) It is sometimes present if the right Fallopian tube is distended by infection or ectopic pregnancy. A very useful sign that should not be ignored.

14. Hyperaesthesia in the right iliac fossa can sometimes be demonstrated and is a useful confirmatory sign.

INVESTIGATIONS

A white-cell count may be helpful in doubtful cases if observation at home is particularly desired. Patients with a raised count should be observed in hospital.

DURATION

Variable. At one extreme, acute appendicitis may progress rapidly to perforation and general peritonitis in under 12 hours. At the other, many mild cases settle after a period of pain (1 to 48 hours) only to recur in a few weeks or months. Recurrent attacks are common.

COMPLICATIONS

The family doctor should aim to avoid the following:

1. General peritonitis

Pointers include rising pulse rate, vomiting and absent peristaltic sounds. Paralytic ileus and death may follow.

2. Appendix abscess

Pointers include the continued passage of mucus or loose stools with fever and a 'boggy' tender mass felt in front of the rectum.

3. Pelvic abscess

Pointers include the continued passage of mucus or loose stools with fever and a 'boggy' tender mass felt in front of the rectum.

(Practice experience: in 10 years of practice, three cases of general peritonitis following perforation were encountered: (1) a teenager whose parents went to work, and who perforated an appendix while he was alone in the house, before I was called; (2) a patient who was diagnosed as acute gastroenteritis and who perforated while under my care at home; (3) a patient who had been admitted to hospital with pneumonia, and who developed symptoms of acute appendicitis and perforated while in the medical ward. All these patients were young males.)

MISLEADING FEATURES AND PITFALLS

1. Hospital admission of patients with acute appendicitis may be delayed through fear of sending trivial cases into hospital. This fear is created by two factors: (a) the implication in teaching hospitals that general practitioners tend to admit patients unnecessarily; (b) the failure to realise that the G.P.'s aim in this instance is not that of accurate diagnosis but to ensure that no patient with acute appendictis is ever allowed to perforate outside hospital. Remember that conclusions drawn by surgeons inside hospital are often based

on a later clinical picture than that encountered before admission.

2. One of the two main clinical pointers (i.e. abdominal pain and right-sided abdominal tenderness) is ignored.

3. Vomiting, diarrhoea or abdominal pain are mistakenly diagnosed as acute gastroenteritis. In such cases, the presence of right-sided tenderness (abdominal or rectal) suggests acute appendicitis.

4. Frequency, dysuria and abdominal pain are mistakenly taken to indicate an acute infection of the urinary tract. This error is avoided if the urine is examined for pus cells. Absence of pus cells in the urine suggests that the patient should be admitted to hospital. (Practice experience: occasional pus cells have been noted in patients of all ages in whom operation has later revealed an acute appendicitis.)

5. Patients with acute appendicitis are mistakenly kept at home overnight.

> EXAMPLE 1. A doctor's wife was seen at midnight 2 hours after the onset of abdominal pain when signs and symptoms were slight. She was not revisited that night. A check examination 2 hours later might well have revealed the classic picture of acute appendicitis. The next morning a mass could be felt in the right iliac fossa and an acutely inflamed appendix wrapped in omentum was removed.
>
> EXAMPLE 2. A 19-year-old girl with abdominal pain was seen after evening surgery. A pulse rate of over 100 was ignored and the patient kept at home but not revisited that night because the doctor had other commitments. Operation on the following day revealed a gangrenous but not apparently perforated appendix. This patient died in hospital 6 weeks later from a subphrenic abscess.

A. DIFFERENTIAL DIAGNOSIS — CHILDREN

Diseases that may be confused with acute appendicitis:

Acute tonsillitis

Similar features: abdominal pain; right-sided tenderness; fever; vomiting.

Distinguishing features: contact cases; flushed face; high temperature; inflamed pharynx.

> NOTE. In children under 7 years, with tonsillitis the throat is often not painful.

Acute mesenteric adenitis

Similar features: abdominal pain; right-sided tenderness; fever; vomiting.

Distinguishing features: the clinical picture is like that of acute tonsillitis but absence of throat inflammation may make differentiation from acute appendicitis difficult; admission to hospital may be indicated (see also *periodic syndrome* p. 296).

Acute gastroenteritis

Similar features: abdominal pain; right-sided tenderness; fever; vomiting; diarrhoea.

Distinguishing features: vomiting and diarrhoea are repeated; stools are watery, not merely loose; abdominal pain is related to onset of vomiting or defaecating and is relieved by them; hospital admission may be indicated.

Acute pyelitis and pyelonephritis

Similar features: abdominal pain; right-sided tenderness; fever; vomiting; frequency and dysuria; occasional pus cell.

Distinguishing features: fever is high; right flank or loin pain is common; pallor; urine contains many pus cells after the first 5 hours; differentiation sometimes extremely difficult; hospital admission may be indicated.

B. DIFFERENTIAL DIAGNOSIS — WOMEN

Diseases that may be confused with acute appendicitis:

Acute pyelitis and pyelonephritis

Similar features: abdominal pain; right-flank tenderness and guarding; frequency and dysuria; fever; urine contains an occasional pus cell.

Distinguishing features: rigors and high fever common; nocturia and urinary symptoms marked; loin tenderness common; urine contains many pus cells; differentiation may be difficult especially if urine is not examined for pus cells.

Ovulation syndrome (mittelschmerz)

Similar features: abdominal pain with history of previous attacks; right iliac fossa tenderness and guarding; low fever; tenderness to right side on rectal examination.

Distinguishing features: onset and previous history of pain, at midpoint of menstrual cycle; differentiation sometimes impossible without operation; hospital admission may be indicated.

Ectopic gestation and ruptured ectopic

Similar features: abdominal pain; right iliac fossa tenderness with guarding and rigidity; tenderness to right on rectal examination.

Distinguishing features: Ectopic gestation — history of one missed period common; other signs of early pregnancy (i.e. nausea, nocturia and breast changes); brown vaginal discharge; cervix acutely tender on rectal examination. Ruptured ectopic — as above, but with added evidence of acute pelvic peritonitis; severe pain and shock; immediate admission to hospital indicated.

Twisted ovarian cyst
Similar features: abdominal pain with history of previous attacks; vomiting; right iliac fossa tenderness with guarding; low fever.

Distinguishing features: a rounded tender swelling lying in the pouch of Douglas is felt on rectal examination; immediate admission to hospital is indicated.

Acute salpingitis
Similar features: abdominal pain; right iliac fossa tenderness with guarding; fever.

Distinguishing features: uncommon; history of recent vaginal discharge; fever usually high; cervix acutely tender on rectal examination; admission to hospital may be indicated.

Acute cholecystitis
Similar features: abdominal pain; right-flank tenderness and guarding; low fever.

Distinguishing features: rarely confused with appendicitis; history of previous flatulent dyspepsia and upper abdominal pain; pain radiates to shoulders; gall bladder is acutely tender.

Acute gastroenteritis
See under children, above.

C. DIFFERENTIAL DIAGNOSIS — MEN

Duodenal ulcer, gastroenteritis, pyelonephritis and cholecystitis occasionally simulate acute appendicitis. If abdominal pain and right-sided tenderness are present together, a diagnosis of appendicitis is most likely. Doubtful cases are watched in hospital.

D. DIFFERENTIAL DIAGNOSIS — ELDERLY PATIENTS

Elderly patients tend to develop acute abdominal conditions very quietly, thus an acute appendicitis may perforate and a paralytic ileus develop before the doctor is aware of the gravity of the situation. Elderly patients who complain of abdominal pain suggestive of appendicitis, should not be watched at home.

E. OTHER RARE DISORDERS OCCASIONALLY CONFUSED WITH APPENDICITIS

Acute pancreatitis, regional ileitis and acute diverticulitis (including Meckel's). Investigation in hospital is needed to differentiate these conditions.

MANAGEMENT OPTIONS

Prevention: Early diagnosis with early admission is the aim. Patient education is required to reduce delays. This requires that reception staff and doctors themselves show increased understanding of the patient's fears and of the problems involved.

Suspected appendicitis: (a) immediate hospital admission; (b) observe.

MANAGEMENT SAFEGUARDS:

1. A routine is established that calls from patients who complain of abdominal pain are visited as soon as possible.

2. It is impossible to lay down fixed rules about those cases of suspected acute appendicitis that can be watched at home. In my practice it is considered in the following circumstances:

- The duration of pain is less than 2 hours. Such cases must be revisited within 2 to 4 hours.
- The abdominal pain has stopped before the doctor's visit and right-sided tenderness (rectal or abdominal) is slight or doubtful.
- The abdominal pain is of more than 36 hours duration and the diagnosis is still in doubt.

(Practice experience: average duration of pain before the doctor was called was 17 hours for proven cases and 49 hours for non-proven cases; indicating the need for patient education.)

3. When a patient with possible acute appendicitis is to be watched at home, the following precautions are taken:

- The possible nature of the pain is explained to the patient or parent.
- The patient is told to call the doctor if the pain returns or if other symptoms develop.
- The patient is put to bed on fluids.

4. In my practice adult males with clinical features suggesting appendicitis are not watched at home. Experience has shown that symptoms of acute appendicitis are easily disregarded by both patient and doctor.

5. Follow up and case discussion of all patients admitted.

ABDOMINAL HERNIAS

Any weakness in the muscles or supporting tissues that enclose the abdominal contents may be followed by protrusion (i.e. herniation) of these contents.

CLASSIFICATION

According to the anatomical sites:

1. Inguinal hernia.
2. Femoral hernia.

3. Umbilical hernia.
4. Oesophageal hernia (syn. hiatus hernia).
5. Incisional hernia.
6. Other rare hernias — obturator, epigastric, etc.

AETIOLOGY

The abdominal contents behave as a liquid and tend to push into and enlarge any weak spot in the walls of the abdominal cavity. For this reason the common hernias are in the lower part of the abdomen where the hydrostatic pressures are greatest. Most of these weak points are situated where structures leave the abdominal cavity.

INGUINAL HERNIA

Classification: ICHPPC 550 (RCGP 2720)

AETIOLOGY

Inguinal hernia arises at the point where the spermatic cord leaves the abdomen. An indirect inguinal hernia follows the oblique inguinal canal. A direct hernia pushes straight through the abdominal wall at the site of the external inguinal ring, a result of trauma. The two types have a similar external appearance. The weakness may be congenital or acquired.

DIAGNOSTIC RANGE (rates per 1000 patients per year)

Personal: Suspected 4.8. Probable 4.4. *National*: 5.5 (includes femoral) (Ref. 0.2). Many cases are adequately controlled by a truss and the patients rarely report to the doctor.

AGE INCIDENCE

All ages. Congenital hernias are usually seen under 2 years.

SEX INCIDENCE

Males are especially liable.

CLINICAL POINTERS

1. High risk factors: (a) unaccustomed lifting; (b) known hernia previously.

2. History of trauma or strain. This may be so slight that it passes unnoticed. Later when the patient thinks back, or when the question of compensation arises, a specific incident of strain is incriminated.

3. Swelling in the inguinal region (80%) arises from the external inguinal ring close to the pubic tubercle, and is soft and easily

reduced at first; later it enlarges and pushes into the scrotum.

4. Pain (65%) is felt as an ache in the groin, made worse by standing, and in the early stages is common.

5. Cough impulse is helpful in hernias without obvious swelling. A finger is placed in the external ring and the rupture is felt tapping the tip of the finger when the patient coughs.

DURATION

The condition persists indefinitely if not treated.

COMPLICATIONS

Obstruction and strangulation are not uncommon (see p. 482).

MISLEADING FEATURES AND PITFALLS

Hernias which present with pain in the groin but show neither a visible swelling nor cough impulse may cause diagnostic difficulty in the early stages.

DIFFERENTIAL DIAGNOSIS

It may be difficult to distinguish between a femoral and an inguinal hernia. Identification of the inguinal ligament and pubic tubercle makes the position clear.

MANAGEMENT OPTIONS

Prevention: Avoid high risk factors.

Established hernia: Refer for surgery.

FEMORAL HERNIA

Classification: ICHPPC 553 (RCGP 2725)

Femoral hernias arise at the point where the femoral vessels leave the abdomen and push under the inguinal ligament.

DIAGNOSTIC RANGE (rates per 1000 patients per year)

Personal: Probable 0.5. The diagnosis was rarely in doubt.

AGE INCIDENCE

Adults. The incidence increases with age.

CLINICAL POINTERS

1. High risk factors: (a) females especially liable; (b) unaccustomed lifting is occasionally a trigger.

2. Swelling in the inguinal region is situated below and lateral to the inguinal ligament. It is smaller and less easily reduced than the swelling of an inguinal hernia. It bears no relation to the

external inguinal ring which can be identified medial to the femoral hernia.

3. Pain may be felt locally or as abdominal colic.

DURATION

The condition persists indefinitely if not treated.

COMPLICATIONS

Strangulation and symptoms of intestinal obstruction tend to occur with femoral hernia.

DIFFERENTIAL DIAGNOSIS

Enlarged inguinal lymph nodes are sometimes confused with a femoral hernia.

MANAGEMENT OPTIONS

As for inguinal hernia.

UMBILICAL HERNIA

Classification: ICHPPC 553 (RCGP 2735)

An obvious swelling with eversion of the navel. The swelling is soft and easily reduced. It varies in size and is common in young babies. As the baby grows the hernia usually disappears. The condition is rare in adults. Operation or truss are only very rarely indicated, although worried parents will often try to persuade the doctor to give active treatment.

DIAGNOSTIC RANGE (rates per 1000 patients per year)

Personal: Probable 0.9.

COMPLICATIONS

Rare.

MISLEADING FEATURES

The hernia appears when the baby cries and the parents become convinced that it is causing pain. They put pressure on the doctor for surgical intervention.

INCISIONAL (VENTRAL) HERNIA

Classification: ICHPPC 553 (RCGP 2735)

Arises at any point of weakness in an abdominal incision. Deformity and swelling (usually reducible) of an abdominal operation scar are obvious.

DIAGNOSTIC RANGE (rates per 1000 patients per year)
Personal: Probable 6.0. Diagnosis rarely in doubt.

COMPLICATIONS
Obstruction and strangulation can occur.

MANAGEMENT OPTIONS
Established hernia: (a) Nil (b) Strapping or truss (c) surgery.

CARCINOMA COLON

Classification: ICHPPC 151 (RCGP 0415)

This is usually a slow-growing cancer with a good prognosis if diagnosed early. Colirectal Carcinoma — one of the commonest curable cancers.

AETIOLOGY
Unknown. Often follows polyposis of the colon. Geographical variations in incidence suggest that diet is crucial. Diets high in animal fat may be causal, while a high fibre diet is protective.

DIAGNOSTIC RANGE (rates per 1000 patients per year)
Personal: Suspected 1.2. Probable 0.85. *National*: 0.5 (Ref. 0.2).

AGE INCIDENCE
Adults, especially over 50 years.

SEX INCIDENCE
Men affected more than women.

CLINICAL POINTERS

1. High risk factors: (a) family history; (b) previous polyposis — (single and multiple); (c) ulcerative colitis; (d) high fat/low fibre diets.
2. Change of bowel habit in a patient of cancer age. Constipation occurs. Less often there is diarrhoea.
3. Abdominal pain is colicky. A vague abdominal discomfort is less common. A relationship between the pain and opening the bowels is often noticed.
4. Symptoms and signs of large bowel obstruction, i.e. marked abdominal colic with distension, absolute constipation and vomiting. Annular growths may present in this way.

5. Abdominal mass is sometimes mobile and is said to be palpable in a third of cases.
6. Anaemia. Unexplained anaemia in middle-aged patients.
7. The passage of frank blood or mucus.
8. Rectal examination is often negative. Occasionally a mass can be felt in the pouch of Douglas.

INVESTIGATIONS

1. Double enema test if large bowel obstruction is suspected.
2. Estimation of haemoglobin and sedimentation rate. The ESR is often unaltered (see p. 681).
3. Sigmoidoscopy combined with radiological contrast studies.
4. Barium enema is useful but may fail to outline growths in the lower and sigmoid colon.

DURATION

In the untreated or inoperable patient a duration of 3 years from onset of symptoms is not uncommon.

MISLEADING FEATURES AND PITFALLS

1. The doctor fails to take an adequate history or check up on a patient with 'constipation' or 'piles'. An easy but often disastrous omission.
2. Carcinoma of colon is sometimes associated with bouts of fever.

DIFFERENTIAL DIAGNOSIS

Diseases that may be confused with carcinoma colon:

Constipation

Similar features: history of pain; abdominal mass.

Distinguishing features: long history; an enema removes mass and relieves symptoms.

Chronic diverticulitis

Similar features: symptoms of partial or acute obstruction; abdominal mass; passage of blood; fever occasionally present in carcinoma.

Distinguishing features: fever is common; attacks usually subside in 1 to 3 days; previous attacks likely; hospital investigation indicated.

Any cause of large bowel obstruction or severe constipation

Similar features: colicky pain; distension; absolute constipation.

Distinguishing feature: in all cases of large bowel obstruction a full immediate hospital investigation is indicated.

The diagnosis of carcinoma of colon has to be considered in a wide variety of chronic diseases in which a poor appetite has produced constipation.

These diseases include growths in other parts of the body, pernicious and hypochromic anaemias, chronic alcoholism and pulmonary tuberculosis. Hospital investigation is indicated.

MANAGEMENT OPTIONS

Prevention: (a) early diagnosis and eradication of polyps; (b) low fat/high fibre diets considered to be protective.

Established disease: (a) early discovery and referral are the main aim; (b) surgery.

Post hospital: (a) discussion and 'whole person' support; (b) patient education (Ref. 18.1); (c) family support; (d) self-help groups (See cancer — general comments: Chapter 9; p. 206 *et seq.*).

ACUTE INTESTINAL OBSTRUCTION

Classification ICHPPC 579 (RCGP 2755)

Acute intestinal obstruction may affect either the large or small bowel. The clinical picture of the two types is different, and although hospital admission is indicated the G.P. should have some knowledge of the likely causes and clinical features of each type.

The main causes of a high intestinal obstruction are: strangulated hernia (0.4 per 1000 patients per year), adhesions and very rarely volvulus or ileitis.

The main causes of a low intestinal obstruction are: carcinoma and diverticulitis.

DIAGNOSTIC RANGE (rates per 1000 patients per year)

Personal: Suspected 1.6. Probable 0.6.

CLINICAL POINTERS

1. Sudden onset. The onset is less sudden if the large, not the small gut is affected.
2. Colicky abdominal pain.
3. Vomiting is marked in high obstruction and occurs early in children. It is followed by dehydration and rapid deterioration.
4. Absolute constipation. Absence of flatus or motions — characteristic of a low obstruction. A double enema test confirms.
5. Visible peristalsis and borborygmi. Occasionally a portion of bowel in spasm can be felt at the height of a pain.

6. Smooth, tense, tender swelling at one of the hernial orifices indicates strangulation. Any attempts to reduce the hernia should be firm, not vigorous.

INVESTIGATIONS

Straight X-ray of abdomen for fluid levels.

DURATION

Mild intermittent obstructive symptoms often precede complete obstruction by many months.

COMPLICATIONS

Gangrene of gut, paralytic ileus and death follow rapidly if the obstruction is not relieved.

DIFFERENTIAL DIAGNOSIS

Occasionally cases in which there are symptoms of partial obstruction may be confused with appendicitis or carcinoma. Admission to hospital is indicated.

MISLEADING FEATURES AND PITFALLS

1. Attempts to reduce a strangulated hernia are said to involve two risks:

- Reduction of the hernia *en masse* without relieving the strangulation.
- A piece of gangrenous gut is pushed back into the abdomen.

2. Reduction may occur if the foot of the bed is raised while waiting for the ambulance.

3. Despite hospital training it is very easy for a general practitioner to get out of the habit of examining the hernial orifices.

MANAGEMENT OPTIONS

Early diagnosis and referral for surgery.

INTUSSUSCEPTION

Classification: ICHPPC 579 (RCGP 2755)

AETIOLOGY

Various factors may act as a trigger:

- A change of diet
- Lymphoid patches are most profuse where intussusceptions usually start (terminal ileum). Lymphoid enlargement and intussusception may follow the pattern of tonsillitis until the lumen of the bowel becomes too wide at 2–3 years.

DIAGNOSTIC RANGE (rates per 1000 patients per year)
Personal: Suspected 0.6. Probable 0.1. Decreasing in our area.

AGE INCIDENCE
Babies aged between 6 and 12 months are said to be most liable, but the condition may occur at any time between birth and school age.

> NOTE. With older babies or toddlers the onset is less acute, and there is a greater likelihood of recurring attacks lasting days or even weeks, instead of a few hours.

SEX INCIDENCE
Male babies said to be especially liable.

CLINICAL POINTERS

1. Sudden onset. The mother can usually fix an exact time when the illness started.

2. Attacks of pain (100%). Even with young babies the mother is able to distinguish the anguished and shrill cry of acute pain; a clear history of repeated spasms of pain is nearly always obtained. In babies these attacks occur 2 to 3 times every hour. In older children the pain is less frequent and less regular. The bout of pain lasts for several moments and cannot be stilled by nursing, rocking or feeding.

3. Intestinal haemorrhage. Evidence of haemorrhage is common and is said to occur in 60% of all cases. A history of passage of blood or a red currant jelly stool is sometimes given. Melaena occasionally occurs in older children. More commonly blood is found on the examining finger after rectal examination.

A rectal examination should always be performed if the diagnosis is suspected.

4. Pallor with the attacks of pain is noticed by the mother who often volunteers the information.

5. Features that may be present but are difficult to assess: (a) vomiting; (b) a history that the child draws up its legs with the spasms of pain — common in other painful disorders; (c) *signe de dance*, i.e. emptiness of the RIF to palpation.

6. An abdominal mass. A sausage-shaped mass can often be felt. It is usually in the right flank, under the liver or in the hypochondrium, and sometimes hardens as the spasm of colic begins. Palpating a mass in a baby or toddler is never easy and the doctor must be prepared to take at least 15 minutes.

INVESTIGATIONS

A barium enema and tests for occult blood in the stools may be performed after admission to hospital.

DURATION

In babies the condition may progress rapidly to death in 2 to 3 days. In toddlers and older children a state of partial obstruction develops and recurrent attacks of colic may continue for days or even weeks. Sometimes an intussusception will reduce itself spontaneously.

COMPLICATIONS

Gangrene, peritonitis and death may occur if the condition is not treated.

MISLEADING FEATURES AND PITFALLS

1. In the early stages of intussusception the baby may be perfectly normal between spasms of pain.

2. Apparent attacks of abdominal pain with associated pallor may precede a vomit from any cause in babies.

3. The baby's ear drums are examined during a crying spell; crying causes the ear drums to be red; the doctor mistakenly ascribes the attacks of pain to acute otitis media, because it is much more common. The doctor may then fail seriously to consider the diagnosis.

DIFFERENTIAL DIAGNOSIS

Diseases that may be confused with acute intussusception:

Feeding problem

Similar features: sudden onset; spasms of colicky pain; vomiting.

Distinguishing features: spasm of pain only occurs once or twice; baby settles if nursed in mother's arms; no abdominal mass or blood on rectal examination..

Impacted faeces

Similar features: spasms of colicky abdominal pain; mass in LIF.

Distinguishing features: older children affected; history of constipation; pain not severe and child easily comforted; mass of hard faeces on rectal examination.

Acute gastroenteritis

Similar features: spasms of colicky abdominal pain; vomiting; passage of blood per rectum.

Distinguishing features: attacks of pain are of short duration and associated with the passage of a loose watery stool; fever; no abdominal mass.

Acute otitis media

Similar feature: spasms of acute severe pain not relieved by nursing.

Distinguishing features: differentiation may be difficult in babies, especially if eardrums cannot be seen; fever; respiratory illness common; no abdominal mass or bowel symptoms; hospital admission may be indicated in doubtful cases.

> NOTE. Teething may make babies restless and irritable, but does not cause pain. In older children, i.e. 2 to 5 years, the condition of intussusception is less acute and may be simulated by Henoch's purpura, acute appendicitis or acute pyelitis. Hospital admission is indicated in such cases.

MANAGEMENT OPTIONS

Early diagnosis and referral.

ACUTE GASTROENTERITIS

Classification: ICHPPC 008 (RCGP 0015)

The term acute gastroenteritis is a useful diagnostic label because in spite of the different pathogens that may be responsible, the clinical picture and treatment vary little.

AETIOLOGY

In Britain the common identifiable organisms are as follows:

A. Bacterial pathogens

1. *Shigella sonnei* — the commonest pathogen.
2. *Shigella flexneri* — occasionally encountered, produces a severe disease. *Shigella dysenteriae* never occurs in UK.
3. *Salmonella typhimurium* and *Sal. enteritidis* — these bacteria produce gastroenteritis. Contaminated food is usually responsible. Imported dried foods such as egg and coconut are often responsible. Incubation period 24 to 48 hours.
4. *Clostridium welchii* causes explosive outbreaks of food poisoning and is rarely confused with the milder disease of enteritis. Incubation period 12 to 24 hours.
5. *Staphylococcus aureus* — a common cause of food poisoning. Incubation period 4 to 6 hours.

B. Campylobacter organisms

Campylobacter jejuni — recently (1977) identified as causing 7–10%

of enteritic food poisoning. *Incubation*: 2–5 days. *Duration*: Self limiting. *Pointers*: Illness rarely severe, prodromal fever with abdominal pain lasting 1 day leads to diarrhoea for 2–3 days. Vomiting rare. Abdominal pain common, can mimic surgical emergencies in babies and children. 10% of cases may need admission. Organisms sensitive to Erythromycin but this is rarely indicated.

C. Viral pathogens

In some cases of acute gastroenteritis no obvious pathogens can be isolated. Enteroviruses have been shown to be responsible for many such cases. Rotaviruses often cause infantile attacks.

D. Protozoal pathogens

1. *Entamoeba histolytica* (amoebic dysentery) must be considered in patients from endemic areas.

2. *Lamblia intestinalis* (giardiasis) is occasionally found in cases of dysentery. The extent of its pathogenicity is uncertain. Infections are common in some countries, e.g. Russia.

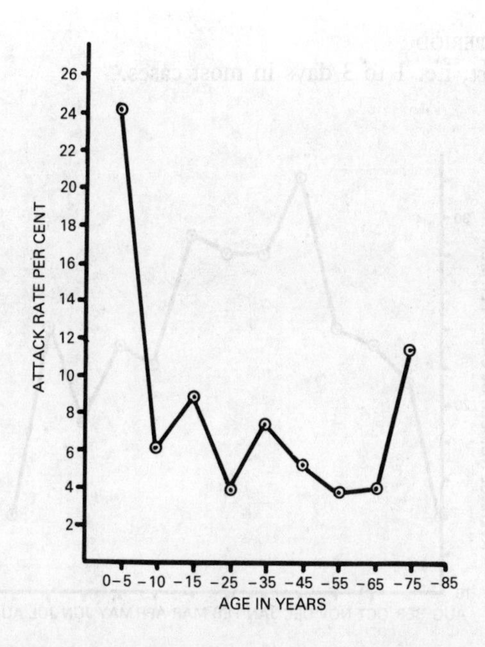

Fig. 47 Acute gastroenteritis. Age incidence curve of 298 consecutive cases encountered in 1 year.

MODE OF SPREAD

Many outbreaks of gastroenteritis occur in communities that eat together, i.e. households, schools and works canteens. Apart from *salmonella* it is rarely possible to incriminate any specific foods and the disease probably spreads in households by direct contamination of hands and food from the nose or faeces of active cases and carriers.

DIAGNOSTIC RANGE (rates per 1000 populations per year)

Personal: Suspected 77.84+. *National*: 51.7 (Ref. 0.2). Many cases are never reported.

AGE INCIDENCE

All ages are liable, but children under 10 are especially prone (Fig. 47).

SEASONAL INCIDENCE

Though outbreaks of acute gastroenteritis are said to occur in the summer rather than winter, the overall picture in this practice is one of a fairly steady incidence, with a peak in the winter (Fig. 48). Sonne dysentery is a disease of winter and is probably responsible for this peak.

INCUBATION PERIOD

This is short, i.e. 1 to 3 days in most cases.

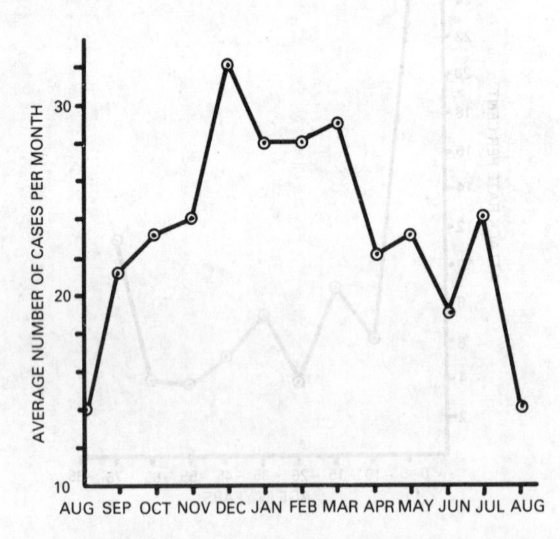

Fig. 48 Acute gastroenteritis. Seasonal incidence of 1433 consecutive cases reported over 5 years.

CLINICAL POINTERS

1. High risk groups: (a) contact cases; (b) poor household hygiene; (c) low socio-economic groups; (d) recent possible source — restaurants, hospital canteens, etc.; (e) recent travel (especially foreign).

2. Other members of household (or community) affected.

3. Diarrhoea (100%). The motions may be loose and light, often green and watery or containing mucus. In a small proportion (5%) the motion contains blood. The number passed in 24 hours may vary from two to 20. Flatus is excessive and offensive.

4. Vomiting (45%) is more common in babies and children than in adults. It may precede the diarrhoea by several hours causing difficulties in diagnosis.

5. Abdominal pain (40%) is colicky and not localised. It is characteristically relieved by passing a motion or flatus. Occasionally the abdominal pain is continuous or is not related to opening of the bowels. Such cases may be difficult to distinguish from acute appendicitis.

6. Fever (30%) may vary between normal and 39°C.

7. Abdominal tenderness is maximal over the descending colon but tenderness in the right iliac fossa may render distinction from acute appendicitis difficult.

8. Anorexia, malaise and headache occur in severe cases.

INVESTIGATIONS

Stool culture. If a serious epidemic is suspected or if a particularly vulnerable community is at risk, i.e. an old peoples' home or babies' hospital, a faecal specimen or rectal swab is essential. In widespread outbreaks contamination of food or water must be considered.

DURATION

The condition may persist for several days or weeks if it is not treated.

COMPLICATIONS

1. Dehydration. Severe loss of fluid and electrolytes occasionally occurs. Babies are especially prone to this complication if gastroenteritis is inadequately treated. Fatalities in such cases are fortunately now rare. Occasionally tetany may follow excessive vomiting.

2. A chronic carrier-state is probably more common than is generally realised, and will remain so until more extensive bacteriological investigation is practical.

3. Recurrences are common but may merely reflect the widespread nature of the disease. Toddlers are sometimes troubled by a recurring enteritis that may last several months.

MISLEADING FEATURES AND PITFALLS

1. Diarrhoea with intermittent colicky abdominal pain occurs in acute appendicitis. Right-sided abdominal tenderness and a continuous abdominal pain, not related to passing a motion, may occur in acute gastroenteritis and cause confusion. Many G.P.s have made the serious mistake of treating a case of acute appendicitis as one of acute gastroenteritis. A pelvic abscess should be remembered as an occasional cause of persistent diarrhoea in an ill patient.

2. Apparent attacks of acute gastroenteritis are sometimes caused by well-meaning parents who give their children a laxative and then do not tell the doctor, because they are afraid that they have done the wrong thing.

DIFFERENTIAL DIAGNOSIS

Diseases that may be confused with acute gastroenteritis:

Acute appendicitis

Similar features: colicky abdominal pain; right-sided tenderness; vomiting; low fever.

Distinguishing features: history of previous attacks; pain precedes diarrhoea; pain not related to (or relieved by) passing a motion; stool not watery or profuse; motion merely unformed; descending colon and left flank are not usually tender; release sign positive; contact cases absent; distinction can be difficult and hospital admission may be indicated.

Ulcerative colitis

Similar features: attacks of diarrhoea; little systemic disturbance.

Distinguishing features: history of recurrent attacks common; diarrhoea fails to clear with treatment; stool culture is negative; distinction may be difficult in the early stages of colitis.

Acute intussusception

Similar features: attacks of colicky abdominal pain in a baby; vomiting; passage of blood per rectum.

Distinguishing features: loose motions not a feature; attacks of colic are severe; fever absent; abdominal mass; no contact cases.

Carcinoma of rectum

Similar feature: diarrhoea with colicky abdominal pain.

Distinguishing features: diarrhoea is of morning type and consists of mucus; preceding history of several weeks altered bowel habit; diarrhoea fails to clear with antibiotics; rectal mass palpable.

Occasionally serious diseases such as typhoid or a fulminating ulcerative or bacterial colitis may also have to be considered.

MANAGEMENT OPTIONS

Prevention: (a) adequate public health measures relating to food, water, sewage and public eating; (b) adequate health education regarding — personal and household hygiene, food storage and preparation; (c) identify and treat carriers, if feasible.

Established disease: (a) rest; (b) fluids; (c) explore and treat contacts and possible sources of infection; (d) avoid antibacterials where possible.

DIVERTICULITIS (AND DIVERTICULOSIS)

Classification: ICHPPC 562 (RCGP 2760)

Diverticulosis is caused by numerous small diverticulae arising in the distal half of the colon during middle age. The condition is symptomless and is not uncommon. It is discovered incidentally, during barium enema examination.

Diverticulitis develops if colonic diverticulae become chronically infected. Acute exacerbations are frequent and can simulate carcinoma of the colon closely.

AETIOLOGY

Diverticulosis

Considerable evidence suggests that 'Western' low fibre diets are a cause of both diverticulosis and its preceeding constipation.

Diverticulitis

The causes of the inflammation are unknown.

DIAGNOSTIC RANGE (rates per 1000 patients per year)

Personal: Suspected 1.6. Probable 0.4. Many cases are never reported.

AGE INCIDENCE

Over 40 years. The incidence of diverticulitis increases with age.

SEX INCIDENCE

Sexes are said to be equally affected.

CLINICAL POINTERS

Diverticulitis

1. High risk groups: (a) previous attacks; (b) previous chronic constipation; (c) low fibre diets.
2. Long history of recurring attacks of abdominal pain.
3. Long symptom-free periods.
4. Attacks of colicky abdominal pain. The pain is usually left-sided; lasts 1 to 3 days and settles rapidly with bed rest.
5. Attacks of diarrhoea or rectal bleeding are common.
6. Abdominal tenderness usually left-sided.
7. Abdominal mass. A tender mass may be felt in the left iliac fossa or in the pouch of Douglas on rectal examination.
8. A low fever is occasionally present.

INVESTIGATIONS

Barium enema (including double contrast studies). Diverticulae are clearly seen and if diverticulitis is present, narrowing of the lumen and loss of haustration occur.

Sigmoidoscopy or laparotomy are often needed to differentiate diverticulitis from carcinoma.

DURATION

The disease progresses slowly unless it is treated surgically.

COMPLICATIONS

1. Obstruction of the pelvic or descending colon.
2. Perforation and fistula formation are said to occur.

DIFFERENTIAL DIAGNOSIS

Diseases that may be confused with diverticulitis:

Carcinoma of colon

Similar features: left-sided colicky abdominal pain; symptoms of low intestinal obstruction (see p. 482); diarrhoea; passage of blood per rectum; fever; tender mass felt per abdomen or rectum; barium enema does not always distinguish; hypochromic anaemia; raised ESR.

Distinguishing features: symptoms usually steadily progressive; long symptom-free periods rare; sigmoidoscopy or laparotomy needed to differentiate.

Ulcerative colitis

Similar features: attacks of diarrhoea associated with the passage of blood per rectum; history may cover several years.

Distinguishing features: younger age affected; diarrhoea with loose frequent motions; pain slight or absent; sigmoidoscopy and barium enema differentiate.

MANAGEMENT OPTIONS

Prevention: (a) high fibre diet; (b) avoid stimulant laxatives — BNF 1.6.2 (Ref. 0.1)

Established disease: (a) bed rest; (b) light diet; (c) advice re bulk-forming laxatives — BNF 1.6.1.

ULCERATIVE COLITIS

Classification: ICHPPC 555 (RCGP 2745)

AETIOLOGY

Mainly a disease of 'Western' societies, diet appears to play a crucial role. High fibre diets may protect. Pregnancy aggravates attacks. Psychosomatic influences may play a causative role.

DIAGNOSTIC RANGE (rates per 1000 patients per year)

Personal: Suspected 1.0. Probable 0.4, *National*: 0.37.

AGE INCIDENCE

Young adults are liable. It is rare in the elderly and young children.

SEX INCIDENCE

Both sexes are said to be equally affected. In my practice women were affected more than men (10:1).

CLINICAL POINTERS

1. High risk factors: (a) previous attacks; (b) positive family history; (c) low fibre diets.

2. Onset is insidious. In most cases the diagnosis is only made after several attacks of apparent enteritis. Occasionally the onset is acute; in these cases the disease may be rapidly progressive and even fatal.

3. History of recurring attacks of diarrhoea is common.

4. Passage of blood, pus and mucus in the stool may be associated with either loose or comparatively normal stools.

5. Absence of systemic disturbance. A mild depression or low fever may be the only early systemic signs.

6. Abdominal pain is slight or absent.

7. Proctoscopy may reveal a granular proctitis that bleeds on examination.

INVESTIGATIONS

1. Stool culture: pathogens absent.

2. Barium enema: loss of normal haustration occurs late. The ulceration may be visible as slight blurring of the normal outline. Double contrast studies.

3. Sigmoidoscopy and colonoscopy in the early stages is the best way of confirming the diagnosis. The mucous membrane is granular, red, bleeds easily and may be ulcerated. Biopsies can be taken.

4. Blood tests: the ESR (see p. 681) may be considerably raised and hypochromic anaemia is common.

DURATION

In most proven cases the disease progresses slowly as the attacks are repeated. Gradually the symptoms become continuous; mild cases are often encountered in which the diagnosis remains in doubt for long periods. Less often the disease progresses rapidly.

COMPLICATIONS

Mild cases may subside after a few years. Severe cases if not treated may progress rapidly until perforation results in death. Haemorrhage, polyp formation and carcinomatous changes may occur.

Ankylosing spondylitis, iritis and liver disease are associated.

MISLEADING FEATURES AND PITFALLS

The initial attacks of diarrhoea are often widely separated in time. Both patient and doctor can easily forget the previous attacks if these are not recorded.

DIFFERENTIAL DIAGNOSIS

Diseases that may be confused with ulcerative colitis:

Carcinoma of colon and rectum

Similar features: blood in motions; passage of mucus (often confused by patient with diarrhoea); negative stool culture.

Distinguishing features: older patients affected; symptoms usually steadily progressive; constipation common; colicky pain; morning passage of slime; but no true diarrhoea; palpable abdominal or rectal mass may be present; hospital investigation indicated.

Functional enteritis and mucous colitis

Similar features: repeated attacks of diarrhoea often related to emotional disturbance; negative stool culture.

Distinguishing features: attacks are of shorter duration; passage of blood in motions absent; diarrhoea often related to constipation or taking purgatives; differentiation may be difficult without hospital investigation.

MANAGEMENT OPTIONS

Prevention: High fibre diet may play an important preventive role, especially in high risk groups.

Established disease: (a) local steroid enemas BNF 1.7.2 (Ref. 0.1); (b) oral steroids (if severe) BNF 6.3.2; (c) sulphasalazine BNF 1.5; (d) bulk forming laxatives BNF 1.6.1. and high fibre diets between attacks; (e) referral usually needed; (f) Ileostomy and surgery if rapidly progressive; (g) regular follow up.

After ileostomy or severe attacks: Education and support by (a) self-help groups (Ref. 18.2); (b) district nurse and doctor; (c) family. All are vital but easily omitted.

NOTE. Diverticulitis and polyps of the colon or rectum may cause the occasional passage of blood per rectum. Such cases may be confused with ulcerative colitis and hospital investigations with double contrast studies are indicated.

FUNCTIONAL INTESTINAL DISORDERS

Classification: ICHPCC 5640 (RCGP 2770)

CLASSIFICATION

1. Constipation and impacted faeces.
2. Mucous colitis } irritable bowel syndrome.
3. Spastic colon }
4. Functional diarrhoea (nervous diarrhoea) — little is known about the aetiology of this group.

CONSTIPATION

Classification: ICHPPC 5640 (RCGP 2765)

AETIOLOGY

Perhaps the commonest of all the so called 'Western diseases' there is considerable evidence that diet rather than sedentary life is responsible. High fibre diets and bulk forming laxatives are certainly the best cure and may protect individuals against many other diseases e.g. piles, diverticulosis, colitis and colon-cancer.

Two aetiological types are described:

1. Colonic constipation. The passage of faeces through the colon may be delayed for the following reasons.

• Inadequate food intake. A patient who is not taking solid food may not open his bowels for long periods (28 days recorded in one patient).

• Inadequate peristalsis as in myxoedema.

• Partial obstruction of the colon either from within as in carcinoma or from without as in pregnancy.

2. Simple constipation (dyschezia). Habitual difficulty in evacuation of the rectum may follow:

• Poor childhood training and persistent failure to respond to desire to defaecate;

• Lack of roughage in the diet;

• Fear of painful evacuation, e.g. fissure in ano;

• Change of domicile with different food and water.

DIAGNOSTIC RANGE (rates per 1000 patients per year)

Personal: Probable 12.1+. *National*: 7.5. Many patients never report to the doctor.

AGE INCIDENCE

All ages. The condition is common at the extremes of age.

CLINICAL POINTERS OF SIMPLE CONSTIPATION

1. High risk factors: *Babies*: (a) underfeeding; (b) bottle feeding; (c) febrile illness.

Children and adults: (a) low fibre diet; (b) lack of fluid; (c) changes in water supply.

Elderly: (a) inactivity; (b) diminishing, inappropriate or changed diet; (c) chronic illnesses, especially hypothyroid.

2. Failure to open the bowels regularly [100%].

3. History of previous similar difficulty.

4. Abdominal pain is common (50%) especially in children. Further elaboration (sometimes investigation) always indicated.

5. A full rectum. A rectal examination is indicated if there is doubt about the diagnosis or if the patient is of carcinoma age.

INVESTIGATIONS

An enema can be used to confirm the diagnosis. A double enema test can be performed if there is possibility of acute obstruction.

DURATION

The tendency may be lifelong, if dietary measures are ineffective.

COMPLICATIONS

1. Impaction of faeces (see below).

2. Fissure in ano.

MISLEADING FEATURES AND PITFALLS

1. In carcinoma of colon the first symptom is frequently one of increasing constipation. The patient rarely realises the significance of the changed bowel habit. It is extremely easy for the general practitioner to accept the patient's evaluation of the symptoms and overlook the carcinoma.

2. The pain of acute appendicitis is attributed to constipation. The inflammation is aggravated by giving purgatives.

MANAGEMENT OPTIONS

Prevention: (a) high fibre (or vegetarian) diets; (b) physical exercise (jogging, etc.); (c) early training in childhood may be important; (d) education of high risk groups.

Established condition: Start by (a) excluding serious causes; then (b) high fibre high fluid diet; (c) Increase activity; then (d) bulk forming laxatives — BNF 1.6.1 (Ref. 0.1); then (e) faecal softeners — BNF 1.6.3 and rectally administered laxatives — BNF 1.6.5; (f) stimulant laxatives — BNF 1.6.2 and osmotic laxatives — BNF 1.6.4 are best avoided for regular or daily use. *Remember that by encouraging a regular change to a high fibre diet you may be preventing many other diseases.*

IMPACTED FAECES

Classification: ICHPPC 579 (RCGP 4670)

DIAGNOSTIC RANGE (rates per 1000 patients per year)

Personal: Suspected 1.0. Proven 0.5. Diagnosis sometimes difficult.

AGE INCIDENCE

All ages. Toddlers and the elderly are especially prone.

CLINICAL POINTERS

1. High risk groups: (a) Under 6 years; (b) elderly and chronically ill if confined to bed; (c) previous history of constipation.

2. Faecal incontinence. In the elderly this may take the form of spurious diarrhoea — looseness of the bowels follows a purgative but does not relieve the impaction. It must be distinguished from the similar picture of faecal impaction with diarrhoea which is produced by a partially obstructing rectal carcinoma.

3. Urinary incontinence may follow faecal impaction in the elderly.

4. Abdominal mass. A nobbly mass in the pelvis usually the LIF. Unlike the mass of an intussusception it is felt easily.

5. Rectal examination should never be omitted. The hard mass of faeces is easily distinguished by its consistency.

MISLEADING FEATURES AND PITFALLS

1. The diagnosis is easily overlooked in elderly bedridden patients.

2. The rectum is not examined in a confused elderly patient with incontinence of urine.

DIFFERENTIAL DIAGNOSIS

Diseases that may be confused with faecal impaction:

Intussusception

Similar features: colicky abdominal pain in toddlers, associated with an abdominal mass; pallor occurs with spasm of colic.

Distinguishing features: babies commonly affected; history of constipation absent; vomiting likely; pain is severe; abdominal mass difficult to feel and usually on the right side of the abdomen; rectal examination — faeces absent, blood may be present; symptoms not relieved by an enema.

Carcinoma of rectum

Similar features: constipation with abdominal pain in adults over 35; mass in abdomen; spurious diarrhoea.

Distinguishing features; constipation of recent onset; passage of morning slime unassociated with purgatives; rectal examination may reveal growth; enema does not relieve; referral indicated.

Megacolon

Similar feature: history of constipation in a child with abdominal mass and full rectum.

Distinguishing features: difficult to differentiate in early stages; repeated attacks of impaction; hospital investigation usually required.

MANAGEMENT OPTIONS

Prevention: appropriate high fibre diet and exercise in high risk groups.

Established impaction: (a) enemas after softening; (b) manual removal; (c) treat constipation.

IRRITABLE BOWEL SYNDROME

Classification: ICHPPC 558 (RCGP 2770)

Epidemiology suggests that this is another of the so called 'Western

Diseases' which is probably precipitated by diets low in fibre. It includes two syndromes:
Mucous Colitis in which a middle aged or elderly person becomes preoccupied with their bowel habit. Indiscriminate use of stimulant (BNF 1.6.2) laxatives or enemas leads to attacks of both diarrhoea and constipation. There are often vague abdominal pains with the passage of mucus.
Spastic Colon. Symptoms are similar but the tightly contracted descending colon may be palpable and tender.

DIAGNOSTIC RANGE (rates per 1000 patients per year)
Personal: Suspected 1.2

DURATION
Often intractable but no complications.

MANAGEMENT OPTIONS
Prevention: (a) high fibre diets.
Established condition: (a) attempt to wean patient from previous habits; (b) high fibre diets, (c) bulk forming laxatives — BNF 1.6.1 (Ref. 0.1).

FUNCTIONAL DIARRHOEA (NERVOUS DIARRHOEA)

Classification:

The tendency to pass a loose motion when nervous, frightened or anxious has been experienced by most of us. Few cases are reported to the doctor because it rarely causes inconvenience.

CARCINOMA RECTUM

Classification: ICHPPC 151 (RCGP 0420)

AETIOLOGY
Unknown. Epidemiology suggests that as with colonic cancer patients on 'Western' low fibre diets may be vulnerable.

DIAGNOSTIC RANGE (rates per 1000 patients per year)
Personal: Suspected 0.7. Probable 0.5. *National*: 0.4 (Ref. 0.2).

AGE INCIDENCE
Adults — usually over 35 years.

SEX INCIDENCE
Men are said to be affected twice as often as women.

CLINICAL POINTERS

1. Change of bowel habit. Diarrhoea is usual, but constipation may occur.

2. The passage of blood per rectum is said to occur in 50% of cases — an early symptom.

3. The passage of 'slime' or mucus per rectum. Another early symptom. The slime is usually noticed in the morning and for many months may be the only complaint.

4. Pain may range from a vague feeling of abdominal discomfort to pain in the rectum. A colicky pain suggests obstruction of the bowel. Occasionally the pain is related to food; further questions reveal a relation between the pain and defaecation.

5. Anaemia.

6. Loss of weight and appetite are late symptoms.

7. A palpable mass in the rectum. A hard craggy mass with a definite edge — may be mobile or fixed.

25% of rectal growths lie beyond the reach of the examining finger.

INVESTIGATIONS

1. Proctoscopy is of little help.
2. Sigmoidoscopy is the only certain method of diagnosis.
3. Barium enema rarely helps diagnosis.
4. Double contrast radiology may be helpful.
5. Sedimentation rate is rarely altered at first.
6. Haemoglobin estimation.

DURATION

Slow growth is usual — in the untreated or inoperable case a duration of 3 years is not uncommon. A curable cancer.

COMPLICATIONS

Liver metastases, low bowel obstruction and death.

MISLEADING FEATURES AND PITFALLS

1. Failure to perform a rectal examination in an adult who complains of persistent bowel or rectal symptoms. If cancer is present this disastrous omission will soon become apparent to patient and relatives.

2. Failure to examine the upper rectum with a sigmoidoscope. The doctor fears the fuss of referral to a surgeon or is lulled into false security by a negative rectal examination.

3. The assumption that bowel symptoms are due to piles.

> NOTE. Piles may arise as a result of a developing carcinoma or a carcinoma may start in a patient with longstanding piles.

4. Failure to investigate frequent attacks of so called gastroenteritis in a patient of cancer age.

DIFFERENTIAL DIAGNOSIS

Diseases that may be confused with rectal carcinoma:

Internal piles

Similar feature: painless passage of blood per rectum.

Distinguishing features: bleeding usually occurs after or at the end of defaecation; there is no passage of slime; a long preceding history of similar attacks is likely; sigmoidoscopy may be needed to differentiate.

Ulcerative colitis

Similar feature: recurring passage of blood and slime per rectum.

Distinguishing feature: differentiation can only be made by sigmoidoscopy and barium enema examination.

Functional disorders of colon (spastic colon, mucous colitis, nervous diarrhoea, etc.)

Similar feature: repeated attacks of diarrhoea.

Distinguishing features: symptoms are preceded by a long suggestive history; sigmoidoscopy, barium enema and full surgical opinion are probably required before the patient accepts the harmless nature of his symptoms.

MANAGEMENT OPTIONS

As for Carcinoma of colon (p. 482).

ANAL FISSURE

Classification: ICHPPC 565 (RCGP 2785)

AETIOLOGY

Overstretching of the sphincter by a constipated motion may occur in the following circumstances:

1. Babies — after a change of food.
2. Toddlers — when the child is old enough to disregard the call to stool.
3. Adults — constipation, a bout of diarrhoea, pregnancy or piles may precipitate a fissure. Low fibre diets.

DIAGNOSTIC RANGE (rates per 1000 patients per year)

Personal: Probable 4.9. *National*: 1.4 (Ref. 0.2). Diagnosis rarely in doubt.

CLINICAL POINTERS

1. High risk factors: (a) constipation; (b) hard motions.
2. Pain on defaecation (95%) is often severe and followed by throbbing or burning.
3. A visible fissure (30%). This may be difficult to identify with certainty. The anal canal is opened for inspection by separating the buttocks on either side. A vertical slit can then be seen lying between the anal creases. Granulation tissue is absent.
4. The passage of blood per rectum (30%) in babies and toddlers.
5. A history of constipation (30%).

DURATION

The disorder may last many weeks or months. Stretching the sphincter under a general anaesthetic often produces early relief but may have to be repeated in adults.

COMPLICATIONS

Recurrences are uncommon in babies and toddlers; the disorder may lead to difficulty over bowel habit.

Recurrences are common adults.

DIFFERENTIAL DIAGNOSIS

Toddlers — the disease is confused with a behaviour problem.

Adults — differentiation from internal piles is sometimes difficult and may require examination under anaesthetic.

MISLEADING FEATURES AND PITFALLS

1. The pain causes anal spasm which renders the fissure invisible.
2. Piles and fissure occur concurrently in an adult; the obvious piles mask the less obvious fissure.

MANAGEMENT OPTIONS

Prevention: (a) high fibre diet may prevent.

Established fissure: (a) analgesic suppositories — BNF 1.7.1. (Ref. 0.1); (b) stretching under anaesthetic; (c) referral for surgery if intractable; (d) high fibre diet.

ANAL FISTULA

Classification: ICHPPC 565 (RCGP 2785)

AETIOLOGY

An ischiorectal abscess drains into the rectum and a chronically infected fistula develops. The condition is said occasionally to be associated with tuberculosis, local malignancy colitis or ileitis.

DIAGNOSTIC RANGE (rates per 1000 patients per year)
Personal: Probable 0.2.

CLINICAL POINTERS
A chronic sinus in the anal region that may discharge faeces as well as pus.

MANAGEMENT OPTIONS
Prevention: early treatment of perianal abscess.
Established disease: referral for surgery as healing unlikely.

ISCHIO-RECTAL ABSCESS

Classification: ICHPPC 565 (RCGP 2785)

AETIOLOGY
The tissues in the region of the anus contain much fat and few vessels. As a result once a superficial infection has arisen it is difficult to eradicate.

DIAGNOSTIC RANGE (rates per 1000 patients per year)
Personal: Probable 0.8.

CLINICAL POINTERS
1. Throbbing, often intense pain near to the anus.
2. Red, tense area of cellulitis.
3. Scars of previous infections or operations.

COMPLICATIONS
Recurrences are common. The abscess may track into the rectum, causing a fistula if not treated by early incision.

MISLEADING FEATURES AND PITFALLS
The abscess may be deep and signs of cellulitis appear late. The doctor is thus tempted to await the effects of systemic antibiotics and the abscess discharges into the rectum.

MANAGEMENT OPTIONS
Early referral for surgery. Antibiotics not indicated as an alternative to referral.

CHRONIC CHOLECYSTITIS SYNDROME

Classification: ICHPPC 574 (RCGP 2815)

This clinical term covers three related and overlapping clinico-pathological entities:

1. Acute cholecystitis (ICHPPC 574; RCGP 2820);
2. Chronic cholecystitis ICHPPC 574; (RCGP 2815)
3. Cholelithiasis (gallstones) (ICHPPC 574; RCGP 2815).

The terms acute and chronic cholecystitis suggest that the basic aetiology is a simple and progressive infection. This is not so and other factors are involved.

Chronic cholecystitis is the name given to the condition of flatulent dyspepsia which is associated with a tendency to stone formation and the pathological appearances of chronic inflammation in the gall bladder.

Acute cholecystitis occurs only after chronic cholecystitis has been present for some time and it rarely arises unless the outflow of bile from the gall bladder is obstructed by a stone.

It is simpler for the primary physician to regard the three diseases as components of a single complex and to leave the surgeons and pathologists to work out the details of an artificial classification.

AETIOLOGY

The aetiology of the syndrome is probably multifactorial with age, sex, diet and infection all playing a part. Obesity and diabetes are often associated. Cholesterol stones are related to overnutrition and are less likely to develop on diets high in unrefined carbohydrate and fibre.

After chronic cholecystitis has started, the subsequent clinical and pathological course is decided by the relative extent of: (a) infection; (b) stone formation; (c) obstruction of cystic or common bile ducts.

DIAGNOSTIC RANGE (rates per 1000 patients per year)

Personal: Suspected 4.8. Probable 1.9. *National*: 1.1 (Ref. 0.2). Many patients have few symptoms and do not report.

AGE INCIDENCE

Adults — a peak of incidence is reached between 50 and 70.

SEX INCIDENCE

Women are said to be affected 20 times more than men. (Practice experience 5:1.)

CLINICAL POINTERS

1. High risk factors: (a) obesity; (b) previous attacks; (c) diabetes; (d) multiparity; (e) middle aged women.

2. History of flatulent dyspepsia: (a) abdominal discomfort after meals, i.e. slight upper abdominal pain and feeling of distension;

(b) belching of wind; (c) aggravation of symptoms by fatty or fried foods; (d) little or no relief from alkalis; (e) absence of periodicity. This background complaint of flatulent dyspepsia is probably related to the chronic inflammatory changes in the gall bladder and it is present in the majority (87%) of proven cases.

3. Attacks of upper abdominal pain (100%) is the symptom that brings the patient to the doctor. It may be felt centrally or in the right hypochondrium. Gall stones are sometimes discovered at operation or post-mortem in patients who have had no pain. The abdominal pain is of three types: (a) severe intermittent pain which is referred to as gall-stone colic and follows impaction of a stone; (b) severe continuous pain with evidence of acute inflammation; acute cholecystitis is the symptom complex of severe, continuous pain, low fever and gall-bladder tenderness; (c) pain is less severe and less well defined and may be due to impaction of a stone or impaction plus infection.

4. Radiation of the abdominal pain. Classically this is to one or both shoulders, such characteristic pain is uncommon (25% of proven cases). Pain is also felt substernally or in the back. The disease may thus simulate myocardial ischaemia or peptic ulcer.

5. History of recurrent attacks of pain (75%). These are more severe and tend to be less frequent than those of peptic ulcer.

6. Tenderness over the gall bladder under the right costal margin (75%). Sometimes this is absent or felt on deep inspiration (Murphy's sign). The gall bladder may be palpable.

7. Fever during an attack of pain (37%) is rarely over 38°C. Occasionally high temperatures or a rigor are noted.

8. Jaundice (5%) becomes obvious in the sclerotics or urine one to 2 days after the onset of colic from impaction in the common duct.

9. Associated diseases. Coronary artery disease and peptic ulcer are both thought to occur more often in patients with chronic cholecystitis.

INVESTIGATIONS

1. Examination of the urine for bile salts and pigments.

2. Serum bilirubin, Alkaline phosphatase and SGPT may be indicated.

3. A straight X-ray of abdomen reveals opaque stones.

4. A cholecystogram can be performed as an out-patient.

5. Ultrasound gives helpful information about stones and gall bladder walls.

6. A cardiograph, chest X-ray or barium meal may be indicated.

DURATION

The disease continues indefinitely until cholecystectomy.

COMPLICATIONS

1. Empyema of gall bladder. The immediate treatment of an acute attack of cholecystitis is conservative in most cases. Sometimes an empyema of gall bladder develops while the doctor is waiting for the acute attack to subside. Fever and tenderness in the right hypochondrium persist. Admission to hospital is indicated.

2. Impaction of a gall stone in the common duct. Progressive jaundice and liver damage occur if the obstruction is not relieved. Admission to hospital is indicated.

MISLEADING FEATURES AND PITFALLS

1. A myocardial infarct may occur in a patient with chronic cholecystitis. Both patient and doctor may ascribe the symptoms of the infarct to the known gall bladder disease.

2. A peptic ulcer and chronic cholecystitis may arise in the same patient. Straight abdominal X-ray or cholecystogram reveal the gall bladder disease. The more extensive barium meal investigation is not performed because the patient's symptoms are ascribed entirely to the cholecystitis.

DIFFERENTIAL DIAGNOSIS

Diseases that may be confused with chronic cholecystitis:

Peptic ulcer and ulcer dyspepsia

Similar features: long history of indigestion with acute exacerbations; attacks of upper abdominal pain, aggravated by fried foods; pain may radiate to back; vomiting and belching; upper abdominal tenderness.

Distinguishing features: periodicity marked; symptom-free periods; symptoms relieved by taking further food and alkalis; fever and jaundice absent; Murphy's sign absent; cholecystogram and barium meal differentiate.

Reflux oesophagitis

Similar features: attacks of substernal pain related to meals; fat women liable.

Distinguishing features: pain often daily and aggravated by lying down; history of flatulent dyspepsia absent; fever and jaundice absent; Murphy's sign absent; cholecystogram and barium meal differentiate.

Myocardial infarction and angina pectoris
Similar features: attacks of acute substernal pain; fever and leucocytosis (on 2nd and 3rd day of myocardial infarct); meals may precipitate angina.

Distinguishing features: *myocardial infarction* — history of flatulent dyspepsia absent; pain is continuous and radiates to arms, fingers, neck and chin; shock and fall in blood pressure; cardiac arrhythmias occur; Murphy's sign absent; electrocardiogram differentiates *Angina pectoris* — pain related to exertion and radiates to arms, fingers, neck or chin; pain relieved by trinitrini or amylnitrite; Murphy's sign absent.

Acute appendicitis
Similar features: recurrent attacks of right-flank pain and tenderness; vomiting; low fever; raised pulse rate; leucocytosis.

Distinguishing features: history of flatulent dyspepsia absent; pain does not radiate to shoulders or back; differentiation may only be possible at operation; admission to hospital indicated.

Carcinoma of colon
Similar features: colicky abdominal pain (often severe); low fever; tender mass under liver; Murphy's sign positive.

Distinguishing features: history of flatulent dyspepsia absent; recent alteration of bowel habit; pain is abdominal and does not radiate above diaphragm; passage of blood in stool; large bowel obstruction; admission to hospital indicated.

NOTE. If jaundice is present, the possibility of other serious disease is raised and hospital investigation is indicated.

MANAGEMENT OPTIONS

Prevention: (a) high fibre diets may protect against cholesterol stone formation.

Established disease: most cases are best referred for either surgery or occasional bile acid dissolution — BNF 1.9.1 (Ref. 0.1).

Table 27 Less common diseases of the digestive system

Disease and distinguishing clinical pointers	Incidence per 1000 patients per year Suspected	Confirmed
Mixed parotid tumour Progressive painless enlargement of salivary gland. Refer.	—	1 in 10 years
Salivary calculus Adults; sudden onset while eating; swelling, often transient, of parotid or submandibular gland; pain and tenderness of gland; calculus or plug of debris often visible at duct mouth; obstruction can often be dislodged and followed by jet of saliva; X-ray usually negative	0.9	0.5
Acute infections of salivary glands	0	0
Malignant epithelioma of lip Persistent ulcer with hard rolled edge	—	1 in 10 years
Malignant epithelioma of tongue Patients over 30, persistent ulcer with hard rolled edge, growth may be wart like, usual site — edge of tongue	—	1 in 10 years
Achalasia Gradual onset under 40, dysphagia, regurgitation, pain absent, barium swallow. Refer.	0	1 in 10 years
Plummer-Vinson syndrome Dysphagia, severe hypochromic anaemia	0	0 in 10 years
Paralytic ileus Symptoms of intestinal obstruction. Refer.	0	0 in 10 years
Mesenteric infarction Left-sided heart disease, sudden onset, severe abdominal pain, vomiting, repeated diarrhoea with passage of blood, shock	—	1 in 10 years
Volvulus Sudden onset, intestinal obstruction	0	0 in 20 years
Regional ileitis Gradual onset of intestinal obstruction	0	2 in 10 years
Pilonidal sinus Young adults, midline swelling over sacrum, infection with intermittent pain and discharge may occur. Surgery indicated.	0.4	0.4
Peritoneal adhesions Previous abdominal operation, symptoms (often mild) of intestinal obstruction, often used as a scapegoat diagnosis to explain abdominal symptoms that persist after an operation	0.6	—
Rectal prolapse Young children and adults after piles or pregnancy; soft round pink or purple mass at anus, recurrences frequent. High fibre diet indicated.	0.3	0.3

Table 27 cont'd

Disease and distinguishing clinical pointers	Incidence per 1000 patients per year Suspected	Confirmed
Carcinoma of gall bladder and pancreas Progressive jaundice, upper abdominal pain, loss of weight. Before jaundice appears there may be several weeks of vague abdominal discomfort and entirely negative investigations.	—	2 in 10 years
Cirrhosis of liver (*portal*) Onset gradual after 45, portal hypertension (anorexia, indigestion, splenomegaly, ascites, gastrointestinal haemorrhage, anaemia), hepatic failure bleeding tendency, muddy complexion, palpable liver. Alcoholics.	0.3	0.1
Acute haemorrhagic pancreatitis Picture resembles that of a perforated peptic ulcer but previous indigesion absent, vomiting and shock marked. Early referral.	0.2	0.2

19

Diseases of the urinary system

Please read introduction for explanation of figures and analyses.

GLOMERULONEPHRITIS (BRIGHT'S DISEASE)

A disease for specialists. A *few* uncommon clinical entities of *uncertain* aetiology may *occasionally* progress to *a rare* but treatable end point. The rare but treatable end point is chronic glomerulonephritis (p. 526) now sensibly called End Stage Renal Disease (ESRD). It is clinically characterised by evidence of renal failure and is treatable by renal dialysis or transplant. The national incidence of ESRD is 0.1 per 1000 population. The various uncommon clinical entities of uncertain aetiology which may eventually progress to ESRD are:

— Acute (proliferative) glomerulonephritis (p. 511) characterised by haematuria, occasionally related to streptococcal infections.
— The nephrotic syndrome (p. 526) characterised by extensive proteinuria and oedema.
— Renal disease of diabetic origin.
— Chronic pyelonephritis which sometimes develops after recurrent renal infections of many years standing (p. 520).
— Severe hypertension.
— Polycystic disease (p. 526).
— Systemic lupus (SLE p. 626) and Periarteritis (PAN p. 626)

Many of these disease are either reversible or preventable with immunotherapy, antibiotics, antihypertensives or insulins. Much expensive terminal treatment of ESRD can be avoided through the sensitive early clinical awareness of the family doctor. This involves early diagnosis, early referral combined with appropriate explanations, support and follow up of patients at risk. Blood pressure, kidney function, infection and heart, as well as drug treatment may all require monitoring.

ACUTE PROLIFERATIVE GLOMERULONEPHRITIS

Classification: ICHPPC 580 (RCGP 2900)

AETIOLOGY

Streptococcus pyogenes (especially type 12) plays a part. A throat infection precedes the nephritis. The exact relationship between the two diseases is uncertain but autoimmune processes are probably involved.

DIAGNOSTIC RANGE (rates per 1000 patients per year)

Personal: Suspected 0.4. Probable 0.2. In this practice the incidence has decreased steadily in the past few years.

AGE INCIDENCE

All ages. Children and adolescents are especially prone.

CLINICAL POINTERS

1. High risk factors history of preceding streptococcal infection. A history of sore throat 1 to 4 weeks previously is common.
2. Painless haematuria (100%). The urine is pink, red or smoky.
3. Symptoms of systemic disturbance are rarely marked and include headache, malaise, vomiting and low fever.
4. Evidence of oedema usually absent, but the face may be puffy and pale.
5. Hypertension is said to occur.

INVESTIGATIONS

1. Routine throat swabs and urine microscopy is confined to cases of tonsillitis with possible nephritis.
2. Proteinuria is present in most cases.
3. Renal biopsy and renal function tests occasionally indicated.

DURATION

Most patients recover within 1 to 4 weeks. A small proportion are said to show evidence of permanent renal damage and later develop chronic glomerulonephritis.

COMPLICATIONS

Chronic glomerulonephritis, heart failure, renal failure and death after many years.

MISLEADING FEATURES AND PITFALLS

Beetroot, senna, rhubarb, phenolphthalein and cheap dyes used in ice cream and other food stuffs may colour the urine red

DIFFERENTIAL DIAGNOSIS

Disease that may be confused with acute glomerulonephritis:

Angioneurotic oedema

Similar feature: facial oedema and periorbital puffiness.

Distinguishing features: haematuria and systemic signs absent; tongue and lips are swollen; urine normal.

Acute GU tract infections

Similar features: painless haematuria; fever; loin tenderness and systemic disturbance.

Distinguishing features: frequency and dysuria are usual in adults; haematuria subsides rapidly and pyuria persists.

Renal calculi

Similar features: painless haematuria can occur.

Distinguishing features: recurring attacks of haematuria in adults; renal colic is usual; hospital investigation indicated.

Tuberculosis of kidney

Similar features: painless haematuria; fever.

Distinguishing features: urinary symptoms are persistent and chronic; adults mainly affected; evidence of pulmonary TB sometimes present; hospital investigation indicated.

Papilloma of bladder or renal tract

Similar features: painless haematuria.

Distinguishing features: haematuria is persistent and recurrent; adults mainly affected; cystoscopy and hospital investigation indicated.

Hypernephroma, carcinoma of bladder

Similar feature: painless haematuria.

Distinguishing features: haematuria is persistent or recurrent; children not affected; hospital investigation indicated.

Congenital defects (*e.g. aberrant vessels or polycystic kidney*)

Similar feature: painless haematuria.

Distinguishing features: haematuria is persistent or recurrent; kidney sometimes palpable; all ages affected; rare; hospital investigation indicated.

MANAGEMENT OPTIONS
Referral for investigation and diagnosis.

INFECTIONS OF THE KIDNEYS, URETER AND BLADDER

Classification

The accepted classification of this group of diseases is simple and sensible:

1. Acute pyelonephritis (or pyelitis). } — Upper urinary tract
2. Chronic pyelonephritis. }
3. Acute cystitis. — Lower urinary tract.

Accurate diagnosis of a urinary tract infection and the correct allocation into one of these groups is a difficult practical problem for the following reasons:

A. CRITERIA OF DIAGNOSIS ARE UNSATISFACTORY

1. Clinical criteria. The salient clinical features of urinary infections are dysuria and frequency. Unfortunately these symptoms are common in patients with cystocele and functional frequency and are often absent in the urinary infections of childhood.

2. Therapeutic criteria. The response of symptoms to sulphonamides and antibiotics can be used, but is unsatisfactory.

3. Bacteriological criteria. Accurate assessment of the infection can be made by isolation of pathogenic bacteria or by bacterial counts. Unfortunately these methods are often impractical in general practice because fresh specimens are needed.

4. Proteinuria is only found in heavy infections.

5. Pyuria. Microscopy of a specimen shows pus cells. This test is quick and reasonably accurate and if performed as part of the routine physical examination, prevents much needless clinical doubt. A clean mid-stream specimen (uncentrifuged) is placed under the microscope; two or more pus cells in six random high-power fields are taken to indicate infection.

6. Many doctors use one of the 'quick culture' slides which can be incubated overnight in the surgery.

B. DIFFICULTIES IN DIFFERENTIATION BETWEEN UPPER AND LOWER URINARY TRACT INFECTIONS

Confirmation of the exact site of the infection is rarely possible because instrumentation is contra-indicated, pyelograms show little and post-mortems in the acute phase of the infections are exceedingly rare. It is therefore difficult to ascertain how much of the tract is actually involved in each type of infection.

These difficulties apply especially in children.

In adults it is feasible to differentiate clinically between acute cystitis and acute pyelonephritis.

AETIOLOGY OF URINARY TRACT IN INFECTIONS

The aetiology of all urinary tract infections is probably similar.

1. The infection ascends from rectum via urethra and bladder.

2. Infection is bacterial. *Escherichia coli* is usually involved but Staphylococci, Proteus, Pseudomonas or *Streptococcus faecalis* are often isolated.

3. Pregnancy. The upper urinary tract is especially prone to infection during pregnancy. The excessive dilatation of ureters and tendency to stasis of urine in the upper tract during the latter half of pregnancy is thought to be responsible. Urinary infections in pregnant women are often symptomless.

4. Sexual intercourse often acts as a trigger factor in women.

5. Obstructions or mechanical defects of the urinary tract. Enlargement of the prostate, congenital defects or calculi in the pelvis ureter or bladder are frequently associated with recurrent or chronic urinary infections.

6. Diabetes mellitus. Diabetics are especially prone to recurring urinary tract infection.

7. Blood-borne infection may occur occasionally.

ACUTE UPPER URINARY TRACT INFECTIONS IN ADULTS

Classification: ICHPPC 5901 (RCGP 2910)

DIAGNOSTIC RANGE (rates per 1000 patients per year)

Personal: Suspected 15.9. Probable 10.3. *National*: 6.6 (Ref. 0.2). Many cases are never reported.

AGE INCIDENCE

Peaks of incidence occur in the under 5's and in sexually active, and elderly, women (Fig. 49).

Recently sexual freedom has led to an increased attack rates in 15–25 year old girls.

SEX INCIDENCE

Women affected more than men (10:1).

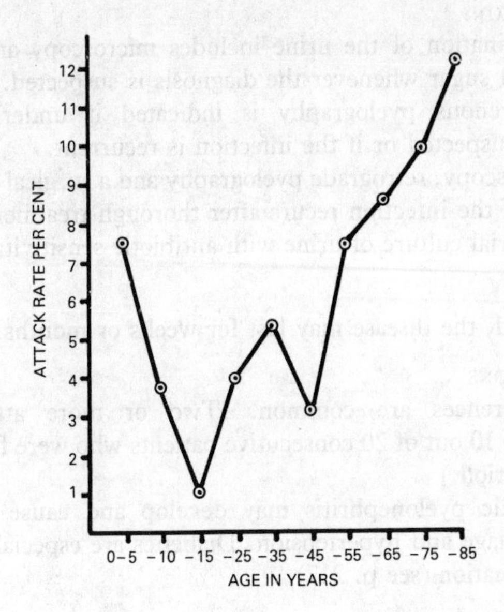

Fig. 49 Acute pyelonephritis and urinary tract infections. Age incidence curve of 147 consecutive cases encountered in 1 year.

CLINICAL POINTERS

1. High risk factors: (a) previous attacks; (b) sexual intercourse; (c) pregnancy; (d) multiparity; (e) diabetes; (g) old age; (h) prostatic enlargement; (i) congenital defects.

2. Frequency of micturition (75%). Recent nocturia is a reliable pointer in most cases.

3. Dysuria (35%). A burning pain in the lower urethra is felt during micturition. This symptom suggests possible infection of the urinary tract, but it is absent in some upper urinary tract infections. This observation suggests that dysuria may be due, not to the upper urinary tract infection, but to an associated cystitis.

4. Loin pain (75%) and loin tenderness (65%) distinguish upper urinary tract infections from cystitis. They may be present together or separately. Sometimes the pain and tenderness are felt in the flank and distinction from acute appendicitis may be difficult.

5. Rigors (25%).

6. Fever (70%) may be high but it is often slight or absent.

7. Pyuria (65%) is the most helpful finding and confirms the clinical diagnosis in most cases.

INVESTIGATIONS

1. Examination of the urine includes microscopy and tests for protein and sugar whenever the diagnosis is suspected.
2. Intravenous pyelography is indicated if underlying renal disease is suspected or if the infection is recurrent.
3. Cystoscopy, retrograde pyelography and a surgical opinion are indicated if the infection recurs after thorough treatment.
4. Bacterial culture of urine with antibiotic sensitivities.

DURATION

If untreated, the disease may last for weeks or months.

COMPLICATIONS

1. Recurrences are common. (Two or more attacks were recorded in 10 out of 20 consecutive patients who were followed for a 3 year period.)
2. Chronic pyelonephritis may develop and cause permanent kidney damage and hypertension. Diabetics are especially liable to this complication (see p. 217).

MISLEADING FEATURES AND PITFALLS

1. Small amounts of pus are occasionally found in women suffering from other diseases. An acute abdominal emergency may thus be mistakenly diagnosed as an acute urinary tract infection.
2. Haematuria with pyuria sometimes occurs at the onset of a urinary tract infection.
3. Catheterisation may introduce infection.
4. Patients often tell the doctor that they suffer from kidney trouble. This often means that they have a recurring backache.
5. In the last few months of pregnancy patients sometimes develop an almost symptomless pyelitis.

DIFFERENTIAL DIAGNOSIS

Diseases that may be confused with upper urinary tract infections:

Acute cystitis

Similar features: pyuria; women commonly affected; frequency; nocturia; dysuria; haematuria; slight fever.

Distinguishing features: dysuria at end of micturition; systemic disturbance slight; rigors absent; loin pain and tenderness absent; fever rarely high; differentiation often impossible.

Pregnancy (early)

Similar features: sudden onset; frequency; nocturia; vomiting.

Distinguishing features: amenorrhoea; breasts heavy and tender; dysuria absent; pyuria and fever absent; pregnancy tests positive.

Prolapsed uterus

Similar features: frequency; dysuria.

Distinguishing features: nocturia and loin tenderness absent; stress incontinence; cystocele appears on coughing; pyuria; no fever.

Acute appendicitis

Similar features: right-sided abdominal pain and tenderness; frequency; nocturia; dysuria; vomiting and fever.

Distinguishing features: fever rarely over 38°C; loin tenderness absent; rebound and rectal tenderness to right common; pyuria absent; differentiation sometimes difficult; hospital admission indicated in doubtful cases.

Ectopic pregnancy

Similar features: frequency; nocturia; dysuria; abdominal pain; fever.

Distinguishing features: history of missed period; brown vaginal discharge; acute persistent abdominal pain; cervix acutely tender on vaginal examination; pyuria absent; acute salpingitis or a twisted ovarian cyst may give a similar history; gonadotrophin test positive.

Other renal diseases (e.g. tuberculosis and calculi)

Similar features: frequency; nocturia; dysuria; abdominal pain; haematuria; pyuria.

Distinguishing features: *Renal tuberculosis* — history of contact or previous pulmonary TB; long history of frequency and dysuria common; response to routine treatment slight or absent; pyelography distinguishes; *Renal calculus* — haematuria common; pain usually marked, often colicky; history of gravel; pyelography.

MANAGEMENT OPTIONS

Prevention: case finding and early treatment in high risk groups.

Established disease: 5–7 days co-trimoxazole or sulpha — BNF 5.1.8 (Ref. 0.1).

Recurrences: (a) bacteriological and other investigations after 2nd or 3rd recurrence; (b) appropriate antibiotic — BNF 5.1; (c) intractable cases may need referral or even prolonged antibiotics.

ACUTE GENITO-URINARY TRACT INFECTIONS IN CHILDREN

DIAGNOSTIC RANGE (rates per 1000 patients per year)

Personal: Suspected 9.8. Probable 5.9.

AGE INCIDENCE

Children under the age of 5 years are especially liable (Fig. 49).

SEX INCIDENCE

Girls are affected more than boys.

CLINICAL COURSE

The infection starts as an acute febrile illness. Dysuria and frequency are rarely present and for this reason the urinary origin of the infection is easily overlooked. If the disease is allowed to continue untreated, it becomes subacute. The main characteristics of subacute infections are an indefinite period of malaise, anorexia, vague ill-health, occasional fever and facial pallor.

CLINICAL POINTERS

1. High risk factors: (a) congenital defects of tract; (b) previous attacks; (c) presence of Vesico-ureteric reflux; (d) diabetes.
2. Malaise and anorexia (75%). Both are found in many other diseases of childhood.
3. Unexpected fever (70%). Initially this may be high (over 38.5°C) and associated with delirum. Later a low fever is common.
4. Facial pallor is often marked in the subacute case and is a useful sign because it is easily observed.
5. Abdominal pain (30%) is a confusing sign which raises many diagnostic problems and may make early differentiation from acute appendicitis difficult. The pain is often felt in one flank also.
6. Backache and loin tenderness (15%).
7. Frequency, nocturia and enuresis (35%) are useful pointers when of recent onset but are often caused by other conditions.
8. Dysuria (15%)
9. Pyuria (60%).

INVESTIGATIONS

1. Examination of urine for albumen, sugar and pus cells is a routine procedure.
2. Culture of urine for organisms and antibiotic sensitivities.
3. Intravenous pyelogram.
4. Recurrent cases. Paediatric referral with micturating cysto-urography to exclude ureteric reflux.

DURATION

The disease may be easily cured in the acute stage, but if untreated it may persist for weeks or months; chronic pyelonephritis is said to develop from these persisting infections. Patients with a long history are the most difficult to cure.

COMPLICATIONS

Recurrences occur but are not as common as in adults. [Two or more attacks were recorded in four out of 20 cases followed during a 3-year period.] Chronic pyelonephritis is thought to develop from the subacute case which has been overlooked.

MISLEADING FEATURES AND PITFALLS

1. Pus cells may not appear in the first 6 to 8 hours and differentiation from appendicitis may be difficult.

2. Pus may be absent from the urine for short periods during a long-standing urinary infection.

3. Red cells without pus are sometimes found in the urine in the early stages.

4. Enuresis may be the presenting symptom of a subacute or recurrent urinary infection. The associated malaise and anorexia are easily attributed to psychological causes.

A DIFFERENTIAL DIAGNOSIS OF ACUTE URINARY TRACT INFECTIONS IN CHILDREN

Diseases that may be confused with acute urinary tract infections:

Acute appendicitis

Similar features: abdominal pain; right-sided abdominal tenderness; fever; high pulse rate (out of proportion to fever); vomiting; dysuria; frequency.

Distinguishing features: fever rarely high; rebound tenderness; pyuria and loin tenderness absent; differentiation may be extremely difficult, admission to hospital indicated in doubtful cases.

Acute tonsillitis

Similar features: abdominal pain and tenderness; high fever; rigor; vomiting; tonsillar exudate may be absent in first 2 days; sore throat may be absent in young children with tonsillitis.

Distinguishing features: contact cases; sore throat and tonsillar exudate; offensive breath; cervical adenitis; pyuria absent.

Acute mesenteric adenitis

Similar features: abdominal pain and tenderness; vomiting; fever.

Distinguishing features: history of sore throat; differentiation may be difficult; the doctor is often more concerned with excluding appendicitis than distinguishing between these two diseases.

Early infective hepatitis

Similar features: abdominal pain and right-flank tenderness; fever; vomiting; malaise; anorexia.

Distinguishing features: contact cases; abdominal pain slight; pyuria absent; bile salts and pigment in urine on 2nd to 4th day; stools pale; conjunctivae yellow; liver tender; fever low; pulse slow.

B. DIFFERENTIAL DIAGNOSIS OF SUBACUTE URINARY TRACT INFECTIONS IN CHILDREN

Diseases that may be confused with subacute urinary tract infections:

Behaviour problems and enuresis
Similar features: malaise; anorexia; frequency; enuresis.
Distinguishing features: fever absent; pyuria persistently absent.

Residual aspiration pneumonitis
Similar features: malaise; anorexia; slight fever.
Distinguishing features: history of respiratory illness 1 to 3 weeks previously; cough; persistent adventitious sounds in chest; pyuria absent; chest X-ray confirms the diagnosis.

Acute cervical adenitis
Similar features: malaise; anorexia; slight fever.
Distinguishing features: history of sore throat 4 to 21 days previously; enlarged tender cervical glands.

Tuberculous meningitis and miliary TB
Similar features: malaise; anorexia; slight fever in a baby or child.
Distinguishing features: rare; TB contact; tuberculin test positive; pyuria absent; hospital investigation indicated.

MANAGEMENT OPTIONS

Prevention: case finding, treatment and follow up of vulnerable high risk groups.

Established disease: (a) 5–7 days antibiotics — BNF 5.1 (Ref. 0.1); (b) adequate follow up to check cure — the most vital step; (c) parental education about reporting recurrences.

Recurrent disease: case finding and early treatment of any recurrence are crucial if renal damage and long term complications are to be avoided — (a) referral and investigation of all recurrent cases in children; (b) long term antibiotics and follow up often needed.

CHRONIC PYELONEPHRITIS

Classification: ICHPPC 598 (RCGP 2955)

Many diseases predispose to chronic pyelonephritis. These include diabetes, congenital deformities, calculi, enlarged prostate and inadequately treated acute pyelonephritis. Opinions differ but some evidence suggests that this disease is preventable.

DIAGNOSTIC RANGE (rates per 1000 patients per year)

Personal: Suspected 0.5+. In the elderly the disease is easily overlooked or not reported.

CLINICAL POINTERS

1. High risk factors: (a) repeated attacks; (b) inadequate follow up of recurrent infections; (c) diabetes; (d) other chronic diseases of the urinary tract, as above.
2. Vague ill-health.
3. Periods of malaise.
4. Indefinite symptoms of frequency and dysuria.
5. Occasional low fever.
6. Pyuria.

INVESTIGATIONS

Hospital investigation is indicated.

DURATION

The disease is difficult to eradicate and recurrences are common.

COMPLICATIONS

Hypertension, renal failure and death.

MANAGEMENT OPTIONS

Prevention: case finding in high risk groups leading to early referral and treatment with adequate follow up and education to encourage full compliance subsequently.

Established disease: as for Acute upper urinary tract infections.

RENAL CALCULI AND RENAL COLIC

Classification: ICHPPC 592 (RCGP 2920)

AETIOLOGY

The exact aetiology is uncertain. Recurrent infection of the renal pelvis, low fluid intake and soft water may all contribute. Colic is caused when a stone blocks the ureter.

1. Prolonged bed rest with chronic illness.
2. Congenital deformities of the renal tract.
3. Parathyroid tumours — rare.
4. The pH of the urine governs the type of stone.

   Three types of calculus are common:

a. Calcium oxalate stones are hard and spiky. They cause bleeding and pain when still small.
b. Calcium phosphate stones develop comparatively quickly in alkaline urine and form large smooth stagshorn calculi with few early symptoms.
c. Uric acid crystals are hard, smooth and often multiple.

DIAGNOSTIC RANGE (rates per 1000 patients per year)
Personal: Suspected 2.1. Probable 1.3. *National*: 0.8 (Ref. 0.2).

AGE INCIDENCE
All age groups are liable but the majority (80%) of proven cases arise between the ages of 30 and 50.

SEX INCIDENCE
Males are affected more than females (2:1).

CLINICAL POINTERS
1. High risk factors: (a) previous renal calculi (70% of proven cases had subsequent attacks); (b) low daily fluid intake; (c) long period confined to bed (20% of cases); (d) congenital abnormalities of urinary tract (10%); (e) patient lives in a known stone forming district; (f) Positive family history.

2. Severe pain over kidney or ureter (85%). The pain is felt over one loin and radiates into the flanks down the line of the ureter. Radiation into the scrotum or tip of the penis is a helpful distinguishing feature. The pain is severe and lasts up to several hours. It is continuous or colicky (Typical colic was observed in only 40% of proven cases.) Occasionally the pain is aggravated by deep breathing and movement, and may simulate the pain of pleurisy or lumbago.

3. Haematuria. Macroscopic blood is present in a proportion (40%) of cases. Microscopic evidence of bleeding is present in the urine of the majority (100%) of proven cases.

4. The passage of stones or gravel (15%). After colic the patient should examine every specimen of urine for a possible calculus.

5. Dysuria (20%) and frequency (30%) are helpful features because they confirm the renal origin of the pain. They can however be misleading.

6. Vomiting is common and probably follows the severe pain.

INVESTIGATIONS
1. Microscopic examination of the urine for blood cells.
2. A straight X-ray of the abdomen may exclude large calculi.

3. Intravenous pyelography is indicated in all suspected cases.

4. Retrograde pyelography, cystoscopy and a surgical opinion may be indicated.

DURATION

Each attack of pain if not relieved lasts from a few minutes to several hours. Symptoms recur until the stone is passed or removed.

COMPLICATIONS

1. Recurrences are common [70% (14 out of 20) proven cases recurred over a 4 year period].

2. Pyelonephritis.

3. Hydronephrosis or pyonephrosis may develop if the stone becomes impacted in a ureter.

4. Renal failure may develop if large stones remain indefinitely in both kidneys.

MISLEADING FEATURES AND PITFALLS

1. Small stones are easily overlooked in an X-ray picture. These small stones are especially liable to produce pain and bleeding and may be present for years.

2. Painless haematuria is a confusing but not uncommon presenting feature.

DIFFERENTIAL DIAGNOSIS

The site, character and severity of the pain, combined with haematuria, make the diagnosis straightforward in most cases. Occasionally if the stones are large, the pain is less and the picture resembles chronic pyelonephritis. A pyelogram differentiates.

MANAGEMENT OPTIONS

Prevention: (a) ensure large fluid intake especially in high risk groups; (b) avoid stone forming districts.

Established colic: (a) pethidine or Diconal — BNF 4.7.2 (Ref. 0.1) by injection, suppository or tablet; (b) monitor urine for passage of stone or blood; (c) admit or refer if pain persists or diagnosis in doubt; (d) operation occasionally indicated.

ACUTE CYSTITIS (IN ADULTS)

Classification: ICHPPC 595 (RCGP 2935)

DIAGNOSTIC RANGE (rates per 1000 patients per year)

Personal: Suspected 22.4. Probable 14.5. *National*: 20.4 (Ref. 0.2).

AGE INCIDENCE
The susceptibility increases with age (see Fig. 49).

SEX INCIDENCE
Women are especially liable (6:1).

CLINICAL POINTERS
1. High risk factors: (a) previous attacks (85% of attacks were recurrent); (b) adult women; (c) sexual intercourse; (d) pregnancy; (e) multiparity; (f) prostatic enlargement; (g) catheterisation.
2. Dysuria (85%). A burning sensation is felt in the urethra on passing water. Characteristically this pain continues for a few moments after micturition.
3. Frequency of micturition (80%) occurs by both night and day. Nocturia of recent onset suggest cystitis. Urgency also occurs.
4. Suprapubic pain and tenderness (20%).
5. Haematuria (20%). Blood may be observed with naked eye or on microscopy.
6. Fever (20%) is low or absent.
7. Pyuria (70%) is the most significant finding and confirms the clinical diagnosis in most cases.
8. Other conditions which predispose to urinary infections (20%) include chronic cervicitis, diabetes, urinary calculi, congenital abnormalities of GU tract and other obstructive lesions.

INVESTIGATIONS
1. The urine is examined routinely for pus. Microscopy and tests for protein and sugar are performed. Cultures and bacterial sensitivities may be done.
2. Intravenous pyelography, cystoscopy, retrograde pyelography and a surgical opinion are indicated after recurrent attacks or if underlying disease is suspected.

DURATION
The infection may last for weeks if not treated.

COMPLICATIONS
Recurrences are extremely common. [Two or more attacks were recorded in 85% (17 out of 20) cases followed for a 5 year period.] Recurrences are often caused by reinfection as well as failure of initial treatment.
Acute and chronic pyelonephritis.

MISLEADING FEATURES AND PITFALLS
1. Failure to examine the urine microscopically leads to many diagnostic mistakes.

2. Failure to realise that a patient has already had several attacks of urinary infection. This mistake is easily made if records are inadequate or if previous records are not consulted.

3. An unnecessary cathetarisation introduces an infection.

DIFFERENTIAL DIAGNOSIS

As for acute pyelonephritis in adults. Occasionally the dysuria which follows vaginitis or excoriation of the labia is confused with cystitis. This difficulty is avoided if the patient is questioned about the exact site of the soreness and if the labia are inspected.

MANAGEMENT OPTIONS

As for Acute upper urinary tract infections. (p. 517).

NON-SPECIFIC URETHRITIS (SEE CH. 8 p. 194)

URINARY INCONTINENCE

Classification: ICHPPC 618, 7883 (RCGP 4690)

The Family doctor encounters three types of urinary incontinence.

1. Stress incontinence affects women mainly. Onset is usually after childbirth. There is a momentary incontinence on coughing, laughing or sneezing. There may be an associated cystocele or prolapse uteri. Middle aged obese multiparae mainly affected.

The condition can be both annoying and intractable. Many minor cases often never reported. Management — surgical referral if symptomatic treatment is unacceptable.

2. Overflow incontinence may affect any individual with acute retention. The bladder can be felt above the pubic symphysis, despite the repeated and uncontrollable passage of small amounts of urine. Management — hospital referral for treatment of acute retention.

3. Senile incontinence affects elderly patients, usually with evidence of cerebral arteriosclerosis. Intractable cases are cared for at home, by means of disposable and absorbent pads. Management — catheters should be avoided at all costs. Referral to a geriatric unit is often effective with co-operative patients. The family doctor should learn the local retraining programme so that this can be reinforced at home.

DIAGNOSTIC RANGE

Difficult to assess accurately. Intractable incontinence in the elderly is said to account for the occupancy of more institutional beds than any other single complaint.

Table 28 Less common diseases of the urinary system

Disease and distinguishing clinical pointers	Incidence per 1000 patients per year Suspected	Confirmed
Carcinoma of kidney Painless haematuria, palpable renal mass, anaemia	—	1 in 10 years
Nephrotic syndrome Insidious onset; massive oedema affecting face, limbs and serous cavities; proteinuria; serum proteins; blood urea. Children affected.	—	1 in 10 years
Chronic glomerulonephritis (see also p. 510) Onset insidious, age usually over 40, history of previous kidney disease, polyuria, thirst, headaches, bleeding tendency, anaemia, hypertension, retinitis, proteinuria, uraemia, haemoglobin and blood urea estimation	—	3 in 10 years
Congenital polycystic kidneys Disease may be discovered at any age, bilateral palpable kidneys, haematuria, hypertension, retinitis, uraemia. Refer.	—	1 in 10 years
Renal dwarfism and renal rickets Chronic renal disease, dwarfism or bony deformity	—	1 in 10 years
Uraemia — see ESRD page 510 Chronic renal disease, drowsiness, vomiting, hiccup, diarrhoea, muscle twitchings, convulsions, coma, bleeding tendency, dry brown tongue, uraemic breath, blood urea and haemoglobin estimation. Refer.	—	4 in 10 years
Pyonephrosis Obstructive urinary tract lesion, loin pain, persistent fever, tender mass in flank, pyuria, leucocytosis	—	2 in 10 years
Perinephric abscess Loin pain, tenderness and swelling, fever	0	0 in 10 years
Hydronephrosis Obstructive urinary tract lesion, renal mass	0.3	0.3
Carcinoma of bladder Painless haematuria. Cytology may show malignant cells.	—	1 in 10 years
Papilloma of urinary tract Painless, intermittent, haematuria. Refer.	0.2	0.2
Urethral stricture Adult males with history of trauma or inadequately treated gonorrhoea, dysuria, poor stream, straining needed to pass urine (differentiates from prostatic obstruction), dribbling. Refer early.	—	3 in 10 years
Urethral caruncle Females, dysuria, small red area of granulation at urethral meatus. Conservative treatment.	—	2 in 10

Table 28 cont'd

Diseases and distinguishing clinical pointers	Incidence per 1000 patients per year Suspected	Confirmed
Acute retention of urine Males usually over 50, frequency and incontinence with overflow, difficult micturition, suprapubic pain and cystic mass, evidence of prostatic obstruction on rectal examination, drugs precipitate (guanethidine). Early referral.	—	4 in 10 years

20

Diseases of the male genital organs

Please read introduction for explanation of figures and analyses. The shyness, fears and taboo which exist in the lay mind concerning disease of this type occasionally cause misunderstandings or delay in reporting. The clinical problems are seldom difficult.

BENIGN HYPERTROPHY OF THE PROSTATE

Classification: ICHPPC 600 (RCGP 2960)

AETIOLOGY
The aetiology is unknown. Two hypotheses have been put forward: (a) it is a benign overgrowth; (b) it is due to androgen/oestrogen imbalance.

DIAGNOSTIC RANGE (rates per 1000 patients per year)
Personal: Suspected 1.5. Probable 0.8. *National*: 2.5 (Ref. 0.2). Recent work suggests that 80% of men over 40 have some degree of enlargement. 50% over 50 are said to have some symptoms.

AGE INCIDENCE
After the age of 50 the incidence increases steadily.

CLINICAL POINTERS

1. High risk groups — males over 50.
2. Frequency of micturition. Nocturia is the first symptom, gradually the frequency becomes diurnal and may be associated with urgency.
3. Decreasing size and force of the urinary stream.
4. Difficulty in starting (hesitancy) and stopping micturition. Urine may dribble for a little while after the patient has tried to stop urinating. Dribbling of urine causes the patient most annoyance because clothes are stained and become offensive. The symptom is due to collection of urine in the lax posterior urethra and can frequently be cured by the simple measure of teaching the patient

to 'milk' the residual urine forward from the posterior urethra every time he finishes micturition.

5. Deterioration in general health. A pool of stagnant urine collects in the bladder behind the prostate and becomes chronically infected. Ill-health follows.

6. Rectal examination. One or both lateral lobes of the prostate may be expanded by a diffuse firm (but not hard) regular swelling. The median groove is never obliterated by simple hypertrophy. In some patients the prostate feels normal in size and shape and symptoms are caused by expansion of the middle lobe or a fibrous prostatic bar inside the bladder.

7. Acute retention of urine may arise suddenly in a patient with few previous symptoms. It may be precipitated by an over distended bladder, fever, bed rest or alcohol. Clinical pointers include: suprapubic discomfort; continual desire to micturate; overflow incontinence; bladder that is palpable suprapubically and dull to percussion.

INVESTIGATIONS

1. The urine is examined routinely. Pus in the urine of an elderly male may indicate prostatic hypertrophy with infection of residual urine.

2. Pyelography and referral is indicated for patients with infection of the residual urine or persistent symptoms.

3. Acid serum phosphatase to exclude prostatic carcinoma.

DURATION

Symptoms are intermittent at first and gradually become continuous. Hesitancy is a frequent sign that may indicate the need for operation.

COMPLICATIONS

Chronic basal cystitis; hydronephrosis; acute retention; uraemia and death may then follow. Increased libido, with resultant misdemeanours, is occasionally associated with hypertrophy — probably a result not of the hypertrophy, but of the hormonal changes associated with it.

MISLEADING FEATURES AND PITFALLS

Carcinoma of prostate may present with the clinical picture of benign hypertrophy. The doctor may delay referral to a surgeon because the condition is thought to be benign. Routine investigation of the acid serum phosphatase indicates metastatic spread and may help to avoid this mistake. A normal test does not rule out malignant prostatic disease.

DIFFERENTIAL DIAGNOSIS

In the early case with slight hypertrophy and transient symptoms, the diagnosis may be difficult, but it is rarely in doubt when the disease is fully developed.

Diseases that may be confused with benign prostatic hypertrophy:

Acute cystitis

Similar features: frequency; dysuria; difficult micturition; pyuria.

Distinguishing features: symptoms are transient and improve with treatment; prostate is not enlarged; differentiation may be difficult because the diseases may be associated.

Carcinoma of prostate

Similar features: frequency; dysuria; difficult micturition.

Distinguishing features: normal architecture of prostate is altered; median groove is obliterated; gland may be hard and craggy; early secondary deposits in the bones may be visible on X-ray; raised acid serum phosphatase; operation or biopsy may be indicated.

MISTAKES AND PITFALLS

The following commonly used drugs may aggravate the condition: (a) anticholinergics — BNF 1.2 (Ref. 0.1); (b) ephedrine — BNF 3.1 and 1.2; (c) tricyclics (BNF 4.3.1) and MOAI (BNF 4.3.2) antidepressants.

MANAGEMENT OPTIONS

Early disease: Initially symptoms may be controlled by (a) emptying posterior urethra after passing water (see above); (b) limited fluid intake before retiring; (c) discuss future; (d) stress that surgery will not affect libido.

Indications for referral: (a) marked hesitancy; (b) embarrassing dribbling; (c) rapid progression of symptoms; (d) evidence of kidney or bladder infection; (e) acute retention or its possibility; (f) possible malignant disease or renal damage.

PHIMOSIS

Classification: ICHPPC 605 (RCGP 2985)

The orifice of the prepuce is unduly small and retraction of the foreskin over the glans penis is impossible. The disorder is congenital and may lead to balanitis. In babies stretching the orifice with a pair of Spencer-Wells forceps usually enables the foreskin to be fully retracted. Circumcision is occasionally indicated.

DIAGNOSTIC RANGE (rates per 1000 patients per year)
Personal: Probable 2.3. Diagnosis rarely in doubt.

PARAPHIMOSIS

Classification: ICHPPC 605 (RCGP 2985)

A disorder that arises in toddlers if a tight foreskin is allowed to remain retracted. The small preputial orifice acts as a constricting tourniquet behind the glans penis. The portions of foreskin and penis distal to the constriction become rapidly oedematous, making it difficult or impossible to pull the foreskin forward again. The resulting cherry-like swelling at the tip of the child's penis may stimulate a worried parent to put in an urgent call couched in mysterious or euphemistic terms. Circumcision usually indicated.

DIAGNOSTIC RANGE (rates per 1000 patients per year)
Personal: Probable 0.2. Diagnosis rarely in doubt.

MALE INFERTILITY

Classification: ICHPPC 606 (RCGP 2990)

This disorder is discovered during routine investigation of subfertility. Causes may be as follows:

1. Aspermia or oligospermia. The production of sperms is absent or under average as a result of cryptorchism, mumps and other infections.
2. Impotence. Psychological or congenital deformities may be responsible. Other causes such as alcoholism, depression, diabetes, etc. must be excluded (See p. 262).
3. Obstructions in the vas deferens. Gonorrhoea is usually responsible.

DIAGNOSTIC RANGE (rates per 1000 patients per year)
Personal: Suspected 0.6. Oligospermia and not aspermia was present in most cases and it is of interest that half the patients considered to be subfertile on the evidence of sperm counts eventually conceived successfully.

MISLEADING FEATURES AND PITFALLS
These patients may want advice or help about artificial insemination and the family doctor should know his own mind on this subject.

MANAGEMENT OPTIONS

Prevention: measures controlling spread of gonorrhoea (p. 191) may prevent some cases.

Suspected cases: semen to laboratory.

Established sperm deficiency: (a) full discussion alone and then with spouse; (b) counter guilt reactions; (c) discuss with couple long term i.e. adoption, A.I. Donor, etc.

Probable (psychological): (a) counselling alone and with partner; (b) encourage enjoyment of physical contact without intercourse; (c) short period of abstinence; (d) general sex education — Sex Problems (for patients) in Reader's Digest Family Medical Adviser (Ref. 0.3); (e) squeeze technique for premature ejaculation; (f) referral.

ULCERS OF PREPUCE AND URETHRAL MEATUS

Classification: ICHPPC 607 (RCGP 3000)

Toddlers and babies frequently spend the night soaked in ammoniacal urine, ulceration of the prepuce or urethral meatus may arise and is managed as a nappy rash.

BALANITIS

Classification: ICHPPC 605 (RCGP 2995)

The space between the foreskin and the penis becomes infected.

DIAGNOSTIC RANGE (rates per 1000 patients per year)

Personal: 3.1 Diagnosis rarely in doubt.

CLINICAL POINTERS

1. Soreness of the penis, especially when the foreskin is retracted.
2. Discharge usually profuse, occasionally slight.
3. Excoriation and redness of foreskin or glans penis.

DURATION

Untreated the infection may persist for long periods.

MISLEADING FEATURES AND PITFALLS

1. Balanitis is sometimes an early sign of diabetes mellitus. In these cases the discharge is usually slight.

2. An acute gonococcal urethritis or primary chancre may be overlooked because the doctor is reluctant to examine the penis of a patient with balanitis or urethral discharge.

MANAGEMENT OPTIONS

Prevention: circumcision prevents, but is only advised if there are other reasons.

Established disease: (a) exclude serious disease; (b) local cleansing and antibiotics; (c) circumcision occasionally indicated.

Table 29 Less common disease of the male genital organs

Disease and distinguishing clinical pointers	Incidence per 1000 patients per year Suspected	Confirmed
Carcinoma of prostate Symptoms of prostatism, hard prostate with median groove obliterated, acid serum phosphatase raised if metastasised.	—	2 in 10 years
Acute prostatitis Middle-aged males; sensation of perineal heaviness; dysuria; frequency slight or absent; fever or rigor; on rectal examination prostate is tender and boggy, seminal vesicles tender and enlarged; urethral smear contains pus after prostatic massage; urethroscopy. Referral usual.	0.4	0.2
Hydrocele Painless fluctuant cystic swelling in scrotum, upper pole can be defined and thus distinguished from hernia, swelling transilluminates. Infants and elderly males affected. Tapping. Surgery.	0.8	0.8
Acute epididymo-orchitis Recent urinary tract infection or instrumentation, fever, rigors, scrotal pain that radiates to the flank, tender swelling of one epididymis (and testis). Antibiotics with supporting strap.	0.8	0.8
Incomplete descent of testes The testes of babies should be examined routinely at birth and boys at other suitable opportunities to exclude this disorder. Refer — before 6 years, operate before 12, to achieve fertility.	0.5	0.5
Mastitis of puberty in boys Tender hard disc (2 to 3 cm diam.) under one or both nipples; transient, lasts for 2 to 6 months. Reassurance only indicated.	0.4	0.4

21

Diseases of the female genital organs

Please read the introduction for explanation of figures and analyses.

CARCINOMA OF BREAST

Classification: ICHPPC 174 (RCGP 0465)

AETIOLOGY

Unknown. Epidemiology suggests several possible causes: genetic, socio-economic, hormonal and dietary; from a family doctor's view point the last three may have some relevance (see high risk factors below).

The commonest cancer in women; many cases are curable, but despite advances in diagnostic and therapeutic skills the survival rates are the same as 50 years ago. This suggests that prognosis is more dependent on the type of cancer than on early diagnosis.

DIAGNOSTIC RANGE (rates per 1000 patients per year)

Personal: Suspected 1.2. Proven 1.1. *National*: 1.1 (Ref. 0.2)

AGE INCIDENCE

Women of menopausal age are especially liable. Cancer of the breast occurs but is uncommon in women under 35 years.

CLINICAL POINTERS

1. High risk factors: (a) previous cancer of breast or elsewhere; (b) positive family history; (c) childlessness or first child after 30; (d) late menopause; (e) low socio-economic groups; (f) high fat/low fibre diets may predispose.

2. A lump in the breast (100%). Any lump is suspect and should be referred for surgical opinion. The observation that a lump cannot be felt with the flat of the hand in no way rules out carcinoma.

3. The quadrant of breast. 60% of malignant growths arise in the upper outer quadrant or axillary tail.
4. The following classical signs develop late:
   - Axillary node enlargement.
   - Retraction of the nipple.
   - Pain. An occasional ache or tenderness. Pain at period times usually suggests a benign origin.
   - Involvement of the muscle and skin. The growth spreads locally and is fixed to pectoralis major and skin (peau d'orange).
   - Discharge from nipple. (A blood stained discharge suggests either duct papilloma or duct carcinoma.)
   - Evidence of distant metastases, e.g., pathological fractures.
   - Systemic symptoms, e.g. anorexia and loss of weight.

INVESTIGATIONS

Removal with histological examination of the lump. Self examination, thermography and mammography (X-rays) have been extensively used as screening routines. These may increase survival rates but evidence is lacking.

DURATION

The prognosis with treatment is fairly good. The patient with inoperable carcinoma dies 1 to 2½ years after onset.

COMPLICATIONS

Recurrences in the remaining breast are not unusual. Metastases in bones or brain may develop.

MISLEADING FEATURES AND PITFALLS

The family doctor may be lulled into a false sense of security because:

1. A lump seems to decrease in size at consecutive examinations.
2. The youthful age of the patient raises doubt about the diagnosis.
3. Previous removal of benign growths.

DIFFERENTIAL DIAGNOSIS

All lumps in the breast, which persist for 14 days or more, should be regarded as malignant until proved otherwise by removal.

Different types of breast carcinoma occur at different ages and have different prognoses:

— Scirrhus (66%): mainly in middle-age. Prognosis often fair to good.

— Anaplastic medullary (18%): 25 to 35 years and especially in large breasts. Prognosis poor.
— Duct carcinoma (8%): middle-age.
— Mastitis carcinoma (2%): with pregnancy.
— Paget's disease of nipple (1%): over 50.

MANAGEMENT OPTIONS

Prevention: despite inconclusive evidence two preventive measures should be considered (a) using every opportunity to encourage and teach women over 35 to make regular examination of their breasts; (b) encourage high fibre diets.

Established lumps: referral within 14 days.

Treated cases: (a) discuss prosthesis; (b) encourage patient to ask the significant questions about diagnosis and prognosis; (c) encourage patient, family and friends to have an optimistic attitude; (d) self help groups often helpful (Mastectomy Association — Ref. 21.1) (e) tactful follow up; (f) general measures discussed in chapter 9 — page 207 *et seq*.

CHRONIC MASTITIS, FIBROADENOSIS, CYSTIC DISEASE AND OTHER PERSISTENT LUMPS IN THE BREAST

Classification: ICHPPC 610 (RCGP 3020)

Attempts to differentiate clinically between benign and malignant tumours of the breast eventually lead to disaster and unnecessary loss of life.

There is one rigid rule for all tumours of the breast:

Every lump in a breast is observed for not more than 14 days; the patient is referred for a surgical opinion if the lump is still present at the end of this time.

ACUTE MASTITIS

Classification: ICHPPC 611 (associated with pregnancy 676) (RCGP 3025, 3460)

Acute mastitis is usually associated with lactation and is difficult to distinguish from an early breast abscess. During lactation it is probably a wise policy to regard every patient with evidence of inflammation in a breast as having a potential breast abscess.

AETIOLOGY

One of the mammary ducts becomes blocked and the segment of breast which it drains becomes infected. *Staph. aureus* is usually responsible. Both blockage and infection are especially liable to occur during lactation.

DIAGNOSTIC INCIDENCE

Minor degrees of mastitis are common and may not even be reported to the doctor. As the infection progresses it is difficult to distinguish from a breast abscess. Figures for incidence, based on clinical findings are therefore inaccurate.

CLINICAL POINTERS

1. Lactation.
2. Pain in the breast may be severe.
3. Cellulitis of breast. A segment becomes hard, red, swollen and acutely tender. Often a relatively late occurrence.
4. Fever is common.

COMPLICATIONS

Breast abscess.

MISTAKES, PITFALLS AND MANAGEMENT OPTIONS

See Breast Abscess.

HORMONAL MASTITIS

Classification: ICHPPC 611 (RCGP 3030)

A tender lumpiness of one or both breasts may arise during early pregnancy, occasionally at period times, at the menopause, or at puberty when it affects boys as well as girls. The condition settles in a few weeks.

BREAST ABSCESS

Classification: ICHPPC 611 (pregnancy 676) (RCGP 3025, 3460)

AETIOLOGY

As for acute mastitis.

DIAGNOSTIC RANGE

0.3 to 0.5 per 1000 patients per year. This is equivalent to 1.0 per 50 pregnancies.

CLINICAL POINTERS

1. Lactation. 80% of acute mastitis and abscesses develop in the first months of lactation.
2. Persistent severe pain; often an early sign.
3. Persistent cellulitis of breast. Tenderness, redness and indu-

ration lasting more than a day suggest abscess formation. Red overlying skin appears late — a result of infection deep in the breast.

4. Fever may be present.

DURATION

The abscess in its early stages may clear up with antibiotic treatment. Often it progresses steadily for a few days until thorough surgical drainage is required.

COMPLICATIONS

Recurrences are common with subsequent lactation.

MISLEADING FEATURES AND PITFALLS

1. The classical signs of inflammation and abscess formation become apparent late, and abscess formation is overlooked.
2. The infection can arise in a breast which is not lactating.
3. The possibility of a mastitis carcinoma is not considered.

MANAGEMENT OPTIONS

Prevention: (a) adequate preparation and hardening of nipples in antenatal period; (b) adequate support of mother in early lactation; (c) early antibiotics — BNF 5.1 (Ref. 0.1) for mastitis.

Established mastitis: (a) support breast; (b) early antibiotics — BNF 5.1; (c) continue breast feeding if possible.

Established abscess: refer early for surgery.

ACUTE SALPINGITIS

Classification: ICHPPC 614 (RCGP 3035)

The disease enters into the differential diagnosis of both acute appendicitis and tubal pregnancy. Although still relatively uncommon it must be frequently considered because of the increasing incidence of venereal disease.

AETIOLOGY

The infection may follow pregnancy, gonorrhoea, septic abortion, or operations on the uterus. Infection without obvious cause occurs.

DIAGNOSTIC RANGE (rates per 1000 patients per year)

Personal: Suspected 0.3. Probable 0.1. *National*: 1.1 (Ref. 0.2) — includes chronic salpingitis.

AGE INCIDENCE

Women of child-bearing age liable.

CLINICAL POINTERS

1. High risk factors: (a) recent abortion or termination; (b) recent delivery; (c) Possibility of Sexually transmitted disease — page 190.

2. Bilateral or unilateral lower abdominal pain; tenderness may be diffuse, central or in one iliac fossa; pain may be intermittent or continuous; it is often associated with rebound tenderness and, unlike appendicitis, may build up over 2 or 3 days before it is reported.

3. Vaginal discharge of recent onset.

4. Intense pain on moving the cervix uteri during vaginal examination. This is a very suggestive sign but it also occurs with a tubal pregnancy.

5. Fever is usually high (38° to 39.5°C).

6. Treatment should start before tubal enlargement occurs.

DURATION

The inflammation tends to settle in a few days with conservative treatment and antibiotics.

COMPLICATIONS

Chronic salpingitis, pyosalpinx and infertility.

MISLEADING FEATURES AND PITFALLS

Menstrual irregularities are often associated with acute salpingitis and confusion with a tubal pregnancy may occur.

DIFFERENTIAL DIAGNOSIS

The disease is easily confused with appendicitis, ectopic pregnancy and other acute abdominal conditions. Acute salpingitis is comparatively uncommon and usually settles after the acute phase; the diagnosis should therefore only be made after exclusion of other acute abdominal conditions which are more likely and require immediate operation.

MANAGEMENT OPTIONS

Prevention: case finding and early treatment in high risk groups.

Established disease: (a) Exclude other disease requiring emergency operation; (b) bed rest; (c) antibiotics — BNF 5.1 (Ref. 0.1); (d) analgesics — BNF 4.7 if diagnosis is certain.

CHRONIC SALPINGITIS

Classification: ICHPPC 614 (RCGP 3035)

AETIOLOGY

A true chronic salpingitis with pyosalpinx is surprisingly rare. More commonly a diagnosis of chronic salpingitis is made in a woman of childbearing age to explain a recurring pain of moderate severity in the lower abdominal or sacral areas. Varying degrees of chronic pelvic inflammatory disease undoubtedly occur but in most instances the diagnosis is hard to substantiate.

DIAGNOSTIC RANGE (rates per 1000 patients per year)

Personal: Probable 0.1 + *National* 1.1 (Ref. 0.2) — includes acute salpingitis.

AGE INCIDENCE

Childbearing age, usually over 30.

CLINICAL POINTERS

1. High risk groups: as for acute salpingitis.
2. Insidious onset.
3. Chronically recurring pain of varying severity in lower abdomen and low back.
4. Pain may be worse just before or during periods.
5. Dyspareunia.
6. Vaginal discharge said to be present.
7. Cervix tender on vaginal examination with palpable tender tubes.

INVESTIGATIONS

Laparoscopy may be helpful. Leukocytosis sometimes present.

MISLEADING FEATURES AND PITFALLS

1. The diagnosis is incorrectly used to explain a recurrent low back or abdominal pain. As a result after repeated failure of antibiotics, surgical intervention may be advised. The physician should remember that there is a four-fold increase in the incidence of depression within 3 years of a hysterectomy.

2. Chronic tuberculous salpingitis is not common but should be remembered because it is treatable.

DIFFERENTIAL DIAGNOSIS

Similar to endometriosis but the diagnosis should always be used with caution.

MANAGEMENT OPTIONS

Prevention: as for acute salpingitis.

Established disease: Often unsatisfactory because diagnosis uncertain. Conservative treatment if possible. Avoid referral when possible.

OVARIAN TUMOURS

CLASSIFICATION

Ovarian tumours are classified, as follows, according to their pathology, unfortunately this does not help their early recognition:

1. Retention cysts, i.e. dilated glandular structures, are common but rarely large (ICHPPC 629, RCGP 3065).

2. Neoplastic cysts may grow to an enormous size and their contents are either serous or pseudomucinous. Histology reveals that they can be benign or malignant (ICHPPC 180, RCGP 0480 — malignant; ICHPPC 229, RCGP 0565 — benign).

3. Dermoid cysts — benign or malignant.

4. Solid ovarian tumours — benign or malignant.

5. Para-ovarian cysts arise in the broad ligament. They are rarely large but are liable to torsion.

A clinical classification of ovarian tumours is of greater practical value to the family doctor.

- Small ovarian cysts and tumours that produce symptoms which are localised to the pelvic organs.
- Ovarian and para-ovarian tumours that twist, and present as an acute abdomen.
- Ovarian cysts that are silent until their large size produces symptoms of pressure and displacement in the abdomen.

SMALL OVARIAN TUMOURS THAT PRODUCE SYMPTOMS WHICH ARE LOCALISED TO THE PELVIC ORGANS

These tumours are usually harmless retention cysts but should be referred for a surgical opinion to exclude malignancy.

DIAGNOSTIC RANGE (rates per 1000 patients per year)

Personal: Suspected 1.0. Probable 0.7.

AGE INCIDENCE

Women of menstrual age are liable to develop the common retention cyst. Malignant primary ovarian tumours tend to arise after the age of 50, but younger age groups are occasionally affected. Secondary metastatic ovarian tumours are said to arise in younger women.

CLINICAL POINTERS

1. Gradual onset (80%).

2. Intermittent lower abdominal pain (100%). A dull ache that is situated in one iliac fossa or the suprapubic region. Occasionally the pain is felt in the groin or in the rectum.

3. Relationship of the pain to the menstrual cycle (70%). A characteristic and useful distinguishing feature. Pain may be related to a period or ovulation time. Menstrual irregularities are uncommon.

4. Dyspareunia is a less constant but suggestive sign.

5. Palpable pelvic mass (70%). A rounded tender mobile mass is felt in the pouch of Douglas or in one fornix. A rectal as well as vaginal examination is helpful.

DURATION

Small benign ovarian cysts may persist for years without symptoms. Malignant ovarian tumours may progress rapidly.

COMPLICATIONS

These include torsion, rupture and malignancy.

MISLEADING FEATURES AND PITFALLS

The pain and discomfort from a small ovarian cyst is overlooked because it is regarded by patient and doctor as a part of the normal menstrual cycle.

DIFFERENTIAL DIAGNOSIS

Diseases that may be confused with small ovarian cysts:

Acute appendicitis

Similar features: recurrent attacks of lower abdominal pain; tenderness in RIF.

Distinguishing features: differentiation often difficult; attacks not related to menstrual cycle; pelvic examination fails to reveal ovarian tumour.

Ovulation syndrome

Similar features: recurrent attacks of lower abdominal pain; tenderness in lower abdomen and on pelvic examination; relationship of pain to ovulation time.

Distinguishing features: differentiation often difficult; pelvic examination fails to reveal ovarian tumour; pain is associated with ovulation but not with periods.

Endometriosis (and chocolate cyst)
Similar features: recurrent attacks of lower abdominal pain and tenderness; relationship of pain to period and defaecation; dyspareunia; ovarian or pelvic mass.

Distinguishing features: differentiation difficult; often only possible at operation or laparoscopy; pain sometimes severe.

TWISTED OVARIAN TUMOUR

Small tumours and cysts — especially para-ovarian cysts which arise from structures in the broad ligament — are liable to twist and produce a characteristic acute abdominal syndrome.

DIAGNOSTIC RANGE (rates per 1000 patients per year)
Personal: Suspected 0.7. Probable 0.3.

CLINICAL POINTERS

1. Sudden onset.
2. Severe lower abdominal pain situated centrally or in one iliac fossa. The pain is usually intermittent and occasionally radiates through to the buttocks or rectum.
3. Vomiting is common.
4. A low fever may cause confusion with acute appendicitis.
5. A tender smooth round swelling is felt in the pelvis. The mass usually lies in the pouch of Douglas and is therefore best examined per rectum.
6. Menstrual irregularities and a constant relationship of attacks to the menstrual cycle are uncommon.

DURATION
The disorder may progress until signs of pelvic peritonitis indicate the need for operation. Sometimes the cyst untwists and the symptoms suddenly cease.

COMPLICATIONS
Recurrences are common if the cyst is not removed.
Rupture and gangrene are said to occur.

DIFFERENTIAL DIAGNOSIS
Diseases that may be confused with a twisted ovarian cyst:

Acute appendicitis

Similar features: recurring attacks of acute abdominal pain; tenderness in RIF; vomiting; low fever; frequency of micturition.

Distinguishing features: pelvic examination fails to reveal the characteristic smooth tender mass; admission to hospital indicated.

Twisted or degenerating fibroid

Similar features: sudden onset; severe lower abdominal pain; tender mass in pelvis; attacks may suddenly stop and later recur.

Distinguishing features: the tender pelvic mass is part of the uterus; admission to hospital indicated.

Ectopic tubal pregnancy

Similar features: intermittent severe lower abdominal pain and tenderness; low fever; tenderness in pouch of Douglas.

Distinguishing features: menstrual irregularities and signs of early pregnancy; brown or red vaginal discharge; vaginal examination reveals acutely tender cervix; ovarian mass absent; tubal mass may be felt; admission to hospital indicated. Pregnancy tests positive.

Endometriosis

May simulate a twisted cyst, when the pain is not related to the period.

MANAGEMENT OPTIONS

Suspected: early referral for surgery

LARGE OVARIAN CYSTS

Diagnostic range (rates per 1000 patients per year)

Personal: Proven 0.2.

AGE INCIDENCE

Women aged 30 to 60 are liable.

CLINICAL POINTERS

1. Swelling of the abdomen is noticed by the patient.

2. Pressure symptoms include dyspnoea, frequency and oedema of ankles.

3. A large cystic abdominal mass is distinguished from obesity, ascites, pregnancy and other pelvic tumours by palpation and bimanual examination. Percussion reveals peripheral abdominal resonance.

4. Menstrual irregularities are often associated but are probably coincidental because cysts are common about the menopause.

DURATION

Symptomless cysts may grow slowly for years.

COMPLICATIONS

Rupture and torsion are said to occur.

MISLEADING FEATURES AND PITFALLS

A large ovarian cyst may be ignored by both patient and doctor because the symptoms are ascribed to obesity.

Such cysts may be malignant.

PROLAPSED OVARY

Classification: ICHPPC 629 (RCGP 3070)

Normal ovaries, like the testes, are tender to pressure and an ovary which slips down into the pelvis may cause pelvic pain, low backache and dyspareunia. Symptoms are especially prominent during ovulation or menstruation. Conservative management advised.

CHRONIC CERVICITIS

Classification: ICHPPC 622 (RCGP 3040)

Chronic cervicitis and cervical erosion are probably closely related. The aetiology, symptomatology and management are the same.

The condition is often associated with a recurrent cystitis and occasionally with dyspareunia.

Cervical biopsy is the only certain way of making this diagnosis.

CERVICAL EROSION

Classification: ICHPPC 622 (RCGP 3075)

Comparatively little is known about this common disorder. Cervical erosions are said to be present in 85% of all women but such statements are difficult to confirm.

AETIOLOGY

Cervical erosions are mainly noted in women who have borne children.

DIAGNOSTIC RANGE (rates per 1000 patients per year)
Personal: Suspected 6.9+. Many erosions go undiscovered because they are symptomless.

AGE INCIDENCE
Women of child-bearing age.

CLINICAL POINTERS
1. Typical cervical lesion (100%). Inspection of the cervix with a vaginal speculum reveals the characteristic red granulating appearance at the cervical os. The lesion is covered with epithelium from the cervical canal.
2. Low back pain (65%). A dull ache in the lumbosacral region.
3. Low abdominal pain. A dull ache in either iliac fossa.
4. Vaginal discharge (30%). A yellow, green or brown vaginal discharge may be noted. It is probably due to an associated chronic cervicitis and is sometimes observed draining from the cervical canal.

INVESTIGATIONS
A cervical smear should be taken for bacteriology as well as cytology.

DURATION
A cervical erosion persists indefinitely unless treated.

COMPLICATIONS
Women with a cervical erosion are prone to cystitis. [Cystitis was noted in 30% (six out of 20) consecutive cases of cervical erosion that were followed for 3 years.]

MISLEADING FEATURES AND PITFALLS
1. The significance of cervical erosion is difficult to assess because it is not known how often it is present without symptoms.
2. Cervical carcinoma is mistaken for cervical erosion.

DIFFERENTIAL DIAGNOSIS
A cervical smear is indicated and differentiates the disorder from carcinoma.

MANAGEMENT OPTIONS
Established erosion: essentially conservative. Cautery may be used.

CARCINOMA OF UTERINE CERVIX

Classification: ICHPPC 180 (RCGP 0470)

The prognosis for this type of carcinoma is fairly good provided that treatment is started early.

AETIOLOGY

Multiparous women are more susceptible than nullipara. Epidemiology suggests an association with: (a) parity; (b) increased promiscuity. Cervical malignancy and premalignancy are therefore often regarded as sexually transmitted diseases. There may be a relationship with genital herpes.

DIAGNOSTIC RANGE (rates per 1000 patients per year)

Personal: Suspected 0.5. Probable 0.2. *National*: 0.6 (Ref. 0.2).

AGE INCIDENCE

Post-menopausal women are most susceptible, but younger women are liable especially if parity is great. The average age of presentation is falling, e.g. from 50 in 1967 to 35 in 1977 in one survey.

CLINICAL POINTERS

1. High risk factors: (a) coitus at an early age; (b) coitus with many partners; (c) use of non-barrier contraceptives; (d) multiparity.

2. Vaginal haemorrhage. In post-menopausal women the slightest loss of blood from the vagina is always suggestive of carcinoma. Before the menopause the loss may be confused with the periods. Careful questioning usually reveals the separate origin of the blood. In carcinoma of the cervix the bleeding occurs irregularly between periods, after intercourse, defaecation, or after vaginal examination. Loss is rarely heavy.

3. Vaginal discharge may be the first sign of carcinoma of cervix and may precede vaginal haemorrhage by several months. It is usually offensive and mucopurulent but may be clear and watery or brown.

4. Pain is a late symptom and is likely to confuse rather than clarify the diagnosis.

5. Vaginal examination.

• Bimanual examination reveals the mobility of the cervix. A fixed cervix always suggests carcinoma but is a late sign. An irregular cervix is usually due to child-bearing, but may be a late sign of carcinoma. The spread of a growth to the vaginal walls may occasionally be noted.

• With a vaginal speculum. Carcinoma should be suspected when the cervix bleeds after inspection with a duck-billed speculum. Large unhealthy cervical erosions sometimes bleed in this way. All lesions which bleed are referred to a gynaecologist for a second opinion. A cervical growth that can be clearly diagnosed with a vaginal speculum is usually far advanced.

SPECIAL INVESTIGATION

1. Cervical smears are examined for malignant cells.
2. Referral for possible cone biopsy in all doubtful cases.

DURATION AND COMPLICATIONS

An untreated carcinoma progresses steadily to death in 12 to 24 months. For the purpose of assessing prognosis, four stages of development are recognised:

Stage I. Prognosis very good — only the cervix is affected. It is freely mobile. This group includes premalignancy (cancer in situ).

Stage II. Prognosis moderately good — affects cervix, parametria, broad ligament and upper vagina, but the growth has not extended to the pelvic walls. The cervix is still mobile.

Stage III. Prognosis poor — the growth has spread to the pelvic walls or lower vagina. The cervix is fixed.

Stage IV. Prognosis bad — evidence of distant metastases or spread to bladder, rectum or structures outside the pelvis. The cervix is fixed.

MISLEADING FEATURES AND PITFALLS

1. It is easy to confuse the haemorrhage of cervical carcinoma with menstrual irregularities from other causes.

2. Hormonal replacement therapy for symptoms of the menopause may lead to withdrawal bleeding when oestrogens are stopped. Bleeding from a uterine carcinoma is overlooked.

3. Women are reluctant to be examined vaginally. If they are also losing blood per vagina they may fail to report back for examination.

4. Women of high parity and low income are most prone, yet they are often least able to report for examination or cervical smears.

5. Questions about previous sexual promiscuity though relevant, can cause much guilt and suffering.

DIFFERENTIAL DIAGNOSIS

Diseases that may be confused with carcinoma of the cervix:

Dysfunctional uterine haemorrhage
Similar features: irregular vaginal loss in women approaching the menopause; vaginal examination may be normal.

Distinguishing features: periods are heavy and intermenstrual loss is usually continuous with the period; post-coital bleeding absent; vaginal examination reveals a bulky uterus with normal cervix; distinction may be impossible without cervical biopsy.

Uterine fibroids
Similar features: irregular vaginal loss in women approaching the menopause.

Distingusihing features: loss between periods uncommon; periods are heavy; post-coital bleeding absent; vaginal examination reveals uterus expanded by the fibroid; gynaecological opinion indicated.

Cervical erosion and chronic cervicitis
Similar features: vaginal loss following coitus and vaginal examination; vaginal discharge.

Distinguishing features: all women of child-bearing age liable; gynaecological opinion indicated in doubtful cases; cervical smear negative.

MANAGEMENT OPTIONS

Prevention: (a) avoidance of high risk factors of promiscuity; (b) barrier contraceptives sometimes indicated; (c) Cervical screening and case finding programmes are being aimed at progressively younger age groups. Many family planning clinics check routinely. All women over 35 (possibly 30) should be checked regularly every 3 to 5 years.

Established disease or premalignancy: immediate referral.

Treated patients: (a) encourage patients to ask the significant questions about the diagnosis and prognosis; (b) encourage patient, family and friends to look forward; (c) self-help group helpful; (d) regular follow up (see p. 207 *et seq*.).

CARCINOMA OF THE BODY OF THE UTERUS

Classification: ICHPPC 180 (RCGP 0475)

AETIOLOGY

Unknown. Post-menopausal women are mainly affected. Nulliparous women are especially liable. Strong epidemiological associations have been noted with obesity and to a lesser extent with early menarche, late menopause, maturity onset (NIDD) diabetes and hypertension.

In the USA recent increased incidence may possibly be related to increased prescribing of oestrogens post menopausally (HRT).

DIAGNOSTIC RANGE (rates per 1000 patients per year)
Personal: Suspected 0.2. Proven 0.

AGE INCIDENCE
A peak of incidence is said to occur in the mid-fifties. Only a small proportion of cases arise in women under 50.

CLINICAL POINTERS

1. High risk factors: (a) post menopause; (b) nullipara, (c) obesity and maturity onset diabetes; (d) prolonged hormone replacement therapy (HRT) after menopause (not proven).
2. Vaginal haemorrhage.
3. A brown offensive discharge.
4. Vaginal examination may reveal an expanded uterus and blood may be seen emerging from the cervical os.

INVESTIGATIONS
A diagnostic curettage is indicated in all suspected cases.

DURATION
The prognosis of the treated case is good provided that the disease is diagnosed reasonably early.

MISLEADING FEATURES AND PITFALLS
Unmarried nulliparous patients may be reluctant to be examined. They can be referred straight to a gynaecologist.

DIFFERENTIAL DIAGNOSIS
Similar to that for carcinoma of the cervix uteri.

MANAGEMENT OPTIONS

Prevention: The disorder is rare and epidemiological associations are unproven. Avoidance of high risk factors therefore justified on general grounds only. Screening programmes are inappropriate.

Established disease: as for Cervical Carcinoma (See p. 549).

UTERINE FIBROIDS

Classification: ICHPPC 218 (RCGP 0560)

A benign fibromyoma of the uterine muscle.

AETIOLOGY
Unknown. Fibroids atrophy after the menopause suggesting that oestrogens may be a cause of both the atrophy and the carcinoma of uterine body that is occasionally associated with it.

DIAGNOSTIC RANGE (rates per 1000 patients per year)
Personal: Suspected 1.9. Probable 0.3. *National*: 1.0 (Ref. 0.2).

AGE INCIDENCE
30 to 50 years.

CLINICAL POINTERS
1. High risk factors: (a) nulliparity; (b) previous myomata.
2. Menorrhagia (75%). The patient may delay reporting to the doctor for many months. Metrorrhagia is uncommon and suggests a submucous fibroid or carcinoma of uterus.
3. Uterine enlargement or mass (65%). The tumour is felt on bimanual vaginal examination as an irregular or diffuse expansion of the uterus. Large tumours can be felt abdominally.
4. Pain (45%) is a late sign which sometimes brings the patient to the doctor. It is rarely severe and may be pelvic or sciatic. Dysmenorrhoea may occur.
5. Anaemia. Simple hypochromic anaemia may be marked after prolonged menorrhagia.

INVESTIGATIONS
1. Haemoglobin estimation.
2. Inspection of cervix and vaginal vault by speculum in conjunction with bimanual pelvic examination.
3. Diagnostic dilatation and curettage.

DURATION
Myomata may be present for many years.

COMPLICATIONS
Hypochromic anaemia. Red degeneration and sarcomatous changes are said to occur.

MISLEADING FEATURES AND PITFALLS
1. Confusion with pregnancy.
2. The bleeding from a carcinoma of uterus is overlooked.
3. A hysterectomy is performed when a more conservative operation is preferred by the patient.

DIFFERENTIAL DIAGNOSIS
Diseases that may be confused with uterine myomata:

Pregnancy
Similar feature: expansion of uterus.

Distinguishing features: menorrhagia unlikely; vomiting and breast changes; pregnancy tests positive.

Threatened or complete abortion
Similar features: expansion of uterus; continued or excessive loss; pregnancy tests may be negative (if abortion is complete).

Distinguishing features: prolonged loss unlikely; vomiting and breast changes indicate pregnancy; pregnancy tests may be positive; hospital investigation may be indicated.

Metropathia haemorrhagica (dysfunctional uterine haemorrhage)
Similar features: menorrhagia; bulky uterus.

Distinguishing features: prolonged bleeding common; hospital investigation indicated.

Endometriosis
Similar features: menorrhagia; bulky uterus.

Distinguishing features: long history common; dyspareunia; rectal pain or bleeding; pelvic mass; hospital investigation may be indicated.

Carcinoma uterus
Similar features: menorrhagia; bulky uterus.

Distinguishing features: metrorrhagia more likely than menorrhagia; hospital investigation indicated.

MANAGEMENT OPTIONS

Established myomata: referral re conservative treatment (myomectomy) and hysterectomy. The family physician is wise to discuss appropriate options with patient before referral.

VULVO-VAGINITIS IN CHILDREN

Classification: ICHPPC 6161 (RCGP 3045)

AETIOLOGY

The infection is usually non-specific. Gonococcal epidemic infections are said to occur in schools and institutions. Masturbation, bacteria, monilia and threadworm infestations are precipitating factors.

DIAGNOSTIC RANGE (rates per 1000 patients per year)
Personal: Suspected 1.8.

AGE INCIDENCE

Girls before the menarche are liable. Two-thirds of cases occurred between the ages of 5 and 12.

CLINICAL POINTERS

1. High risk factors: (a) monilia; (b) threadworm; (c) foreign bodies.
2. Irritation or soreness of the vulva.
3. Slight vaginal discharge.
4. Redness of vulva is always present.

DURATION

The untreated case may persist.

COMPLICATIONS

Recurrences may occur but are not common.

MISLEADING FEATURES AND PITFALLS

The association with a threadworm infestation may be overlooked.

MANAGEMENT OPTIONS

Established disease: (a) exclude and treat bacteria, thrush, threadworms and foreign bodies; (b) general hygiene; (c) cotton panties; (d) local oestrogen creams — BNF 7.2.1 (Ref. 0.1) if above, ineffective after 14 days.

VAGINITIS IN WOMEN

Classification: ICHPPC 6161 (RCGP 3045)

AETIOLOGY

Vaginitis may be caused directly or indirectly by many different high risk factors (see below), which are often difficult to identify with certainty.

DIAGNOSTIC RANGE (rates per 1000 patients per year)

Personal: Suspected 2.4+. *National*: 23.9 (Ref. 0.2). Numbers of cases depend on criteria of classification. In 50% of patients the infection was caused by monilia — in 25% post-menopausal changes were responsible.

AGE INCIDENCE

Vaginitis of infective origin arises in women of child-bearing age. Senile vaginitis seldom occurs under the age of 60.

CLINICAL POINTERS

1. High risk factors: (a) monilia (50%); (b) trichomonas infestation; (c) gonococcal infection; (d) senile vaginitis (25%); (e) physical and mechanical irritants, e.g. foreign bodies, retained tampons, pressaries, douches, lubricants, etc.; (f) birth pill and oral antibiotics may encourage monilia; (g) tights, tight jeans and vaginal deodorants may increase vulnerability.

2. Vaginal discharge. In Trichomonas infections the discharge may be profuse, frothy and offensive. In gonococcal vaginitis there may be urethritis or Bartholinitis. A tampon or condom causes a very offensive discharge (if overlooked) after 1 to 3 weeks.

3. Irritation or soreness of the vulva.

4. Inflammation of the vagina.

- In thrush vaginitis — loosely adherent patches of white exudate are scattered over the reddened vaginal walls.
- In other infective forms of vaginitis — the vagina appears red and granular.
- In senile vaginitis — areas of granular or ulcerated epithelium are seen. The thickened white epithelium of leukoplakia is occasionally observed.

INVESTIGATIONS

A high vaginal or urethral swab is taken for bacteriological examination. If gonorrhoea is suspected, special steps must be taken to ensure survival of the bacteria during transport to laboratory.

A therapeutic test may be helpful if gonorrhoea is not suspected:

For thrush infections — local antifungals: Nystatin etc. — BNF 7.2.2 (Ref. 0.1).

For Trichomonas — systemic metronidazole — BNF 5.4.3.

DURATION

The untreated case persists.

COMPLICATIONS

Recurrences are common.

MISLEADING FEATURES AND PITFALLS

1. Many women develop a moderate degree of vaginal discharge after marriage or pregnancy. Differentiation from true vaginitis may be difficult.

2. The vaginal discharge of acute gonorrhoea may be confused with that from simple vaginitis.

NOTE re gonorrhoea in the female. Classically there is evidence of infection in urethra, Bartholin's glands or vagina, but some women with gonorrhoea have no symptoms. The family doctor's knowledge of a patient's background may then assist diagnosis.

3. Reinfection occurs because the sexual partner has not been treated or is non-compliant.
4. Diabetes is not excluded as a cause of monilia.

MANAGEMENT OPTIONS

Prevention: patient education regarding high risk factors (see above).

Established condition: (a) identify, modify and treat appropriate high risk factors; (b) identify infective causes (Gonococcal — penicillin — BNF 5.1.1.1 (Ref. 0.1); other *bacterial* — BNF 5.1; *thrush* — local antifungals — BNF 7.2.2; *Trichomonas* — systemic trichomonacides — BNF 5.4.3.

UTEROVAGINAL PROLAPSE (PROCIDENTIA)

Classification: ICHPPC 618 (RCGP 3060)

Prolapse of the uterus is a form of hernia that follows damage to the pelvic floor following childbirth. Mild degrees are common in middle-aged women and may lead to much discomfort and suffering.

CLASSIFICATION

1. Grade I procidentia — the cervix descends into the vagina.
2. Grade II procidentia — the cervix drops to the level of the vulva.
3. Grade III procidentia — the cervix shows outside the vulva.
4. Cystocele — the anterior vaginal wall bulges into the vulva.
5. Rectocele — the posterior vaginal wall bulges into the vulva.

AETIOLOGY

Uterine prolapse is uncommon in nulliparous women. The two main causes are: (a) parturition; (b) general regression of the sexual organs after the menopause. Sometimes the onset is related to a strain.

DIAGNOSTIC RANGE (rates per 1000 patients per year)

Personal: Suspected 6.4. Probable 2.0. *National*: 4.0 (Ref. 0.2). (45% of the suspected cases were cystoceles — 15% were rectoceles — 40% were procidentias of varying degree.)

AGE INCIDENCE

The majority of cases are in women over 50. A transient prolapse is sometimes evident during the early pregnancy of multipara.

CLINICAL POINTERS

1. High risk factors: (a) multiparity (95%); (b) over 50 (65%) or post menopause; (c) history of 'straining'.

2. A sensation of something coming down (65%). The patient complains that her inside is dropping and that there is a lump in her vagina.

3. Stress incontinence (50%). A slight leakage of urine occurs when the patient coughs, laughs or strains.

4. Sacral or low back pain (25%). A dull ache which is aggravated by standing or walking. Occasionally pain is felt in the groins.

5. Vaginal examination confirms the diagnosis. A cystocele (45%) or rectocele (15%) pushes into the vulva if the patient coughs.

DURATION

In the absence of treatment prolapse tends to recur and becomes gradually worse. In mild cases, symptoms may be intermittent.

COMPLICATIONS

Grade II and Grade III procidentias are often associated with ulceration of the protruding cervix.

MISLEADING FEATURES AND PITFALLS

1. Patients with a cystocele have an associated residual urinary infection that may pass unnoticed if the urine is not examined. Treatment of the cystitis may alleviate many of the symptoms of a mild prolapse.

2. The hard cervix at the vulva may make the patient fear a growth — this fear may not be mentioned to the doctor.

3. The doctor forgets that women are vulnerable to depression after any pelvic operation.

MANAGEMENT OPTIONS

Prevention: — often crucial — involves at all deliveries (a) avoidance of 'pushing' before cervix is dilated; (b) avoidance of prolonged second stage; (c) avoidance of fundal pressing to expel placenta; (d) careful layer by layer repair of tears and episiotomies; (e) early ambulation; (f) teaching and full compliance with pelvic floor, puerperal exercises.

Established condition: (a) conservative if symptomless; (b) adequate operative repair; (c) Hodge or ring pessaries if operation inappropriate; (d) full explanation and support of patient.

RETROFLEXION OF THE UTERUS

Classification: ICHPPC 629 (RCGP 3070)

Retroflexion of the uterus (called retroversion if cervix as well as body is rotated) is a common and usually symptomless disorder.

AETIOLOGY

The malposition may be congenital or may follow a pregnancy. A congenital retroflexed uterus may also be poorly developed.

DIAGNOSTIC RANGE (rates per 1000 patients per year)

Personal: Suspected 1.8+. The diagnosis was rarely in doubt. A few [two out of 18] required surgical treatment.

CLINICAL POINTERS

1. Backache. It is difficult to assess the extent to which retroflexion causes backache.
2. Pelvic examination reveals the retroflexed uterus and indicates if the retroflexion is mobile or fixed. When it is fixed, the possibility of endometriosis or chronic pelvic sepsis may have to be considered.

INVESTIGATIONS

Ring test. The uterus is replaced and kept in position with a Hodge pessary; if symptoms are relieved, referral and occasionally surgery may be indicated.

COMPLICATIONS

A retroflexed gravid uterus may become impacted in the pelvis during the 3rd month and cause acute retention of urine. (No cases encountered in 10 years of practice.)

Sterility and pain are not now considered to follow retroflexion.

MISTAKES AND PITFALLS

A retroflexion is discovered routinely in a patient with sterility or backache. The patient is told this may be a cause of symptoms and understandably develops a 'fixation' which may then lead to needless operation.

MANAGEMENT OPTIONS

Established retroflexion: (a) patients should be encouraged to regard retroflexion as a 'normal finding' that is unlikely to cause symptoms; (b) endometriosis or chronic pelvic sepsis may indicate referral.

ENDOMETRIOSIS

Classification: ICHPPC 629 (RCGP 3055)

A pelvic mass develops which bears an histological resemblance to endometrial tissue. Chocolate cysts of the ovary probably have the same origin.

AETIOLOGY
The aetiology is uncertain.

DIAGNOSTIC RANGE (rates per 1000 patients per year)
Personal: Suspected 0.6. Probable 0.1. An unknown number are symptomless.

AGE INCIDENCE
Women aged 30 to 40 chiefly affected.

CLINICAL POINTERS
1. High risk groups: (a) delayed parity or nullipara; (b) previous menstrual irregularity; (c) fibroids often associated.
2. Lower abdominal or sacral pain that occurs 2 to 7 days before and continues during a period. The pain is continuous, severe, and may be associated with discomfort in the rectum, on micturition or defaecation.
3. Heavy periods.
4. Dyspareunia.
5. Rectal bleeding, as well as rectal pain, is said to occur.
6. Abdominal tenderness and guarding may be present at the height of the attack.
7. A tender pelvic mass may be felt in the pouch of Douglas. A fixed tender chocolate cyst of the ovary may be felt behind the uterus.

DURATION
Each attack settles after the period.

INVESTIGATIONS
Laparoscopy and sometimes laparotomy may be indicated.

COMPLICATIONS
Bleeding (or rupture of a chocolate cyst) may produce severe abdominal pain. Laparotomy may be performed.

MISLEADING FEATURES AND PITFALLS
1. The disease is easily overlooked because the symptoms are wrongly ascribed to a spasmodic dysmenorrhoea.

2. The pain is not always clearly associated with menstruation.

DIFFERENTIAL DIAGNOSIS

Diseases that may be confused with endometriosis:

Spasmodic dysmenorrhoea

Similar feature: chronic severe dysmenorrhoea in nulliparae.

Distinguishing features: onset at puberty; periods normal; vaginal or rectal examination normal.

Acute appendicitis

Similar features: repeated attacks of lower abdominal pain; tenderness in RIF; guarding and rigidity of lower abdomen.

Distinguishing features: relationship of pain to periods indefinite; menorrhagia and dysmenorrhoea absent; pelvic mass unlikely in early stages; admission to hospital indicated.

Twisted ovarian cyst

Similar features: repeated attacks of lower abdominal pain; tenderness in RIF; tender mass in pelvis.

Distinguishing features: relationship of pain to periods indefinite; pelvic mass is mobile and smooth; differentiation may be difficult and hospital admission is indicated.

MANAGEMENT OPTIONS

Suspected disease: referral is usually wise to: (a) establish diagnosis; (b) decide appropriate treatment — the options are many, i.e. combinations of sex hormones, surgery and radiotherapy.

DISORDERS OF MENSTRUATION

Classification: ICHPPC 6260–6269 (RCGP 3100–3139)

The common menstrual disorders include:

— Dysmenorrhoea (painful periods)
— Menorrhagia, metrorrhagia and polymenorrhoea (excessive loss)
— Amenorrhoea and oligomenorrhoea (absent or small loss).

Confusion arises because these terms are used loosely to describe both a symptom and a disease. Thus — the term dysmenorrhoea may be used to describe both the primary disorder of spasmodic dysmenorrhoea and the symptomatic dysmenorrhoeas that are secondary to disorders such as endometriosis.

The common primary diseases of menstruation also described are:

— Spasmodic dysmenorrhoea
— Hormonal amenorrhoea (and oligomenorrhoea)
— Dysfunctional uterine haemorrhage, i.e. all cases of menorrhagia, polymenorrhoea and metrorrhagia in which there is no other primary disease. Sometimes called essential uterine haemorrhage.

PRIMARY AMENORRHOEA

Classification: ICHPPC 6260 (RCGP 3115)

Menstruation may start normally between 9 and 16 years (mean age 13). In about 1% onset is delayed beyond 16 and the many possible serious causes of primary amenorrhoea must be considered. Once psychological conditions, such as anorexia nervosa, can be excluded, an early gynaecological or paediatric opinion is usually wise.

DIAGNOSTIC RANGE (rates per 1000 patients per year)
Personal: Probable 0.1.

SECONDARY AMENORRHOEA

Secondary amenorrhoea is associated with many diseases:

1. Wasting disorders such as anorexia nervosa, advanced tuberculosis and cancer.
2. Endocrine disorders such as Simmond's disease, Cushing's syndrome, acromegaly and myxoedema.

HORMONAL AMENORRHOEA

This term covers those cases of amenorrhoea which are not physiological, primary or secondary. The condition is usually transient, is easily confused with pregnancy and does not affect fertility.

AETIOLOGY
Aetiology is unknown. It may arise after the menarche, marriage, puerperium, after stopping the contraceptive pill or before the menopause.

DIAGNOSTIC RANGE (rates per 1000 patients per year)
Personal: Suspected 3.5.

MANAGEMENT OPTIONS

Suspected condition: (a) waiting; (b) full explanation and reassurance.

OLIGOMENORRHOEA AND HYPOMENORRHOEA

Classification: ICHPPC 6260 (RCGP 3120)

The periods may be scanty and regular (oligomenorrhoea) or the interval between periods may be prolonged (hypomenorrhoea). Mild degrees of these disorders are common and may be associated with sub-fertility.

MANAGEMENT OPTIONS

Established condition: (a) full explanation and reassurance; (b) wait; (c) occasional referral is indicated.

SPASMODIC DYSMENORRHOEA

Classification: ICHPPC 6260 (RCGP 3100)

AETIOLOGY

The pain is in part due to a tight cervix which may be cured by the stretching of pregnancy. Delivery by Caesarean section does not relieve the pain. The pain only occurs after ovulation and may be absent with a girl's first few periods or after taking the contraceptive pill.

DIAGNOSTIC RANGE (rates per 1000 patients per year)

Personal: 5.7+. *National*: 8.4 (Ref. 0.2). Many cases are never reported.

AGE INCIDENCE

The majority of cases (77%) occur in young nulliparous women. Of these nearly half were under the age of 20.

CLINICAL POINTERS

Pain at period times (100%) is sometimes severe and is worse at the start of the period. It eases after 1 or 2 days. Pain thresholds are easily lowered by worry, unhappiness, conflicts and boredom.

DURATION

The ailment persists until cured by natural or artificial dilatation. In a few women it persists in spite of repeated pregnancies.

COMPLICATIONS

In membranous dysmenorrhoea a mucous caste of the uterus is shed causing much pain. (No cases encountered in 10 years of practice.)

DIFFERENTIAL DIAGNOSIS

Diseases that may be confused with spasmodic dysmenorrhoea:

Endometriosis and chocolate cyst of ovary

Similar features: dysmenorrhoea; nulliparous women liable.

Distinguishing features: women over 30 affected; periods often heavy and irregular; dyspareunia; pain on defaecation; infertility; tender pelvic mass may be palpable on vaginal examination.

Fibroid of uterus

Similar feature: dysmenorrhoea.

Distinguishing features: dysmenorrhoea usually associated with large fibroids; vaginal examination clarifies diagnosis; women over 30 affected; menorrhagia.

Chronic salpingitis or pelvic sepsis

Similar feature: dysmenorrhoea.

Distinguishing features: teenagers rarely affected; history of precipitating abortion or delivery; dyspareunia; fever; tender pelvic mass may be palpable on vaginal examination.

MISLEADING FEATURES AND PITFALLS

1. Often difficult to assess severity. Parents and doctors (especially male) can cause inappropriate reactions in teenage girls by both underestimating or overestimating the severity of the pain.

2. Teenage girls sometimes say they suffer dysmenorrhoea when they are afraid to ask for the contraceptive pill.

MANAGEMENT OPTIONS

Established condition: (a) minimise patient anxiety by empathetic explanation; (b) encourage normal activities which raise pain thresholds; (c) analgesics — BNF 4.7.1 (Ref. 0.1) and myometrial relaxants — BNF 7.1.2; (d) Hormonal suppression of ovulation — BNF 7.3; (e) referral and even surgery are occasionally indicated.

CONGESTIVE DYSMENORRHOEA

This is the name given to dysmenorrhoea which is secondary to other pelvic disorders.

OVULATION SYNDROME (MITTELSCHMERZ)

Classification: ICHPPC 6253 (RCGP 3100)

AETIOLOGY

Ovulation. Slight pain may occur with normal ovulation. Intraperitoneal bleeding arises from the rupture of a Graafian follicle and causes the syndrome.

DIAGNOSTIC RANGE (rates per 1000 patients per year)

Personal: Suspected 1.9. Probable 0.7. *National*: 0.5 (Ref. 0.2).

AGE INCIDENCE

All women capable of menstruation are liable, but adolescents, young or recently married women are especially prone.

CLINICAL POINTERS

1. High risk factors: (a) adolescent girls; (b) recently married women.
2. Abdominal pain (100%). The site of the pain varies, in most cases (75%) the pain is in one of the iliac fossae or flanks — in others (20%) it is felt suprapubically or centrally. Pain is occasionally felt in the sacral or loin regions.
3. Symptoms at the midpoint of the menstrual cycle (85%). Ovulation usually occurs between the 12th and 16th day of the menstrual cycle, but a wider range is not uncommon.
4. Abdominal tenderness (65%) is felt suprapubically or in one iliac fossa.
5. Tenderness on rectal or vaginal examination (20%). Movement of the cervix or pressure in the lateral or posterior fornices may be painful.
6. Fever may be due to ovulation itself or to blood in the peritoneal cavity. It may be as high as 38.0°C. The pulse rate is rarely increased.
7. Painful and tender breasts (10%) suggest that ovulation has occurred.

DURATION

Symptoms subside in 1 to 4 days.

COMPLICATIONS

None unless the disorder is mistaken for an acute abdomen and laparotomy performed.

MISLEADING FEATURES AND PITFALLS

1. Ovulation may not always occur at the usual midperiod point.

The relationship to the periods may be especially hard to identify in those women whose periods are irregular.

2. An ectopic gestation or acute appendicitis can be so closely simulated that laparotomy is the only method of differentiation.

3. The doctor omits to ask if the woman is taking the birth pill.

DIFFERENTIAL DIAGNOSIS

Diseases that may be confused with the ovulation syndrome:

Acute appendicitis

Similar features: abdominal pain and tenderness in suprapubic or right iliac fossa regions; tenderness to right on vaginal or rectal examination; low fever; history of previous attack.

Distinguishing features: attacks are not related to midpoint of periods; tenderness or pain in breasts absent; ovulation in right ovary may be indistinguishable from early acute appendicitis; admission to hospital indicated.

Ectopic gestation

Similar features: lower abdominal pain and tenderness localised in either iliac fossa; tenderness on palpating the cervix uteri; low fever.

Distinguishing features: history of one missed period is usual but not invariable; pain is severe even before rupture occurs; patient appears ill and drawn; sleep is lost; vomiting, anorexia and increased pulse rate common; admission to hospital indicated in doubtful cases. Rupture makes the diagnosis disastrously clear. Pregnancy tests positive.

Acute pyelonephritis

Similar features: pain and tenderness in one flank; pain in loin or back; low fever.

Distinguishing features: frequency; dysuria; pyuria; fever, usually high; rigors common.

MANAGEMENT OPTIONS

Suspected condition: (a) rest and observe; (b) refer if doubt remains.

DYSFUNCTIONAL UTERINE HAEMORRHAGE

Classification: ICHPPC 6269 (RCGP 3135)

Dysfunctional uterine haemorrhage refers to any disorder in which there is excessive uterine bleeding and no obvious primary disease.

It includes patients with menorrhagia, polymenorrhoea, metrorrhagia and metropathia haemorrhagica. The diagnosis is only made after all serious causes have been excluded.

Unfortunately the term dysfunctional uterine haemorrhage is cumbersome and is seldom used. Instead the disorders are referred to by their shorter but ambiguous symptomatic names, i.e. menorrhagia, polymenorrhoea. Sometimes called Essential Uterine haemorrhage.

AETIOLOGY

Hormonal disturbances are thought to be responsible. Women are liable in the few years before the menopause or occasionally for short periods after the puerperium.

DIAGNOSTIC RANGE (rates per 1000 patients per year)

Personal: Suspected 12.1. Probable 9.7.

AGE INCIDENCE

The majority (65%) of patients are of menopausal age.

CLINICAL POINTERS

1. Excessive uterine bleeding (100%). Excessive loss (menorrhagia); loss which occurs abnormally often (polymenorrhoea); loss between periods (metrorrhagia); continuous or excessively prolonged loss following periods of amenorrhoea (metropathia haemorrhagica).
2. Absence of other possible causes of bleeding.

DURATION

Variable. The loss may clear up in a few months or continue intermittently for several years, until the menopause.

INVESTIGATIONS

Curettage may help diagnostically and therapeutically.

COMPLICATIONS

Hypochromic anaemia.

MISLEADING FEATURES AND PITFALLS

Carcinoma of uterus, myxoedema and hypochromic anaemia are all treatable conditions that are easily confused with dysfunctional uterine haemorrhage.

DIFFERENTIAL DIAGNOSIS

Diseases that may be confused with dysfunctional uterine haemorrhage:

Fibroid of uterus
Similar features: menorrhagia; anaemia; women of 30 to 50 liable.

Distinguishing features: fibroids large enough to cause menorrhagia are usually palpable on bimanual vaginal examination.

Endometriosis
Similar features: menorrhagia and polymenorrhoea; anaemia; women of 30 to 50 liable.

Distinguishing features: nulliparous women especially liable; dysmenorrhoea; dyspareunia; pain or bleeding on defaecation; vaginal examination reveals pelvic mass; distinction may be difficult.

Carcinoma of cervix
Similar features: metrorrhagia; women of 30 to 50 liable.

Distinguishing features: patient can distinguish between bleeding of carcinoma and menstrual loss; bleeding after coitus; metrorrhagia common; free bleeding after examination of cervical canal; offensive yellow or bloodstained discharge; speculum examination may reveal growth; cervical smear positive.

Carcinoma of body of uterus
Similar features: metrorrhagia.

Distinguishing features: nulliparous and post-menopausal women mainly affected; metrorrhagia; irregular or continuous loss; distinction may be difficult. Diagnostic curettage differentiates.

Other anovulatory causes
Abortion (threatened, incomplete, etc.), ectopic pregnancy, IUD's, blood disorders, chronic pelvic inflammation and *thyroid disease* may all have to be considered and excluded.

MANAGEMENT OPTIONS

Suspected dysfunction: exclude and treat other serious or primary causes.

Established dysfunction: (a) curettage may be curative; (b) a course of progestogens — BNF 6.4.1.2. (Ref. 0.1); repeated for several cycles; (c) antifibrinolytics — BNF 2.11; (d) referral for surgery is occasionally indicated; (e) full explanation (Ref. 0.3 — Period Problems). Patient threshold to pain, anxiety and depression are often lowered by any chronic pelvic complaint. Understanding and support by medical personnel and husbands are then crucial.

INTERMENSTRUAL BLEEDING (METRORRHAGIA)

Classification ICHPPC 6269 (RCGP 3135)

This is a symptom not a disease, therefore serious causes must be excluded as early as possible. Unfortunately it is often difficult to be sure if a reported loss is intermenstrual or a part of an irregular cycle.

The position is further confused if the patient is already taking sex hormones for other purposes.

Diagnostic curettage is usual if there is doubt.

PREMENSTRUAL SYNDROME (PMS)

Classification ICHPPC 6269 (RCGP 3105)

Often called premenstrual tension, this combination of physical and psychological symptoms is clearly recognised by 80 to 95% of healthy women of reproductive age. In a proportion of cases the symptoms are severe and interfere considerably with the sufferer's life.

AETIOLOGY

Uncertain — probably many factors are involved. A number of different hormones may play a part. PMS like pregnancy, the menopause and the menarche all demonstrate similar combinations of physical and psychological symptoms in otherwise healthy women.

DIAGNOSTIC RANGE (rates per 1000 patients per year)

Personal: Reported 0.9+. Many other cases were probably reported incidentally.

AGE INCIDENCE

Most cases report to the doctor between 20 and 35 years. Symptoms stop at the menopause.

CLINICAL POINTERS

1. High risk factors: (a) parity; (b) menstrual irregularity; (c) women with marital or emotional upsets; (d) boredom or fatigue; (e) high social class (work in our practice suggests that in lower social classes other more serious social problems displace patient awareness of PMS); (f) positive family history.

2. Onset is usually during the 5 (occasionally 10) days before the period starts.

3. Physical symptoms include; swelling or bloatedness, tender breasts, gastrointestinal or bladder symptoms and occasionally joint pains.
4. Psychological symptoms include; headache, weepiness, irritability, depression and fatigue.

DURATION
Symptoms decrease as the period starts and are usually gone by the third day.

COMPLICATIONS
Very occasionally antisocial acts may occur.

MISTAKES AND PITFALLS
1. Occasionally patients or their lawyers may use PMS as a legal defence for antisocial acts. The lack of clear clinical definition is likely to put the patient's doctor in a dubious legal position.
2. Blunt statements that symptoms are imagined or due to 'nerves' especially if made by a male doctor are likely to aggravate symptoms.

MANAGEMENT OPTIONS
Prevention: as with the symptoms of pregnancy and the menopause, active case finding is likely to be counter productive.
Reported PMS: (a) exclude serious disease e.g. depressive illness and hyperthyroidism; (b) full empathetic explanation and understanding with encouragement of full normal activities; (c) physical symptoms — symptomatic treatment; (d) psychological symptoms as for simple anxiety and tension (pp. 243 and 246). Various hormonal treatments have been tried with dubious effect.

THE FEMALE CLIMACTERIC OR MENOPAUSE

Classification: ICHPPC 627 (RCGP 3150)

The female climacteric, or 'change', is the physical and mental condition of women when the ovaries cease to stimulate menstruation. The symptoms are thought to be due to overaction of the anterior lobe of the pituitary. The menopause refers to cessation of the periods. The menopause has many similarities with pregnancy and other 'normal' processes such as menstruation, PMS and simple anxiety. Each occur routinely in healthy individuals, each is associated with physical and psychological symptoms that can upset the patient and confuse the doctor but are rarely harmful; the symptoms are often aggravated by emotional upsets, worry, boredom and fatigue; doctors (especially male) vary greatly in their understanding and management of the psychological symptoms.

DIAGNOSTIC RANGE (rates per 1000 patients per year)
Personal: Suspected 12.8. Probable 6.2. *National*: 11.0 (Ref. 0.2). This represents 5–10% of women of menopausal age.

AGE INCIDENCE
Women aged 40 to 55 years (80%).

CLINICAL POINTERS

1. Amenorrhoea or irregularities of menstruation are usual.
2. Hot flushes (flashes) (80%).
3. Emotional lability, depression, fatigue, dizziness, headache and recurring fears about health or possibly pregnancy are reported. A history of marital or sexual difficulty is common (40%).
4. Abdominal swelling or sensations of bloatedness.
5. Associated diseases which may be aggravated by the menopause include migraine, obesity, and vague arthritic pains.
6. Some women report more illness to the doctor after the menopause; but apart from a general tendency to be more depressed, sleep more lightly, and develop symptoms of simple anxiety (p. 243), no specific constellation of psychological symptoms is associated with the menopause.

DURATION
The symptoms of the female climacteric may start several years before the periods cease and occasionally continue for as long as 10 years afterwards. Most patients eventually learn to live with the discomfort.

COMPLICATIONS
Psychoses sometimes arise; the vagina becomes dry; there is increased vulnerability to osteoporosis (with back pain) and carcinoma of the uterine body; occasionally libido is decreased.

MISLEADING FEATURES AND PITFALLS

1. Women are often afraid of the 'change'. They may have been upset by the tales of other women and may feel old or worried by fear of losing libido. Such fears are groundless in most instances.
2. It is easy for both doctor and patient to attribute symptoms of organic disease to the 'change'.
3. The feeling of bloatedness often leads women to fear a growth.

DIFFERENTIAL DIAGNOSIS

Diseases that may be confused with the menopause:

Pregnancy

Similar features: amenorrhoea; feeling of abdominal distension.

Distinguishing features: nocturia and frequency of micturition; tenderness and swelling of the breasts; nausea and vomiting; pregnancy tests are positive.

Hormonal amenorrhoea

Similar features: amenorrhoea.

Distinguishing features: a variable period of unexplained amenorrhoea may occur after a pregnancy or towards the end of a woman's menstrual life; flushes are usually absent.

Simmond's disease (Sheehan's syndrome)

Similar feature: amenorrhoea.

Distinguishing features: rare; history of precipitating pregnancy with severe post-partum haemorrhage; amenorrhoea is permanent; lassitude; slight loss of weight; loss of pubic hair.

NOTE. Anorexia nervosa, prolonged fever, advanced tuberculosis, severe anaemias and cancer may lead to amenorrhoea. Evidence of serious disease differentiates.

MANAGEMENT OPTIONS

Prevention: Many needless fears about the 'change' can be avoided if timely health education is provided. Unfortunately those most likely to be helped are often the most reluctant to obtain such assistance.

Physical symptoms:

1. Flushes (a) clonidine — BNF 4.7.4.2 (Ref. 0.1); (b) hormone replacement therapy, — BNF 6.4.1. — not indicated routinely.
2. Osteoporosis, oestrogens — BNF 6.4.1.1 may help to arrest this.
3. Dry vaginitis, local oestrogens — BNF 7.2.1.
4. Contraception — barrier type for initial 2 years.

Psychological symptoms: (a) full empathetic explanation and counselling; (b) drugs — as for simple anxiety (p. 246) and depression (p. 257).

FEMALE STERILITY

Classification: ICHPPC 606 (RCGP 3155)

AETIOLOGY

In the majority of cases the cause is not obvious even after a full investigation. The known causes include the following.

1. Congenital defects in the female passages.

2. Inadequate development of uterus or ovaries. (Irregular periods, masculine distribution of hair and obesity are characteristically associated with this type of sterility.)

3. Acquired mechanical defects in the female passages, e.g. salpingitis, pelvic peritonitis or ectopic pregnancy.

4. Diseases of the uterus, e.g. uterine fibroids, carcinoma and chronic cervicitis.

5. Psychological difficulties such as vaginismus, frigidity or anxiety (see p. 263).

DIAGNOSTIC RANGE (rates per 1000 patients per year)

Personal: Suspected 3.0±. [A 3-year follow-up showed that 43 per cent (13 out of 30) patients who were suspected of being infertile and were referred to the infertility clinic subsequently conceived.]

MANAGEMENT OPTIONS

Suspected: (a) full discussion (with couple), giving likely possibilities; (b) outline plan involving following steps: checking husband; 6–18 months trial of relaxed pre-ovulation intercourse; referral for hospital investigation and treatment *after* trial period (see male infertility — p. 532).

Proven: (a) counsel couple together; (b) counter guilt feelings of wife; (c) discuss options of adoption, *in vitro* fertilization etc.; (d) appropriate education — Sex problems (for patients) (Ref. 0.3); (e) follow up; (f) referral.

Table 30 Less common diseases of the female genital organs

Disease and distinguishing clinical pointers	Incidence per 1000 patients per year	
	Suspected	Confirmed
Carcinoma of vulva Persistent ulcer with hard rolled edge	—	1 in 10 years
Bartholin's abscess Tender red swelling of posterior third of labia	0.4	0.4
Haematocolpos Primary amenorrhoea at puberty, severe lower abdominal pain and backache at monthly intervals, malaise between attacks, suprapubic or pelvic mass, imperforate hymen. Refer.	—	1 in 10 years

22

Family planning, complications of pregnancy, childbirth and the puerperium

Please read the introduction for explanation of figures and analyses.

The problems of early diagnosis that face the family doctor are similar to those facing the consultant obstetrician who runs an antenatal clinic.

All new entrants into practice require three essentials from their previous obstetric training in hospital:

1. A practical working knowledge of the normal antenatal (prenatal) period including prevention, diagnosis and management of the common abnormalities.

2. A full working experience of the assessment and management of normal labour including the prevention, diagnosis and management of the common deviations from the normal.

3. A clear assessment of their own limitations (knowledge, skills and attitudes) in relation to the obstetric field.

This experience should be acquired in hospital and can be applied directly to the primary situation. Details are therefore outside the scope of this book.

An excellent concise guide to prescribing in pregnancy and breast feeding is given in the introductory Guidance to Prescribing section of the BNF (Ref. 0.1).

Contraception, tubal and early pregnancy are discussed because they may present special problems of diagnosis to the family doctor.

FAMILY PLANNING, CONTRACEPTIVE ADVICE AND PREVENTION OF PREGNANCY

Classification: ICHPPC V250–V256 (RCGP 6350–6400)

Contraceptive advice is the third most frequent reason for patients to report to the doctor in Britain (Appendix VII).

The problems are not those of diagnosis but of management and appropriateness of method.

MANAGEMENT OPTIONS

All family doctors should have a working knowledge of the advantages and disadvantages of all methods (summarised in Table 30). The knowledge is rapidly changing and every doctor should make a point of monitoring progress in the field from the Family Planning Association (Ref. 22.1) and Catholic Marriage Advisory Council (Ref. 22.2).

EARLY PREGNANCY

The early symptoms and signs of pregnancy are easily confused with some diseases.

DIAGNOSTIC RANGE (rates per 1000 patients per year)

Personal: Proven 38.2

CLINICAL POINTERS

1. Amenorrhoea.
2. Vomiting and nausea start during the first 6 weeks and may occur at any time of day.
3. Nocturia and frequency of micturition start in the first 2 to 4 weeks. They may be noted before the first period has been missed.
4. Tenderness, tingling or heavy feeling in the breasts is usually noted in the first 2 to 4 weeks.
5. Vaginal examination reveals a soft cervix; after the eighth week the fundus can be felt as a mobile rounded mass (5 cm diam.) lying above the soft cervix (Hegar's sign).

INVESTIGATIONS

Tests for gonadotrophic hormone in the urine are quick and accurate. The tests are positive about 10 days after the date of the first missed period.

MISLEADING FEATURES AND PITFALLS

Women who fear pregnancy may suppress information about amenorrhoea, vomiting or nausea.

ECTOPIC TUBAL PREGNANCY

Classification: ICHPPC 633 (RCGP 3305)

An ectopic pregnancy occurs when the ovum is fertilised and develops outside the uterine cavity. Such abnormal conceptions almost invariably arise within one of the ovarian tubes. The term ectopic pregnancy is often used loosely to describe these tubal pregnancies.

The ovum develops without symptoms for 3 to 6 weeks.

AETIOLOGY

Previous infection in the ovarian tubes may prevent the ovum from reaching the uterus. In many cases the cause is not obvious.

DIAGNOSTIC RANGE (rate per 1000 patients per year)

Personal: Suspected 0.4. Proven 0.2.

AGE INCIDENCE

Women of child-bearing age.

CLINICAL POINTERS

1. High risk factors: (a) previous history of ectopic; (b) previous history of tubal sepsis; (c) positive family history.

2. Abdominal pain is intermittent at first and situated suprapubically or in one iliac fossa. It may be severe enough to wake the patient at night. It is aggravated by movement and may radiate to vagina or leg.

3. History of one missed period is a classical feature. It is not always present.

4. A brown vaginal discharge or slight loss is common. It is sometimes mistaken for a normal period.

5. Irritation of other pelvic viscera. As with pelvic infections, dysuria, frequency or slight diarrhoea may occur.

6. Abdominal tenderness is maximal in one iliac fossa.

7. Pelvic examination. Palpation, especially movement, of the cervix produces acute pain.

8. Temperature and pulse are normal in the early stages. A moderate fever may be noted after 1 or 2 days of pain.

DURATION

The duration and severity of the intermittent abdominal pain varies. (In this practice durations of 1 to 21 days have been recorded.) In the untreated case the disorder terminates in one of two ways:

1. The ovum dies and a tubal mole develops — rare.
2. Rupture, haemorrhage and occasionally death occur.

COMPLICATIONS

Rupture of the ovarian tube causes a dramatic change in the patient's condition. The pulse rate rises in a few minutes to 120 or over. The patient becomes rapidly shocked and may faint. Blood collects in the peritoneal cavity and may track up to the diaphragm causing shoulder pain.

MISLEADING FEATURES AND PITFALLS

The early stages of an ectopic gestation are easily confused with an acute salpingitis and may be mistakenly treated conservatively at home. Provided the possibility of the diagnosis is borne in mind most patients can be admitted to hospital before rupture occurs. (Two out of three cases ruptured while being observed in hospital.)

DIFFERENTIAL DIAGNOSIS

Diseases that may be confused with an ectopic tubal pregnancy:

Acute pelvic appendicitis

Similar features: abdominal pain; frequency of micturition; low fever; right-sided abdominal tenderness; release sign positive; rectal tenderness to the right.

Distinguishing features: differentiation may be extremely difficult; previous attacks; menstrual irregularities absent; signs of early pregnancy and vaginal discharge absent; uterine cervix is hard and can be moved without discomfort; gonadotrophin test negative.

Acute salpingitis

Similar features: low abdominal pain and tenderness in one iliac fossa; vaginal discharge; menstrual irregularities; fever; acute discomfort on moving uterine cervix.

Distinguishing features: differentiation may be extremely difficult; signs of early pregnancy absent; vaginal discharge offensive; fever high; hospital admission indicated in doubtful cases; gonadotrophin test negative.

Septic abortion

Similar features: low abdominal pain and tenderness; menstrual irregularities and signs of early pregnancy; vaginal discharge; low fever; acute discomfort on palpation of uterus.

Distinguishing features: differentiation may be difficult; patient's statements may be unreliable; uterus enlarged; cervix uteri soft and may be open; products of conception sometimes apparent.

Twisted (small) ovarian cysts

Similar features: intermittent severe low abdominal pain and tenderness; tender mass in pouch of Douglas.

Distinguishing features: previous attacks; menstrual irregularities uncommon; signs of early pregnancy and vaginal discharge absent;

characteristic smooth rounded mass in pouch of Douglas; gonadotrophin test negative.

MANAGEMENT OPTIONS

Prevention of rupture: should be the aim of the family doctor. This inevitably involves admitting doubtful cases.

Suspected cases: immediate admission.

Post hospital: Full discussion re further attacks and possible infertility (see p. 571).

Table 31 Contraceptive methods — advantages and disadvantages
If a normal young woman has regular intercourse without using any sort of contraception, there is an 80–90% chance that she will get pregnant within a year. All types of contraception have some limitations or disadvantages. (For up to date Family Planning Information see Ref. 22.1 and 22.2.)

Breast Feeding
Reliability:Poor
Advantages:No preparation before intercourse.

Douche
Reliability:Poor
Advantages:No preparation before intercourse.

Natural family planning (rhythm method)
Reliability:Fair
Advantages:No artificial aids required. No preparation before intercourse.
Disadvantages:Needs careful calculation, probably by more than one method. Limits occasions when intercourse may occur. Requires male co-operation. (see Ref. 22.2)

Withdrawal
Reliability:Fair
Advantages:No preparation before intercourse.
Disadvantages:Satisfaction reduced. Requires male co-operation.

Spermicide only (suppositories, foaming tablets, etc. BNF 7.3.3. (Ref.0.1)
Reliability:Fair
Advantages:Easily available
Disadvantages:Requires preparation before intercourse.

Progestogen-only pill
BNF 7.3.2 (Ref. 0.1)
Reliability:Good
Advantages:Can be taken while breast feeding, and by women over 35. No preparation before intercourse. Male co-operation not required. All ages.
Disadvantages:Must be taken every day. Periods irregular.

Progestogen injection
BNF 7.3.2 (Ref. 0.1)
Reliability:Good.
Advantages:Lasts up to 3 months. No preparation before intercourse. Male co-operation not required.
Disadvantages:Irreversible for 3 months. Periods irregular.

Combined pill BNF 7.3.1. (Ref. 0.1)
Reliability:Very good.
Advantages:Predictable, light periods with few cramps. No preparation before intercourse. Now considered safe for women over 35 (as well as under 35) if they are non-smokers.
Disadvantages:Must be taken regularly. Can have side effects. Contra-indicated in women who smoke, are obese, have diabetes or hypertension.

Condom (sheath)
Reliability: Fair to good.
Advantages:Easily available. Protects against V.D. Disadvantages:Requires male co-operation. May interfere with satisfaction.

Diaphragm (cap)
Reliability: Fair to good.
Advantages:No side effects. Easily available. Male co-operation not required.
Disadvantages:Needs to be fitted first, by a doctor or nurse. Requires preparation before intercourse.

Intra-uterine device (loop, coil, etc.)
BNF 7.3 (Ref. 0.1)
Reliability:Fairly good
Advantages:Once inserted no further preparation needed. Male co-operation not required.
Disadvantages:Needs to be fitted by doctor or nurse. Unsuitable for women with heavy periods or those who have not had children.

Vasectomy (sterilisation for men)
Reliability:Very good.
Advantages:No preparation before intercourse.
Disadvantages:Irreversible, minor operation. Only for men who want no more children.

Tubal ligation (sterilisation for women)
Reliability:Very good
Advantages:No preparation before intercourse. Male co-operation not required.
Disadvantages:Irreversible, minor operation. Only for women who want no more children.

Hysterectomy
Reliability:100%.
Advantages:Totally reliable. No preparation before intercourse.
Disadvantages:Major operation. There must be other reasons apart from contraception. Irreversible.

For Health Education purposes the patient can be referred to Ref. 22.1 or 22.2

23

Diseases of the skin and cellular tissue

Please read introduction for explanation of figures and analyses.

RECOGNITION OF SKIN DISEASES IN PRIMARY CARE

Recognition of skin diseases is similar to the diagnostic process in other systems. Despite this, many experienced physicians confess to feelings of inadequacy in relation to dermatology. A highly competent doctor will comment 'if it doesn't improve with topical clioquinol and hydrocortisone I refer'. This attitude is largely unnecessary.

The appropriate visual experience of common skin conditions may be difficult to obtain. The ideal method is to work for a time in the 'skin department' of a hospital. An alternative or supplementary method is to use a good atlas of dermatology in your clinic. This latter method is practical and allows continuous updating.

Some basic knowledge and equipment is required:

1. EQUIPMENT

Plenty of light and a book on dermatology with good illustrations of common skin diseases. I use *Dermatology — an Illustrated Guide* by Lionel Fry (Ref. 0.7).

I find that an auriscope without a speculum provides excellent, always available, lighted magnification.

A suitable solution of 10% potassium hydroxide, a microscope, and a sterilized skin biopsy set can be added if these are found to be necessary.

2. HISTORY

As with other areas of primary care 70 to 90% of the clinical information which leads to a diagnosis comes from the history not the examination or tests. Once this fact is realised, dermatology becomes an easier subject.

Some special information may have to be collected:

— *Background information* regarding previous attacks, occupation, contact with chemicals, etc., drugs and medicines taken for other reasons.
— *Emotional influences* are said to aggravate skin conditions but rarely help to make a diagnosis. In fact, if a doctor cannot distinguish between eczema, scabies and psoriasis, the patient's mental state is unlikely to assist the diagnosis.
— *Symptom elaboration* follows the routine BASTARD catechism.* The physician should always ask about any irritation.

THE DISTRIBUTION AND TYPE OF LESION

These are the two pieces of information that allow the primary physician to sift efficiently the likely diagnostic possibilities.

Thus the common skin diseases can be grouped under the following four headings (see Table 32, p. 582):

I Single lesions that may occur at any site.
II Larger skin lesions (often multiple) that affect a single area — any site.
III Larger skin lesions that are characteristically localised to a particular site.
IV Rashes that affect many sites or the whole body.

A brief glance at the table concerned shows that with little dermatological experience it is possible to group the 70 common skin diseases into manageable small groups of less than 10 possibilities. A short study of the appropriate text then allows the inexperienced doctor to identify from the history the most likely diagnoses.

Once this has been done it becomes feasible for the doctor to use a skin atlas (Ref. 0.7) while consulting. In 1 or 2 minutes the physician can, with an appropriate excuse to the waiting patient, retire and match up a lesion with possible illustrations from his atlas.

Many primary physicians become skilled dermatologists by using this simple method of clinic identification and self-learning. In primary care nearly twice as many patients report with skin complaints (7.4%) as with cardiovascular conditions (4.6%). Therefore the time spent on this self-learning process is rarely wasted and

*Bodily location; Area and size; Start; Timing and duration; Aggravating and Alleviating factors; Related phenomenon especially itching; general Description.

the extra skill adds considerably to the physician's satisfaction and effectiveness.

EXAMINATION AND DESCRIPTION OF LESIONS

Description of a skin lesion is an essential part of diagnostic recognition. Therefore the doctor must have a working knowledge of the terms used to describe common dermatological lesions:

Erythema — redness, no clearly defined edge.

Papule — a little lump or spot.

Macule — a mark, usually red with a well defined edge which can be seen but not felt; a stain or freckle.

Maculo-papule — a useful descriptive term for any lesion with a well defined colour edge that is also raised.

Vesicle — a little blister containing serum.

Pustule — a blister containing pus.

Bulla — a large blister.

Nummular (coin-shaped) or discoid — a round, well-defined circular patch of varying size (2–30 cm). Patches may become confluent, large and irregular but are still often referred to as nummular or discoid.

Plaque — a well defined plate of tissue with a distinctive appearance or consistency.

Excoriation — evidence of linea scratch marks.

Scaling may be centripetal (free edge of scale to centre of lesion) or centrifugal (free edge of scale pointing towards the periphery of lesion).

Guttate (drop-like — any rash with many small isolated round patches — usually 2–15 mm diameter.

Applications to practice

If the doctor decides to develop his technique of consulting room recognition he should start with the following routine:

1. Take the history and examine all the lesions.

2. Consult Table 32 and decide in which of the four groups the lesion is likely to be found. This is best done in a room away from the patient.

3. Consult the appropriate text in this book to identify the *one* or *two* most likely possibilities. This step soon becomes unnecessary.

4. Look up the appropriate alternatives in an atlas of dermatology.

At first there will be difficulty in matching but as the physician sees more skin lesions and becomes accustomed to a particular atlas, accuracy, skill and confidence rapidly increase.

RODENT ULCER (BASAL CELL EPITHELIOMA)

Classification: ICHPPC 173 (RCGP 0455)

AETIOLOGY

Exposure to sunlight for long periods — especially strong sunlight.

DIAGNOSTIC RANGE (rates per 1000 patients per year)

Personal: Suspected 1.5+. *National*: 0.6 (Ref. 0.2). In sunny or tropical districts inhabited by large numbers of fair skinned people rates may be strikingly increased.

AGE INCIDENCE

Over 40 years.

SEX INCIDENCE

Men are affected more than women (2:1)

CLINICAL POINTERS

1. High risk factors: (a) prolonged or intense exposure to sunlight; (b) fair skin; (c) facial lesion.

2. The ulcer, A small white painless pimple breaks down centrally and may be covered with a scaly crust. In the early stages the crust only is seen and the lesion looks like a spot with a scab often white and scaly. Sometimes the lesion forms a purple rounded wart-like growth with a smooth mottled surface (button or cystic type). Growth is slow and the lesion may be present for many years before a doctor is consulted.

3. The site. Face (or scalp) (70%). Multiple lesions sometimes develop on the trunk.

4. Less commonly a firm infiltrating slightly red plaque (morphoeic type) or a red scaly patch with raised pearly edge (superficial type) usually found on the trunk. Both types spread slowly without deep erosion and are easily overlooked by both patient and doctor. Confusion with nummular eczema, granuloma annulare and lupus vulgaris is easy. A biopsy is always indicated if there is scarring or if a lesion has been present for over 4 months.

DURATION

The untreated case is slowly progressive. The ulcer is easily treated although a second ulcer may develop.

Table 32 Seventy common skin conditions

I. SINGLE LESIONS THAT MAY OCCUR AT ANY SITE

Viral warts (p. 585)	Junctional naevus	Easily distinguished by colour (red, purple or pigmented) and shape.
Viral warts (plantar) (p. 585)	Pigmented naevus (mole) (p. 584)	
Senile seborrhoeic warts (p. 586)	Capillary haemangioma (port wine stain) (p. 584)	
Basal celled epithelioma (p. 581)	Immature haemangioma (strawberry mark) (p. 584)	
Keratoacanthoma (p. 625)	Keloid scarring	
Squamous cell epithelioma	Boil (p. 590)	
Malignant melanoma (p. 625)	Granuloma (Orf, etc.) (p. 625)	
Granuloma annulare (p. 624)	Acquired haemangioma (pyogenic granuloma) (p. 625)	
	Spider naevus (p. 583)	
	Campbell de Morgan spots	

II. LARGER SINGLE OR MULTIPLE LESIONS AT ANY SITE

Cellulitis (p. 593)	Tinea corporis (p. 587)
Herpes zoster (p. 159)	Contact eczema (p. 602)
Molluscum contagiosum (p. 623)	Nummular eczema (p. 602)

III. LARGER SKIN LESIONS THAT CHARACTERISTICALLY ARISE AT A PARTICULAR SITE

A. Scalp
- Ringworm (tinea capitis) (p. 586)
- Alopecia areata (p. 617)
- Seborrhoea capitis (dandruff) (p. 596)
- Psoriasis of scalp (p. 609)
- Pediculosis capitis (p. 199)

B. Face
- Acne vulgaris (p. 620)
- Impetigo (Strep.) (p. 593)
- Impetigo (Staph.) (p. 593)
- Erysipelas (p. 204)
- Sycosis barbae (p. 619)
- Herpes simplex (p. 162)
- Acne rosacea (p. 607)
- Lupus vulgaris (p. 203)
- Lupus erythematosus (p. 626)
- Rodent ulcer (face) (p. 581)

C. Back of neck, face, arms, legs and sites available to hands
- Neurodermatitis (p. 625)
- Pompholyx (p. 602)
- Dermatitis artefacta (p. 624)
- Erythema serpens (erysipeloid) (p. 624)

D. Groins, axillae, beneath breasts pudendal and perianal areas
- Tinea cruris (p. 587)
- Pruritus ani & vulvi (p. 613)
- Intertrigo — monilia (p. 196, 622)
- Nappy rash (p. 606)
- Pediculosis pubis (p. 200)

E. Shins and lower leg
- Varicose eczema and ulcer (p. 371)
- Erythema nodosum (p. 624)
- Dermatitis artefacta (p. 624)

F. Feet, between toes and dorsum
- Tinea pedis — Athlete's foot (p. 588)

G. Nails of feet & hands
- Chronic paronychia (bacterial) (p. 593)
- Chronic paronychia (fungal) (p. 589)
- Onychogryphosis (Toenails only) (p. 625)

IV. SKIN LESIONS THAT AFFECT MANY SITES OR WHOLE BODY

COMPLICATIONS

A locally malignant growth that does not metastasise.

MANAGEMENT OPTIONS

Prevention: fair skinned people should use ultra violet barrier creams (sunscreens) — BNF 13.8.1 (Ref. 0.1) when prolonged exposure to sun is likely.

Suspected condition: (a) referral for confirmation and decision about appropriate treatment, e.g. excision, radiotherapy, curettage etc.; (b) full explanation stressing non-metastatic natural history.

NEUROFIBROMATA

Classification: ICHPPC 216 (RCGP 0590)

Pedunculated harmless growths with a narrow stalk that arise on the trunk, especially the axillae. They may cause annoyance by their size (1 to 20 mm diam.). Simple removal is then indicated.

DIAGNOSTIC RANGE (rates per 1000 patients per year)
Personal: Probable 2.1.

SPIDER NAEVI

Classification: ICHPPC 216 (RCGP 0550)

Small spider-like capillary dilatations (2 to 3 mm diam.) They characteristically disappear on tensing the skin. High risk factors: (a) facial site; (b) children; (c) pregnancy; (d) liver disease. No treatment.

PORT WINE NAEVI (MATURE CAPILLARY NAEVI)

Classification: ICHPPC 216 (RCGP 0570)

Purple birthmarks that may cover a large area of face or body. They are due to capillary dilatation of the skin. The surface of the lesion is smooth: occasionally it is roughened or raised. High risk factors: (a) face and neck; (b) eye and brain occasionally involved. Much distress is caused.

Management: Referral for advice regarding: (a) laser treatment; (b) plastic surgery; (c) camouflage.

STRAWBERRY NAEVI (IMMATURE CAPILLARY NAEVI)

Classification: ICHPPC 216 (RCGP 0570)

Small raised purple birthmarks which appear soon after birth and can be emptied of blood by pressure and rarely reach diameters of more than 2 to 5 cm. They tend to clear centrally and disappear as the child grows up.

Management: Reassure and leave to cure itself in 2–5 years.

PIGMENTED NAEVI (MOLES)

Classification: ICHPPC 216 (RCGP 0550)

Occasionally grow to a large size and have a superficial resemblance to a senile wart. They may be hairy. Occasionally they undergo malignant change and metastasise rapidly.

The small jet-black moles and those in which there is surrounding pigmentation of the skin are said to be most likely to undergo malignant change. Induration of the base, bleeding, ulceration and increasing size indicate the need for immediate removal and biopsy; otherwise reassure and leave alone.

LIPOMA

Classification: ICHPPC 214 (RCGP 0545)

A harmless subcutaneous, soft, smooth, often loculated swelling of variable size. *Aetiology*: Unknown. Adults mainly women (4:1) affected. Swellings are not fixed and occasionally tender. *Duration*: There is a slow increase in size. *Management*: Reassure and leave unless causing annoyance.

DIAGNOSTIC RANGE (rates per 1000 patients per year)
Personal: Probable 1.54. The diagnosis was rarely in doubt. Many are never reported.

VIRUS WARTS

Classification: ICHPPC 0781 (RCGP 0170)

AETIOLOGY
A DNA virus is responsible. Warts are infectious and are spread by close contact, i.e. shaking hands and walking about on bare feet in changing rooms. (The incidence of plantar warts, in this practice, doubled after the opening of a new school with emphasis on swimming and sport involving showers.)

DIAGNOSTIC RANGE (rates per 1000 patients per year)
Personal: Suspected 17.4. Probable 12.6.

AGE INCIDENCE
The majority (72%) are school children or teenagers.

CLINICAL POINTERS

1. High risk factors: (a) school children; (b) communal washing or changing rooms; (c) family or household contacts; (d) sexual contacts.
2. The lesion. Many fleshly columns of cells are packed tight to make up a solid tumour that varies in size from 1 to 10 mm diameter. On the plantar surface of the foot, the lesion may be difficult to distinguish from a corn. Plantar warts have a punctate surface and are countersunk in the skin of the sole. Crops of minute flat warts sometimes appear on the face or hands. Similar crops of warts sometimes appear on the genitals and a veneral origin is likely.
3. The common sites are: fingers and hands (60%), plantar surface of foot (33%), rest of body (7%).
4. Pain is common with plantar warts.

DURATION
Lesions progress slowly for years. Warts may suddenly spread or disappear for no obvious reason.

COMPLICATIONS
Localised bacterial infection. This sometimes cures the wart.

MANAGEMENT OPTIONS
Prevention: (a) avoid barefoot walking in communal situations; (b) treat and isolate household (and sexual) contacts.

Established warts: (a) avoid radical treatment for extensive multiple lesions; (b) local applications — BNF. 13.7 (Ref. 0.1); (c) radical treatments include: cryotherapy, curettage and cautery; (d) facial warts — salicylic collodion (BNF 13.7).

SENILE (SEBORRHOEIC) WARTS

Classification: ICHPPC 709 (RCGP 3785)

Senile warts are often seen on the backs of elderly patients. They are larger than ordinary warts and diameters of 20 mm are not unusual. The surface is like that of a wart but they have a characteristic flattened, stuck on appearance and may be pigmented. They cause no symptoms, do not become malignant and require no treatment.

FUNGUS INFECTIONS OF THE SKIN

Classification: ICHPPC 110 (RCGP 0220)

Many morphologically different fungi cause skin lesions. Ringworm is the name given to the common lesions.

Different fungi have a predilection for different portions of the skin. A simple anatomical classification is therefore possible:

1. Ringworm of scalp.
2. Ringworm of body (tinea corporis).
3. Ringworm of groin (Dhobie's itch, tinea cruris).
4. Ringworm of feet (athlete's foot, tinea pedis).
5. Ringworm of nails.

AETIOLOGY

The fungus can be detected under a microscope in scrapings from ringworm lesions. This quick standard method of confirming the diagnosis can easily be carried out in any consulting room. Skin scrapings are placed on a slide in a drop of 10% Pot.. hydroxide and examined (low power) after 30 minutes for hyphae. Scrapings can also be taken for culture.

RINGWORM OF SCALP (TINEA CAPITIS)

DIAGNOSTIC RANGE (rates per 1000 patients per year)

Personal: Probable 0.2. Scrapings failed to confirm the diagnosis in any of the suspected cases.

AGE INCIDENCE
Children.

CLINICAL POINTERS
1. High risk factors: (a) school children; (b) family and household contacts.
2. The lesion is a scaly round bald patch with visible stumps of many broken diseased hairs.

INVESTIGATIONS
1. Scrapings examined by microscope or culture (see above).
2. Wood's lamp reveals phosphorescence of affected hairs.

DIFFERENTIAL DIAGNOSIS
Differential diagnosis is from alopecia areata and may require scrapings or a Wood's lamp investigation.

MANAGEMENT OPTIONS
Prevention: measures to prevent spread to contacts.
Established disease: griseofulvin only — BNF 5.2 (Ref. 0.1).

RINGWORM OF THE BODY OR GROINS (TINEA CRURIS)

DIAGNOSTIC RANGE (rates per 1000 patients per year)
Personal: Suspected 2.9. Probable 1.5.

AGE INCIDENCE
All ages.

CLINICAL POINTERS
1. High risk factors: contacts.
2. The lesion is a round, red, scaly ring with well-defined edge and clear centre; it gradually grows outwards.
3. Characteristic sites are the trunk or face. If the groins are affected, the disorder is called Dhobie's itch or Tinea cruris.
4. Irritation is slight or absent.

INVESTIGATIONS
1. Therapeutic test with fungicidal applications.
2. Scrapings for mycelia and possible culture.

DIFFERENTIAL DIAGNOSIS
Diseases that may be confused with ringworm of the body:

Granuloma annulare
Similar features: ring lesions with clear centre.

Distinguishing features: hands and feet liable; failure to respond to fungicides.

Pityriasis rosea
Similar features: round, red patches with well-defined edge and clear centre; irritation.

Distinguishing features: herald patch; numerous lesions — do not increase in size; free edge of scales face the centre of lesion; fungicides ineffective.

Nummular eczema
Similar features: round, red patch with well-defined edge; irritation.

Distinguishing features: centre of lesion active; vesicles and weeping may occur; fungicides aggravate the lesion.

Intertrigo
Similar feature: red patch affecting skin of groins.

Distinguishing features: surface of lesion is uniform; fissuring may occur; irritation absent; fungicides ineffective. If monilia is the cause there will be satellite lesions and the rash will clear with topical antifungals — BNF 13.10.2 (Ref. 0.1).

MANAGEMENT OPTIONS

Prevention: prevent spread to household (and 'changing room') contacts.

Established tinea: (a) topical antifungals — BNF 13.10.2; (b) systemic antifungals — BNF 5.2 if topical treatment ineffective.

RINGWORM OF FEET (TINEA PEDIS OR ATHLETE'S FOOT)

DIAGNOSTIC RANGE (rates per 1000 patients per year)
Personal: Suspected 6.0. Probable 2.0

AGE INCIDENCE
All ages, young adult males are especially prone.

CLINICAL POINTERS

1. Contact cases can rarely be traced.

2. The lesion starts as a soggy mass of white skin between the toes; a rash with clear cut edge, scales and vesicles then spreads on to the dorsum of the foot or instep. The lesion is not so symmetrical or red as ringworm of the body; it does not heal centrally and may blister.

3. Typical sites are between toes, dorsum of feet and soles.
4. Irritation is slight.

INVESTIGATIONS

1. Therapeutic test with topical fungicides — BNF 13.10.2 (Ref. 0.1).
2. Scrapings for mycelia and possibly culture are rarely indicated.

DIFFERENTIAL DIAGNOSIS

Differential diagnosis is from intertrigo and contact eczema. The lesions are similar but contact eczema usually affects the hands not feet. Secondarily infected ringworm may resemble impetigo. Tests with antibiotic and fungicidal ointments usually indicate the diagnosis.

MANAGEMENT OPTIONS

Prevention of recurrences is often difficult: (a) frequent changes of socks; (b) frequent washing and drying of feet; (c) avoid long periods of standing.

Established condition (a) treat sweaty feet (p. 620); (b) topical antifungals — BNF 13.10.2 (Ref. 0.1); (c) systemic antifungals — BNF 5.2 — if topical are ineffective.

RINGWORM OF THE NAILS (TINEA UNGUIUM)

Ringworm of the nails causes a very chronic troublesome infection.

DIAGNOSTIC RANGE (rates per 1000 patients per year)

Personal: Suspected 0.3. (Hospital investigation failed to confirm the diagnosis in any of the suspected cases.)

AGE INCIDENCE

Adults.

CLINICAL POINTERS

1. High risk factors: (a) previous attacks; (b) excessive immersion of hands in water.
2. The nail becomes chronically ridged, thickened, stunted and fragile.

INVESTIGATIONS

Nail clipping for microscopy and culture.

DURATION

Recurrences are common.

MANAGEMENT OPTIONS

Established disease: systemic antifungals — BNF 5.2.

BOILS (FURUNCLES) AND CARBUNCLES

Classification: ICHPPC 680 (RCGP 3600)

A boil is a superficial abscess with a single discharging centre. A carbuncle has more than one point of discharge.

AETIOLOGY

Many varying factors are involved:

1. *Staphylococcus aureus* (*pyogenes*). Household cross-infection appears to be a potent source of spread. (In a series of 440 households one in 10 reported boils, carbuncles or similar staphylococcal lesions in a single year. In 55% of the affected households there was clinical evidence of household cross infection.)

2. Individual susceptibility. Certain individuals appear to be especially prone — the male with a tendency to seborrhoea, the fat female and the adolescent. In staphylococcal households certain individuals may remain strikingly free while others are continually affected.

3. The source of infection. Nasal, skin and occasionally vaginal carriage; also discharge from lesions.

4. Site of lesion.

[A consecutive series of 180 boils and carbuncles were distributed as follows: ear and external auditory meatus, 17% (31); back of neck, 15% (27); scalp and face (excluding styes), 14% (25); arms and hands (excluding fingers), 13% (23); legs and feet (excluding toes), 12% (21); nose, 10% (18); buttocks and perineum, 7% (13); axillae, 6% (11); trunk, 6% (11).]

5. Personal and household hygiene.

DIAGNOSTIC RANGE (rates per 1000 patients per year)

Personal: Reported 24.2+, *National*: 12.1 (Ref. 0.2). The diagnosis was rarely in doubt but many cases are never reported.

AGE INCIDENCE

There is a peak in adolescence (Fig. 50).

SEX INCIDENCE

After adolescence men report boils a little more than women.

SEASONAL INCIDENCE

Six hundred consecutive cases during four years showed a peak in October, November and December (Fig. 51).

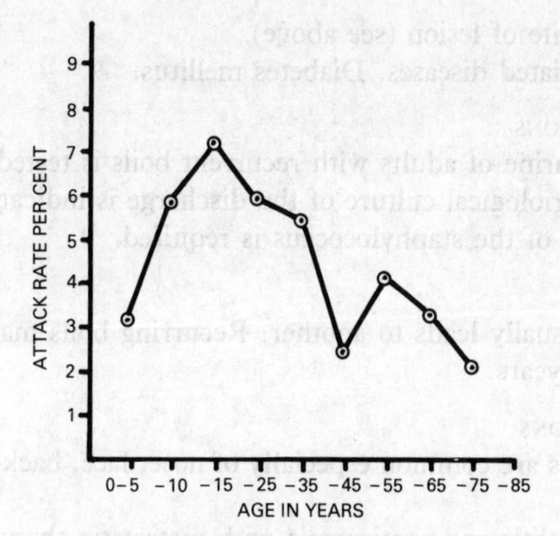

Fig. 50 Boils. Age incidence of 120 consecutive cases reported in 1 year.

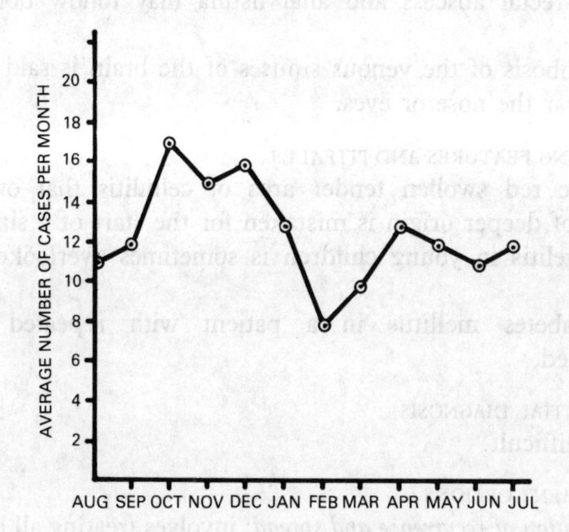

Fig. 51 Boils. Seasonal incidence of 600 cases reported over 4 years.

CLINICAL POINTERS

1. High risk factors: (a) household contacts; (b) nasal or skin carriage; (c) previous attacks; (d) recent stay in a hospital or an infected household; (e) teenage or young adult; (f) diabetes.

2. The lesion. An area of tenderness. A red area of cellulitis becomes fluctuant in the centre and is said to 'point'. After 1 to 4 days a yellow head appears and then discharges. After a further 2 to 5 days a central purulent slough — the core — may be discharged. The lesion then heals in a few days.

3. The site of lesion (see above).
4. Associated diseases. Diabetes mellitus.

INVESTIGATIONS

1. The urine of adults with recurrent boils is tested for sugar.
2. Bacteriological culture of the discharge is indicated when the phage type of the staphylococcus is required.

DURATION

One boil usually leads to another. Recurring boils may persist for months or years.

COMPLICATIONS

Recurrences are common especially of nose, face, back of neck and axillae.

Osteomyelitis and septicaemia with metastatic abscess formation are rare.

Ischio-rectal abscess and anal fistula may follow boils of the buttocks.

Thrombosis of the venous sinuses of the brain is said to follow a boil near the nose or eyes.

MISLEADING FEATURES AND PITFALLS

1. The red swollen tender area of cellulitis that overlies an abscess of deeper origin is mistaken for the start of a simple boil. Osteomyelitis in young children is sometimes overlooked in this way.
2. Diabetes mellitus in a patient with repeated boils is overlooked.

DIFFERENTIAL DIAGNOSIS

Rarely difficult.

MANAGEMENT OPTIONS

Prevention of recurrence and spread: involves treating all household members — a tedious procedure that is rarely justified unless severity or upset is sufficient to ensure compliance. Procedure: (a) nasal (and lesion) swabs from all household members; (b) carriers treated with Naseptin — BNF 12.2.3 (Ref. 0.1) until free; (c) all household members must comply with general hygienic measures involving, washing and use of own towels, etc.; (d) household use of skin disinfecting soaps and solutions — BNF 13.11 (e) regular follow up and swabbing.

Established lesions: (a) local rest; (b) local heat; (c) simple analgesics — BNF 4.7.1.1; (d) incision (occasionally); (e) antibacterials rarely indicated.

WHITLOWS AND PARONYCHIA

Classification: ICHPPC 680 (RCGP 3605)

Fingers and toes are liable to septic staphylococcal lesions.

A whitlow is an infection of the finger pulp. The pulp is a rigidly confined space and the abscess is unable to discharge. Pain is acute and the terminal phalanx may be damaged if the pressure is not relieved by incision.

Paronychia is an infection in the region of the nail. The drainage of the abscess is often poor and in adults the lesion may become chronic if the overlying portion of nail is not removed. Young babies are especially liable to mild paronychia.

AETIOLOGY

See Boils.

DIAGNOSTIC RANGE (rates per 1000 patients per year)

Personal: Probable 11.5+. *National*: 7.2. Many lesions are not reported.

AGE INCIDENCE

All ages.

MANAGEMENT OPTIONS

As for boils but earlier surgical intervention is indicated.

CELLULITIS

Classification: ICHPPC 680 (RCGP 3615)

A tender red swollen area of inflammation which sometimes progresses to a boil. The origin is usually obvious, i.e. an insect bite or previous infection — occasionally no cause is apparent. An associated lymphangitis or lymphadenitis is not unusual. *Treatment*: symptomatic.

IMPETIGO

Classification: ICHPPC 684 (RCGP 3625)

AETIOLOGY

Streptococcus pyogenes. Cases due to *Staphylococcus pyogenes* are increasing.

Impetigo is a household disease. Close personal contacts, trauma and dislike of washing make the school child especially susceptible.

DIAGNOSTIC RANGE (rates per 1000 patients per year)
Personal: Suspected 9.0. Probable 8.4. *National*: 8.0 (Ref. 0.2).

AGE INCIDENCE
All ages. There is a peak of incidence in the first 3 years of school (Fig. 52).

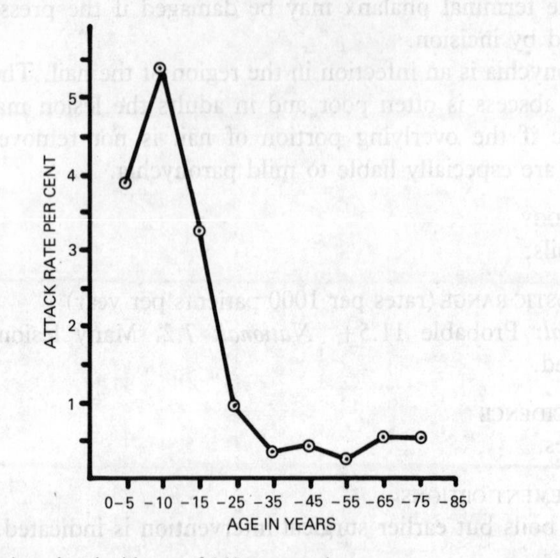

Fig. 52 Impetigo. Age incidence of 149 consecutive cases.

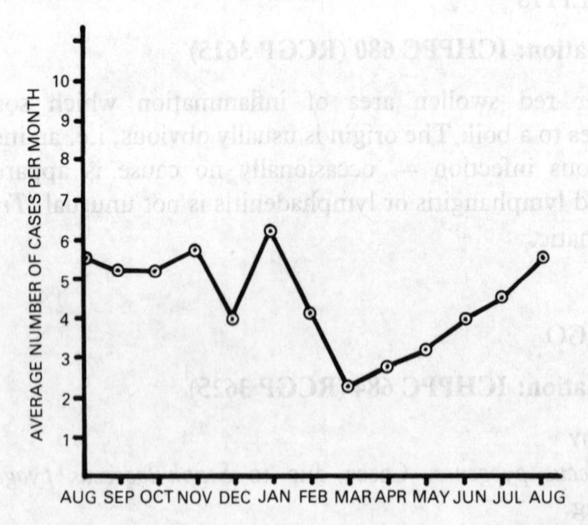

Fig. 53 Impetigo. Seasonal incidence of 212 consecutive cases reported over 4 years.

SEASONAL INCIDENCE

The infection is prevalent at all times of the year but is lowest in the spring and early summer (Fig. 53).

CLINICAL POINTERS

1. High risk factors: (a) household and school contacts; (b) children.

2. The lesion. A superficial spreading yellow crust. The streptococcal lesion — an irregular outline with well-marked yellowish-brown crust. The circinate lesion — crusting is less marked and the lesion initially bullous, bursts to form a raw circular discharging area with a clearly defined spreading edge. Circinate impetigo forms satellite lesions, is often difficult to treat and is usually due to *Staph pyogenes*.

3. The site. Usually on the face or head. Asymmetrical.

4. Itching is occasionally noted.

5. Poor personal or household hygiene.

INVESTIGATIONS

Swabs for bacteriological investigations are occasionally needed.

DURATION AND COMPLICATIONS

Recurrences and household spread may occur. There is no scarring.

DIFFERENTIAL DIAGNOSIS

Herpes simplex or an infected eczema may be confused but this rarely affects management.

MANAGEMENT OPTIONS

Suspected impetigo: (a) topical antibacterials — BNF 13.10.1.1 (Ref. 0.1); (b) systemic antibacterials — BNF 13.10.1.2 and 5.1 occasionally indicated, after swabbing, if resistant.

PYODERMA

Classification: ICHPPC 685 (RCGP 3635)

Multiple purulent vesicles in an area of skin already affected by eczema or fungus infection.

THE SEBORRHOEIC STATE

Classification: ICHPPC 690 (RCGP 3645)

At puberty the skin becomes thicker and more oily and the sebaceous glands become hypertrophied and more active. These changes are marked in the face and hairy regions. The seborrhoeic state is probably an exaggeration of these normal physiological changes. The skin desquamates excessively and dandruff (seborrhoea capitis) forms. There is an increased tendency to develop the typical scaly pink rash of seborrhoeic dermatitis, chronic blepharitis and acne vulgaris. The relationship between infantile and adult seborrhoea is uncertain, as is the aetiology of the condition as a whole. Hormonal influences may play a part.

SEBORRHOEA CAPITIS (DANDRUFF)

DIAGNOSTIC RANGE (rates per 1000 patients per year)

Personal: Probable 6.6+. Many patients never report the disease.

AGE INCIDENCE

Adults are liable — the disorder tends to develop soon after puberty. A severe degree of seborrhoea capitis is often noted over the unclosed fontanelle of young babies (Cradle cap).

CLINICAL POINTERS

1. Dandruff (10%).
2. Slight irritation is common; often absent.
3. Associated disorders include seborrhoeic dermatitis, chronic blepharitis, otitis externa, acne vulgaris and rosacea.

DURATION

The tendency is lifelong.

COMPLICATIONS

Furunculosis.

DIFFERENTIAL DIAGNOSIS

Dandruff may also be a feature of other skin diseases of the scalp, i.e. eczema and psoriasis. Evidence of these diseases elsewhere in the body usually makes the diagnosis clear.

MANAGEMENT OPTIONS

Prevention: shampoos and scalp lotions containing tar, salicylic acid or a diluted corticosteroid — BNF 13.9 (Ref. 0.1) two to three times a week.

Active: as for prevention, but use daily.

Cradle cap: (a) apply olive oil; (b) *half strength* shampoos as for adults above if cap is excessive — BNF 13.9. Use for short periods only.

SEBORRHOEIC DERMATITIS

DIAGNOSTIC RANGE (rates per 1000 patients per year)
Personal: Suspected 9.1. Probable 6.6. *National*: 4.4 (Ref. 0.2).

AGE INCIDENCE
Adults are liable but the disease is rare in the elderly. A post-auricular seborrhoeic dermatitis which resembles that of adults is found in babies and young children (35% of all suspected cases). The aetiology of this lesion is uncertain.

CLINICAL POINTERS
1. The typical lesion. A patch of bright skin with a slight brown tinge and a clearly defined edge. The patch has a uniform appearance and varies from 1 to 20 cm in diameter. Scales of dandruff are evident especially at the periphery of the lesion. The vesicles and weeping areas of a true eczema are absent although exudation may occur from fissures especially when the lesion is behind the ears.
2. Characteristic sites of the rash are: behind the ears (55%), scalp and hair margin (35%), flexures (30%). Numerous small scattered lesions sometimes appear on the trunk and simulate pityriasis rosea.
3. Slight irritation.
4. Associated disorders include seborrhoea capitis, recurrent styes, chronic blepharitis, furunculosis, otitis externa, acne vulgaris and rosacea.

DURATION
The rash clears easily with treatment.

COMPLICATIONS
Sepsis of affected areas may lead to fissuring, exudation and pustule formation, which resembles an infected eczema.

Recurrences are common (20% of patients observed for 3 years had more than one attack.)

DIFFERENTIAL DIAGNOSIS
Diseases that may be confused with seborrhoeic dermatitis:

Pityriasis rosea
Similar features: numerous small scaly pink macules over trunk; slight irritation.

Distinguishing features: herald patch; oval lesions following lines of dermatomes on the back; lesions tend to clear centrally; free edges of scales point to centre of lesions; recurrences absent; differentiation may be difficult.

Intertrigo
Similar features: red patch with clear-cut edge; flexures are affected; slight irritation; concurrent monilial infection.

Distinguishing features: skin surfaces damp and soggy; scales absent; other signs of seborrhoeic state absent; response to treatment poor.

Tinea cruris and corporis
Similar features: red patch with clear-cut edge; groins affected; slight irritation.

Distinguishing features: lesion gets slowly larger and clear centrally; other signs of seborrhoeic state absent; rapid response to fungicidal ointment.

Contact dermatitis of scalp as from hair dye, etc.
Similar features: diffuse scaly lesion of scalp with secondary sepsis; exudate.

Distinguishing features: history of contact; previous seborrhoea absent; lesion may become generalised; vesicles; post-auricular region not especially prone; differentiation may be difficult.

MANAGEMENT OPTIONS

Prevention: not cost-effective.

Established or recurrent attacks: topical steroids — BNF 13.4 (Ref. 0.1). Mild potency; water-mixable creams allow further dilution; short courses only.

ALLERGIC DERMATOSES

CLASSIFICATION
The various types of allergic dermatoses are poorly defined because the aetiology is obscure.

1. Urticaria (including angioneurotic oedema). ICHPPC 708 (RCGP 3775).

2. Eczema. The terms dermatitis and eczema are interchangeable. ICHPPC 692 (RCGP 3655, 3665). This group is sometimes divided into eczemas in which there is an obvious contact factor called the exogenous eczemas or extrinsic dermatitis and those in which there is presumed hereditary factor with no obvious contact the atopic, endogenous or intrinsic eczemas. Several different types of endogenous eczema are described. In each the basic lesion is the same but the bodily distribution and age of patient affected are

different (see p. 602). The extrinsic and intrinsic groups may overlap in one individual and clear-cut definition may not be practical.

3. Drug eruptions and similar allergic rashes. The clinical definition is difficult because the suspected drug or food cannot be continued for the purpose of confirming the diagnosis.

4. Allergic rashes that follow bacterial infection. The rash of scarlet fever and the circinate urticarial rash of rheumatic fever are probably of this type. It is not known if the rashes of measles and rubella are due to allergic reactions or to the presence of virus in the skin.

GIANT URTICARIA (SYN. NETTLE RASH) AND ANGIONEUROTIC OEDEMA

Irritant urticarial weals (giant urticaria) and swelling of the face, tongue and elsewhere (angioneurotic oedema) often develop simultaneously.

AETIOLOGY

Allergy probably plays a large part but an obvious causal agent is only noted in a proportion (30%) of cases. Nervous reactions may affect the rash.

DIAGNOSTIC RANGE (rates per 1000 patients per year)

Personal: Probable 4.0+. Many cases are never reported.

AGE INCIDENCE

Adults and older children liable.

CLINICAL POINTERS

1. The typical lesion is a round urticarial weal which may vary from 5 to 100 mm in diameter. The weal is whiter than the surrounding skin but may be reddened by scratching or rubbing. The patient often refers to the lesion as a lump. In severe cases a blister may form. Characteristically the lesions come and go in a few hours. Lesions may become confluent.

2. Situation of the lesion. Any part of the skin may be affected.

3. Irritation (100%) may be intense at the onset.

4. Swelling of the face (45%). The periorbital tissues or lips, occasionally the tongue, palate and glottis are affected. Swelling of wrists and ankles may occur.

5. Associated diseases (20%). There is sometimes a history of

other allergic diseases — eczema, asthma, hay fever and serum sickness. Erythema multiforme (iris form) is an associated urticarial disease (hands often affected).

DURATION

An attack may last from a few hours to several days. Recurrences can often be modified by antihistamine drugs. The attacks may cease suddenly after causing years of annoyance.

COMPLICATIONS

Oedema of the glottis and tongue may be so severe that suffocation causes death — a frightening complication that is fortunately very rare (no cases encountered).

MANAGEMENT OPTIONS

Prevention of attacks: (a) avoidance of known allergens; (b) prophylactic systemic antihistamines — BNF 3.4.1 (Ref. 0.1) — often ineffective; (b) specific desensitising vaccines are rarely advisable.

Established attack: (a) systemic antihistamines — BNF 3.4.1; (b) topical antipruritics — BNF 13.3 (avoid topical antihistamines).

ECZEMA (SYN. DERMATITIS)

Eczema is the commonest skin disease. It has many variations because different individuals react to irritant stimuli in many ways.

AETIOLOGY AND CLASSIFICATION

The exact aetiology is uncertain but it is probable that two main factors are responsible:

1. *External irritants or allergens*. There are three main groups:

• Simple physical irritants such as, exposure to cold, to wind or irritant chemicals — diesel, bleaches, detergents, formalin, cleaners, soda, solvents, flour, etc. The eczema reaction is usually localised to the point of contact and disappears if skin is protected or the irritant removed. Nappy rash (p. 606), housewives' hand and the mild non-recurrent patch of eczema on babies' faces, are all common examples.

• True allergic contact eczema. There is often a widespread delayed reaction not related to the point of contact. Many industrial dermatoses are examples.

• Photosensitive reactions — often aggravated by specific drugs or cosmetics. There is a characteristic distribution on face, hands, neck and upper sternum.

2. *Endogenous constitutional factors* possibly involving immunological defects or T-lymphocyte deficiencies. Several clinical types are described in the following sections:

— Atopic eczema: affecting toddlers, children and young adults (p. 602)
— Seborrhoeic eczema: affecting infants and adults (p. 597)
— Nummular (discoid) eczema affecting young adults (p. 602)
— Neurodermatitis (p. 625) affecting adults
— Pompholyx eczema affecting adults (p. 602)

Correct assessment of the interplay of constitutional and irritant factors influences treatment.

DIAGNOSTIC RANGE (rates per 1000 patients per year)
Personal: Suspected 35.7. Probable 29.0. *National*: 38.4 (Ref. 0.2). Many mild cases are probably never reported.

CLINICAL POINTERS

1. High risk factors: (a) contact with known irritants; (b) family history of allergy; (c) previous history of allergy; (d) age of patient and site of lesions — vulnerability varies with age (see above) and site (see below).

2. The basic lesion. It has long been known that when normal skin is rubbed with an irritant the following events occur:

• The area becomes red and slightly swollen. If no further application is made, the redness subsides and desquamation with scaling occurs. The skin then returns to normal.

• If the application is continued, the redness becomes more marked, the patch becomes slightly oedematous and small vesicles appear. This is the onset of the acute weepy stage.

• Irritation causes scratching, and the acute stage of ruptured vesicles or diffuse oozing from the raw surfaces. Crusts of coagulated serum develop. Local oedema may be marked.

• The lesion may gradually heal by passing through a stage of fine epithelialisation and scaling with occasional vesicle formation.

• If the local application continues, a similar rash may affect other parts of the body symmetrically and it is then postulated that the skin of the body has developed an allergy to the irritant.

One or more of these stages can be observed in every case of eczema. The lesions vary according to the individual reactions, but the above sequence probably represents the behaviour of the basic unit of eczema.

3. The extent of the disease varies greatly. This depends upon the interplay of constitutional and external (trigger) factors giving rise to the following types:

• *Mild extrinsic (non-recurrent) eczema* (35%). One or two small patches of roughened skin appear. Vesicles are not obvious and the lesion is limited to a small rounded scaly patch with a clear-cut edge which disappears after a week or two. Irritation is slight and many such lesions probably go unnoticed. This type is commonly seen on the faces of babies. Reassurance and bland treatment only are needed.

• *Mild extrinsic contact eczema* (25%). One or two isolated patches of irritant vesicles appear over the contact areas. The patch often has a clearly defined edge and may be red, scaly or weeping. The hands and face are common sites but suspender or brassière buckle areas may be affected. These patients are resistant to treatment unless the irritant is removed. Continued scratching may cause a lichenified patch of neurodermatitis.

• *Generalised extrinsic eczema* in which there is an obvious physical trigger stimulus (10%). A specific irritant — penicillin, or light (actinic dermatitis) — may precipitate an attack of generalised eczema. The part of the body that is most severely affected may suggest the physical cause, e.g. in actinic dermatitis, the rash is worst over the face and hands.

• *Recurrent generalised atopic (intrinsic) eczema* in which there is no obvious physical trigger stimulus (20%). Asthma and other hereditary factors may be noted. The lesions are usually symmetrical and often affect the flexures. Mild cases give a history of an occasional irritant vesicular rash. In severe cases large areas of the body are covered by rash and remissions are less common.

• *Nummular or discoid (intrinsic) eczema*. One or more lesions are scattered over the body in a series of dry or weeping round patches. Rare under 20, it is commonest in young or middle aged adults. Lasts a few months and clears. Relapse rate is low.

• *Pompholyx* is a localised form of eczema affecting palms of hands and soles of feet where the vesicular features of eczema are modified by the thick skin. The lesions dry up and desquamate after a few days or weeks; weeping and exudation are less common. Dyshidrosis, stress and tinea pedis infections are all said to be causative agents.

The picture of eczema is complicated because the clinical types merge and because any lesion may be seen in the dry (scaly), vesicular, weeping or healing stage.

4. Irritation is usually present, often severe and varies in intensity.

5. Associated diseases (20%). Asthma, hay fever, and other allergic disorders.

INVESTIGATIONS

When a specific contact is suspected, a patch test or series of scratch skin tests can be performed.

DURATION

Some (50%) of patients with mild eczema clear up completely within 2 or 3 weeks; in others recurrences are common and the disease may be chronic.

COMPLICATIONS

Secondary infection may confuse the clinical picture. Yellow purulent crusting develops and pustules form in the skin. Secondary infection may lead to cellulitis or erysipelas.

MISTAKES AND PITFALLS

The simple rule of treatment — when acute, handle gently, when chronic treat vigorously — is ignored.

A. DIFFERENTIAL DIAGNOSIS OF A LOCALISED PATCH OF ECZEMA

Diseases that may be confused with a localised patch of eczema:

Tinea corporis and pedis (and monilia)

Similar features: circumscribed lesions affecting flexures, hands or feet; scratched vesicles sometimes present on dorsum of foot or hand; irritation.

Distinguishing features: *Tinea pedis* — usually affects dorsum of feet rather than hands; lesion gradually spreads outwards; evidence of tinea between toes; responds to fungicides; *Tinea corporis* — clearly defined circinate edge of lesions with clear centre; responds to fungicides. *Monilia* — small satellite lesions just outside the patch.

Impetigo

Similar feature: weeping lesion with crusting exudate and clearly defined edge.

Distinguishing features: face usually affected; crusting marked; differentiation between impetigo and secondarily infected eczema may be difficult.

B. DIFFERENTIAL DIAGNOSIS OF GENERALISED ECZEMA

Diseases that may be confused with generalised eczema:

Seborrhoeic dermatitis
Similar features: recurring scaly rash; flexures liable; irritation; exudation.

Distinguishing features: dandruff, blepharitis and other signs of seborrhoeic state; rash is reddish brown with clearly defined edges; vesicles are not seen and exudate (if any) arises from fissures; differentiation in severe cases difficult.

Sweat rashes and papular allergic rashes
Similar feature: papular irritant rash covering large area of the body.

Distinguishing features: short duration; vesiculation, weeping and scaling absent.

Scabies
Similar features: generalised irritant vesicular rash; tops of vesicles are scratched.

Distinguishing features: scratch marks, beheaded papules and vesicles are main lesions; burrows occasionally visible; typical sites are rim of navel, genitalia, buttocks, hands and webs of fingers; contact cases; responds to antiscabetics.

Psoriasis
Similar feature: scattered patches of scaly purple or red rash.

Distinguishing features: lesions have typical silvery foam-like scales with free edge of scales facing outwards; irritation, vesiculation and weeping absent; typical sites are extensor surfaces of knees and elbows; psoriatic pitting of nails; psoriatic lesions of scalp.

MANAGEMENT OPTIONS

Prevention: Extrinsic and intrinsic eczema: (a) avoidance of allergen; (b) physical protectives including: extraction fans, protective garments, barrier preparations — BNF 13.2.1 (Ref. 0.1); (c) breast feeding protects against atopic eczema.

Established extrinsic and intrinsic eczemas: Acute phase: handle gently using plain emulsifying ointment, physiological saline and bland drying lotions.

Subacute and chronic: (a) gradual introduction of dilute then full strength fluorinated topical steroids — BNF 13.4 — use weakest strengths for shortest periods that are effective; (b) topical tar preparations — BNF 13.5 and oral antihistamines — BNF 3.4.1, if itching is marked or causing insomnia; (c) if secondarily infected, anti-infective skin preparations —BNF 13.10 — may be used topically (and orally); (d) occlusive bandages if resistant — BNF 13.4 and 13.5; (e) all immunisations (except smallpox) are safe for atopics; (f) self help groups — National Eczema Society (Ref. 23.1) information (+ magazine) especially for school children; raises funds also.

DRUG ERUPTIONS AND SIMILAR ALLERGIC RASHES (EXCLUDING URTICARIAL RASHES)

AETIOLOGY
Uncertain.

DIAGNOSTIC RANGE (rates per 1000 population per year)
Personal: Suspected 29.7+. Many rashes are not reported to the doctor.

CLINICAL POINTERS

1. High risk factors: Any drug whether used systemically or topically is suspect. Certain incrimination is difficult but suspected cases should be reported to health authorities.

2. The rash. The majority (70%) of patients have a fine punctate papular red rash, which resembles that of scarlet fever but without its background flush. In the remainder (30%), the rash consists of blotchy red, often confluent macules and resembles measles rather than scarlet fever, this latter type is commonly associated with drugs, e.g. penicillin, sulpha or bromides.

2. Site of rash. The rash is usually generalised.

3. Irritation is common but not invariable. It may be intense and scratching may raise added urticarial weals.

DURATION
Rarely longer than 14 days. Occasionally a drug rash persists for several weeks after withdrawal of the offending agent.

COMPLICATIONS
None if drug is stopped.

MISTAKES AND PITFALLS
Ampicillin is given to a patient with mononucleosis.

DIFFERENTIAL DIAGNOSIS
Diseases that may be confused with drug eruptions, etc.:

Scarlet fever
Similar feature: punctate fine red papular rash affecting whole body.

Distinguishing features: contact cases; sore red throat (with or without exudate); fever; diffuse bright pink flush of skin; circumoral pallor; furred tongue; offensive breath.

Rubella
Similar features: morbilliform rash of the whole body; fever absent.
Distinguishing features: contact cases; low fever; occipital, cervical or post-auricular adenitis; distinction may be impossible.

Measles
Similar feature: confluent morbilliform rash of whole body.
Distinguishing features: contact cases; cough always present; Koplik's spots; fever; children affected; distinction rarely difficult.

Secondary syphilis
Similar features: macular rash affecting whole body; patient may be taking sulpha or penicillin for concurrent gonorrhoea.
Distinguishing features: background information about patient may help; history of possible contact or primary sore; fever; generalised or inguinal adenitis; snail track changes in mouth; serology becomes positive soon after rash developes.

MANAGEMENT OPTIONS
Suspected rash: (a) stop suspected agent; (b) record sensitivity on front of patient's record; (c) notify central health authority (yellow card); (d) follow up; (e) antipruritics — BNF 13.3 and sedatives — BNF 4.1.

NAPKIN (DIAPER) ERUPTIONS
Classification: ICHPPC 6910 (RCGP 3650)

AETIOLOGY
There are many different causes (see below).

DIAGNOSTIC RANGE (rates per 1000 patients per year)
Personal: Suspected 5.7+. Many parents treat the condition without consulting the doctor.

CLINICAL POINTERS
1. High risk factors: (a) infrequent changing especially overnight; (b) insufficient rinsing of nappies after washing; (c) use of plastic outside pants; (d) deficient socio-economic conditions; (e) change of diet, especially to meat.
2. The eruption affects the napkin area and varies in appearance:
— a fine red papulo-vesicular rash suggests contact with a mild irritant such as soap, detergent or urine.
— well defined punched out ulcers (10 mm diam.) suggests ammonia burns resulting from prolonged contact with alkaline urine as in older, weaned babies.

— large red confluent patches suggest seborrhoeic intertrigo. If there are small satellite areas at its edges, monilia is likely (see Moniliasis — p. 196).

DURATION

The rash clears rapidly with treatment.

MISTAKES AND PITFALLS

1. Topical preparations are prescribed without ensuring either avoidance of plastic waterproofing or more frequent nappy changes.

2. Powerful topical steroids are used over long periods and may cause atrophy of skin.

MANAGEMENT OPTIONS

Prevention: patient education in the antenatal period.

Established eruption: (a) avoid plastic pants; (b) ensure sufficiently frequent changing of nappies; (c) encourage long periods 'open to the air'; (d) check adequate rinsing of nappies; (e) protective creams — BNF 13.10.5 (Ref. 0.1) — simple petroleum jelly is often best; (f) topical antifungals if monilial — BNF 13.10.2.

ROSACEA

Classification: ICHPPC 709 (RCGP 3685)

AETIOLOGY

Unknown. Overbusy, overanxious, overconscientious types of people and rich foods are all said to contribute. There is no real evidence for any of these causes.

DIAGNOSTIC RANGE (rates per 1000 patients per year)

Personal: Probable 1.6+. Many cases are probably never reported.

AGE AND SEX INCIDENCE

Middle age; women especially liable.

CLINICAL POINTERS

1. The lesion starts as a chronic facial flush and progresses to acne-like papules in the purple red skin.

2. Characteristic site. The butterfly area of the cheeks and bridge of nose. The rash is usually symmetrical.

3. Associated disorders. Chronic conjunctivitis, seborrhoea, chronic alcoholism and rhinophyma.

DURATION

Once established the disorder tends to persist for many years. Remissions occur in mild cases.

COMPLICATIONS

Corneal ulceration and keratitis. Said to arise in 50% of cases.

DIFFERENTIAL DIAGNOSIS

Lupus erythematosus also starts with a red rash of the butterfly area but lesions are deeper with scaling, a firm plaque and scarring.

MANAGEMENT OPTIONS

Established disorder: (a) 6 + weeks tetracyclines twice daily — BNF 5.1.3 (Ref. 0.1); (b) metronidazole — BNF 5.1.11.1; (c) avoid trigger factors — rarely identifiable; (d) relapses after stopping treatment common.

PSORIASIS

Classification: ICHPPC 6961 (RCGP 3695)

AETIOLOGY

Unknown. Trauma, mental strain and streptococcal infections are said to precipitate attacks. There is an increased turnover (desquamation) time in the affected skin layers. Two per cent of population said to be affected.

DIAGNOSTIC RANGE (rates per 1000 population per year)

Personal: Probable 5.0+. *National*: 3.5 (Ref. 0.2).

AGE INCIDENCE

The rash starts in young adults and persists indefinitely.

CLINICAL POINTERS

1. High risk vulnerability factors: (a) family history (positive in 40%); (b) skin trauma; (c) infections; (d) cold weather; (e) drugs — lithium; antimalarials; (f) mental conflict — possibly.

2. The lesion [100%] is easily recognised by the following features: a slightly raised papule or plaque 5 to 100 mm diameter; clear-cut discoid sometimes irregular outline; deep red almost purple colour; central scale with typical silvery colour and firm foam-like appearance; the scale usually covers most of the lesion and has a free peripheral edge — a distinctive characteristic; absence of scarring when the lesion heals.

3. The site of the lesions. The extensor surfaces of knees and elbows are common; but the lesions may arise anywhere on the trunk or limbs. The face is rarely affected. The distribution varies — there may be many small lesions (guttate psoriasis) or fewer lesions of greater individual size (sometimes circinate).

4. The tendency of the disease to come and go but never clear completely.

5. Associated lesions: (a) scalp — a thick matted plate of dandruff with some loss of hair; (b) nails may be thimble pitted, ridged, greatly thickened or show early separation with loss of pink nail-bed colour. Arthritis especially of distal interphalangeal joints.

6. Absence of irritation.

DURATION

Treatment may shorten the life of individual lesions but rarely leads to permanent cure. Remissions may occur.

COMPLICATIONS

A rheumatoid type of arthritis occasionally develops in patients with psoriasis. The terminal phalanges are especially affected. As the aetiology is unknown there is no indication whether the psoriasis complicates the rheumatoid lesions or vice versa. (Practice experience: this condition arose in 0.8 per 1000 patients and was treated in a similar way to rheumatoid arthritis.)

MISLEADING FEATURES AND PITFALLS

Patients are traditionally told that there is no cure for this disease — a statement which does little to help; in fact the family doctor can do a great deal to ameliorate the symptoms.

DIFFERENTIAL DIAGNOSIS

Difficulties arise with:

— Guttate psoriasis when the differential diagnosis is similar to that of Pityriasis rosea (see next section).
— Scalp psoriasis. There may be large plaques of severe thick scurf and no other evidence of psoriasis.
— Nail psoriasis may simulate fungal nail infections.

MANAGEMENT OPTIONS

Established psoriasis: (a) full explanation and support to counter commonly held gloomy views; (b) avoid where possible, high risk trigger factors; (c) sun bathing and UV lamp; (d) topical keratolytics — salicyclic acid, tar, dithranol, etc. — BNF 13.5 (Ref. 0.1); (e) topical fluorinated steroids (potency II or III) — BNF 13.4 — are pleasant and effective but are expensive and have certain risks: with prolonged use, effectiveness lessens and risks increase; (f) referral if intractable for PUVA, cytotoxics (methotrexate) — BNF 8.1.3, etc.; (g) support from patient groups — Psoriasis Association (Ref. 23.2).

PITYRIASIS ROSEA

Classification: ICHPPC 6963 (RCGP 3700)

AETIOLOGY

Unknown. Some features of the disorder suggest a virus origin. Occasionally two members of the same household are affected.

DIAGNOSTIC RANGE (rates per 100 patients per year)

Personal: Suspected 2.0. Probable 1.1. *National*: 1.6.

AGE INCIDENCE

School children and young adults.

SEX INCIDENCE

Females affected more than males.

CLINICAL POINTERS

1. Herald patch (40%). A large macule (10 to 50 mm in diameter) clearing in the centre with scaly edge, is noted by the patient 1 to 3 weeks before the main eruption.

2. The rash (100%) has the following characteristics:

- Bright red or brown macules which vary from 2 to 20 mm diameter.
- Macules are round or oval — a collar of centrally directed scales surrounds a clearer centre.
- The macules are symmetrical and arranged in a characteristic pattern which is usually apparent on the back — the longitudinal axis of the oval macules lie in the line of the ribs and dermatomes.

3. The distribution of the rash is symmetrical and mainly on the trunk. The face, scalp and hands are usually spared.

4. Irritation is slight (70%).

INVESTIGATIONS

A serological test to exclude syphilis is taken when the rash is clearing in adults.

DURATION

Varies from 2 to 12 weeks. Recurrences rare but do occur.

COMPLICATIONS

None.

MISLEADING FEATURES AND PITFALLS

The rash is sometimes localised to a comparatively small area.

Mild malaise, low fever and slight generalised lymphadenopathy may confuse the diagnosis. Two members of a household may be affected simultaneously.

DIFFERENTIAL DIAGNOSIS

Diseases that may be confused with pityriasis rosea:

Secondary syphilis

Similar features: red or purple macular rash of trunk which lasts 2 to 6 weeks; fever, malaise and lymphadenopathy.

Distinguishing features: history and background knowledge of patient; fever; malaise and lymphadenopathy marked; rash does not irritate; snail track changes in mucous membranes of mouth; evidence of recent primary; serology distinguishes.

Drug eruptions

Similar features: red or purple irritant macular rash of trunk which lasts 2 to 6 weeks.

Distinguishing features: history of drugs being taken, e.g. barbiturate, bromide, sulpha, penicillin or phenophthalein; individual lesions do not clear centrally; scaling is absent and coalescence may occur; staining of skin may persist.

Seborrhoeic dermatitis

Similar feature: orange-red rash persists for weeks.

Distinguishing features: evidence of seborrhoea in scalp and elsewhere; history of previous attacks; the scales of seborrhoeic lesion point outwards and not centrally.

Tinea corporis

Similar features: red rash; lesions on trunk which clear centrally.

Distinguishing features: confusions occur with the herald patch and early lesions; the individual lesions increase in size and rash is not general.

Guttate psoriasis

Similar feature: red macular rash of trunk; several weeks duration.

Distinguishing features: confusion unlikely; lesions are raised; extensor limb surfaces often affected; scaling is silvery and free edge of scale points outwards; evidence of psoriasis elsewhere; irritation absent; previous attacks.

Rubella and glandular fever

Similar features: macular rash; malaise, low fever and lymphadenopathy.

Distinguishing features: contact cases; rash lasts less than a week; lesions are smaller; confusion unlikely.

MANAGEMENT OPTIONS

Prevention: None. Symptomatic treatment only.

Irritation: (a) topical calamine — BNF 13.3; (b) oral antihistamines for sleep — BNF 3.4.1. (Ref. 0.1).

GENERALISED PRURITUS

Classification: ICHPPC 698 (RCGP 3720)

AETIOLOGY

Unknown.

DIAGNOSTIC RANGE (rates per 1000 population per year)

Personal: 1.4.

AGE INCIDENCE

Adults. Elderly patients are especially prone.

CLINICAL POINTERS

1. High risk factors: (a) diabetes; (b) thyroid disease; (c) contraceptive pill and pregnancy; (d) old age; (e) psychogenic; (f) liver and renal disease; (g) the reticuloses; (h) certain drugs.
2. Generalised irritation of skin. Sometimes severe.
3. Absence of lesions.

INVESTIGATIONS

Blood tests: ESR, FBC, Phosphatase, etc. Urine tests.

DURATION

May be transient or persistent.

COMPLICATIONS

Neurodermatitis.

DIFFERENTIAL DIAGNOSIS

Diabetes mellitus, a blood disease, early jaundice or a reticulosis may cause general irritation without rash.

MANAGEMENT OPTIONS

Established pruritus: (a) exclude high risk trigger factors; (b) oral antihistamines — BNF 3.4.1; (c) topical antipruritics — BNF 13.3 (Ref. 0.1).

PRURITUS ANI AND VULVAE

Classification: ICHPPC 698 (RCGP 3710, 3715)

AETIOLOGY

Unknown. Psychological factors appear to play a part in perpetuating the complaint. No obvious 'triggers' in most cases.

DIAGNOSTIC RANGE (rates per 1000 patients per year)

Personal: Probable 4.5.

AGE INCIDENCE

Adults.

CLINICAL POINTERS

1. High risk factors: (a) sedentary job in sweaty conditions; (b) poor hygiene occasionally.
2. Irritation (often intense) of the vulva, anal or pubic regions.
3. Absence of lesions. Sometimes excoriation of the perianal skin follows scratching.

INVESTIGATIONS

The urine is examined for sugar.

DURATION

Symptoms may be continuous or intermittent and the disorder may last for many years.

COMPLICATIONS

None.

MISLEADING FEATURES AND PITFALLS

Itching of the anal or vulval region is an early sign of diabetes.

DIFFERENTIAL DIAGNOSIS

Diseases that may be confused with pruritus ani and vulvae:

Diabetes mellitus

Similar feature: recurring irritation and excoriation of perianal region.

Distinguishing features: thirst; polyuria; weight loss; glycosuria.

Threadworms

Similar feature: recurring irritation of anus of vulva.

Distinguishing features: children mainly affected; contact cases; irritation mainly in bed; worms visible outside anus at night and in motions; tests for ova.

Piles
Similar feature: recurring irritation of anus.
Distinguishing features: blood loss per rectum; prolapse of piles; skin tags suggesting piles on rectal examination.

Vaginitis and leucorrhoea
Similar feature: recurring irritation of vulval region.
Distinguishing features: vaginal discharge; vaginal walls inflamed.

Tinea cruris and Monilia
Similar feature: recurring irritation of perineal region.
Distinguishing feature: typical rash with circinate edge slowly spreading outward from perineal region. Monilia — satellite lesions.

MANAGEMENT OPTIONS
Established condition: (a) astringent antipruritics (0.5% phenol) — BNF 13.3 (Ref. 0.1); (b) frequent cleansing and change of pants; (c) topical steroids — BNF 13.4 as a last resort (encourage intermittent use).

PAPULAR URTICARIA

Classification: ICHPPC 698 (RCGP 3775)

AETIOLOGY
Probably a hypersensitivity to insect or mite bites. Rarely is it possible to identify the source.

DIAGNOSTIC RANGE (rates per 1000 patients per year)
Personal: Suspected 25.2. Probable 18.8. (The high rates indicate a young practice.)

AGE INCIDENCE
Half the patients are under 5 years and most of the remainder are under 10 (Fig. 54).

SEASONAL INCIDENCE
Autumn and spring (Fig. 55).

CLINICAL POINTERS
1. High risk factors: (a) previous attacks; (b) household contacts.
2. The rash (100%). Crops of small urticarial weals, 5 to 10 mm diameter, that may have a central punctum or vesicle — often scratched away. Lesions may be general but usually occur in localised crops, especially on the trunk, and resemble flea bites or scabies, from which the condition may be difficult to distinguish.

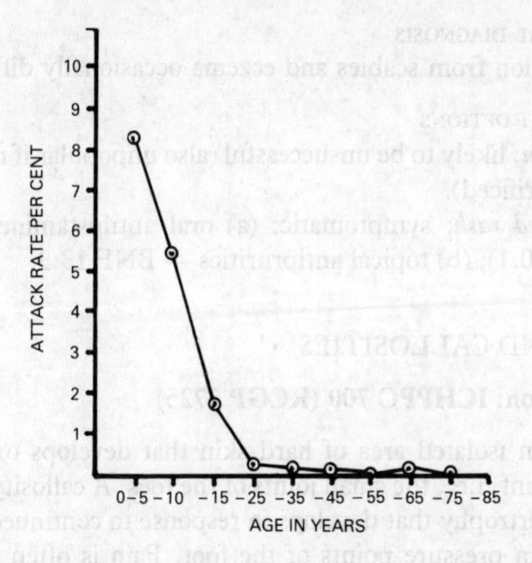

Fig. 54 Papular urticaria. Age incidence of 65 consecutive cases in 1 year.

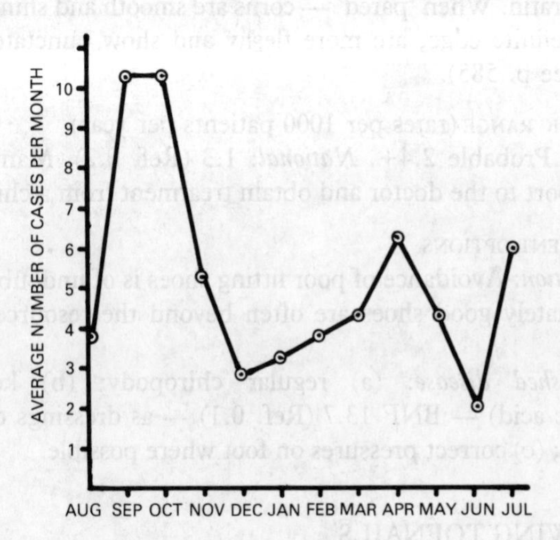

Fig. 55 Papular urticaria. Seasonal incidence of 248 consecutive cases reported over 4 years.

3. Irritation (100%) is intense and worse at night.

DURATION

Up to 4 weeks. Recurrences are common and certain children report each year at the same season. Attacks cease after 3 or 4 years.

DIFFERENTIAL DIAGNOSIS

Differentiation from scabies and eczema occasionally difficult.

MANAGEMENT OPTIONS

Prevention: likely to be unsuccessful (also unpopular if much loved pets are sacrificed).

Established rash: symptomatic: (a) oral antihistamines — BNF 3.4.1 (Ref. 0.1); (b) topical antipruritics — BNF 13.3.

CORNS AND CALLOSITIES

Classification: ICHPPC 700 (RCGP 3725)

A corn is an isolated area of hard skin that develops over a small pressure-point, i.e., the small joints of the toes. A callosity is a wider area of hypertrophy that develops in response to continued pressure, i.e. the main pressure points of the foot. Pain is often associated. Corns may be difficult to distinguish from plantar warts because both are painful, both may arise over the pressure points and cause excess keratin. When 'pared' — corns are smooth and shiny — warts have a definite edge, are more fleshy and show punctate capillary points (see p. 585).

DIAGNOSTIC RANGE (rates per 1000 patients per year)

Personal: Probable 2.4+. *National*: 1.3 (Ref. 0.2). Many patients never report to the doctor and obtain treatment from a chiropodist.

MANAGEMENT OPTIONS

Prevention: Avoidance of poor fitting shoes is of undoubted value. Unfortunately good shoes are often beyond the resources of poor families.

Established disease: (a) regular chiropody; (b) keratolytics (salicyclic acid) — BNF 13.7 (Ref. 0.1) — as dressings or plasters may help; (c) correct pressures on foot where possible.

INGROWING TOENAILS

Classification: ICHPPC 703 (RCGP 3740)

The nail grows into the underlying nail bed, causing pain.

DIAGNOSTIC RANGE (rates per 1000 population per year)

Personal: Probable 2.4+. Many cases not reported.

MANAGEMENT OPTIONS

Prevention: avoid ill fitting shoes and treat 'sweaty feet' (see p. 620).

Established condition: (a) *conservative*: teach patient to raise the nail with pledget of cotton wool, discourage patient from 'digging' or cutting back the nail edge; (b) Treat hyperhidrosis; (c) 'dress' toe frequently; (d) surgical removal of nail or nail bed if condition interferes with activity.

ALOPECIA AREATA

Classification: ICHPPC 704 (RCGP 3745)

AETIOLOGY

Unknown; possible autoimmunity; may run in families.

DIAGNOSTIC RANGE (rates per 1000 patients per year)

Personal: Probable 3.0+.

AGE INCIDENCE

Older children and adults are liable.

CLINICAL POINTERS

1. High risk factors: (a) previous attacks; (b) other patches; (c) positive family history (20%).
2. The lesion (100%). A small bald patch of the scalp is suddenly noticed. The smooth bald area may slowly enlarge or other smaller patches may develop. There is no irritation.
3. A few single short hairs with an unnatural 'reverse tapering' (*exclamation mark* hairs) at the edge of the patch.

INVESTIGATIONS

Illumination under a Wood's lamp and microscopic examination of scrapings for mycelia distinguish the lesion from ringworm.

DURATION

The patch expands for a week or so — after about 6 to 10 weeks fine hairs grow again. In 90% cure is complete in 2 to 4 months.

COMPLICATIONS

The new hair is sometimes light in colour. Considerable areas of scalp may be affected and occasionally after repeated attacks the alopecia may be permanent. In those patients with recurring lesions of the hair margin a total alopecia may develop.

DIFFERENTIAL DIAGNOSIS
Distinction from tinea capitis may be difficult. Numerous broken hairs or obviously diseased hair follicles suggest a fungus infection.

MANAGEMENT OPTIONS
Established condition: (a) reassurance and explanation; (b) most local treatment of doubtful effect; (c) systemic or intralesional steroids encourage growth but do not cure; (d) bland applications probably better than topical steroids; (e) referral may help reassure.

GENERAL PARTIAL ALOPECIA

Classification: ICHPPC 704 (RCGP 3745)

A self-limiting disorder affecting young and middle-aged adults which may be related to a period of ill-health or a confinement.

AETIOLOGY
Unknown.

DIAGNOSTIC RANGE (rates per 1000 patients per year)
Personal: Suspected 0.9+.

CLINICAL POINTERS
The patient, usually a woman, complains that she is losing large quantities of hair. Examination reveals little evidence of this temporary moult. Reassurance of complete recovery is all that is required.

SCARRING ALOPECIA

Classification: ICHPPC 704 (RCGP 3745)

A severe form of permanent generalised alopecia often of unknown aetiology that affects patients over 30 years old. It leads to partial or even complete baldness and may be very distressing. The affected areas show diminution of hair follicles with little sign of new hair growth. Management: (a) none effective; (b) wig.

DIAGNOSTIC RANGE (rates per 1000 patients per year)
Personal: Probable 0.4.

SENILE ALOPECIA

Classification: ICHPPC 704 (RCGP 3745)

A slowly progressive baldness that affects men and occasionally elderly women. There is a characteristic thinning of the hair over temples and crown.

DIAGNOSTIC RANGE

This is the commonest type of alopecia but few cases are reported.

MANAGEMENT OPTIONS

(a) Acceptance; (b) wig.

PUSTULAR FOLLICULITIS

Classification: ICHPPC 704 (RCGP 3745)

A large number of adjacent hair follicles become infected with staphylococci and develop small yellow vesicles. The lesion may develop spontaneously, following chemical irritation or in the skin around a boil or under adhesive plaster.

MANAGEMENT OPTIONS

(a) Remove irritant; (b) simple skin disinfectants — BNF 13.11 (Ref. 0.1); (c) antibacterials topical (BNF 13.10.1.1) and systemic (BNF 5.1 or 13.10.1.2) if resistant.

SYCOSIS BARBAE

Classification: ICHPPC 704 (RCGP 3745)

The irritation of shaving causes a number of staphylococcal lesions to coalesce and form a crusted raised purulent folliculitis.

MANAGEMENT OPTIONS

As for Pustular folliculitis; stop shaving until clear.

MULTIPLE PIN-HEAD PUSTULES

Classification: ICHPPC 704 (RCGP 3745)

The small lesions (milia) appear on the faces of many small babies. The spots clear spontaneously in a few weeks. Reassurance only.

SWEAT RASH

Classification: ICHPPC 705 (RCGP 3750)

A fine irritant papular rash may appear on the skin after unusual exertion and sweating. The sites of maximum skin frictions are affected — trunk, inside of thighs and anus. No treatment indicated.

DIAGNOSTIC RANGE (rates per 1000 patients per year)
Personal: Suspected 1.6+. Many cases are never reported.

HYPERHYDROSIS (EXCESSIVE SWEATING)

Classification: ICHPPC 7808 (RCGP 4530)

A common, often trying, condition that affects both sexes, (usually 15 to 30 years) and is often difficult to treat except by: (a) frequent bathing and showers; (b) use of loose non-irritant cotton clothing, socks and shoes which are changed frequently; (c) antiperspirant lotions — Aluminium chloride, — BNF 13.12 (Ref. 0.1).

ACNE VULGARIS

Classification: ICHPPC 7061 (RCGP 3760)

AETIOLOGY
The hormone changes of puberty cause sebaceous glands to enlarge and keratinise. Blockage, infection (*Propionobacterium acnes*) and local inflammation of the gland follow. If local reaction is excessive scarring and cyst formation occur.

DIAGNOSTIC RANGE (rates per 1000 patients per year)
Personal: Probable 8.8. *National* 6.5 (Ref. 0.2).

85% of adolescents are probably affected. About 15% are bad enough to seek medical advice.

AGE INCIDENCE
Adolescents and young adults are mainly liable.

SEX INCIDENCE
Both sexes are affected. Scarring is greater in males, but girls report the lesions more often because they are more sensitive about their appearance.

CLINICAL POINTERS

1. High risk factors: (a) puberty; (b) greasy skin; (c) certain drugs, e.g. barbiturates, INA, bromides and large doses of steroids; (d) menstruation.
2. Pustules and blackheads (100%).
3. Sites. Face (100%), back (20%) and nape of neck.
4. Scarring and pitting of varying degree follows the active lesion.
5. Onset at puberty.

6. Associated diseases. Seborrhoea capitis and dermatitis (10%); recurrent boils and styes (25%).

DURATION
The tendency to develop acne is greatest in youth but occasionally persists throughout adult life.

COMPLICATIONS
Scarring and disfigurement can cause many personal and emotional problems.

MANAGEMENT OPTIONS
Prevention: enthusiastic, active treatment of early cases even when severe, can do much to prevent later distress caused by prolonged inflammatory reaction.

Established condition: (a) full explanation of factors involved; (b) frequent washing may help remove sebum and blockage; (c) UV light and sunlight causes a helpful erythema and scaling; (d) detergent antiseptics and keratolytic agents (benzoyl peroxide) — BNF 13.6 (Ref. 0.1); (e) systemic antibacterials (tetracyclines, erythromycin, etc. — BNF 5.1.3 and 5.1.5; (f) abrasives — BNF 13.6 — dietary changes ineffective.

SEBACEOUS CYST

Classification: ICHPPC 7062 (RCGP 3765)

Rounded subcutaneous cysts, filled with white lard-like material, that arise when the mouth of a sebaceous gland becomes blocked. They are commonly found on the scalp, nape of neck or trunk.

DIAGNOSTIC RANGE (rates per 1000 patients per year)
Personal: Probable 4.7.

SEX INCIDENCE
Males more than females (2 : 1).

COMPLICATIONS
Secondary infection. Recurrences and multiple cysts are common in certain individuals.

MANAGEMENT OPTIONS
Leave. Excise if causing annoyance.

EXCORIATION OF SKIN

Classification: ICHPPC 709 (RCGP 3785)

A combination of trauma, minor sepsis and irritation may lead to excoriation of skin. The skin surrounding the nose or anus is liable. Nappy rash (see p. 606) is a specialised example.

DIAGNOSTIC RANGE (rates per 1000 patients per year)
Personal: Probable 0.3+.

MANAGEMENT OPTIONS
(a) remove cause; (b) protect skin if this is impractical; (c) treat monilia if present — BNF 13.10.2.

INTERTRIGO

Classification: ICHPPC 709 (RCGP 0240)

Close contact between two damp skin surfaces may lead to intertrigo. The skin becomes reddened and the superficial layers appear soggy and white. Common sites are the groins, between the buttocks and under the breasts of obese women. Irritation and excoriation of the skin are sometimes associated. Satellite lesions suggest added monilia.

DIAGNOSTIC RANGE (rates per 1000 patients per year)
Personal: Probable 1.1+. Many cases are never reported.

MANAGEMENT OPTIONS
(a) 'cleanse dry' and if possible separate surfaces; (b) astringent skin lotions — BNF 13.11 (Ref. 0.1); (c) topical antifungals — BNF 13.10.2.

CHAPPED HANDS

Classification: ICHPPC 709 (RCGP 5235)

The hands become roughened and sore in cold weather. The disorder is aggravated by washing. In a few individuals deep cracks appear in the thick skin which overlies the finger pulp. Similar fissures are occasionally noted in the thick skin of the foot in menopausal women.

DIAGNOSTIC RANGE (rates per 1000 patients per year)
Personal: Probable 0.4+. Many cases are never reported.

MANAGEMENT OPTIONS

Emollient barrier creams instead of hand washing — BNF 13.2 and 13.11 (Ref. 0.1).

ICHTHYOSIS

Classification: ICHPPC 709 (RCGP 3785)

A congenital often familial disease of unknown aetiology, with a characteristic generalised scaly roughening of the skin. Face and flexures are exempt but the skin may appear dirty, with consequent self-consciousness.

DIAGNOSTIC RANGE

Personal: Probable 1.2+. Many mild cases never reported.

DURATION

Onset is in infancy and persists indefinitely.

COMPLICATIONS

Patients are prone to secondary eczema and skin infections.

MANAGEMENT OPTIONS

10% Urea creams — BNF 13.2 — may help if used daily.

Table 33 Less common diseases of the skin and cellular tissue

Diseases and distinguishing clinical pointers	Incidence per 1000 patients per year Suspected	Confirmed
Multiple neurofibromata (*Von Recklinghausen*) Pedunculated pigmented tumours (can be pushed into pit at the base of its stalk), associated lesions in nervous and skeletal system	—	1 in 10 years
Chronic omphalitis In adults: obese women, chronic red irritation	0.6	0.6
Acute omphalitis In newborn: local signs slight, serious systemic infection	0	0
Molluscum contagiosum Contacts, small raised pearl-like lesions, debris can be expressed from umbilicated top. Treat with curettage.	—	3 in 10 years
Dermatitis herpetiformis Young adults, rash — crops of vesicles, intense irritation — scratching obscures vesicular lesions and causes rash to look like scabies, i.e. headless papules and scratch marks, many weeks duration. In pregnancy a related disease sometimes develops Healed lesions often pigmented.	0.3	0.1

Table 33 Less common diseases of the skin and cellular tissue

Diseases and distinguishing clinical pointers	Incidence per 1000 patients per year Suspected	Confirmed
Erythema multiforme	0.2	0.2
Children and young adults; Pleomorphic rash — (a) red macule (5 to 10 mm diam.) some with central flea bite petechiae, (b) macules with vesicle, (c) pink circinate lesions (5 to 15 mm diam.) with raised urticarial edge (iris); site of lesions — limbs mainly; aphthous ulcers in mouth or vagina; conjunctivitis; fever; malaise; multiple joint pains; 1 to 4 weeks duration; recurrences common. Symptomatic treatment.		
Erythema nodosum	0.4	0.4
Young adults; lesion — red tender induration (1 to 10 cm diam.) resembling area of cellulitis; site — front of both shins, several lesions usual; fever, transient joint pains and raised ESR may indicate associated rheumatic fever, sarcoidosis or tuberculosis (rare); 1 to 4 weeks duration; chest X-ray; ESR; tuberculin test. Symptomatic treatment.		
Erythema serpens (*erysipeloid of Rosenbach*)	0.3	0.3
Puncture wound (of hand usually) by fish, fowl or meat bone followed in 2 to 4 days by spreading, purple-red lesion with raised edge suggesting erysipelas or cellulitis. Systemic disturbance unusual. Duration 2 to 6 weeks. Symptomatic treatment only.		
Lichen planus	0.3	0.3
Adults, rash — lilac, colour fading to sepia, polygonal flat topped papules (1 to 2 mm diam.) with fine creases (Wickam's lines) just visible on top of papule, papules may coalesce and hypertrophy, skin surrounding long-standing lesions is blotchy brown or dull red, intense irritation, white reticulum on buccal mucous membranes (3 to 10 mm diam.), duration — 2 to 6 months, recurrences and chronic cases occur. Referral often wise.		
Granuloma annulare	0.3	0.3
Ring like lesions with raised edge resembling ringworm; no scales; white, red or pink; single or multiple; dorsum of hands and feet usual; grows for 3–6 months then disappears; aetiology uncertain. No treatment — refer if in doubt.		
Dermatitis artefacta	0.2	—
Adults usually; lesion — small irregular fresh red scab or open granulating areas (usually over 1 cm diam.), site — accessible parts of face or limbs, insecure often inscrutable personality. *Management*: occlusive bandage or dressing — BNF 13.13. Consider motivation and personality disorders.		

Disease and distinguishing clinical pointers	Incidence per 1000 patients per year Suspected	Confirmed
Onychogryphosis Elderly patients unable to cut toenails; typical deforming hypertrophy usually of big toenail. Remove if annoying.	0.2	0.2
Brittle nails Adults, nails thin and easily cracked; excessive washing (with detergents)	0.2	0.2
Bedsore Debilitated, bedridden patients; site: pressure points.	0.2	0.2
Granuloma pyogenicum (Haemangioma) Dome-shaped, vascular, granulation; bleeds easily and often on slight trauma (10 to 20 mm diam.). Curette or cauterise — not pyogenic.	0.2	—
Orf Small papule becoming umbilicated to form a pox virus granuloma with raised edge up to 20 mm diameter, fingers usually affected, duration up to 8 weeks, contact with sheep. Heals without treatment.	—	1 in 10 years
Flea bites Incidence not recorded. Crops of irritant lesions occurring on different areas of the trunk. Fresh crops usually noted in the mornings.	—	—
Kerato acanthoma Single painless lesion (2–20 mm. diam.) usually on face, rolled edges with central plug. Looks malignant; grows for 3 months, static for 3 months, disappears in 3 months. Biopsy usually indicated.	0.4	0.4
Malignant melanoma Single lesion (2–20 mm. diam.) brown or black colour usual; malignancy suggested by: halo of pigment in adjacent skin; recent increased size; bleeding. Early referral or biopsy if suspected.	0.1	0.1
Vitiligo Flat white irregular patches, any size, mainly adults. Harmless. Refer for PUVA if annoying.	?	?
Tinea Versicolour Large patches of red/brown slightly scaly skin. Upper trunk is usual site. Causes loss of pigment. Topical anti-fungals.	?	?
Neurodermatitis (lichen simplex) Lesion — dark brown purple area with deep skin creases caused by constant rubbing following irritation. Sites: nape of neck, inside thighs and backs of hands. Duration: years.	0.7	0.7

24

Diseases of the bones and organs of movement

Please read the introduction for explanation of figures and analyses.

The so called rheumatological diseases are arbitrarily grouped together because connective tissues, joints and bones are the main target areas. These are further divided into, Inflammatory, Metabolic and Degenerative Groups.

A. INFLAMMATORY DISEASES OF JOINTS AND BONES

1. Acute Septic Arthritis (p. 652) and Osteomyelitis (p. 635).
2. Rheumatic fever and acute rheumatism (p. 334).
3. Disseminated lupus erythematosus (DLE). Scarring butterfly facial rash, arthritis, myalgia, pulmonary, renal pericardial, endocardial and neurological symptoms and signs may occur. Hepatomegaly and typical LE cells in the blood clinch the diagnosis. (Practice experience: one case in 10 years.)
4. Polyarteritis nodosa (PAN) p. 375. Systemic symptoms; fever, weight loss and raised ESR are common; pulmonary, cardiac and arthritic lesions produce pain in the affected organs. Peripheral neuritis and microscopic haematuria are characteristic. Biopsy clinches diagnosis. (Practice experience: one case in 10 years.)
5. Rheumatoid arthritis (p. 627).
6. Scleroderma. Skin becomes hard, rigid, shiny, and thickened — on hand resembles skin scarred by extensive burns. Face, hands and trunk may be totally affected. Dysphagia and dyspnoea are common. (Practice experience: one case in 20 years.)
7. Dermatomyositis. Non-suppurative polymyositis, dermatitis and oedema. (Practice experience: no cases in 10 years.)
8. Polymyalgia rheumatica (p. 634) and temporal arteritis may also be included in this group.
9. Reiter's Syndrome (p. 194) and several other rare diseases. The aetiology of most of these diseases is uncertain but may involve genetic and immunological as well as inflammatory factors.

B. METABOLIC DISEASES OF JOINTS AND BONES
Such as gout (see p. 219)

C. DEGENERATIVE DISEASES OF JOINTS AND BONES
1. Osteoarthritis (p. 631) or Osteoporosis (p. 640)
2. Diseases of wear and tear such as Synovitis, bursistis, etc.

RHEUMATOID ARTHRITIS

Classification: ICHPPC 714 (RCGP 3905)

AETIOLOGY
Uncertain. Current views suggest that the following aetiological processes occur:

1. An altered immune response.
2. Persistent antigenic stimulation in genetically determined individuals.

An auto antibody (IgM — rheumatoid factor) is formed which destroys connective tissue in the target area. What initiates this process is not known.

DIAGNOSTIC RANGE (rates per 1000 patients per year)
Personal: Suspected 9.4. Probable 5.9 *National*: surveys suggest higher figures than this. Many early or mild cases are probably not reported.

AGE INCIDENCE
All ages are liable, but the disease is rare in patients under 35 years.

SEX INCIDENCE
The majority (70%) are women.

CLINICAL POINTERS
1. Onset. Usually insidious with exacerbations and remissions. Symptoms are sometimes slight and limited to vague complaints of stiffness in joints and muscles. At first one joint only may be affected. Careful records reveal that in most cases there have been attacks of joint pains or muscle stiffness on several occasions before the disease is even suspected. Occasionally the onset is acute with fatigue, malaise sweating, fever, tachycardia, joint pains and raised ESR. The course is then likely to be rapid and the prognosis poor.

2. Characteristic arthritis (100%). Any joint may be involved, but the metacarpophalangeal joints are usually affected with conse-

quent deformity — the ulnar drift (65%). Knees, elbows, shoulders and joints of the feet may also be involved early. The lesions are often symmetrical.

3. Stiffness of joints and muscles (100%). The patient complains that, on walking, one or more joints are stiff and slightly painful. Muscles also feel stiff and there may be numbness or tingling of hands and feet. These symptoms are worse on getting up in the morning.

4. Pain (100%). As the disease progresses, one or two joints become increasingly painful and may feel hot and inflamed.

5. Limitation of movement. Inability to put the hands on the nape of neck or to arrange the hair is a typical early sign.

6. Swelling and deformity (25%). The swelling of the knuckle joints with ulna deviation and spindling of fingers is characteristic. Periarticular swelling of knee or elbow joints is accentuated by wasting of those muscles which act on the joints. Symmetrical joint involvement is characteristic.

7. Systemic disturbances (20%). Anorexia, weight loss, malaise, fever, tachycardia and raised ESR may occur in the early stages. Sometimes the patient is investigated as a pyrexia of unknown origin if the early joint symptoms are minimal or atypical.

8. Carpal tunnel syndrome is a common early symptom.

9. The following early features suggest a poor prognosis: raised ESR and positive serology, low haemoglobin levels, poor hand grip and a large number of affected joints. To a lesser extent being underweight, in an older age group and early erosions on radiology are also poor prognostic signs.

INVESTIGATIONS

1. The ESR (see p. 681) is raised when the arthritis is active.

2. Rose-Waaler or latex fixation tests are said to be positive in 85% of patients. Unfortunately these tests may not become positive until the disease has lasted several years and in some cases the test becomes negative after only a short period of positive or high titres. Initially high or steadily progressing titres are bad prognostic signs.

3. Haemoglobin levels are often low.

4. X-ray show decalcification, erosions and joint disorganisation.

DURATION

In about a third of cases the disease progresses relentlessly by repeated attacks. Joints, especially those of the hands and knees, become deformed and disorganised. After many years the activity may subside.

Benign multiple arthritis
Describes the 30% of patients with symptoms of mild early rheumatoid arthritis that never becomes established and in whom the clinical and serological evidence of the disease never develops.

COMPLICATIONS

1. The knees may become fixed in partial flexion and the patient keeps his hips flexed on walking — this leads to a typical bent Z posture.
2. A number of systemic complications may arise and affect the following sites: skin, peripheral nerves, eye, pericardium, pleura, lungs, and kidneys. Hypochromic anaemia is common.

MISLEADING FEATURES AND PITFALLS

1. Hypochromic anaemia is easily overlooked.
2. As with asthma and other chronic remitting diseases depression may be marked and recurring.

DIFFERENTIAL DIAGNOSIS

Diseases that may be confused with rheumatoid arthritis:

Rheumatic fever
Similar features: polyarthritis; intermittent disease; evidence of joint inflammation; fever; tachycardia; ESR raised; responds to salicylates.

Distinguishing features: children and young adults liable; history of acute rheumatism previously; joint pains are fleeting and less constant; metacarpophalangeal joints not affected; Rose-Waaler and latex fixation tests negative.

Osteoarthritis
Similar features: arthritis affecting one or more joints in latter half of life; small joints of hands may be affected.

Distinguishing features: joints rarely affected symmetrically; cause of joint wear and tear may be obvious, e.g. old trauma, obesity, etc.; ulnar drift absent; systemic disturbances absent; ESR, Rose-Waaler and latex fixation tests negative; X-ray of joint shows osteoarthritic changes.

Gout
Similar features: arthritis affecting one or more joints; hands and feet commonly involved; acute joint inflammation apparent; middle age-groups liable; fever and ESR raised; responds to salicylates.

Distinguishing features: men more liable than women; attacks of joint pain very severe but only last a few days; big toe joint commonly affected; tophi may be apparent on rim of ears; serum uric acid raised in attacks; Rose-Waaler and latex fixation tests negative; typical X-ray changes apparent in hands and feet of long-standing cases.

Reiter's syndrome

Similar features: subacute polyarthritis of several weeks duration affecting peripheral limb joints; fever; tachycardia and raised ESR.

Distinguishing features: young men mainly affected; history of urethritis, bacillary dysentery or conjunctivitis; skin lesions may arise.

Carpal tunnel syndrome

Similar features: chronic pain and stiffness in one or both hands; numbness and tingling of hands.

Distinguishing features: symptoms are limited to hands and forearms; systemic disturbances absent; ESR normal; median nerve lesions demonstrable. The two diseases are associated.

Psoriatic arthritis

Similar features: adults mainly affected; small joints of hand affected.

Distinguishing features: other psoriatic lesions in skin, nails and scalp; terminal interphalangeal joints affected; little systemic upset; X-ray of hands; serology.

Disseminated lupus erythematosus is associated with an arthritis which is clinically similar to rheumatoid arthritis. The characteristic skin lesions and blood tests make the distinction clear.

MANAGEMENT OPTIONS

Prevention: amelioration of the destructive effects is all that is possible.

Suspected disease: (a) careful and repeated investigation; (b) referral (c) maintain an optimistic attitude as long as evidence of joint disease is minimal.

Established disease: (a) physician must develop a patience to match that needed by the patient — as in diabetes a long and caring relationship is developed; (b) involve rheumatologist early; (c) full explanations and education to enable patient to carry out own treatment; (d) physical exercise well within the limits of pain; (e) non-steroidal anti-inflammatory drugs (NSAID) — BNF 10.1.1.2 and BNF 10.1.1.1. (Ref. 0.1); (f) daily living assessments to establish appropriate aids in the home; (g) physiotherapy — a great morale booster; (h) frequent follow ups to encourage and monitor progress, also to check for anaemia and depression, etc.; (i) group therapy; literature, information and support from British Rheumatism and Arthritis Society (Ref. 24.1 and Ref. 13.1 for aids in the home); (j) regular visits to rheumatologist for guidance concerning physiotherapy, surgery and alternative drugs (e.g. gold, penicillamine, antimalarials, immunosuppressives, etc.)

OSTEOARTHRITIS (OSTEOARTHROSIS)

Classification: ICHPPC 715 (RCGP 3950)

A degenerative joint disease that arises if any joint is unable to meet the mechanical stress placed on it. There is loss of articular cartilage with new bone formation (osteophytic lipping) at the edges of the joint. It is extremely common and radiological signs start to show in many joints after the age of 30 years, although symptoms are unusual before 50.

AETIOLOGY

1. Previous trauma. Joints which have been damaged by injury or operation are affected early — secondary osteoarthritis.
2. Unaccustomed wear. The knees and weight-bearing joints of middle-aged women who put on weight are liable to osteoarthritis.
3. Sex. (Practice experience: in 193 consecutive cases, women were affected three times more than men — possibly due to the tendency of middle-aged women to put on weight) Elderly women are liable to osteoarthritis of the hands (Heberden's nodes).
4. The menopause. Women at the menopause are especially prone. The association is difficult to confirm because both the menopause and osteoarthritis are common and ill-defined.

DIAGNOSTIC RANGE (rates per 1000 patients per year)
Personal: Suspected 32.6. Probable 22.6. *National*: 20.3 (Ref. 0.2). The diagnosis was sometimes difficult to confirm.

AGE INCIDENCE
The majority (65%) are over 50 years. Younger patients may develop osteoarthritis in a joint that has been injured.

SEX INCIDENCE
Females more than males [3:1].

CLINICAL POINTERS

1. High risk factors: (a) increasing age; (b) previous injury, operation or disease of a joint; (c) obesity causing increased load; (d) menopause.

2. Insidious onset.

3. Attacks of pain and stiffness on movement in one or more joints (100%). As the disease becomes established the pain sometimes becomes continuous. The joint is often tender.

4. The site. Every joint can develop osteoarthritis, but unless injury has rendered a joint susceptible, the disease has a predilection for certain sites. [Practice experience: a series of 193 consecutive cases showed: knee joints, 39.0% (75); shoulder, 17.5% (34); spine, 10.5% (20); hands, 10.0% (19); hips, 8.0% (15); other, 15.0%(30).]

5. Crepitus (45%).

6. Swelling and deformity of the joint. Nodular swelling on the back and sides of the interphalangeal joints (Heberden's nodes) give the hands of the elderly a gnarled look.

7. Recurring effusions occasionally develop in a joint with severe osteoarthritis.

8. Symmetrical joint involvement is characteristic of a primary degenerative osteoarthritis or rheumatoid disease.

INVESTIGATIONS

Radiography shows loss of joint space, lipping and bony osteosclerosis around joint.

DURATION

The disease is slowly progressive but a proportion of patients (40%) after an initial attack of pain are symptom free for many years.

COMPLICATIONS

Disuse atrophy of the surrounding muscles.

MISLEADING FEATURES AND PITFALLS

1. Osteoarthritis is common and can easily become a diagnostic rag-bag to account for all the aches and pains of a patient with an ageing skeletal system.

2. Rheumatoid arthritis is easily confused with osteoarthritis.

DIFFERENTIAL DIAGNOSIS

Diseases that may be confused with osteoarthritis:

Rheumatoid arthritis

Similar features: pain and stiffness on moving joints; knees, shoulders, elbows and hips affected; disease is slowly progressive.

Distinguishing features: younger age-group liable; wrists, metacarpo and interphalangeal joints usually affected; deformity and ulnar deviation of fingers marked; Heberden's nodes absent;

evidence of systemic disease — fever, malaise, raised ESR see p. 681; Rose-Waaler and latex fixation tests positive; hypochromic anaemia.

Fibrositis
Similar features: pain on moving joints.
Distinguishing features: younger ages liable; pain is muscular not in joints; disease is not progressive; local tenderness of affected muscles; distinction rarely difficult.

Psoriatic arthritis
Similar features: terminal interphalangeal joints swollen chronically in middle age groups. Skin lesions often minimal or absent.

Distinguishing features: other psoriatic lesions in skin, nails and scalp, X-rays of hand.

MANAGEMENT OPTIONS

Prevention: rarely possible apart from avoiding obesity and overload of a vulnerable joint.

Established disease: conservative measures, mainly; (a) simple aspirin type analgesics — BNF 10.1.1.1. (Ref. 0.1); non-steroidal anti-inflammatory analgesics — BNF 10.1.1.2, have few advantages and are more costly; (b) protect joint with stick or splint; (c) modify daily living (Ref. 13.1); (d) physiotherapy; (e) referral if severe for surgery and joint replacement, etc.

ANKYLOSING SPONDYLITIS

Classification ICHPPC 714 (RCGP 3985)

AETIOLOGY
Uncertain; autoimmunity and familial factors are likely. Young males are mainly affected. Pain and stiffness is followed after months or years by ossification affecting the ligaments of spine. Lumbar and sacroiliac spine first then upper spine and sternum. Pokerback develops. X-ray shows sacro-ileitis (early) and Bamboo spine (late).

MANAGEMENT OPTIONS
Symptomatic only: (a) anti-inflammatory (non-steroid) analgesics — BNF 10.1.1 (Ref. 0.1); (b) physiotherapy; (c) support and advice about modifying life style in severe cases (Ref. 13.1). (Practice experience: one case in 10 years).

ACUTE FIBROSITIS

Classification: ICHPPC 728 (RCGP 4075)

This disorder is ill defined and is a diagnostic rag-bag.

AETIOLOGY
Unknown. Patients with anxiety are prone to fibrositic aches and pains, possibly because they have a lowered pain threshold (see pp. 77 and 243).

A proportion of cases are probably due to nerve root pain.

DIAGNOSTIC RANGE (rates per 1000 patients per year)
Personal: Suspected 36.2. It was impossible to confirm the diagnosis and there may have been many causes for the varied complaints.

CLINICAL POINTERS
1. Pain on muscle contraction.
2. Local tenderness.
3. Absence of other cause of the pain.

DURATION
Recurrent attacks are common. Symptoms clear up in 2 to 4 days.

MISLEADING FEATURES AND PITFALLS
Serious organic disease may be mistakenly labelled fibrositis.

MANAGEMENT OPTIONS
Symptomatic treatment only: simple analgesics or a local depot steroid injection are occasionally needed — BNF 10.1.2.2 (Ref. 0.1).

POLYMYALGIA RHEUMATICA

Classification: ICHPPC 725 (RCGP 4025)

DIAGNOSTIC RANGE
Three patients in 10 years.

CLINICAL POINTERS
1. Patients; usually over 60.
2. Onset usually sudden.
3. Pain and stiffness in muscles and joints of back of neck, shoulder and pelvic girdles. Muscle weakness, atrophy and deformity slight or absent.
4. ESR raised see p. 681.
5. Dramatic relief from steroids.

DURATION

6 months to 6 years.

COMPLICATIONS

Temporal arteritis. Recurrences are common.

MISLEADING FEATURES AND PITFALLS

Easily overlooked. Patient liable to consider symptoms rheumatic.

MANAGEMENT OPTIONS

Established disease: (a) oral corticosteroids — BNF 10.1.2.1 (Ref. 0.1) — gradually reduce drugs once ESR and symptoms are controlled; (b) follow up essential.

TEMPORAL (GIANT-CELL) ARTERITIS

Classification: ICHPPC 459 (RCGP 2235)

A rare condition related to Polymyalgia rheumatica. Giant cell arteritis may affect arteries other than temporal. Main danger is that some cases may develop a sudden partial or complete, irreversible visual loss if not treated. (No cases in 20 years.)

Headache, local tenderness of the artery and a raised ESR are characteristic. Immediate referral and biopsy indicated. Drug treatment as for polymyalgia (see above).

ACUTE OSTEOMYELITIS

Classification: ICHPPC 739 (RCGP 4095)

The term acute osteomyelitis covers inflammation of the marrow, the bone cortex (osteitis) and periosteum (periostits).

AETIOLOGY

Staphylococcus pyogenes. The infection is blood-borne and the primary source is not always obvious. Trauma may start the disease by introducing bacteria or causing local bone damage. A common site is near the junction of the epiphysis and diaphysis of a long bone.

DIAGNOSTIC RANGE (rates per 1000 patients per year)

Personal: Suspected 0.6. Proven 0.2.

AGE INCIDENCE

Children and adolescents.

CLINICAL POINTERS

1. High risk factors: (a) growing children; (b) history of trauma; (c) growing end of long bones vulnerable.
2. Previous injury or source of infection. Not always obvious.
3. Sudden onset.
4. Localised pain and tenderness. Often severe and maximal over the site of lesion.
5. Movements limited by pain.
6. Rigors.
7. High fever.
8. Local swelling of bone. Not always obvious.

INVESTIGATIONS

Immediate hospital admission for white cell count, ESR and blood culture.

Osteomyelitis may not show on X-ray until 10 days after onset.

DURATION

Early drainage shortens the illness. If an abscess is allowed to persist, the infection tends to spread inside the bone — it then becomes difficult to eradicate and may become chronic.

COMPLICATIONS

Chronic osteomyelitis and retardation of bone growth.

MISLEADING FEATURES AND PITFALLS

In young children and in patients with a subperiosteal abscess when the pus is not under tension, the onset is sometimes gradual; pain and systemic disturbance may be slight; symptoms are attributed to trauma and diagnosis delayed with disastrous consequences.

DIFFERENTIAL DIAGNOSIS

Diseases that may be confused with an acute osteomyelitis:

Acute rheumatic fever

Similar features: sudden onset; acute localised pain and tenderness in the region of a joint; high fever; tachycardia; children liable.

Distinguishing features: previous streptococcal illness; pain and inflammation is related to a joint not a bone; bony tenderness absent; several joints may be affected; differentiation may be difficult.

Acute septic arthritis

Similar features: sources of primary infection; sudden onset; acute localised pain and tenderness in the region of a joint; high fever; children mainly affected.

Distinguishing features: pain is related to a joint which is held in the position of comfort and may be swollen, hot and sometimes red; differentiation may be difficult; early admission to hospital for joint aspiration indicated.

MANAGEMENT OPTIONS

Suspected disease — immediate referral.

CHRONIC OSTEOMYELITIS

Classification: ICHPPC 739 (RCGP 4095)

AETIOLOGY

Inadequately treated osteomyelitis and trauma, e.g. compound fractures, gunshot wounds, etc.

DIAGNOSTIC RANGE (rates per 1000 patients per year)

Personal: Proven 1.2. The diagnosis was rarely in doubt.

CLINICAL POINTERS

1. History of acute osteomyelitis or trauma at the same site.
2. Recurring incidents of localised pain, tenderness and inflammation at site of previous infection or bone injury.
3. Discharging sinuses. Pieces of dead bone (sequestra) may be discharged.
4. Systemic disturbances occur if free drainage is obstructed.

INVESTIGATIONS

X-rays indicate the extent of the infection and show sequestra.

DURATION

The disease may relapse after many years of apparent cure. Recurrences and chronic discharging sinuses may continue in spite of antibiotic and surgical treatment.

COMPLICATIONS

Spread of infection and amyloid disease are rare.

MANAGEMENT OPTIONS

Prevention: early treatment of acute osteomyelitis is vital.

Established disease: (a) referral for adequate surgical excision and drainage; (b) appropriate antibacterials — BNF 5.1 (Ref. 0.1); (c) appropriate assessment and modification of daily living; (d) early reporting and treatment of recurrent attacks; (e) amputation occasionally needed; (f) follow up.

OSTEITIS DEFORMANS (PAGET'S DISEASE OF BONE)

Classification: ICHPPC 739 (RCGP 4100)

AETIOLOGY

Unknown. Skull, spine, pelvis, femur and tibia are usually affected. There is a familial tendency.

DIAGNOSTIC RANGE (rates per 1000 patients per year)

Personal: Suspected 0.9+. The diagnosis was rarely in doubt but the disease was noted in two types of patients: (a) patients aged 40 to 50 years in whom the disease was localised and symptomless — discovered by incidental X-ray; (b) patients over 70 with clinical evidence of the disease.

AGE INCIDENCE

The disease probably starts between 40 and 60 but does not become clinically apparent for 20 years. Surveys suggest that 3 per cent of population over 50 and 9 per cent over 85 years have radiological evidence of the disease.

SEX INCIDENCE

Men more than women (3:2).

CLINICAL POINTERS

1. Pain in the bone is dull and continuous and aggravated by walking. It is often ascribed to rheumatism or osteoarthritis by both patient and doctor. Symptoms are rare under 60 years.
2. Deformity of the bone. Bowing of legs (usually tibia or fibula, occasionally arms); the characteristic broadening of the skull and upper forehead is insidious and is usually only noted after diagnosis.
3. Radiology for other reasons in patients over 50 may reveal incidental Paget's disease in skull, long bones, spine or pelvis.

INVESTIGATIONS

1. X-rays show a typical increase in density with a cotton wool blurring of the normal bony structure.
2. The serum (alkaline) phosphatase is raised.

DURATION

Indefinite and slowly progressive over many years.

COMPLICATIONS

Gross deformity of bones, Sarcoma, Osteoarthritis, pathological fractures or collapse of vertebrae can all occur.

MISLEADING FEATURES AND PITFALLS

The early radiological appearance of the disease may resemble those of early secondary prostatic metastases. A serum acid phosphatase test will distinguish the malignant condition.

DIFFERENTIAL DIAGNOSIS

Early Paget's disease may be confused with osteoarthritis.

MANAGEMENT OPTIONS

Established disease: symptomatic: (a) simple analgesics — BNF 4.7.1.1. and 10.1.1.1 (Ref. 0.1); (b) drugs for hypercalcaemia — BNF 6.6; (d) appropriate modification of daily living (Ref. 13.1).

OSTEOCHONDRITIS (OSTEOCHONDROSIS)

Classification: ICHPPC 732 (RCGP 4105)

Several diseases of uncertain aetiology are classified together because of certain common features:

1. Growing bones or epiphyses are affected; children and adolescents are liable.
2. A period of active disease lasting several months causes bony deformity and is followed by spontaneous healing.
3. Radiological appearances suggest that deformity is due to use not destruction of bone.
4. A single bone (or group of bones) is affected.
5. Early diagnosis and decreased weight bearing is essential if deformities are to be avoided.

DIAGNOSTIC RANGE (rates per 1000 patients per year)

Personal: Suspected 1.2. Probable 0.2.

AGE INCIDENCE

Children and adolescents.

CLINICAL POINTERS

These depend on the bone affected:

Osteochondritis of hip (Perthes' disease)

Affects children between 5 and 10 years, occasionally as early as 3 or as late as 16 years. Pain in a hip with a limp is characteristic.

Osteochondritis of spine (Scheuermann's disease)

Affects dorsal spine of children between 10 and 16 years. A rapidly increasing dorsal kyphosis with slight pain develops after a month or two. It is said to be the commonest cause of kyphosis (three cases in 10 years).

Osteochondritis of tibial tubercle (Osgood-Schlatter's disease)
Affects children between 10 and 16 years. The tubercle becomes tender and swollen. Localised pain is aggravated by exercise and jumping.

Other bones that are said to be affected are os calcis (Sever's disease), scaphoid tarsal bone (Kohler's disease). Other tarsal or carpal bones may also be affected.

INVESTIGATIONS
X-ray.

COMPLICATIONS
If the effects of compression are not prevented by rest, deformity may be followed by osteoarthritis.

DIFFERENTIAL DIAGNOSIS
Tuberculosis is easily confused. X-rays differentiate. Osteochondritis of the tibial tubercle may simulate a traumatic osteitis of the patella or tubercle (p. 653); they may be the same disease.

MANAGEMENT OPTIONS
Suspected disease: early referral and treatment vital.

SENILE OSTEOPOROSIS

Classification: ICHPPC 7330 (RCGP 4110)

This condition is becoming increasingly common and is easily overlooked in the elderly. Patients on long-standing steroid therapy are prone.

AETIOLOGY
Uncertain.

DIAGNOSTIC RANGE (rates per 1000 patients per year)
Personal: Suspected 1.0+.

SEX INCIDENCE
Women over 60 mainly affected.

CLINICAL POINTERS
1. High risk factors: (a) post-menopausal elderly women; (b) prolonged courses of oral steroids; (c) lack of movement (either general or local); (d) slightly built individuals with small bone mass;

(e) intestinal diseases with deficient calcium absorption.

2. Root pains usually affecting trunk, back or legs.

3. Pain is eased by rest. Many cases revealed by X-ray are symptom free.

INVESTIGATION

X-ray of spine usually distinguishes the disease from disc lesions, oesteoarthritis, secondary deposits and other serious spinal disease. Biochemical tests are negative.

MANAGEMENT OPTIONS

Prevention: encourage full activity in high risk groups.

Established condition: symptomatic and often unsatisfactory; (a) encourage full activity; (b) simple analgesics — BNF 4.7.1 (Ref. 0.1); (c) oral calcium supplements — BNF 9.5.1 are of doubtful use; (d) vitamin D supplements — BNF 9.6.4 also of dubious value; (e) oestrogens and anabolic steroids are contraindicated.

INTERNAL DERANGEMENT OF THE KNEE JOINT

Classification:

1. Tears of the semilunar cartilages.
2. Tears of the lateral or cruciate ligaments (see p. 653).

TORN SEMILUNAR CARTILAGE

Classification: ICHPPC 717 (RCGP 3965)

The medial cartilage is mainly affected (95%).

AETIOLOGY

Injuries in which the knee is flexed when the foot and tibia are fixed on the ground and the body is rotated on the fixed foot. Football and sports injuries are commonly responsible.

DIAGNOSTIC RANGE (rates per 1000 patients per year)

Personal: Suspected 6.0. Probable 2.4. *National*: 1.2 (Ref. 0.2.).

AGE INCIDENCE

The majority (75%) occur between 20 and 35 years.

SEX INCIDENCE

Men more than women (7:1).

CLINICAL POINTERS

1. High risk factors: (a) any activity (sporting or occupational) that involves body twisting while full weight is on one (or both) feet; (b) history of previous torn cartilage or knee injury (45%).

2. History of characteristic twisting injury to knee (80%).

3. Pain in knee joint (85%) is commonly felt at time of injury. In less severe or repeated injuries pain may be delayed until after the knee has been rested for a few hours. Stiffness of the joint is associated with the pain.

4. History that the knee locks and has to be unlocked by special trick movements (40%).

5. History that the knee clicks (40%) is less suggestive of a cartilage lesion but may be caused by small tears of a cartilage that do not produce actual locking. McMurray test is positive (i.e. extension of the flexed knee while one hand rotates the tibia on the femur and the other feels for 'clicks' over the two menisci in the medial and lateral joint spaces).

6. Tenderness over the cartilage (75%) is felt at the side of the joint over the joint line in the gap between femur and tibia just anterior to the medial or lateral ligaments.

7. Effusion (45%) may occur with any knee joint injury.

INVESTIGATIONS

X-ray of knee joint may be needed to exclude old injuries and osteoarthritis. Cartilage lesions cannot be demonstrated by X-ray. Arthroscopy by expert.

DURATION

Indefinite if the cartilage is not removed.

COMPLICATIONS

Osteoarthritis tends to develop in the joint 10 to 20 years later.

MISLEADING FEATURES AND PITFALLS

Patients sometimes say that a knee has become locked when they mean that it has become stiff after an injury.

DIFFERENTIAL DIAGNOSIS

Diseases that may be confused with a torn cartilage:

Acute traumatic synovitis of knee

Similar features: recent injury; pain in knee; effusion.

Distinguishing features: history of recurrent incidents absent; history of locking and unlocking absent; tenderness over affected cartilage absent.

Torn ligament of knee
Similar features: recent injury; pain; effusion; tenderness over cartilage.

Distinguishing features: (1) Lateral or medial ligament tears; tenderness over whole ligament; marked lateral instability of the fully extended knee joint. (2) Cruciate ligament tears; anterior-posterior instability of the flexed joint; knee can be abnormally over-extended when pain and swelling have subsided.

Osteochondritis dissecans
Similar features: repeated incidents of locking, clicking and effusion into joint, in a young man.

Distinguishing features: long history of faulty knee function; cartilage tenderness absent; X-ray appearances characteristic.

MANAGEMENT OBJECTIVES

Prevention: (a) adequate quadriceps exercises before undertaking high risk activities are of undoubted value; (b) supportive bandages may also help to prevent recurrences if a small tear is suspect.

Established tear: (a) referral for meniscectomy; (b) full post hospital quadriceps exercises before further high risk activities.

PLANTAR FASCIITIS AND CALCANEAL SPUR

Classification: ICHPPC 728 (RCGP 4040)

Aetiology unknown. Calcaneal spur is probably a coincidental finding. The most likely cause of pain and tenderness in the anterior heel. Tenderness on sole and sides of heel.

DIAGNOSTIC RANGE (rates per 1000 patients per year)
Personal: Suspected 0.5.

MANAGEMENT OPTIONS
(a) depot steroid injection — BNF 10.1.2.2 (Ref. 0.1) into tender area from side. Two injections; (b) exclude rheumatoid arthritis.

BUNIONS

Classification: ICHPPC 736 (RCGP 4050)

A characteristic deformity and swelling which develops slowly in the feet of middle aged women. Ill-fitting shoes are probably the cause. The big toe is pushed permanently outwards and a bursa develops over the medial side of first metatarsophalangeal joint which becomes enlarged, painful and disorganised. Infection of the overlying bursa is not uncommon.

DIAGNOSTIC RANGE (rates per 1000 patients per year)
Personal: probable 2.0 *National*: 0.9 (Ref. 0.2).

SEX INCIDENCE
(Female to males: 10:1.)

MANAGEMENT OPTIONS

Prevention: (a) avoid ill fitting (especially pointed) shoes; (b) avoid high heeled shoes.

Severe disease: refer for surgery.

PREPATELLAR BURSITIS (HOUSEMAID'S KNEE)

Classification: ICHPPC 7263 (RCGP 4055)

A painful collection of fluid in the prepatella bursa after trauma or excessive kneeling. There is a well-marked slightly painful swelling on the front of the patella. Occasionally the fluid becomes infected. Recurrences are common.

DIAGNOSTIC RANGE (rates per 1000 patients per year)
Personal: Probable 1.5+.

MANAGEMENT OPTIONS

Established disease: (a) avoid causative trauma; (b) rest; (c) simple analgesics — BNF 4.7.1; (d) aspiration with local injection of depot steroid — BNF 10.1.2.2 (Ref. 0.1) followed by firm bandage; (e) kneeling mats are often helpful.

TENOSYNOVITIS

Classification: ICHPPC 7263 (RCGP 4045)

A painful disorder of tendon sheaths. As with fibrositis, the diagnosis easily becomes a rag-bag.

AETIOLOGY

Unaccustomed use rather than direct trauma is usually the precipitating factor. Wearing new shoes may cause tenosynovitis of the Achilles tendon. Prevention by avoidance is rarely possible.

DIAGNOSTIC RANGE (rates per 1000 patients per year)
Personal: suspected 11.9+. (Confirmation of the diagnosis in the absence of crepitus is difficult.)

DIAGNOSTIC RANGE (rates per 1000 patients per year)
Personal: Suspected 0.5.

AGE INCIDENCE
Sufferers often women are usually 50 to 70 (rarely under 40).

CLINICAL POINTERS
1. Gradual onset over several weeks.
2. Shoulder pain on active and passive movements. Pain is said to be worse at night.
3. Immobility of the joint. Muscle spasm fixes the scapulo-humeral joint. Arm movements are achieved by moving the scapula and humerus together. The scapula must be fixed before the mobility of the humerus is examined. Rotation of shoulder joint is painful from the start of the condition.
4. Wasting of all shoulder muscles may develop — a result of fear of moving the shoulder.

INVESTIGATIONS
Blood tests are normal. X-rays are normal or show osteoporosis.

DURATION
Varies from 2 months to 2 years.

COMPLICATIONS
None. Shoulder mobility may be permanently lessened.

DIFFERENTIAL DIAGNOSIS
Diseases that may be confused with periarthritis of shoulder:

Rheumatoid arthritis and polymyalgia rheumatica
Similar features: pain on passive shoulder movements; fixity of joint; patients in later life affected.
Distinguishing features: shoulder pain clears after a week or so with salicylates; other joints affected; fever; serology and blood sedimentation rate differentiate.

Supraspinatus tendinitis
Similar features: pain on active shoulder movements; pain persists for many months.
Distinguishing features: pain is related to shoulder abduction beyond 45°; no pain on passive shoulder movements; external rotation of shoulder is full.

Osteoarthritis of shoulder
Similar features: pain on passive shoulder movements; elderly patients affected.

CLINICAL POINTERS
1. Onset after unaccustomed activity.
2. Pain associated with movement of a specific tendon.
3. Crepitus on moving the tendon.
4. Local tenderness is usually slight.
5. Sites commonly affected. Hand and wrist (47%), foot and ankle (45%) and Achilles tendon (8%).

DURATION
Usually about 1 to 4 weeks.

COMPLICATIONS
None. Recurrences are common.

DIFFERENTIAL DIAGNOSIS
When crepitus is absent tenosynovitis may be difficult to distinguish from other trivial strains, fibrositis, etc.

MANAGEMENT OPTIONS
Established tenosynovitis: (a) rest; (b) simple splints; (c) anti-inflammatory (non-steroid) analgesics — BNF 10.1.1.1 (Ref. 0.1); (d) local injection of depot steroid (Ref. 13.8) — BNF 10.1.2.2.

TRAUMATIC SYNOVITIS

Classification: ICHPPC 7263 (RCGP 4045)

Synovial fluid collects in a joint after damage.

DIAGNOSTIC RANGE (rates per 1000 patients per year)
Personal: probable 6.2+. *National*: 1.6 (Ref. 0.2). (In many sprains a traumatic synovitis passes unnoticed.)

AGE INCIDENCE
All ages. Adolescents and young adults mainly affected.

CLINICAL POINTERS
1. High risk factors: (a) sport; (b) trauma; (c) previous occurrence. Occasionally no definite history of trauma is obtained.
2. Pain on movement. The joint assumes the position of greatest comfort, i.e. maximum capacity of joint space.
3. A fluctuant effusion is seen and felt bulging between the ligaments of the joint.
4. The joint affected. Usually knee or ankle.
5. Local inflammation. Tenderness, heat and occasionally redness.

INVESTIGATIONS
An X-ray may be needed to exclude bony injury.

DURATION
The effusion absorbs in a few days. After severe injury (or operation) it may persist for months.

MANAGEMENT OPTIONS
Prevention: graduated exercise before starting high risk activities.
Acute synovitis: (a) rest; (b) anti-inflammatory (non-steroid) analgesics — BNF 10.1.1 (Ref. 0.1); (c) graduated exercises once pain has settled.
Chronic synovitis: if above not effective — injection of depot steroids (Ref. 13.8) — BNF 10.1.2.2 may be indicated.

CLICKING RIB AND CLICKING JAW

Classification: ICHPPC 739 (RCGP 4150)

These two disorders are both due to traumatic synovitis.

Clicking rib syndrome. Pain and tenderness over the costochondral junction. Movement aggravates the pain. Examination of the other side negative.

DIAGNOSTIC RANGE (rates per 1000 patients per year)
Personal: Suspected 1.3

Clicking jaw syndrome. Pain and tenderness over the mandibular joint. Movement aggravates the pain. A click can occasionally be felt if patient opens and shuts the jaw.

DIAGNOSTIC RANGE (rates per 1000 patients per year)
Personal: Suspected 0.6.

MANAGEMENT OPTIONS
As for previous condition.

GANGLION

Classification: ICHPPC 7274 (RCGP 4060)

A small cyst filled with clear jelly which develops in adults from the tendon sheaths of the wrist, foot or hand. The tense, occasionally painful swelling is rarely more than 1 cm diameter.

DIAGNOSTIC RANGE (rates per 1000 patients per year)
Personal: probable 2.3+.

MANAGEMENT OPTIONS
Established disease: (a) leave if symptomless — spontaneous disappearance common; (b) disperse by pressure or aspiration; (c) surgical excision if chronically painful.

PERIARTHRITIS OF THE SHOULDER AND OTHER SIMILAR CHRONIC SELF-LIMITING DISEASES OF THE SKELETAL SYSTEM

This group of diseases includes frozen shoulder, supraspinatus tendinitis, tennis elbow and plantar fasciitis (see p. 643). They have several clinical features in common.

- — Aetiology uncertain.
- — Gradual onset unrelated to trauma.
- — Increasing, continuous pain which waxes for several weeks or months and then wanes for a similar period; the pain is aggravated by movement.
- — No local deformity or redness.
- — Treatment often appears ineffective.
- — Pathological findings are said to be those of chronic inflammation with degeneration.

NOTE ON THE ANATOMY OF THE SHOULDER
The shoulder is sometimes described as a joint within a joint. The inner joint between the humeral head and the shallow saucer like glenoid is surrounded and supported by the joint capsule and the broad flat tendons of subscapularis, supraspinatus, infraspinatus and teres minor — the so-called rotator cuff. The outer joint is formed by the subacromial bursa separating the head of humerus and rotator cuff from the coraco-acromial arch and deltoid. Lesions of the cuff are painful as the lesion moves under the arch (the painful arc) on abducting the humerus. Ruptures of the cuff (particularly supraspinatus) destroy the stability of the inner joint, so that the deltoid pulls the humeral head upwards instead of abducting the arm.

CAPSULITIS OF SHOULDER (FROZEN SHOULDER)

Classification: ICHPPC 7260 (RCGP 4030)

AETIOLOGY
Unknown. A few patients give a history of trauma. Some cases of capsulitis probably follow inflammation of the supraspinatus and rotator cuff tendinitis. The capsulitis immobilises the joint.

Distinguishing features: pain does not persist and is rarely severe; other joints often affected; crepitus on passive movements.

Bronchogenic carcinoma (Apical)
Similar features: chronic shoulder pain.
Distinguishing features: full range of active and passive movement; raised ESR.

MANAGEMENT OPTIONS
Established disease: (a) prepare patient for 6 to 12 months duration; (b) anti-inflammatory (non-steroid) analgesics — BNF 10.1.1 (Ref. 0.1); (c) physiotherapy; (d) intra-articular depot steroids (Ref. 13.9) — BNF 10.1.2.2; (e) increase mobility as symptoms decrease; (f) treatment often ineffective and many unsatisfactory and fringe alternatives may be considered.

THE PAINFUL ARC SYNDROME

Classification: ICHPPC 7260 (RCGP 4030)

The syndrome includes:

— Supraspinatus tendon rupture, partial rupture and calcification.
— Subacromial (or subdeltoid) bursitis.
— Other lesions, usually traumatic, affecting the rotator cuff.

AETIOLOGY
Uncertain. (Patients related the onset of symptoms to trauma in half the cases.)

DIAGNOSTIC RANGE (rates per 1000 patients per year)
Personal: Suspected 1.2. Probable 0.9.

AGE AND SEX INCIDENCE
Males between 25 and 55 years mainly affected.

CLINICAL POINTERS
Characteristic shoulder pain is felt when the arm is actively abducted from the side. Pain is absent or less marked on passive abduction or with active movements in the horizontal position. The arm can be held abducted at 90° without pain. Crepitus is sometimes noted.

INVESTIGATIONS
X-rays are normal, but chronic cases may show calcification of the supraspinatus tendon.

DURATION
The complaint clears with symptomatic treatment in 2 to 8 weeks in most cases. Recurrences occur.

COMPLICATIONS
A capsulitis of the shoulder may develop.

DIFFERENTIAL DIAGNOSIS
The characteristic shoulder pain differentiates.

MISLEADING FEATURES AND PITFALLS
The shoulder may appear normal if the patient is examined in the horizontal, not the vertical, position.

MANAGEMENT OPTIONS
As for previous section.

TENNIS ELBOW

Classification: ICHPPC 7263 (RCGP 4035)

DIAGNOSTIC RANGE (rates per 1000 patients per year)
Personal: suspected 1.4. Probable 0.7.

AGE INCIDENCE
Adults over 30 years are mainly affected.

CLINICAL POINTERS
1. Onset is gradual and usually unrelated to trauma.
2. Pain related to movement is felt in a number of places near the joint. The usual site of pain is in the extensor origin of the muscles arising from the lateral epicondyle. The patient can often carry a bag, etc. without pain.
3. Localised tenderness may be acute.
4. Prolonged continuous pain.

INVESTIGATIONS
Radiological investigation is normal.

DURATION
Usually between 1 and 12 months.

COMPLICATIONS
Recurrences may occur.

DIFFERENTIAL DIAGNOSIS
The disorder is distinguished from minor injuries to the elbow and

from rheumatoid arthritis by the continuous and prolonged pain. In rheumatoid arthritis other joints may be affected.

MANAGEMENT OPTIONS

Established condition: (a) prepare patient for annoying complaint because recurrences are common and treatment may be ineffective; (b) anti-inflammatory (non-steroid) analgesics — BNF 10.1.1 (Ref. 0.1.); (c) local injection (at tender site) of depot steroids (Ref. 13.9) — BNF 10.1.2.2; (d) physiotherapy and early movements once symptoms improve.

FLAT FOOT

Classification: ICHPPC 736 (RCGP 4125)

The feet of all babies are flat, but by the age of 16 the foot should have a well-marked longitudinal arch — a result of growth and physical activity. Flat foot is recognised by the low or absent medial longitudinal arch and by the inward bulge of the upper part of this arch and foot eversion. Under 16 years the disorder is reversible, rarely causes pain and usually disappears with full, normal activity. After this the deformity may follow obesity, excessive or unaccustomed walking and gradually becomes irreversible. Secondary bony changes develop and the foot becomes increasingly painful. Cheap, faulty shoes may aggravate the condition.

DIAGNOSTIC RANGE (rates per 1000 patients per year)
Personal: Probable 1.9. Many cases are not reported.

MANAGEMENT OPTIONS

Prevention: (a) physical activity and sport; (b) well fitting shoes.
Established state: *Under 16*: (a) most reported cases are normal and reassurance is all that is needed; (b) heel raising exercises; (c) raised medial edge of shoe; (d) 'Heal seat' to control medial collapse of shoes. *Over 16* as for under 16 but cure is less likely and daily activities may require modification.

METATARSALGIA AND PAINFUL ANTERIOR TRANSVERSE ARCH

Classification: ICHPPC 7263 (RCGP 4040)

A common disorder in middle-aged, obese women, that is difficult to treat. Following inadequate exercise, faulty shoes and obesity, the transverse metatarsal arch splays and flattens. A characteristic tender callous forms under one of the central metatarsal heads.

DIAGNOSTIC RANGE (rates per 1000 patients per year)
Personal: Probable 1.5+. *National*: 1.1 (REF. 0.2). Many patients report to the chiropodist and not the doctor.

Management options

Prevention: (a) plenty of exercise; (b) supportive shoes.

Established condition: (a) foot exercises; (b) metatarsal support with pad; (c) reduce weight if obese.

KNOCK KNEES

Classification: ICHPPC 736 (RCGP 4140)

When a child starts to walk a certain degree of knock knee is inevitable. Some deviation of the tibia may persist until the child goes to school, but permanent deformity is rare. An orthopaedic second opinion is obtained under the following circumstances:

1. The parents cannot be reassured.
2. The deformity is worse at 3 years than it was at 2 (the distance between the malleoli is measured when the child is sitting on an examination couch with extended fully adducted knees);
3. The distance between the malleoli approaches 8 cm (3 inches) when the child is 4 years old.

DIAGNOSTIC RANGE (rates per 1000 patients per year)
Personal: Probable 0.4+.

Table 34 Less common diseases of bones and organs of movement

Disease and distinguishing clinical pointers	Incidence per 1000 patients per year Suspected	 Confirmed
Sarcoma of bone Progressive pain and swelling, early secondaries, rapid deterioration, X-ray	—	1 in 10 years
Acute septic arthritis Picture resembles acute osteomyelitis, joint swelling and tenderness, joint immobilised in position of greatest comfort, source of infection elsewhere (not always obvious).Refer early.	—	2 in 10 years
Acute or irritable hip syndrome Children; short history of limp and pain in hip; low fever; duration 3 to 10 days; X-rays, ESR and white cell count are normal. Symptomatic treatment.	0.6	—

Table 34 Less common diseases of bones and organs of movement

Disease and distinguishing clinical pointers	Incidence per 1000 patients per year Suspected	 Confirmed
Slipped femoral epiphysis Older children, trauma sometimes precedes limp, X-ray. Early referral.	—	2 in 10 years
Osteochondritis dissecans Teenagers, repeated effusions, pain, progressive knee joint destruction, loose bodies, locking, X-ray.	0	0 in 10 years
Steroid osteoporosis Pain and spinal compression, steroids, X-ray	—	1 in 10
Traumatic osteitis of patella A painful lesion at the attachment of the patella tendon; children, usually 10 to 15 years; pain in one or both knees after running, jumping; lower patella is hot and tender; complete recovery with rest in 4 to 12 weeks; X-ray may show osteoporosis of lower patella. Treatment p. 640	— 1 in 10 years	3 in 10 years
Sudek's osteoporosis Chronic painful osteoporosis after trauma. Treatment unsatisfactory		
Torn ligament of knee Severe trauma, pain, effusion, torn lateral ligament gives abnormal lateral mobility to fully extended joint, torn cruciate gives abnormal anteroposterior mobility of flexed joint. Refer early.	—	2 in 10 years
Olecranon bursitis Chronic cystic swelling. Treat as for housemaid's knee — p. 644	0.4	0.4
Semimembranosus bursitis Painful tense cyst over upper medial half of popliteal fossa. Refer .	0.3	0.3
Baker's cyst A popiteal cyst (3 to 6 cm diam.), associated with osteoarthritis. Refer for surgery if annoying.	—	1 in 10 years
Dupuytren's contracture Middle-aged patients, flexion deformity of fingers (usually 4th or 5th) with palpable band and dimpling at the base of the finger. Leave. Treatment often unsatisfactory.	0.3	0.3
Postural deformities of spine May be acute, severe and unexplained in early 'teens'. Refer early.	0.3	0.3
Mallet finger Untreated flexion injury of terminal phalanx. Refer early.	0.2	0.2
Pigeon toes A mild degree of in-toeing may be noted between 2 and 6 years, unless the deformity persists or is excessive no treatment is needed.	0.6	0.6

Table 34 Less common diseases of bones and organs of movement

Disease and distinguishing clinical pointers	Incidence per 1000 patients per year Suspected	Confirmed
Hammer toe Acquired flexion deformity of 2nd, 3rd, or 4th toes. Refer for surgery if annoying.	0.4	0.4
Bowing of tibia Arises normally when a child starts to walk, anterior bowing suggests rickets. Reassure.	—	—
Coccydynia Chronic, recurrent coccygeal pain after sitting. Direct trauma is usually responsible. Patients often female with low threshold of pain. Appropriate decisions about the extent of intervention difficult. Referral often helpful.	0.4	0.4

25

Congenital malformations and certain diseases of early infancy

Please read the introduction for explanation of figures and analyses.

The diagnosis of major congenital deformities is usually obvious at, or soon after, birth. (The figures for the incidence of congenital malformations are difficult to interpret because some patients with deformities die at birth while others report to the doctor every year. Incidence rates are also swollen when several deformities arise in one patient.)

Further discussion of this field is mentioned in Chapter 4.

CONGENITAL ANOMALIES OF HEART

Classification: ICHPPC 746 (RCGP 4225)

1. Fallot's tetralogy, i.e. pulmonary stenosis, interventricular septal defect, dextroposition of aorta overriding the septal defect, and right ventricular hypertrophy. (One proven case in 10 years.)
2. Atrioseptal defect. (One proven case in 10 years.)
3. Interventricular septal defect. The defect is often suspected but rarely proven unless there is disability.
4. Patent ductus arteriosus. (No cases in 20 years.)
5. Coarctation of aorta. (No cases in 20 years.)

AETIOLOGY

Parental rubella during the first 3 months of pregnancy may cause defects. In most cases the cause is not obvious.

DIAGNOSTIC RANGE (rates per 1000 patients per year)

Personal: Suspected 2.0. Probable 0.6. *National*: 0.4 (Ref. 0.2). Many cases with small septal defects are probably never recognised.

CLINICAL POINTERS

1. Cyanosis in congenital heart disease is due to a shunt of blood from the right to the left side of the heart.

Permanent cyanosis indicates either transposition of vessels or pulmonary stenosis with septal defects. All three features occur in Fallot's tetralogy.

Occasionally cyanosis, i.e. at birth or during lung infections, indicates a possible large septal defect or patent ductus. Then a transient right to left shunt with temporary cyanosis is induced by birth or the infection.

2. Failure to gain weight and poor development is common in severe defects.

3. Poor exercise tolerance is marked in severe cases. The child may squat to avoid standing.

4. Cardiac murmurs. The correct assessment of murmurs is a difficult task. The family doctor rarely has enough experience to be able to do more than decide that a murmur is abnormal and then obtain a chest X–ray or second opinion.

5. Absence of the femoral pulse suggests coarctation of the aorta.

6. Clubbing of fingers.

INVESTIGATION

Doubtful cases should be referred for investigation.

DURATION

Indefinite unless treated.

COMPLICATIONS

Lung infections and death.

MANAGEMENT OPTIONS

Prevention: rubella immunisation (with case finding) of females.

Established disease: referral for assessment and surgery if appropriate.

Post hospital: (a) full explanation and support of parents and patient; (b) lay foundations for a long continuous relationship with medical team; (c) regular follow up to monitor progress (d) prophylactic antibacterials — BNF 5.1 (Ref. 0.1) as needed.

CONGENITAL DISLOCATION OF HIP

Classification: ICHPPC 754 (RCGP 4255)

Early diagnosis is the key to treatment. All babies should be examined routinely for possible dislocation at or soon after birth.

DIAGNOSTIC RANGE (rates per 1000 patients per year)

Personal: Suspected 0.2. Probable 0.1. *National*: 1.5 per 1000 live births.

SEX INCIDENCE

Girls are affected six times more often than boys.

CLINICAL POINTERS

1. High risk factors: (a) female baby; (b) positive family history (36%); (c) breech delivery.

2. Ortolani's test. The child is laid on its back with hips flexed to a right angle and knees also flexed. Starting with the knees together the hips are slowly abducted and if one is dislocated, somewhere in the 90° arc of abduction, the head of the femur slips back into the acetabulum with a palpable click. The test can be done at any age but the click is not always produced.

3. Barlow's test. The baby is laid on its back. The hips are flexed to a right angle and both knees are fully flexed.

The middle finger of each hand is placed over the greater trochanter and the thumb of each hand is applied to the inner side of the thigh close but not quite in the groin. The hips are carried into abduction. With the hips in about 70° of abduction the middle finger of each hand in turn exerts pressure away from the examining couch as if to push the trochanter towards the symphysis pubis. In a normal child no movement occurs. If the hip is dislocated, the greater trochanter and the head of the femur with it can be felt to move in the direction in which the pressure has been applied.

4. Barlow's test — part 2. With the hips in the same position as described in the last paragraph, the thumb which is applied over the upper and inner part of the thigh exerts pressure towards the examination couch. In normal children no movement occurs. In a child with a dislocatable hip, the head of the femur can be felt to slip out and to come back immediately the pressure is released.

5. Limited abduction. After 4 or 5 weeks of age the best single sign of subluxation of the hip is limitation of abduction when the hips are flexed to a right angle.

6. Late signs include absence of a buttock fold, late walking, shortening of limb, absence of femoral head from femoral triangle, high position of greater trochanter, radiological evidence and waddling gait.

DURATION

Indefinite unless treated.

MANAGEMENT OPTIONS

Prevention: regular screening of all babies at birth — the primary physician should never assume that tests have been carried out in hospital by someone else.

Established case: referral.

DOWN'S SYNDROME (MONGOLISM)

Classification: ICHPPC 758 (RCGP 4285)

AETIOLOGY

Abnormal amounts of chromosome 21 material are responsible. This extra material may arise in three different ways:

1. Full trisomy (94% of all cases). The ovum of the mother, usually elderly, is abnormal because the two chromosomes of pair 21 fail to separate. The ovum therefore has two 21 chromosomes. Addition of a normal 21 chromosome from the father's sperm leads to trisomy of all patient's cells which all have an extra 21 chromosome (47 in all).

2. Translocation (3.5%). One parent, usually of a younger age, has a chromosome count of only 45 but a normal amount of chromosome material because chromosome 21 is translocated onto chromosome 15. After fertilisation the zygote has a normal number of chromosomes (46) which include three 21 chromosomes. This type of trisomy tends to be familial.

3. Mosaicism (2.5%) as a result of the faulty division of an early embryonic cell. Trisomy 21 occurs only in some of the patient's body cells. These patients are often less severely affected.

DIAGNOSTIC RANGE (rates per 1000 patients per year)

Personal: Suspected 2.0. Probable 1.0. National rates are decreasing. Overall incidence said to be 1 : 660 births, making it the commonest malformation in man.

CLINICAL POINTERS

1. High risk factors: (a) increasing parental age — pregnant women over 37 are involved in three out of five cases; (b) positive family history; (c) a previous Down's baby — there is only a 1–2% chance of a second.

The syndrome is usually obvious but sometimes certain diagnosis is difficult in the early weeks of life. The following pointers may help to support a diagnosis.

2. Mental defect of varying degree (100%). IQ range said to be 25–50%.

3. Characteristically flat facial profile with wide epicanthic folds (90%).

4. Poor Moro ('startle') reflex (85%).

5. Slanted palpebral fissures (80%).

6. Hypotonia and hyperflexibility of joints (80%).

7. Excess skin at back of neck with brachycephaly (80%).

8. Abnormal pelvic bone configuration (70%).
9. Abnormal or absent mid-phalanx of little finger (60%).
10. Simian crease of palms (45%).
11. Abnormalities of shape and ridge patterns (ulnar loops) of hands (85%).

INVESTIGATIONS

(a) Amniocentesis allows parental decisions about continuance of pregnancy; but carries a small (1%) risk. Should be available for all who desire it and understand the risks. (b) Chromosome laboratories are occasionally needed to establish a diagnosis after delivery.

DURATION

Life expectancy is better than 20 years ago, especially if the child is raised with its own family. At birth life expectancy is about 16 years and if the critical first 6 months are survived it increases to 22 to 30 years. Other figures suggest that 25% may die in the first 6 months and 50% in the first 5 years.

COMPLICATIONS

1. Congential heart lesions (40%).
2. Leukaemia (1%).
3. Growth and development are slow throughout life.
4. Males are always infertile; girls may menstruate and can be fertile.
5. Death from intercurrent infection said to be common in early years.

MISLEADING FEATURES AND PITFALLS

1. The doctor delays telling parents because he is uncertain of the diagnosis.

2. The doctor allows taboos and social attitudes towards mental disease to influence his own attitude to such patients. Down's children, in fact, have a great sense of humour, are very affectionate and interesting to care for.

3. The common major criticisms of doctors raised by parents of Down's children are:

• Failure to inform, discuss, explain and prepare in the early days. This includes the failure to discuss amniocentesis during the antenatal period.

• Failure to understand the isolation and guilt in both parents, especially in the first years.

• Failure to discuss problems ahead — further pregnancies;

schooling; reactions of siblings and neighbours; adolescence and sex; institutional versus home care; the need for holiday relief; the strains on the pair bonding between parents; leaving school when parents are in late middle age.

- Tendency of doctors (and friends) to cover their own feelings of inadequacy by telling Down's parents that they are doing a 'wonderful' job without helping them to do it.
- Failure to introduce parents to all available support groups and financial help (Ref. 25.1).

One of the best yardsticks for 'assessing' any primary physician is how, after 5–10 years in practice, he or she has learnt to handle these problems.

MANAGEMENT OPTIONS

Prevention (a) amniocentesis is offered to mothers over 35 and in high risk groups — *ideally all mothers should be offered this but present chromosome laboratories may not be able to carry this load*; (b) if amniocentesis is positive, the pros and cons of termination should be discussed fully and parents helped to reach *their own* decision about continuing the pregnancy; (c) genetic counselling may be helpful.

Established cases: (a) the physician should learn how to deal with the ongoing problems raised above by acquiring sufficient factual knowledge and by discussions with parents and local Society for Mentally Handicapped; (b) arrange continued support of parents at home — this may include arranging attendance allowance and other financial support; (c) arranging home support services; (d) exploring holiday relief services for mentally handicapped; (e) considering possible institutional care in extreme cases; (f) regular follow up; (g) health visitor or social worker often helpful; (h) local and National Support Groups run many facilities — National Society for Mentally Handicapped (MENCAP) — Ref. 25.1.

Table 35 Less common congential malformations and diseases of early infancy

Disease and distinguishing clinical pointers	Incidence per 1000 patients per year Suspected	 Confirmed
Monstrosity (fresh cases)	0.1	0.1
Spina bifida occulta (fresh cases)	0.1	0.1
Meningomyelocele (fresh cases)	0.2	0.2
Hydrocephalus (fresh cases)	—	2 in 10 years
Congenital eye defects— nystagmus, cataract, Retinitis pigmentosa	0.4	0.4
Tuberous sclerosis	—	1 in 10 years
Microcephalus	—	1 in 10 years
Cleft palate and harelip (fresh cases)	0.1	0.1
Congenital pyloric stenosis (see p. 466)	0.1	0.1
Imperforate anus and mega colon (fresh cases)	0.4 0.2	0.2 0.2
Undescended testicle (see p. 533)	0.5	0.5
Polycystic kidney (see p. 526)	—	1 in 10 years
Achondroplasia	0.8	0.8
Major deformities of limbs (fresh cases)*	—	2 in 20 years
Minor deformities of limbs (fresh cases)	0.5	0.5
Haemolytic disease of newborn Rhesus-negative mother, rhesus-positive father, repeated miscarriages or stillbirths, congenital deformities, hydrops, jaundice, severe anaemia, death. Replacement transfusion vital	0.2	0.2 (1 per 200 deliveries)
Haemorrhagic disease of newborn Onset 1 to 3 days after birth; haemorrhages into bowel, skin or brain; death if not treated with vitamin K	0.1	0.1 (1 per 400 deliveries)
Hypospadias Varying degrees of severity, a bunched hood of foreskin alerts the doctor. Urethral valves and meatal stenosis common; orifice difficult to see, usually proximal to vestigial urethral groove; association with undescended testicles suggests intersex; chordae. Early referral wise	0.2	0.2
Pemphigus neonatorum Rapidly spreading often fatal streptococcal infection, pus-filled vesicles and bullae with crusting, acute omphalitis	—	2 in 10 years

* Two fresh cases in 1962 were probably due to thalidomide. The drug was taken between the 30th and 40th days of pregnancy without the knowledge of the family doctor.

26

Injury and other miscellaneous conditions

Please read the introduction for explanation of figures and analyses.

Traumatic disorders rarely present problems of diagnosis.

Occasionally the effects of injury are masked and a fracture or other serious injury is overlooked. The family doctor should always record history and findings fully and obtain X-rays or a second opinion if a diagnosis is in doubt or if an accident is likely to involve legal proceedings.

HYPERTHERMIA

Classification: ICHPPC 7889 (RCGP 5245)

AETIOLOGY

Cold weather and infection, leads to overclothing and over-heated rooms.

DIAGNOSTIC RANGE

One case in 10 years.

AGE INCIDENCE

Infants are usually affected but the condition can occur in toddlers or young children. The condition can occur in adults in hot countries.

CLINICAL POINTERS

1. Febrile illness — respiratory, gastrointestinal etc.
2. Cold weather.
3. The presence of excessive wrappings.
4. Convulsions are said to contribute but these may be a result.
5. Temperatures over 40.5°C (105°F) should suggest the possibility.

COMPLICATIONS

Death or residual mental defects.

MISTAKES AND PITFALLS

Failure to take a temperature in an obviously ill baby or infant.

MANAGEMENT OPTIONS

Prevention: Parental education.

Established condition: (a) reduce clothing; (b) tepid sponging; (c) immediate hospital admission.

ACCIDENTAL HYPOTHERMIA

Classification: ICHPPC 7889 (RCGP 5240)

AETIOLOGY

Cold weather leading to an unusually cold house combined with inactivity, illness or inadequate food intake. Occurs in the very young and the elderly. Rectal temperatures under 32.5°C (90°F) constitute physiological hypothermia but the condition should be considered before this level is reached.

Hypothermia in babies (two cases in 10 years)

AGE INCIDENCE

First few weeks of life.

CLINICAL POINTERS

1. High risk factors: (a) very young babies, (b) prematurity, (c) intercurrent disease, (d) disadvantaged.
2. Apathy and refusal to feed.
3. Very cold weather. Sometimes the room is warm by day and only gets cold in the early hours (02.00 to 06.00 hours). Sometimes there is a history of a recent move to a new house.
4. Cherry red appearance is characteristic.
5. Hard pitting oedema of hands and feet.
6. Lowered rectal temperature. The condition should be suspected and hospital admission considered in all cases where rectal temperatures below 36°C (97°F) are recorded.

COMPLICATIONS

A fatal outcome is common if the condition is not recognised in time. Brain damage and mental deficiency occur.

MISLEADING FEATURES AND PITFALLS

The 'good colour' and a room that is warm by day can both be very misleading. Failure to consider the possibility is the usual mistake.

MANAGEMENT OPTIONS

Immediate referral if suspected.

Hypothermia in the elderly

DIAGNOSTIC RANGE

Three cases in 10 years.

CLINICAL POINTERS

1. High risk factors in elderly patients living alone:

- Liable to fall and unable to get up.
- Liable to take alcohol.
- Poor housing conditions.
- Few friendly neighbours or relatives.
- Unable to get out of house or be fully active.
- Cold weather and low calorie intake.
- Chronic disease — stroke, Parkinson's disease, myxoedema or previously treated hyperthyroid.
- Previous hypothermia incident.
- Lack of money for fuel or food.

2. Many potential cases are symptom free but have oral temperatures of under 35°C (95°F). Possibly 10% of elderly living alone are in this category.

3. Drowsiness and confusion are usually the first signs.

COMPLICATIONS

Coma and death unless rescued. Brain damage and dementia may follow. Too rapid warming may aggravate cerebral damage.

MISLEADING FEATURES AND PITFALLS

Failure to consider the possibility is the usual mistake. This condition should be remembered in every elderly patient living on their own with unusual symptoms or behaviour.

MANAGEMENT OPTIONS

Prevention: encourage neighbours, relatives, wardens and medical team to be aware of high risk factors and visit frequently.

Established state: immediate referral. *Prevention of recurrences* may involve rehousing, sheltered housing, granny flat, day hospital or institutional care.

FRACTURES

Classification: ICHPPC 802–829 (RCGP 5000–5079)

Fractures are named after the anatomical site and the type of fracture — compound (skin broken), comminuted (many breaks), impacted (ends jammed together), greenstick (incomplete) and simple.

	Incidence per 1000 patients per year	
	Suspected	*Confirmed*
Fractured skull	0.6	0.3
nose	0.2	0.2
spine	0.5	0.2
rib	0.9	0.5
pelvis	0.2	0.1
clavicle	0.8	0.5
scapula	0.2	0.2
humerus	1.3	1.1
radius and ulna	5.5	4.1
hand (excluding scaphoid)	3.7	2.2
scaphoid	0.6	0.4
neck of femur	0.3	0.1
femur (other)	0.3	0.2
patella	0.2	0.1
tibia	0.7	0.6
fibula	1.3	0.9
ankle	1.9	0.9
foot	2.1	1.7
Other fractures	0.1	0
Total	21.4	14.3

DIAGNOSTIC RANGE (rates per 1000 patients per year)
Personal: Suspected 21.4. Probable 14.3.

In general practice there are two big groups of fractures.

A. *The classical fracture* in which the diagnosis is obvious at a glance. The history of trauma, followed by pain, immobility, swelling and deformity render the diagnosis obvious to everyone.

B. *The concealed fracture* which can be overlooked.

CLINICAL POINTERS WHICH SUGGEST A CONCEALED FRACTURE

1. High risk factors: (a) history of trauma (95%). Spontaneous fractures occasionally occur in the elderly or patients with carcinomatosis; (b) osteoporosis; (c) confusion in the elderly; (d) alcohol; (e) strokes, especially if aphasia is present.

2. History of pain at the fracture site (100%).

3. Loss of function. A significant pointer that after a day's rest, helps to differentiate fractures from sprains.

4. Persistent local pain. Sprains should not be painful after 3 to 5 days rest.

5. Bruising. Although often present in other injuries, bruising when associated with a sprain suggests a fracture.

6. Local tenderness is almost invariable. If it cannot be tested directly as in an impacted fracture of neck of femur it can be shown by longitudinal compression of a bone. A helpful pointer.

INVESTIGATIONS

An X-ray should be obtained in all doubtful cases or if legal complications are possible.

DURATION

Varies with age and site of fracture. In young patients a small green-stick fracture may heal in as little as 14 days while in an elderly patient a fractured hip may never heal.

COMPLICATIONS

1. Shock at time of fracture may be severe. It is primary or follows blood loss into tissues.

2. Fat embolism is said to arise and affect lungs or brain.

3. Arteries or nerves distal to a limb fracture may be damaged. Sometimes the blood supply to a portion of bone is cut off (avascular necrosis).

4. Hypostatic pneumonia in the elderly.

5. Non-union or poor functional result of treatment — rare in children.

MANAGEMENT OPTIONS

Prevention: Routine accident precautions should be followed in the home, at work, in sport, travel and icy conditions. Failures are most frequent in the home and on holiday.

Suspected cases: (a) Routine X-ray. Repeat may be needed (b) Check for witnesses if compensation possible.

Established fractures: Referral.

Post hospital: (a) Check physiotherapy (b) Appropriate modifications of daily living (c) Aids required (d) Monitor return to full function.

FRACTURED SKULL (see p. 669)

FRACTURES THAT ARE EASILY OVERLOOKED

These include:

- *Fractured skull (Especially in Children)* — pp. 669 and 670.
- *Fractured Nose*
- *Fractured Lumbar Vertebrae (Crush Type Affecting Dorsal or Lumbar Vertebral Body)* Easily overlooked but spinal process always tender; angulation deformity often not obvious.
- *Fractured Scaphoid*
  Tender over anatomical snuff-box. Fracture line may not show on X-ray for 10 days. Necrosis of distal portion may follow interference of blood supply. Caused by fall onto flat of hand.
- *Mallet Finger and Toe*
  Often not reported.
- *Fractured Acetabulum*
- *Fractured Neck of Femur (Firmly Impacted)*
  In the elderly can be caused by trivial falls. Impaction, senile confusion and referral of pain to the knee all may conspire to make these fractures very easy to overlook. In the prone position, the out-turned foot is obvious.
- *Spiral Fracture of Fibula*
- *Avulsion Fractures of Malleoli*
- *Fractured Calcaneum*
  After falling and landing on heels. Both calcaneal bones may be affected. Crush fractures of vertebrae bodies may be associated.
- *March Fractures*
  Affecting small bones of feet. Often only reported after several days.
- *Fractured Ribs*
  Sometimes only reported after a few days or not at all.
- *Greenstick fractures* (in children) at any site.

DISLOCATION OF JOINTS

Classification: ICHPPC 839 (RCGP 5080–5109)

The diagnosis is usually clear because the joint is deformed. Recurrences are common.

DIAGNOSTIC RANGE (rates per 1000 patients per year)
Personal: Dislocated shoulder 0.2. Other dislocations 0.3.

MISLEADING FEATURES
A dislocation may be associated with a fracture.

MANAGEMENT OPTIONS
As for fractures, see above.

SPRAINED JOINTS

Classification: ICHPPC 840–848 (RCGP 5110–5155)

DIAGNOSTIC RANGE (rates per 1000 patients per year)
Personal: Suspected 29.2. Severe 18.6. Many cases never reported.

CLINICAL POINTERS
1. History of trauma.
2. Pain and tenderness of joint. Movement aggravates the pain.
3. Swelling or fluid in the joint.

Joints that are commonly sprained	*Incidence per 1000 patients per year*
Ankle	11.1
Thumb and fingers	3.9
Sacral and lumbar region	2.9
Other back strain	2.6
Wrist and forearm	2.5
Shoulder	2.3
Elbow	1.6
Other	2.3

MISLEADING FEATURES
A small fracture is easily mistaken for a sprain.

MANAGEMENT OPTIONS
Suspected strains: (a) X-ray of all doubtful cases, especially if legal action is a possibility; (b) rest or splint the joint until pain free; (c) graduated return to normal.

HEAD INJURY (RCGP 5160)

There are three main types of head injury. These may occur separately or together.

1. Fractured skull.
2. Bruising of the brain (concussion).
3. Intracranial bleeding with raised intracranial pressure — may be arterial or venous.

FRACTURED SKULL (ICHPPC 802: RCGP 5000)

DIAGNOSTIC RANGE (rates per 1000 patients per year)
Personal: Suspected 0.6. Proven 0.3.

CLINICAL POINTERS

1. History of head injury often associated with unconsciousness (concussion).
2. Bruising of skull.
3. Blood behind eardrum.
4. Blood in posterior pharynx.
5. Local tenderness of skull often absent if fracture is basal.

COMPLICATIONS

Extradural (middle meningeal artery) haemorrhage, and subdural haematoma. It is vital to consider the possibility of intracranial haemorrhage in every head injury especially those in the region of the ear and middle meningeal artery. (See below.)

MISLEADING FEATURES AND PITFALLS

1. A skull fracture is easily overlooked in a baby or toddler — injury may be slight or go unobserved; local bruising and tenderness goes unnoticed, until after a few days a fluctuant swelling appears in the region of the fracture.

2. A skull fracture is easily overlooked in a 'drunk' or concussed patient or in one with a CVA who has fallen.

CONCUSSION (ICHPPC 850: RCGP 5160)

Cerebral contusion may be slight or very severe.

DIAGNOSTIC RANGE (rates per 1000 patients per year)
Personal: Suspected 4.0.

CLINICAL POINTERS

1. High risk activities: (a) driving and motorcycling; (b) work — heavy industry and construction; (c) sport — riding, climbing, skiing, boxing, rugby.

2. History of head injury. External bruising may be slight.

3. Loss of consciousness may be momentary or last for several weeks. A state of automatism may occur before complete recovery.

4. Retrograde amnesia. Memory for events just prior to injury is lost.

5. Cerebral irritability. The patient is restless and irrational. This state is aggravated by alcohol.

COMPLICATIONS

1. Hypostatic pneumonia while unconscious.
2. Post-concussional depression with inability to concentrate or sleep may be marked for several weeks. It may demoralise the patient.

MISLEADING FEATURES AND PITFALLS

1. Concussion is mistaken for drunkenness.

2. The patient is allowed to get up 2 or 3 days after a head injury without being prepared for his lack of concentration and depression — suicide may follow.

3. A concurrent intracranial haemorrhage is overlooked.

MANAGEMENT OPTIONS

Prevention: appropriate headgear when performing high risk activities.

Established case: (a) exclude fracture and internal bleeding; (b) complete bed rest — length dependent on length of unconsciousness; (c) avoid intellectual activities requiring memory and concentration; (d) avoid alcohol; (e) gradual rehabilitation back to full activity — may require several days or weeks; (f) prepare patient for slow convalescence and possible depression.

TRAUMATIC INTRACRANIAL HAEMORRHAGE

A. Arterial bleeding into extradural (epidural) space

An injury fractures the skull and a closely attached artery (usually the middle meningeal) is torn.

DIAGNOSTIC RANGE

One case in 10 years.

CLINICAL POINTERS

1. Head injury. This may be severe but the period of immediate unconsciousness is often short or occasionally absent altogether.

2. Local evidence of trauma — often just bruising at the site of the skull fracture — side of the head, above the ear if middle meningeal artery is involved.

3. Lucid interval — usually only a few hours. In children this may be less than 2 hours duration. In many cases the lucid interval is blurred by a period of general cerebral confusion.

4. Pupil inequalities or abnormalities. Initially on the side of the lesion the pupil *may be* fixed and dilated. Later both pupils may be affected and a contralateral hemiparesis *may* develop.

5. Drowsiness and unconsciousness return. Pulse and respiration slow. Spasticity and some early upper motor neurone lesions (contralateral) may develop as coma deepens. Convulsions are a late sign.

COMPLICATIONS

Death if not treated, in a few hours.

MISLEADING FEATURES AND PITFALLS

1. The lucid interval is mistaken for recovery and the patient is not kept under observation.

2. After the initial trauma there is a period of general cerebral confusion which is erroneously diagnosed as due to concussion, alcohol or cerebrovascular accident.

3. The general practitioner may take immediate action. Despite this it may take at least 2 hours for the patient to be moved to a neurosurgical unit, pass through a casualty department, obtain an X-ray and prepare for operation. Therefore if this diagnosis is suspected the practitioner should alert the neurosurgical department as soon as the patient has been dispatched to hospital or better accompany the patient.

MANAGEMENT OPTIONS

Top priority emergency admission if disorder is suspected. Alert surgeon when arranging ambulance.

B. Venous bleeding in the subdural space

DIAGNOSTIC RANGE

One case in 10 years.

CLINICAL POINTERS

1. Head injury may be slight.

2. Onset may be gradual because venous bleeding alone does not cause raised intracranial pressure. Symptoms may not develop for weeks or months until osmotic absorption has caused the haematoma to swell.

3. Symptoms of gradually increasing intracranial pressure (see p. 278).

4. The clinical picture sometimes closely resembles that of an extradural arterial haemorrhage (see previous section).

MANAGEMENT OPTIONS

Immediate referral if suspected.

INTERNAL ABDOMINAL INJURY

Classification: ICHPPC 959 (RCGP 5165)

DIAGNOSTIC RANGE

Three cases in 10 years.

Rupture of liver, spleen or bowel

Any peritoneal bleeding causes signs of acute peritonitis with evidence of shock (with rising pulse), increasing rigidity and tenderness maximal over the ruptured organ. There is usually a clear history of abdominal injury. Shoulder pain may arise if the patient is prone for long. *High risk activities* are driving, certain sports (rugger, boxing, etc.) drunken brawls, engineering jobs, etc.

Rupture of kidney

Following injury, is usually associated with haematuria. If the haematuria is slight or clearly decreasing, the patient can occasionally be observed at home.

Ruptured urethra

Follows perineal trauma and if complete is associated with acute retention of urine.

MISLEADING FEATURES AND PITFALLS

The extent of the original injury is not realised. This mistake usually occurs with children and drunks.

MANAGEMENT OPTIONS

Immediate surgical referral of all suspected cases.

LACERATIONS

Classification: ICHPPC 889 (RCGP 5170)

The majority are trivial, some require stitches, most are situated on hands, feet or head. Antibacterial and antitetanus precautions must be considered.

DIAGNOSTIC RANGE (rates per 1000 patients per year)

Personal: All reported lacerations 17.0+.

GRAZES AND SUPERFICIAL INJURIES

Classification: ICHPPC 918 (RCGP 5195)

Trivial accidents and dog bites are the usual causes. Many are treated without reporting to the doctor.

DIAGNOSTIC RANGE (rates per 1000 patients per year)
Personal: All reported cases 15.2+.

RUPTURED TENDONS AND MUSCLES

Rupture of tendons or superficial muscle fibres are occasionally encountered. History of trauma is not always given but the lump of muscle fibres that shows up with contraction is characteristic. Immediate surgical referral indicated in most instances.

BRUISES

Classification: ICHPPC 929 (RCGP 5200)

DIAGNOSTIC RANGE (rates per 1000 cases)
Personal: Reported cases 24.0+. Most bruises are not reported.

Note: Bruises are sometimes reported under a 'cover story', this may indicate cases of non-accidental injury (p. 675 *et seq.*) and family violence. The doctor's background knowledge of the appropriate high risk factors may then be vital.

FOREIGN BODIES

Classification: IHCPPC 912–939 (RCGP 5210–5215)

Eye
5.7 per 1000 patients per year. Mostly adult males. Remove under local or refer.

Swallowed
1.0 per 1000 patients per year. Mostly children who have swallowed coins. X-ray and monitor or refer.

Nose
0.6 per 1000 patients per year. Mostly children.
Remove with loop.

Throat
0.7 per 1000 patients per year. Adults with impacted fish bones. Refer or monitor.

Ears
0.6 per 1000 patients per year. Remove with loop or refer.

Other
2.2 per 1000 patients per year.

INHALED FOREIGN BODIES

Intense and continuous coughing with associated cyanosis should always suggest the diagnosis. Top priority emergency admission.

Sudden chest compression by embrace from behind should be considered immediately as an emergency measure.

BURNS

Classification: ICHPPC 949 (RCGP 5220)

DIAGNOSTIC RANGE (rates per 1000 patients per year)
Personal: Reported burns 5.2+.

AGE INCIDENCE
Half the patients are children.

CLINICAL POINTERS

1. High risk factors: (a) toddlers; (b) fires without guards; (c) table cloths; (d) polystyrene foam furniture and sound proofing; (e) kettles and tea pots; (f) flexes of irons and kettles; (g) electric points; (h) smoking households; (i) work.
2. The burn. Flame burns are usually deeper and more destructive than scalds of similar size and appearance.
3. Shock. May need parenteral fluid if area affected is large.

COMPLICATIONS

1. Sepsis.
2. Behaviour problems in young children following admission to hospital or frequent dressings.
3. Contractures.

MANAGEMENT OPTIONS

Prevention: Education re safety at work, in public places and especially safety in the home. The doctor must be prepared to talk to patients (and parents) about the dangers of the high risk factors.

Established burn: Many children with scalds can be kept at home with systemic antibiotics and sofra-tulle dressings at 2 to 4 day intervals and only referred if a larger area of skin is affected or if healing has not occurred after 10 to 20 days.

NON-ACCIDENTAL INJURY

1. Non-accidental Injury (NAI) in Babies (the 'battered baby') and Child Abuse Syndrome

The frequency of NAI is uncertain and probably varies with the deprivation of the community involved. The child abuse syndromes of all kinds follow parental bonding failures. These may have disintegrated or never developed following separation after birth. The family doctor's index of suspicion must always be high.

AGE INCIDENCE

Most NAI cases are under 1 year. An age when physical injury from accidents is not common. Other more subtle forms of deprivation and 'mental battering' may occur in older age groups.

CLINICAL POINTERS

1. High risk factors: (a) socio-economic deprivation; (b) one or both parents are subjected to prolonged stress, i.e. alcoholism, unemployment, mental illness, poverty, violence, etc.; (c) more than one child in the family; (d) mental defect in baby; (e) baby known to be 'unwanted'; (f) previous possible NAI; (g) parental separation causing bonding failures.
2. Excessive crying or evidence of malnutrition in the baby. May be a result or a cause.
3. Inconsistency between parents' story of injury and nature or extent of injuries in baby.
4. Inconsistencies of story given by different witnesses, siblings, neighbours, relatives, friends or another parent.
5. If the above inconsistencies are to be demonstrated all statements and findings should be carefully recorded at the time.

INVESTIGATIONS

Admission of the baby to hospital provides: (a) another opinion; (b) removes the strain on the family; (c) makes a covert situation more overt without threatening any of the participants; (d) prevents further battering temporarily.

COMPLICATIONS

Repetition is not uncommon. Injuries may be of any type or degree of severity. Death occasionally.

MISLEADING FEATURES AND PITFALLS

1. Details of history or findings are inadequately recorded.

2. The family doctor's natural empathy for all parents' problems may blind the doctor to NAI which later becomes obvious.

3. The family doctor's high index of suspicion and subsequent questions and actions threaten a guilty parent (or parents). All trusting communication then ceases or the parents change their doctor.

4. Every patients' natural guilt whenever one of their children is injured may make them distort or minimise the history. The doctor unjustly suspects that NAI has occurred, when it has not.

MANAGEMENT OPTIONS

Prevention: support of those in high risk categories by relatives, friends and social services. The family doctor's role may be crucial here because support is given when it is needed and potentially violent situations are rendered overt in a non-threatening way.

Suspected cases: (a) involve others in a way that is non-threatening i.e. hospital, grandparents, neighbours, friends, health visitor — a doctor's cover story is usually needed; (b) 'pool' knowledge in confidence with other professionals; (c) take steps to gain more information using a non-threatening 'cover' approach; (d) discuss the problem with NSPCC (Ref. 26.1 or 0.6) — it may be helpful to all concerned if names are not given initially; (e) avoid value judgements which depend on your own observations only; (f) keep detailed records under confidential cover.

Probable cases: inform NSPCC, Social Work department or Local Authority

2. Battered Wives

Injuries can be severe, in such cases there is rarely doubt about the husband's part. With lesser injuries wives may be more diffident and report the injury but not the husband's role. The family doctor should have a high index of suspicion because the diagnosis once suspected can usually be confirmed by tactful direct questioning of the wife.

MANAGEMENT OPTIONS

Prevention: usually involves persuading a wife to take action.

Established cases: refer to: (a) Samaritans; (b) 'Battered wives' home or group (address is usually confidential so that husbands cannot discover it); (c) legal opinion; (d) Citizens' Advice Bureau may be helpful; (e) social worker and health visitors very helpful.

3. The Battered Elderly or Infirm

Frequency uncertain. A high index of suspicion may be needed. Once suspected the problem is best referred to the local geriatrician.

DEATH — ICHPPC 7889 (RCGP 8450–8480)

The diagnosis of death is rarely difficult, although in some instances it may be impossible to give the exact causes.

If there is any doubt about the cause of death, the doctor should inform the appropriate legal authorities. See check list below.

Handling the emotional and physical reactions of patients, and their relatives, to impending death and death itself is a complex subject that is dealt with on pages 92 and 207.

Check list of actions in cases of sudden death

1. See the body in all cases
2. Check the following:

— Pulse, heart, breathing and lungs.
— Optic fundi for palisading.
— Note the approximate body temperature.
— Inspect the body (and clothes) for trauma, bruising, etc.
— Note if rigor mortis is present.
— Note any unusual or odd circumstances.

3. Record the best history possible of the terminal events and if not in records, any previous serious disease and hospital admission.
4. Check all tablets and drugs available.
5. Record at the time all positive and negative facts and findings.
6. Check with your local hospital, the coroner or his legal equivalent on the exact criteria for reporting sudden death. These criteria vary in different countries and are for instance different in Scotland

and England. Check also about: (1) cremation; (b) when to sign a death certificate; (c) what to do if you are not certain of the cause of death.

7. Do not assume that absence of trauma means a 'natural' death. Industrial causes, recent operations, accidents and poisoning may all raise special questions.

8. Remember that undertakers and 'funeral directors' can help both you and the relatives in many ways.

Appendix I

Diagnostic services and tests; desirable weights; growth rates

APPENDIX I A
USE OF HOSPITAL DIAGNOSTIC SERVICES

The practitioner should arrange to see the doctor in charge of each service personally.

The following check lists indicate subjects to be discussed:

A. THE HAEMATOLOGY, BIOCHEMISTRY AND PATHOLOGY LABORATORIES

— those tests which the laboratory will perform at the request of the primary physician.
— the nature of the container required and where these are obtained.
— appropriate labelling and forms required by the laboratory.
— the quantity of material required by the laboratory.
— the extent of clinical details required on the form.
— the method of transport to the laboratory.
— delays and difficulties which may render the specimen unsuitable for analysis.
— the ranges of values considered 'normal' by the laboratory.
— special arrangements for cytology, cervical smears and biopsies.
— other steps which may assist the department.

B. THE BACTERIOLOGY AND VIROLOGY LABORATORIES

As for A above but the family doctor should ask specially about:

— special media, etc., required for different organisms, i.e. pertussis, gonococcus, different viruses, amoebae, tricho-

monas, threadworm ova, skin specimens and smears, (blood and cervical).
— special methods and amounts required for different types of specimen, i.e. blood culture, faeces, sputum, urine, etc.
— delays or other local conditions which may cause death of organisms.
— storage of specimen if transport is not immediately available and whether the specimen can be refrigerated.
— recent techniques for rapid identification of viruses.
— other steps which may assist the laboratory.

C. THE RADIOLOGY DEPARTMENT

— X-ray procedures available to the primary physician.
— appointments procedures for: (a) routine; (b) urgent X-rays.
— special preparation of patients that may be needed, e.g. an aperient the night before.
— local procedures for radiology in undiagnosed potentially pregnant women, i.e. in the pre-ovulation period.
— information required (if any) about previous X-rays, i.e. about dates or identifying numbers.
— those areas of diagnostic radiology that the radiologist considers to be used inappropriately by family doctors.
— other radiological techniques available, i.e. scans, etc.
— other steps which may assist the department.

D. OTHER SPECIAL SERVICES AND CLINICS

These may include Ultrasound, EMI Scans, CAT Scans, Amniocentesis (chromosome analysis), myometry, venography, arteriography, gastroscopy, laparoscopy, etc.

In all cases the family physician starting work in an area is wise to see and discuss the correct use of the facility with the doctor in charge.

APPENDIX I B
DIAGNOSTIC TESTS CARRIED OUT IN CLINIC OR AT PRIMARY CONSULTATION

Where the result of a test is required quickly primary physicians often learn to perform tests themselves:

A. ERYTHROCYTE SEDIMENTATION RATE (ESR)

Equipment

Westergren or Wintrobe tubes are cheap, staff can be taught how to set up and read the ESR.

Interpretation

The normal range is skewed according to age and the reader is referred to Ref. 30.1. This work has validated a simple rule for estimating the maximum ESR considered normal for a given age:

Men: Maximum Normal ESR = Age in years ÷ 2
Women: Maximum Normal ESR = (Age in years + 10) ÷ 2

B. PEAK FLOW METER

A Peak Flow Meter is essential for any doctor interested in asthma or obstructive lung disease in either adults or children. It can be used for diagnosis, monitoring or even home monitoring.

Equipment

A Wright Peak Flow meter obtainable from any medical instrument supplier; or Mini Wright Peak Flow Meter which is cheaper and smaller, obtainable from Clement Clarke International Ltd., 15 Wigmore Street, London, W1H 9LA.

Interpretation

The PEFR (Peak Expiratory Flow Rate) is given by the best of three 'blows' and correlates well with the FEV (Forced expiratory volume).

Normal range

Males 450–700 litres
Females 300–500 litres

Diagnostic

If PEFR is increased by 20 per cent after bronchodilators, reversible obstructive lung disease is present and the patient should benefit from bronchodilator therapy.

Monitoring

An adequately treated asthmatic should have a PEFR within the normal range (Ref. 0.5).

(A simple chart relating the normal range of PEFR to a child's height is illustrated in Update, 1st October 1983, p. 905.)

C. ELECTROCARDIOGRAPH

Although expensive an electrocardiograph can provide crucial information to the primary physician. Staff can be taught to set the leads up, but reading the resultant tracing requires constant practise. Many doctors acquire the skill only to lose it as a result of too little experience. If there is a good cardiographic service in your area it may be cheaper and more effective to use this. Another alternative is for one doctor in a group to acquire and then maintain the necessary expertise by reading all cardiographs taken by the group.

D. SIGMOIDOSCOPY

The technique of passing and using a sigmoidoscope is easy to learn and the equipment is within the means of most practitioners. Two disadvantages are largely responsible for its low usage in primary care:

1. In many patients it must be followed by referral for a Barium Enema.
2. Constant practise is required to maintain the user's diagnostic expertise.

E. BACTERIAL CULTURES FOR URINE, ETC., INCUBATED BY PRIMARY PHYSICIANS BEFORE DELIVERY TO LABORATORY

This allows specimens to be collected overnight or at weekends. Several techniques are available which should be discussed with the local bacteriologist.

F. TESTS FOR PREGNANCY

10 days after first missed period (for next 3 months).

APPENDIX I C
DESIRABLE WEIGHTS FOR MEN AND WOMEN

An up to date chart of desirable weights, related to height and build is essential. Several alternatives are available:

— A wall chart obtainable from Medical Instrument Suppliers.
— Tables are provided by Metropolitan Life Insurance Company, New York.
— Tables are also included in many reference books (Refs. 0.4, 0.5).
— Centile charts can be used. One for each individual patient. Obtainable Creasey's Bull, Hertford, England. In Canada and USA from Mead Johnson Laboratories, Belleville, Ontario or Dept. Maternal and Child Health, Harvard School Public Health, Boston, Mass.

APPENDIX I D
GROWTH RATES FOR CHILDREN (REF. 4.1)

Serial measurement is essential to demonstrate failures. Centile charts should be used for each individual patient wherever possible (See Fig. 56).

These charts should be discussed with your local paediatrician and neonatal physician from whom copies can be obtained and then ordered.

Charts should include:

— Head circumference of babies
— Weight and length of babies
— Height and weight centile charts for Boys and Girls.

Other charts and cards:

— Denver Developmental Screening Test Charts. (Obtainable from your local paediatrician or Wm. Frankenburg, M.D. Univ. Colorado, Medical Centre, 4200 East Ninth Avenue, Box C233, Denver, Colorado 80220)
— APGAR Score Card. Obtainable from your local obstetric unit.

A simple list of milestones with an account of child development suitable for parents is given in Ref. 0.3, also Ref. 4.2 and Fig. 57.

National Health Service Number

PAEDIATRIC DEVELOPMENT SHEET

Surname (Block Letters)

Forenames (Block Letters)

Address

Date of Birth

SIGNIFICANT FAMILY HISTORY:

♂ ♀

Sibling name & year of birth ☐ ☐ ☐ ☐

PRENATAL HISTORY:

AT RISK FACTORS such as: Diabetes Toxaemia Jaundice

CONFINEMENT:

BREAST FEEDING Nil ☐ 2/12 ☐ 2-4/12 ☐ 4/12+ ☐

Solids Started Wks.

NEONATAL EXAMINATION

Weight Kg

Skin..........

Spine..........

Hips..........

Feet..........

Digits..........

Skull..........

Palate..........

Ears..........

C/V/S (Femoral pulses)..........

Eyes..........

Tongue..........

Chest..........

Abdo. & Genitalia..........

Hernia..........

Moro Reflex..........

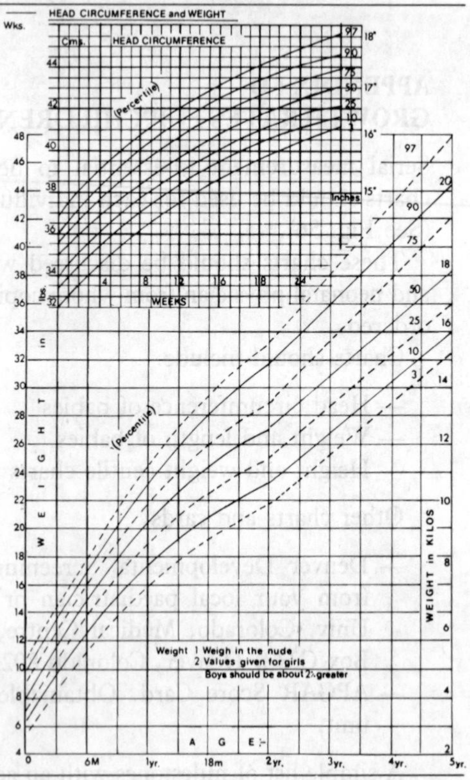

HEAD CIRCUMFERENCE and WEIGHT

Cms. HEAD CIRCUMFERENCE

(Percentile)

97 90 75 50 25 10 3

18" 17" 16" 15" Inches

44 42 40 38 36 34 32

4 8 12 16 18 24 WEEKS

lbs. 48 46 44 42 40 38 36 34 32 30 28 26 24 22 20 18 16 14 12 10 8 6 4

WEIGHT in lbs.

(Percentile)

97 90 75 50 25 10 3

WEIGHT in KILOS 20 18 16 14 12 10 8 6 4 2

Weight 1 Weigh in the nude
2 Values given for girls
Boys should be about 2% greater

AGE:-

0 6M 1yr. 18m 2yr. 3yr. 4yr. 5yr.

Form FP111 K

Fig. 56

DEVELOPMENT CHART

1. Mark "X" for items which child performs.
2. Mark "O" for items which child could not perform.
3. It is suggested that test ages marked ☐ are carried out by the doctor.
4. Record mother's observations and reactions under "Observations".

	TEST Actual Age	6/52	3/12	6/12	9/12	12/12	18/12	2 yrs	4 yrs	Observations	Immunisations
6 weeks	Lifted prone, momentarily holds head in line with body										
	Pull to sit. Head lag partly controlled										
	Hands closed									PKU	
	Grasp reflex +									Hips	
	Smiles									Physical Examination	
	Follows objects side to midline										
3 months	Lifted prone, holds head up										
	Lying prone, lifts head 45–90°										
	Pull to sit – only slight head lag										
	Holds rattle momentarily										
	Supine, watches own hands										
	Follows objects from side to side									Hips	
	Squeals of pleasure										
6 months	Lying prone, back is extended and weight on hands (not arms)										
	Rolls prone to supine										
	Sits up with hands forward for support										
	Weight bearing on legs										
	Transfers cube from one hand to another										
	Reaches out for objects										
	Alert: responds to examiner and mother										
	Smiles and laughs										
	Syllables ba, da, ka										
9 months	Sits steadily										
	Stands up, holding on										
	Creeps on hands and knees										
	Crude thumb-finger grasp										
	Waves "bye-bye"										
	Knows own name										
	Hearing responses at 46cm (18") (Lt. and Rt.) such as rattle, cup and spoon									Hips Squint Examination of Testicles Physical Examination	
12 months	Pivots stably while sitting										
	Walks – one hand held										
	Fine pincer grasp – finger/thumb										
	Plays "Peep-bo"										
	Responds to simple commands										
	Uses 2-3 words with meaning										
18 months	Throws ball without falling										
	Walks upstairs, one hand held										
	Builds 3-4 cubes										
	Feeds without rotating spoon										
	Dry by night mostly										
	Understands simple orders										
	Several intelligible words										
2 years	Kicks ball without overbalancing										
	Walks backwards in imitation										
	Unscrews lids, turns door knobs										
	Builds 6-8 cubes										
	Can put on shoes and socks										
	Asks for food, drink, toilet										
	Joins 2 or 3 words in sentences										
	Hearing responses at 122 cm (4 feet) (Lt. and Rt.)									Hips Squint Physical Examination	
4 years	Hops on one foot									Physical Examination and Pre-school Assessment	
	Can button clothes fully										
	Attends to own toilet needs										
	Imaginative play										
	Tells stories										
	Counts up to ten										
	Questioning at its height										
	Hearing responses at 122 cm (4 feet) (Lt. and Rt.)										

F7024 Gp 3643 Dd 421387 70M 1/76 Swift Ptrs.

Fig. 57

Appendix II

The age/sex register

An accurate Age/Sex register of all patients at risk in any practice, is only possible in countries, such as Britain, where patients register with a primary physician *before* they are eligible for care.

In other countries accurate denominators for patients at risk are difficult to obtain. Sometimes in these countries it is possible to obtain denominator figures in isolated or small communities where a single doctor or group of doctors cares for the whole community. In urban communities where patients choose their family doctor on a more random basis when they feel ill, family physicians are forced to use the less satisfactory method described in the last section of this Appendix (p. 689).

MAKING A REGISTER IN THE NHS

Any card index or foolscap sized loose-leaf method can be adapted for the purpose. Squared sheets are particularly suitable because of the ease of tabulation, but some practitioners prefer overlapping loose-leaf pages with a visible index. Both these methods are probably quicker in use than a card-index file.

1. Two separate pages are used for each year, and the appropriate year is boldly entered in the top right-hand corner or on the visible tag. One of the pages relates to males and the other to females and one of them should bear a distinctive mark for easy recognition — for example, a flash of red ink across the right-hand top corner.

2. Lines are ruled vertically to provide columns for: (a) patient's full name; (b) day and month of birth; (c) date of entry into the practice; and (d) date of departure from it. Some doctors like to have additional columns for address, NHS number, etc.

3. The medical record envelopes are then worked through in sequence, and entries of the details of patients for whom the date of birth is shown are made in the appropriate birth-year pages.

Your local NHS practitioner committee may be prepared to help or provide funds for this.

4. When the year of birth is not recorded on the envelope and cannot be ascertained from consultant's letters inside, the envelope is 'flagged' with a strip of card long enough to protrude conspicuously and so to bring the omission to mind.

5. A list is compiled of the names, last addresses, and NHS numbers of patients whose dates of birth are missing. A copy of this list is sent to your local practitioner committee with a request for as many as possible of the missing dates. The list also is kept in the consulting room or the office in a place such that the practitioner and the receptionist will be reminded to collect the missing dates of birth when patients are seen. A habit should be developed of checking the dates of birth of all patients who attend, because in this way mistakes on the medical record envelopes are detected.

6. Some patients leave the district or change their addresses without notifying the practitioner committee or the general practitioner. If there is no way of tracing them, a list of their names, males and females separately, is kept at the end of the register, and where possible the decade in which they were probably born is indicated. Whenever a census is taken the number of those persons allocated to each decade and the size of the residue for whom no reasonable guess can be made is shown.

MAINTAINING THE REGISTER

1. A secretary should be trained to do this. A specific time every week or month is set aside for bringing the register up to date; new entries are checked, withdrawals are recorded, and the medical records which have been recalled by the local practitioner committee are dispatched.

2. When a new patient registers with the practice the details are immediately entered into the register. The practitioner and the receptionist should develop the habit of obtaining the dates of birth of all new patients.

3. Where several premises are involved, registers are kept at each and the main register is constructed from these.

4. The dates of birth are now usually shown on the medical cards.

5. Withdrawals are indicated by lightly scoring a line through the name of the patient and the dates of birth and entry into the practice, and entering the date of withdrawal in the *Out' column*.

6. Deaths are recorded by entering 'D' alongside the date of death in the 'Out' column. The register can be used similarly to record other events of interest to the doctor, but these should not be too many.

EXTRACTING THE CENSUS

1. A census should be taken at least once a year, on a specific date such as January 1.

Once the register has been amended the census will be the only record of the age/sex structure and available for that particular year.

2. A foolscap sheet is ruled for the following columns: age in years (0, 1, 2, 3, 4, etc.); years of birth (1958, 1957, 1956, etc.); annual number of males; annual number of females; and annual total. Subsequent columns may be used for the doctor's particular requirements — for example, 5-year totals and 10-year totals. (We usually use 5-year totals for adults, this fits the two important milestones — 15 and 65 years — at the beginning and end of adult working life.

A note is made of the number in each decade whose dates of birth are unknown, and of the number of the residue for whom no guess can reasonably be made.

SOME USES OF THE REGISTER

The register can be used to obtain information for many purposes. It is often of interest to compare data from a number of different practices, and, for this, age/sex breakdowns are essential.

Within a single practice it is sometimes desirable to compare the incidence of disease in different age-groups, or, in the same age-group, to compare the two sexes (as has been done throughout Part II of this book). For this a register is essential.

In many investigations it is important to select controls matched with cases for age and sex. These may be obtained simply and in a random manner by the use of the register.

If a census is taken from the register and recorded at regular intervals, it is possible to work out the age incidence of diseases and epidemics several years after they have occurred. In this way the register can be used to provide retrospective information.

In partnership it often happens that one partner only is interested in research, or that the partners have different interests. If a register is maintained, a single member of a partnership can use it for detailed analysis of his own cases of the disease in which he is specially interested. At the same time, if his partners co-operate by recording their cases (without detail), he will have the figures to determine the attack rate in the practice as a whole.

Most preventive medicine involves the examination of population groups at special risk. Age and sex are important in defining such population groups. If a general practitioner wishes to discover which of his patients are in a particular age group — for instance, those in their first year at school — he can do so rapidly by reference to the register.

The occupation of the patient can also be recorded in the register. Unfortunately such information is difficult to obtain and update.

Suitable cards and advice on the use of an age/sex register can be obtained from the Records and Research Advisory Service of the Royal College of General Practitioners, 14 Princes Gate, London.

Recently several programmes have been developed for putting a practice register onto a micro-computer. Practitioners interested in this are wise to visit a practice in which such a programme has been installed and shown to be effective. (Ref. 30.2).

PRACTICES WITHOUT A DEFINED POPULATION

A simple method of obtaining age/sex breakdowns of your practice population is to put a coloured marker on every record. If every patient seen in 1981 has a piece of red scotch tape, every patient seen in 1982, blue, and 1983 yellow, then a census can easily be taken at any time of the practice population seen by the practice in any one year. Also, at the end of 1983 it is possible to remove patients from the active file who have not reported to the office for 1, 2 or 3 years.

As long as you are consistent in using this method, you can compare information from year to year and with other practices using the same method. You can also use this index to obtain controls matched for age and sex.

This register also allows the doctor to isolate high risk groups for screening and preventive purposes.

FAMILY AND HOUSEHOLD REGISTERS

Over long periods family composition changes and names and addresses alter. A family register becomes administratively essential and can also be used for much useful research. Details of such 'F books' can be obtained from Royal College of General Practitioners, 14 Princes Gate, London.

Appendix III

Equipment for primary care

Many excellent articles on this subject are available and the practitioner is wise to consult the literature.

Equipment may be bought or hired and the family doctor should consider the pros and cons of each method in relation to his particular circumstances preferably after discussion with other practitioners who have experience of both methods.

The following is useful check list:

Consulting room

Blinds and curtains.
Towels — cotton, hired or disposable.
Disposable covers for examination couches.
Carpets.
Floor tiles and subfloor finishes — linoleum, vinyl tiles, etc.
Lighting — fluorescent, Anglepoise, standard.
Doctor's desk — should not be too big or threatening to the patient.
Chairs — doctor's, patient's, staff's.
Examination couches — should allow vaginal examinations in lithotomy position. The ends of at least one couch should be clear of walls to allow 'traction' on both head and feet. It is useful to have a couch surrounded by a curtain in the consulting room as well as examination room.
Foot stool or 'step-up' for couch.
Wash basin and towels.
Weighing machines and height standard.
Cupboards — drug cupboards and safes.
Waste bins and waste-paper baskets.
Sound proofing of walls, doors and ceilings.
Wallcharts — normal weight, height, eye testing, etc.
Suitable, friendly pictures.

Examination room

Couch and step up as in consulting room.
Anglepoise, wall-mounted.
Sphygomanometer, wall-mounted.
Wall-mounted auriscope and opthalmoscope.
Wash basin and towels.
Waste bins.
Sound proofing (as above).
Chairs, Mirror, Pegs for hanging clothes.

Office equipment

Files for patients' notes — wood, metal, rotary, lateral or wall.
A4 Records
Other storage files — either hanging or drawer type.
Typists desks and chairs.
Typewriters.
Photocopying machines.
Duplicating equipment.
Adding machine and calculator.
Tape recorders.
Word processor and micro-computer.

Other office equipment

Stationery for appointments system and house calls, diagnostic register, age/sex register, family indentification file, journal storage, patients' records, flow sheets, developmental charts, laboratory and radiological request forms, etc.
Stamps, clips, staplers, treasury tags and small stationery.
Electric clocks.
Tea-making equipment, cooker and food storage.
Crockery for staff and old people's weekly social clinic.
Incinerator and equipment for washing doctor's cars.
Refrigerator.
Steriliser.

Telephones and communications

Telephone systems.
Private and internal extension for intercommunication between staff.

Patient call system.
Radio telephone, pager, etc.

Heating Systems

Gas, Oil, storage and fan heaters.

Standard diagnostic equipment

Stethoscope, auriscope, ophthalmoscope, laryngoscope.
Nasal and vaginal speculum, sigmoidoscope, etc.
Dividers
Disposable gloves.
Tuning forks, etc.
Thermometers.
ECG machine.
Peak flow meter.
Haemoglobinometer.
Centrifuge and urine testing equipment.
ESR tubes.
Specimen cartons and equipment for taking blood, etc.
Microscopes and lamps.
Equipment for estimating blood sugar.

Supplies of emergency drugs and dressings

Standard surgical instruments

Forceps, scalpels, Jobson Horne probes, etc.

Emergency bags

Medical, obstetric, therapeutic. Most doctors will want to work out their own needs which will vary according to the type and area of practice. A tentative list of contents for an urban doctor's bag is given in Ref. 30.3 while the emergency drugs and equipment required for an isolated practice in Canada or Australia is more extensive (Ref. 30.4).

Emergency equipment

Oxygen, defibrillator, glucose, airways, stomach tubes, catheters, intravenous infusions, respirators, etc.

Appendix IV

Practice activity analysis (PAA) and audit

Donebedian has pointed out that there are three levels of data analysis applicable to practice:

1. *The structural level*, i.e. physical data, about premises, equipment, numbers of staff, etc. Inquiry at a structural level would tell you that a doctor owned a cardiograph but not how often he used it or indeed if he knew how to.

Advantages: Such data is very easy to collect.

Disadvantages: Gives little or no information about standards or attitudes towards practice of those providing the data.

2. *The process level*, i.e. the number of patients seen by the staff, for how long, what advice is given, what action is taken. Inquiry at this level would tell you about work loads but not about the effects of the work performed.

Advantages: Such data is relatively easy to obtain. Provides many inferences about the knowledge, skills and attitudes of the doctors and staff providing the service.

Disadvantages: Gives no hard indications of the effects of the care given or of practice activity on the life and health of those attending.

3. *The outcome level*, i.e. the extent to which the activities of the doctor and practice are helping (or hindering) the patients who attend.

Advantages: Provides hard information about the result of the doctors' decisions and whether these are beneficial to patients or not. Extremely influential on doctors' actions.

Disadvantages: Very difficult to measure and obtain. Outcome measures are also extremely difficult to define. Thus we may successfully reduce a patient's blood pressure (? good outcome). If the patient then suffered a stroke due to thrombosis we might consider that our actions had produced an unsatisfactory outcome.

Analysis at outcome level is rarely achievable in primary care and we have to depend largely on the inferences and self criticism generated by monitoring and analysing our activities at process level. The following analysis of practice activity in my own practice indicates the type of data obtainable, some of the inferences about attitudes which can be made and provides a useful measure for comparison with other practices. For instance, our referral rates were twice as high as those for a practice in a city ten miles away. Were our high rates good or bad practice?. We could not answer this question but the comparative figures made us question, in the future, very carefully why? and whom? we referred.

The interested reader is advised to contact the Birmingham Research Unit (Ref. 30.5) for more recent information and advice.

The object of a Practice Activity Analysis (PAA) is to enable the family doctor to be self critical. It should attempt to achieve five aims:

1. Analyse the work of the practice in quantitative terms.
2. Compare these figures with those of other practices.
3. Attempt a retrospective objective assessment of the quality of service in relation to that provided by other practices.
4. Indicate means of improving the service provided by the practice. The analysis should consider:
   - The community that the practice serves and the demands made on the practice.
   - The deployment of the facilities available to meet these demands.
5. Make inferences wherever possible about outcomes and the ultimate standards of care provided.

A. The demands of the community cared for will depend on:

1. Size of practice. This is easily available and allows all rates to be related to the individual or fixed multiples, e.g. 100 or 1000 patients.
2. Age structure of practice. The under 10s and over 65s are more demanding and the proportion of a practice in these two groups should be given. The actual demands of the two groups, i.e. the average yearly *item of service rate* for individuals in each group, is a difficult figure to obtain.
3. Sex structure.
4. Patient-initiated items of service. Because this is out of the doctor's control it is an important item. The information is difficult to collect.
5. Social structure of practice. This may affect demand, i.e. patients from a higher social status might be expected to be more

demanding. Information difficult to collect. Sampling possible.

6. Morbidity as a guide to demand. Theoretically morbidity figures should give a good indication of demand. Thus scabies rates may be high in a young practice and CHF high in an old practice. Unfortunately the vagueness of many diagnoses renders such figures unreliable.

B. The deployment of the facilities available to meet the medical demands of the community will vary considerably for different practices in different areas. The practitioner should be able to monitor and assess some of the major variables in this field:

Number of doctors and items of service provided to each patient per year.

Number of receptionists and items of service provided to each patient per year.

Number of attached nursing staff and items of service provided.

Hours worked by different members of staff.

Appointment system and time spent by patients waiting.

Use of equipment.

Use of diagnostic and hospital services.

Prescribing and dispensing habits.

Use of welfare and other services for treatment and help.

Financial estimates, proportion of gross income spent on equipment, redecoration, telephones, etc.

Some of this information can be collected or sampled from the every day work of most practices.

I have listed below information that is available in this practice so that other practitioners can compare and contrast their own figures. Only in this way will general practitioners be in a position to assess their work objectively and accurately.

SECTION A

PROFILE OF COMMUNITY CARED FOR — DEMANDS MADE ON PRACTICE

PLACE

Redcar, Yorkshire.

TYPE OF COMMUNITY

Urban, dormitory, mainly housing estate.

INDUSTRIES

Heavy — chemical and steel.

GEOGRAPHY AND RELATION TO SURGERY

90 per cent patients live within radius of 1 mile of surgery.

SIZE AND AGE STRUCTURE OF PRACTICE

	1960	*1964*	*1968*	*1969*	*1971*
Total NHS patients	4024	6234	5545	5767	6634
Total private patients	0	0	0	0	0
% NHS patients under 10	19.7	20.6	19.7	21.2	
% NHS patients over 65	5.8	6.7	7.9	7.6	

NOTE. In 1965 one partner left the practice taking 2000 NHS patients.

SEX STRUCTURE OF PRACTICE

Similar to that elsewhere in Britain.

PATIENT-INITIATED ITEMS OF SERVICE

Estimated annual rate patient-initiated consultations per 1000 NHS patients — 1682.

Estimated annual rate patient-initiated house calls per 1000 NHS patients — 579.

(These estimates are based on a single 4 week sample taken in March 1966 and have altered since this time.)

SOCIAL STATUS

Not known accurately. A very small random sample suggests:

Class I	0%
Class II	12.0%
Class III	54%
Class IV	29.9%
Class V	4.1%

Percentage of families with cars — not known.

Percentage of families with telephones — not known.

MORBIDITY

	Rates per 1000 NHS patients per year	
	1969	*1971*
Total diagnoses	2382	2369
1. Communicable diseases	88.6 (3.7%)	65.0 (2.7%)
2. Neoplasms — benign and malignant	20.0 (0.8%)	15.2 (0.64%)
3. Allergic, endocrine and metabolic diseases	102.7 (4.3%)	109.0 (4.6%)

4. Diseases of blood	18.1 (0.76%)	24.5 (1.03%)
5. Mental and behavioural problems	349.3 (14.6%)	304.6 (12.8%)
6. Diseases of nervous system (incl. eyes and ears)	245.3 (10.3%)	167.7 (7.07%)
7. Diseases of circulatory system	110.4 (4.6%)	88.4 (3.7%)
8. Diseases of respiratory system	611.2 (25.6%)	530.0 (22.4%)
9. Diseases of digestive system	214.4 (9.0%)	210.4 (8.9%)
10. Diseases of genito-urinary system	104.5 (4.3%)	118.0 (5.0%)
11. Diseases of skin.	175.3 (7.4%)	181.4 (7.7%)
12. Diseases of locomotor system	135.1 (5.7%)	152.5 (6.4%)
13. Congenital malformations	4.0 (0.17%)	3.5 (0.15%)
14. Trauma etc.	145.7 (6.1%)	142.4 (6.0 %)
15. Pregnancy and complications	19.9 (0.83%)	23.2 (0.98%)
16. Other variable diagnoses	38 (1.4%)	232 (9.93%)
Total	2382 (100%)	2369 (100%)

COMMENTS ON SECTION A

1. The practice is increasing steadily in size; over the 10 years surveyed the annual rate of increase varies from 300 to 500.

2. The proportion of children under 10 has stayed the same.

3. There is a slow steady increase in the proportion of over 65s.

4. Total yearly workload, as would be expected from above, shows a steady increase over the years surveyed. This has been very slightly offset by a slight decrease in the yearly total of deliveries.

SECTION B

THE DEPLOYMENT OF MEDICAL FACILITIES AVAILABLE TO MEET THE MEDICAL DEMANDS OF THE COMMUNITY

	1960	*1964*	*1968*	*1969*	*1971*
Number of patients registered	4024	6234	5545	5767	6634

Number of doctors full-time	2	3	2	2	2
Number of receptionists (full-time)	2	3	2.75	2.5	3
Number of patients per doctor	2012	2078	2772	2883	3317
Number of patients per full-time receptionist	2012	2078	2016	2345	2211

WORK BY DOCTORS

	1960	*1964*	*1968*	*1969*	*1971*
Total items of service per year	20607	32286	21844	21368	25485
Total items of service per doctor per year	10303	10762	10922	10684	12742
Total items of service per patient per year	5.12	5.17	3.93	3.70	3.84
Consulting/visiting ratio	2.06	2.20	3.57	3.52	
Telephone consultation or advice per patient per year	N.R.	N.R.	N.R.	N.R.	N.R.
Repeat prescription without doctor contact per patient per year	N.R.	N.R.	N.R.	0.5	0.43
Maternity deliveries per 1000	22	20	18	15	14
Total number of deliveries year	90	120	100	90	92

DELEGATED WORK

Number of attached nursing staff (full-time)	0	0	1	1.5	2
Number of patients per full-time nurse	0	0	5545	3845	3317
Consultations by attached staff i.e. nurse, health visitor and midwife (rate per patient per annum)	0	0	0.12	0.19	0.23
Visits by nurses (rate per patient per annum)	0	0	0.26	0.24	0.22
Visits by health visitor . . .	N.R.	N.R.	N.R.	N.R.	N.R.
Visits by midwife . . .	N.R.	N.R.	N.R.	N.R.	N.R.

TIME SPENT ON DIFFERENT PRACTICE ACTIVITIES

	1960	*1964*	*1968*	*1969*	*1971*
Average consulting time per consultation	—	—	6.3 min	—	—
Average visiting time per visit	—	—	6.8 min	—	—
Travelling time hours per week	—	—	3⅔ hours	—	—
Administration hours per week	—	—	4½ hours	—	—
Total hours worked per week	—	—	40⅓ hours	—	—

(All these figures were based on a 14 day sample period in March 1968.)

VISITING (HOUSE CALL ANALYSIS)

For every 100 patient-initiated house calls:

28.2 per cent were revisited at home on a later date.
19.7 per cent were referred to surgery.
15.5 per cent were referred to nurse for a further visit.
2.8 per cent were admitted to hospital.
56.3 per cent were in bed when the doctor called.
7.0 per cent were fit enough (in the doctor's view) to have attended surgery.
26.8 per cent could have come to surgery if suitable transport had been available.
74.6 per cent asked for the call between 08.00–10.00 hours.
14.1 per cent asked for the call between 10.00–20.00 hours.
2.8 per cent asked for the call between 20.00–08.00 hours.
(All these figures were based on a 14 day period in March 1968.)

PRESCRIBING

	1960	*1964*	*1968*	*1969*	*1971*
Number of prescriptions per patient per month	0.338	0.348	0.359	0.325	0.325
Average no. of prescriptions per month per patient for doctors in rest of England	0.451	0.375	0.414	0.452	0.457

REFERRALS FOR SPECIALIST ADVICE OR HOSPITAL INVESTIGATION

	Rates per 1000 patients per year		
	1968	*1969*	*1971*
Investigation			
Chest X-ray	43.8	66.5	54.3
Other X-ray	45.2	48.8	72.2
Blood tests	154.1	171.8	160.0
Urine tests	102.2	138.4	155.0
Swabs and cervical smears	50.2	56.4	33.8
Stool culture	6.0	5.3	5.9
Specialist Advice			
Medical and chest	49.7	53.1	50.4
Surgical	82.6	75.0	89.9
Orthopaedic	27.2	29.9	34.4
Obstetrics and gynaecological	54.5	65.6	45.1
ENT and ophthalmological	45.6	39.8	37.2
Physical medicine	8.2	9.2	9.1
Neurosurgical and neurological	5.0	5.5	11.6
Dermatological	18.3	18.3	12.4
Psychiatric	20.0	16.7	20.3
Paediatrics	13.6	18.8	33.6
Plastic	6.7	6.2	4.6
Other	13.4	10.5	10.4
Total	850	795	842

PROPORTION OF GROSS INCOME SPENT ON EXPENSES (EXCLUDING CARS)

	1960	*1964*	*1968*	*1969*	*1971*
Per cent of income spent	25%	30%	25%	23%	25%

COMMENTS ON SECTION B

Many comments are possible. Despite incompleteness it is possible to build up a clear picture, of trends, organisational needs, and the way facilities have been deployed:

1. Total number of patients per doctor steadily increased over 10 years surveyed.

2. Total yearly items of service rendered by each doctor remained

fairly static and did not greatly increase over 1960 level.

3. The increased workload was dealt with by steadily reducing the items of service given to each patient. The yearly items of service were reduced by a total of 1.61 per patient in the 6 years since 1964. The PAA shows how this reduction was achieved:

Delegating visits to nurses	0.24
Delegating surgery consultations to nurses	0.19
Giving repeat prescriptions without seeing patients	0.50
Slight reduction (10 per year) in overall number of deliveries	0.02
Virtual elimination of measles by immunisation	0.04
Other factors	0.62
Total	1.61

The other factors included:

— cutting out 'unnecessary' repeat visits and consultations.

— Ministry of Health policy of discouraging use of doctor for trivia (accurate yearly figures for patient-initiated items of service would give valuable information here).

— greater use of telephone consultation.

4. Although the number of items of service performed by each doctor per year was almost static the consultation/visit ratio was steadily increased over the 10 years from 2.06 to 3.52. The time thus saved undoubtedly reduced the pressure on the doctors and allowed more research work and paramedical activities.

5. Quality of care:

• The number of prescriptions per patient per month remained unchanged throughout the 10 years surveyed. The extra load has not been countered by increased prescribing.

• The 'referral' rate was not increased. The doctors did not appear to be unloading any of the increased work-load on to the hospital.

• There were no great changes in the numbers of diagnoses made per 1000 patients.

• Time studies are insufficient to show how much (if any) of the time saved, by delegation and decreasing the overall number of visits, had been fed back to the patient in longer consultation times. Average consultation times would be of great value.

• There is no positive evidence that the doctors have done anything more than maintain their standards in the face of a steadily increasing workload.

Appendix V

Guidelines and role descriptions given to various members of the practice team

In any practice, whether single handed or larger group, it is helpful to define and describe the roles of the different personnel. This encourages each member to visualise their role and to see their contribution in practical terms. There is always a tendency, especially in small units, for all staff (including doctor) to avoid delegation in an attempt to do everything. This leads to inefficiency and friction between staff. Some flexibility and overlap are always essential, but clear guidelines and descriptions of roles are of great importance. The following are examples.

GUIDELINES LAID DOWN FOR THE MANAGEMENT OF STAFF IN A LARGER SEVEN-DOCTOR URBAN GROUP PRACTICE WITH 21 000 PATIENTS

Some of these outlines and job descriptions could be amalgamated in smaller practices but the principle of defining the basic work unit will be the same.

APPOINTMENT SECRETARIES

One full-time secretary is required to cope with the work-load of two doctors. Each secretary is given her own space at the appointments desk with the names and availability of her doctors.

DUTIES

1. Arrange appointment with enough discipline to make the system effective yet with enough flexibility to keep it human. The secretary is often under conflicting pressure from the patients to give immediate appointments and from the doctors to space them out.

2. When consulting sessions are fully booked, to arrange extra consulting units with the doctors.

3. When a doctor is absent, to get a special form completed by his remaining colleagues so that there are enough consulting units to meet the needs of his patients.

4. Make decisions on the urgency (or non-urgency) of patients' requests to see doctor or nurse.

5. Decide if a patient's needs can be met by the nurse and tactfully channel these needs to her.

6. Advise patients on simple action to be carried out until they can be seen by the doctor or nurse, thus making them feel that their need has been recognised and introducing the idea of the team approach.

7. Process the repeat prescriptions for patients on continuous treatment. This requires the secretary to monitor frequency of previous prescriptions. She will have to know each doctor's prescribing habits so that these can be followed out. A patient may have to be seen or she may be able to prevent an unnecessary doctor/patient contact. Micro computer programmes assist here.

8. Extract case notes from the files and place them in their correct order for the doctor.

9. Refiling of case notes may cause considerable difficulties because:

— mistakes cause chaos
— most staff dislike this boring job.

A simple way of dividing labour is to make one girl responsible for refiling in a particular section of the alphabet.

10. File hospital and other letters in case notes. These should be 'treasury tagged' or summarised in chronological order.

11. Tactful skill in telephone techniques and questioning to:

— ensure that correct, accurate information is fed to the right source of action, i.e. doctor, nurse, etc.
— ensure that the patient does not feel either rejected or thwarted; either effect will cause patients to distort subsequent vital clinical information.
— ensure that no truly 'urgent situation' is overlooked.

12. Guard against over-identification with doctors leading to:

— receptionist taking too much responsibility
— 'dragon at the gate' impersonal authoritarian image
— frustration and aggressive reactions in patients.

This may be a tendency with senior or long-established staff.

13. Guard against over-identification with the patients leading to
— receptionist taking too little responsibility
— sloppy, permissive, administration
— doctor annoyance and frustration.
This may be a tendency with young or freshly appointed staff because reception staff *initially* identify more with patients than they do with the doctors.

14. Listen to all that the patient tells them and to sift from this the vast amount of information that will be of value to the doctor or nurse who may be dealing with the patient.

15. Role — the member of the team who is mainly responsible for controlling the flow of patients and information to doctors and nurses.

THE CLERICAL ASSISTANT

DUTIES

1. Deals with all other telephone communication.
2. Records home visits for doctors and nurses in Day Book.
3. Deals exclusively with: (a) Health Service administration, procedures, e.g. fees for vaccinations, inoculations, temporary residents, maternity services, night visits, etc.; (b) patients joining and leaving doctors' lists; (c) changes of addresses of patients; (d) stocks of prescription pads.
4. Maintains age/sex register.
5. Maintains diagnostic register. Codes illness diagnosed by doctor from day/appointments book into register using international classification of disease. (NOTE: Receptionist in charge of each 'surgery' may be responsible for entering doctor's diagnoses against the patient's name in the day/appointments book.)
6. Maintains 'at risk' register.
7. Keeps practice statistics.
8. Colour codes clinical records.
9. Opens, trims and sorts incoming mail and ensures its distribution to clinical staff.
10. The clerical work involved in clinics.
11. Role — the member of the team largely responsible for the correct recording, monitoring and digestion of factual and written information within the practice.

ACCOUNTS CLERK

DUTIES

1. Paying staff salaries and all that this involves from income tax and stamps to reclaim under reimbursement scheme.
2. Reimbursement of rent and rates claims.
3. Paying accounts.
4. In charge of fees for work outside the Health Service, etc.
5. Keeping accounts in the form that is required by practice accountants.
6. Responsible for petty cash.
7. Role — member of team responsible for all the financial matters of the practice and its members.

MEDICAL SECRETARY

DUTIES

1. Types case notes from electronic notebooks carried by doctors and nurses re all actions taken on home visits, messages for partners, nursing colleagues and other agencies.
2. All hospital appointments, follow-up and other letters.
3. All other typing.
4. Role — the typist member of the team.

THE JUNIOR

DUTIES

1. Filing, other than case notes.
2. Mailing, messages.
3. Coffee making and washing up.
4. Tidying doctors' desks after consulting sessions and restocking with stationery.
5. Maintenance and restocking with syringes and specimen jars of doctors' and nurse's diagnostic and treatment trolleys.
6. Date-stamps and prescription pads.
7. Keeps waiting area tidy, replenishes magazines and health education leaflets, waters plants, feeds fish, etc.
8. Maintenance of practice stationery stocks.
9. Is on one-day release to commercial college.

10. Under supervision can be used effectively as a substitute during sickness and holidays.
11. A training position with a view to promotion.

PRACTICE MANAGER

1. Co-ordinating the activities of the team.
2. Relieving doctors of staff management and routine responsibilities for maintenance, etc.
3. Acts as focal point — necessary in all organisations — where doctors, nurses and staff can make suggestions or voice complaints over a cup of coffee and go away confident that action will be taken.
4. Any distressed, aggressive or disgruntled patients who arrive at the appointments area can be channelled to her office where difficulties can have undivided attention in a quiet atmosphere without embarrassment to either patient, staff or other people waiting.
5. When absences of doctors or staff extend over too long a period from holiday or sickness, arranges payment and details of locums.

Appendix VI

Homes and home background: examination routine

A doctor learns in his training, to search for relevant clinical facts and to carry out a systematic clinical examination. In the same way, a general practitioner must learn to look systematically for relevant social facts. The frequency of home visiting has rightly been reduced but will always be an important part of primary care. The following is a short guide to assessment of home factors.

Many problems presented to the doctor originate in the patient's community environment. A doctor must therefore be prepared with the patient's help to assess empathetically and objectively the origins of such problems.

Knowledge of a patient's home background, working conditions or school may be essential. In the case of the elderly and the disabled, it is especially important to be able to assess difficulties of daily living in the home.

PHYSICAL FACTORS

Physical factors are always less important than the emotional ones in a household. Nevertheless, in many households the obvious physical factors often give surprising insight into the emotional attitudes and problems of family.

1. *Approach and environs* — The doctor is usually aware of the cultural and social implications of each area that he visits. The number of trees, the repair and cleanliness of the roads give a good indication of the income and attitude of the community to this particular area. Rejected communities tend to have few trees, limited, ill-kept gardens, ill-repaired streets often with derelict toys or cars left in the street.

2. *Gateway and approach to the house itself* indicate the attitude of the householder to his community. A house with good outside state of repair, well kept garden but poor internal state of repair might be expected in someone to whom status in the community

was important. The reverse situation often occurs with young couples who will build a beautiful internal home and care little of the external appearances.

3. *Internal appearance*. Living rooms. Are they 'lived in' or just a base for a working couple to sit in? Are their children using them? Are the children allowed to be untidy? Is there a friendly welcoming atmosphere? All these are relevant questions.

Bedrooms may give a good indication of the extent to which the 'home' matters to the couple. This is the only room that the couple feels unlikely to be entered by anyone but themselves and it is essentially their most personal and private-room. The state of bedding and decoration indicate financial problems or those of self care.

Husbands and wives always have their own side of their bed. Each will always use this side if ill or being examined.

Observations about kitchens, bathrooms, and toilets may help the doctor to understand the problems of families with many different life styles.

4. *Material furnishings, decorations and floor coverings* all give a good indication of the TLC (tender loving care) that has been lavished on the household. Floor coverings are perhaps the most sensitive guide here, i.e. have the lowest priority when the family is in financial trouble.

5. *Ornaments and pictures* are of interest because they indicate when the household was put together.

6. *The number of toys* and usage indicate the play and educational patterns of the children. These differ markedly and often give a good indication of the parent/child relationship. Expensive, complex toys indicate a less constructive attitude than crayons or bricks. A single dilapidated 'Teddy bear' beside a child's bed may have deep significance.

7. *Pets* — Dogs, cats, budgies, etc. may all indicate in their own way a householder's need for the give and take of affection.

A large Alsation in a household that is crowded with children may indicate the basic affectionate but feckless attitude that could not resist the tiny puppy but is unable to foresee the devastating effect of a large dog on a crowded household that is short of funds.

The doctor should understand the deep sadness that can follow the loss of a well loved pet.

8. *The general feel of a household*. Outward appearances can be misleading — a house that is too tidy or too clean, or the children

too quiet may indicate excessively authoritarian or even violent home situations.

The feckless household at first overwhelms the outsider with its noise, its untidiness or smell, yet the doctor rarely feels unwelcome.

Much that a doctor observes will give insight that could not be obtained by verbal means; nevertheless, the information is confidential and requires the same empathy and understanding as personal details of any patient's history.

9. *The disabled in the home*. Disabled people, especially the elderly, pose special problems at home. The doctor has a great deal to learn from both occupational and physiotherapists. He should take every opportunity to learn their special contribution:

— the daily living assessment
— the full range of personal 'aides', 'helping hands', tripods, dressing aids, cooking aids, etc.
— the full range of household facilities to increase mobility, hoists, ramps, handles, bath aids, lowered cookers, etc.

Finally he must always be prepared to examine the patient's activities in the home and watch their performance.

The discipline of observing and examining patients in their home may be of far greater relevance than many clinical observations.

IMPORTANT NOTE: **To cope efficiently with a large family, on a low income in a confined space or small house, requires a high level of intelligence and organising ability. This fact should never be forgotten when assessments are made.**

Appendix VII

Analysis of diagnoses — used by 10 family doctors over 4 years — according to frequency and management

This appendix isolates the 475 diagnostic entities used in this book. It aims to help teachers and administrators, interested in primary care, to identify the essential diagnostic vocabulary of current general practice and classify the main problems of the general practitioner according to frequency and management.

The 475 diagnostic labels were used by 10 general practitioners to make on average 2691 diagnoses per doctor per annum for every 1000 patients cared for. To understand fully the magnitude and intellectual scope of the skills involved it is necessary to analyse the doctors' diagnostic vocabulary in terms of five arbitrary subgroups of frequency or commonness (I, II, III, IV and V) and five subgroups of management A, B, C, D and E).

The definition and composition of each of these subgroups together with the teaching and administrative implications is described below and in Tables 36 and 37 (pp. 715–723).

ARRANGEMENT ACCORDING TO RANK ORDER OF FREQUENCY

Group I — Very common — five entities that are responsible for a third (33%) of the diagnoses considered by a G.P. A G.P. might expect to diagnose each of the entities in this group at least 200 times a year.

Group II — Common — 28 entities that are responsible for a further third (33%) of the diagnoses used by a G.P. A brief glance at the contents of this and the previous group reveals how incomplete is the preparation and teaching in the undergraduate and hospital years. A GP. might expect to diagnose each of the entities in this group 40 to 200 times every year.

Group III — Less common — 127 entities that are responsible for a further 29% of diagnoses and together with Groups

I and II (160 entities) are responsible for 95% of all diagnoses made by a G.P. This presents the grey area between primary and secondary care where specialist opinion and hospital based training are of greatest help to both patient and primary physician. A G.P. might expect to diagnose each of the entities in this group four to 40 times every year.

Group IV — Rare — 106 entities that are responsible for a further 4% of diagnoses. Together with the 209 entities in Group V, this group forms the basis of much hospital training. A G.P. would expect to diagnose each of this group less than four times a year.

Group V — Very rare — 209 entities that are responsible for only 1% of the G.P.'s work. A G.P. would expect to diagnose each of this group less than once a year.

SUBCLASSIFICATION ACCORDING TO MANAGEMENT AND DECISION MAKING

The 475 clinical entities (diagnoses) encountered in the primary care situation can be further classified, according to the problems and clinical decision making involved, into five subgroups A, B, C, D and E.

This further classification reflects the clinical contributions of the primary physician and, therefore, has significant administrative as well as Clinical implications:

Subgroup A (11.3% of all primary diagnoses — 33 different entities)

DEFINITION

Minor diseases (mainly short duration) with few problems of diagnosis or treatment e.g. colds, boils, dandruff, etc.

CLINICAL IMPLICATIONS

Many such conditions are never reported. Patients, pharmacists or nurses can safely deal with this group. A small number may need referral to a doctor.

ADMINISTRATIVE IMPLICATIONS

For highly trained doctors to deal with this group is a waste of resources. Para-medical staff with a basic training are perfectly competent to diagnose and treat.

CLINICAL COMPOSITION

(See Tables 36 and 37, pp. 715–723)

Subgroup B (72% of all primary diagnoses — 180 different disease entities)

DEFINITION

Relatively minor diseases that must be carefully watched for complications, recurrences or confusion with more serious disease e.g. migraine, varicose veins, globus, erythema nodosum, etc.

The size and character of this group has tremendous clinical, teaching and administrative implications.

CLINICAL AND TEACHING IMPLICATIONS

1. The majority of these conditions are rarely encountered in hospital. Adequate practical teaching requires considerable exposure to primary care practice outside hospital.
2. The ratio of trivial to serious may be up to 100 times that of the hospital population. The primary physician should not apply blindly, the costly and sometimes dangerous diagnostic and therapeutic methods of hospital to this mass of primary disease. He must develop many other clinical skills to deal with this problem cheaply and effectively.
3. Serious consequences may complicate inadequate primary care e.g. chronic suppurative otitis or glue ear may follow an inadequately treated acute otitis.
4. Complications, etc. in this group only occur in a small proportion of patients. Mistakes and inadequate handling by the primary physician are easily obscured by the less serious disease; primary care physicians need to be trained in the primary care situation to have a high degree of self criticism.
5. The nature and size of this group provide large and almost untapped opportunities for health education and preventive medicine of the most productive kind in the community (See Preventive Management Options throughout Part II.).
6. Presymptomatic screening techniques are still relatively crude. Early symptoms are likely to remain the most effective way of delineating high risk groups. Thus, it is by close watch on this group that early diagnosis of serious disease is most possible, e.g. early pulmonary TB, diabetes in the obese, behaviour problems in children, etc.

ADMINISTRATIVE IMPLICATIONS

1. The straight application of hospital methods of investigation and

treatment to this large primary group can absorb enormous quantities of patient and community resources.

2. Any physician performing primary care must be trained to develop methods that use time, clinical observation, and other means economically to diagnose and treat this large subgroup of diseases.
3. Physicians largely trained and working in hospitals can easily be unaware of both the effort required for, and the enormous potential of, good primary care.
4. A doctor working closely with one, two or three trained practice nurses may perform as effectively as the same number of doctors working on their own.

CLINICAL COMPOSITION

(See Tables 36 and 37, pp. 715–723)

Subgroup C (11.3% of all primary care problems — 144 different disease entities)

DEFINITION

Diseases in which early diagnosis and treatment are essential to prevent serious consequences. Examples: Anaemia, depression, appendicitis, etc.

These are the diseases the primary physician must know however infrequently they occur.

CLINICAL AND TEACHING IMPLICATIONS

1. The primary presentation is often different or less definite than in hospital; acute appendicitis, myxoedema and (pre-ruptive) tubal pregnancy are good examples of this.
2. Such conditions are not too common in primary care and effective teaching situations may be difficult to create even in a 2 year period of primary care training experience.

ADMINISTRATIVE IMPLICATIONS

1. A greater degree of health education in the community about these problems would undoubtedly help to achieve earlier diagnosis.
2. Early diagnosis frequently saves more extensive less costly treatment at a later date.

CLINICAL COMPOSITION

(See Tables 36 and 37, pp. 715–723)

Subgroup D (4.6% of all primary diagnosis — 73 different disease entities)

DEFINITION

Chronic or progressive diseases with major health implication. Treatment is often supportive, partial or otherwise incomplete, e.g. asthma, stroke, alcoholism, arthritis, etc.

The chronic and relatively unpreventable nature of this group of diseases has two main effects:

- early diagnosis is of lesser importance than management.
- despite the proportionately small numbers of patients affected, the number of patient/years in the community over which patients need help is considerable.

CLINICAL IMPLICATIONS

Although much essential treatment and supportive care for these patients is started in hospital, their main needs are for supportive services to enable them to live as near normally as possible in their own community. Thus, for a rheumatoid, good home aid or home help services may be more important over the years than a knee replacement operation.

ADMINISTRATIVE IMPLICATIONS

The concept of the community health team consisting of nurses, physio, occupational therapists, social workers, home helps, meals-on-wheels, holiday relief, laundry services, etc. will only work if doctors are prepared to be fully involved and delegate freely. Methods of payment of health personnel are vital here.

As the services of health professionals become increasingly expensive, there is a parallel need to ensure that wherever possible, the methods of payment encourage not discourage effective delegation to less well paid personnel.

CLINICAL COMPOSITION

(See Tables 36 and 37, pp. 715–723)

Subgroup E (0.8% of all primary diagnoses — 45 different disease entities)

DEFINITION

Life threatening diseases. Diagnosis is expected by both patient and medical profession to be as early as possible, e.g. carcinoma of all kinds, myocardial infarcts, dissecting aneurysm.

CLINICAL IMPLICATIONS

A brief glance at the contents of this group reveals the emotive and spectacular nature of these conditions. A great deal of medical teaching and effort are expended on this small and highly specialised group.

ADMINISTRATIVE IMPLICATIONS

In view of the small numbers of patients affected and the relatively poor return for time and effort spent — the teaching and community approach to this group requires much further study.

Clinical composition

(See Tables 36 and 37, pp. 715–723)

Table 36 Matrix showing distribution in each of the five frequency groups and five management subgroups of the average number of disease incidents encountered (2691) per 1000 patients per year.

	I	II	III	IV	V	Totals
A	72.5 (2.7%)	122.5 (4.6%)	101.0 (3.7%)	7.5 (0.3%)	1.2 (0.4%)	304.7 (11.3%)
B	814.2 (30.3%)	633.1 (23.6%)	431.8 (16.0%)	45.1 (1.7%)	11.4 (0.4%)	1935.6 (72.0%)
C		128.8 (4.8%)	140.0 (5.2%)	25.7 (1.0%)	9.7 (0.4%)	304.2 (11.3%)
D			106.0 (3.9%)	14.8 (0.5%)	4.9 (0.2%)	125.7 (4.6%)
E			4.5 (0.2%)	15.0 (0.5%)	1.3 (0.04%)	20.8 (0.8%)
Totals	886.7 (33%)	884.4 (33%)	783.3 (29%)	108.1 (4%)	28.5 (1.0%)	2691 (11%)
Total number of disease entities in each group	5	28	127	106	209	475

Over 4 years the sample of primary physicians whose clinical material has been analysed in this book, looked after approximately 20 000 patients and made on an average 2691 diagnoses per 1000 patients per year. To do this they utilised a total vocabulary of 475 different diagnostic labels.

TABLE 37

In the list that follows, frequencies are based on the diagnostic frequency rates provided throughout this book. An explanation of how these figures were obtained is given in the introduction. Where two ranges of diagnostic frequency have been given the upper level, i.e. frequency with which a diagnosis is suspected has been used. This slightly inflates the figures as a whole and increases slightly the apparent incidence of those diseases in which a high index of diagnostic suspicion is required.

Figures in brackets after each disease entity:
The first figure represents the overall ranking position of the entity in the total 475 diseases encountered, the second figure represents the frequency with which the entity was suspected per 1000 population per year.

Group I (Rank numbers 1–5 (incl.), 5 entities, responsible for 33% of all diagnoses made)

A. (*Minor diseases — few problems*) — 1 entity — Superficial injuries (5–72.5).

B. (*Relatively minor — but must be watched*) — 4 entities.
— Acute upper respiratory tract infections (1–496.4).

Coughs	133.0
Colds	120.1
Acute tonsillitis	162.7
Acute bronchitis	50.4
Acute tracheitis, etc.	30.2
	496.4

— Simplex anxiety and tension states (2–120.1).
— Contraceptive advice (3–120.0).
— Acute gastroenteritis (4–77.8).

Group II. (Rank numbers 6–33 (incl.), 28 entities, responsible for 33% of all diagnoses made)

A. (*Minor diseases — few problems*) — 5 entities: Chickenpox (14–33.0); Wax in ears (24–26.9); Boils, etc. (26–24.2); Acute gastritis (29–19.6); Styes (30–18.8).

B. (*Relatively minor diseases — must be watched*) — 18 entities. Acute otitis media (6–66.2); Rubella (7–60.0); Mumps (8–50.0); Acute G.U. tract infection (9–48.1); Pregnancy (10–38.2); Prolapsed lumbar I.V. disc (11–36.4); Fibrositis (12–36.2); Eczema (13–35.7); Osteoarthritis (all types) (15–32.6); Red eye (16–32.0);

Obesity (17–30.7); Drug and allergic rashes (19–29.7); Sprains (21–29.2); Sinusitis (max) (23–27.8); Papular urticaria (25–25.2); Scabies (31–18.5); Otitis externa (32–18.4); Influenza (proven) (33–18.2).

C. (*Early diagnosis and treatment of major importance*) — 5 entities. Hypochromic anaemia (18–30.0); Ulcer type dyspepsia (20–29.3); Aspiration pneumonitis (22–28.1); All fractures (27–21.4); Depression (28–20.0).

Group III (Rank numbers 34–160 (incl); 127 entities responsible for 29% of all diagnoses made)

Subgroup A. (*minor diseases — few problems*) — 16 entities. Virus warts (36–17.4); Eustachian catarrh (43–12.4); Dental caries (49–11.7); Blepharitis (58–10.6); Dandruff (76–6.6); Dental extraction (80–6.0); Nappy rash (88–5.7); Muscle cramps (93–5.0); Chilblains (101–4.7); Seb. cysts (102–4.7); Pruritus ani (105–4.5); Nasal polyps (122–3.0); Ingrowing toenails (137–2.4); Ganglion (139–2.3); Herpes stomatitis (145–2.1); Bunions (155–2.0).

Subgroup B. (*Relatively minor — must be watched*) — 64 entities. Insomnia (34–18.0); Acute cervical adenitis (35–17.5); Varicose veins (37–16.7); Migraine (38–16.0); Menopause (40–12.8); Maternal anxiety (41–12.6); Refractive errors (42–12.6); Dysfunctional uterine haemorrhage (45–12.1); Constipation (46–12.1); Tenosynovitis (48–11.9); Herpes simplex (50–11.5); Paronychia, etc (51–11.5); Functional gastritis (55–10.8); Foreign bodies (all sites) (56–10.8); Tonsils and Adenoids (57–10.7); Aphthous ulcer (59–10.5); Allergic rhinitis (64–9.4); Seborrhoeic eczema (66–9.1); Impetigo (67–9.0); Marriage problems (68–9.0); Acne (69–8.8); Acute wheezy bronchitis (70–8.6); Sinusitis (frontal) (72–7.1); Cervical erosion (73–6.9); Dental abscess (74–6.7); Prolapse (78–6.4); Synovitis (79–6.2); Ventral hernia (81–6.0); Tinea pedis (82–6.0); Internal derangement of knee (83–6.0); Faints (84–5.9); Epistaxis (85–5.8); Enuresis (88–5.7); Spasmodic dysmenorrhoea (86–5.7); Teething (89–5.6); Burns (all areas) (91–5.2); Scarlet fever (92–5.0); Congenital cold fingers (Raynaud's) (93–5.0); Psoriasis (95–5.0); Brachial neuralgia (96–5.0); Anal fissure (97–4.9); Herpes zoster (104–4.5); Sleeping problems in children (106–4.4); Giant urticaria (and angioneurotic oedema) (110–4.0); Hormonal amenorrhoea (114–3.5); Balanitis (116–3.1); Hay fever (118–3.1); Threadworms (Pin worms) (120–3.0); Malingering (121–3.0); Alopecia areata (124–3.0); Eating problems (126–2.9);

Tinea corporis (127–2.9); Gingivitis and pyorrhoea (132–2.5); Glossitis (133–2.5); Vaginitis (adult) (135–2.4); Phimosis (138–2.3); Monilia (thrush) vaginal (140–2.2); Tics, etc. (142–2.2); Neurofibromata (147–2.1); Hysterical aphonia, functional laryngitis, etc. (149–2.1); Hypostatic oedema (legs) (150–2.1); Monilia, oral (151–2.0); Pityriasis rosea (153–2.0); Flat-foot (158–1.9); Subconjunctival haemorrhage (160–1.8).

Subgroup C. (Early diagnosis and treatment of major importance) — 27 entities. Piles (39–14.9); Hysteria (44–12.2); Infective hepatitis (47–12.0); Chronic bronchitis (54–10.9); Acute appendicitis (60–10.4); Adult pulmonary tuberculosis (63–10.0); Diabetes mellitus (all types) (87–5.7), [Surveillance (87–4.0, Insulin sensitive (87–0.8), Obese type (87–0.9)]; Inguinal hernia (98–4.8); Chronic cholecystitis (99–4.8); Acute lobar pneumonia (100–4.7); Squint and ocular imbalance (108–4.3); Cataract (109–4.1); Concussion (111–4.0); Myxoedema (112–4.0); Chronic rheumatic heart disease (113–3.7); Reflux oesophagitis and hiatus hernia (115–3.3); Dry pleurisy (117–3.1); Female sterility (123–3.0); Pernicious anaemia (125–3.0); Chronic suppurative otitis media (129–2.8); Acute mesenteric adenitis (134–2.4); Renal calculi (146–2.1); Speech problems (148–2.1); Congenital malformation of circulatory system (154–2.0); Uterine fibroids (156–1.9); Ovulation syndrome (157–1.9); Glandular fever (159–1.9).

Subgroup D. (Chronic, progressive diseases — many problems) — 19 entities. Essential hypertension (52–11.3); Congestive heart failure (53–11.1); Simple asthma (61–10.3); Strokes, Cerebral haemorrhage, thrombosis, etc. (62–10.1); Rheumatoid arthritis (65–9.4); Angina pectoris (71–8.5); Chronic asthmatic bronchitis (COLD) (75–6.7); Duodenal ulcer (77–6.5); Deafness (90–5.2); Atrial fibrillation (107–4.3); Chronic alcoholism (119–3.0); Bronchiectasis (128–2.8); Emphysema (generalised chronic) (130–2.8); Paralysis agitans (131–2.7); Corns and callosities (136–2.4); Hypochondriasis (141–2.2); Gout (143–2.2); Obsessional neurosis (144–2.2); Intermittent claudication (152–2.0).

Subgroup E. (Life threatening diseases) — 1 entity. Myocardial infarct (103–4.5).

Group IV (Rank numbers 161–266 (incl), 106 entities comprising 3.9% of all diagnoses made)

Subgroup A. (Minor diseases — few problems) — 6 entities. Retroflexed uterus (161–1.8); Acne rosacea (169–1.6); Sweat rash

(170–1.6); Lipoma (179–1.5); Tarsal and meibomian cysts (180–1.5); Intertrigo (201–1.1).

Subgroup B. (*Relatively minor but must be watched* — 44 entities. Vulvovaginitis in children (162–1.8); Globus hystericus (171–1.6); Paroxysmal auricular tachycardia (172–1.6); Vitreous opacities (175–1.5); Metatarsalgia (176–1.5); Adenopharyngeal conjunctival virus infection (177–1.5); Prepatellar bursitis (181–1.5), Generalised bursitis (184–1.4); Tennis elbow (185–1.4); Clicking jaw (188–1.3); Quinsy (189–1.3); Angular stomatitis (190–1.3); Clicking rib (192–1.3); Ichthyosis (193–1.2); Tonsillar debris (196–1.2); Supraspinatus tendinitis (199–1.2); Habit cough (203–1.1); Pediculosis capitis (206–1.0); Premenstrual tension. (214–0.9); General alopecia (215–0.9); Whooping cough (217–0.9); Carpal tunnel syndrome (218–0.9); Inadequate personality (220–0.9); Extrasystoles (222–0.9); Salivary calculus (223–0.9); Umbilical hernia (224–0.9); Impotence (227–0.8); Bell's palsy (228–0.8); Deviated nasal spectrum (230–0.8); Hydrocele (232–0.8); Acute epididymo-orchitis (234–0.8); Tantrum (in children) (235–0.7); Sexual behavioural problems of childhood (236–0.7); Neurodermatitis (237–0.7); Sibling jealousy (244–0.6); Male infertility (248–0.6); Chronic omphalitis (250–0.6); Acute hip syndrome (251–0.6); Pigeon toes (253–0.6); Nail biting habit (257–0.5); Continual crying (children) (258–0.5); Frigidity (259–0.5); Frozen shoulder (265–0.5); Plantar fasciitis and calcaneal spur (266–0.5).

Subgroup C. (*Early diagnosis and treatment of major importance*) — 30 entities. Gastric ulcers (166–1.7); Diverticulosis and diverticulitis (174–1.6); Rodent ulcer (177–1.5); Benign hypertrophy of prostate (182–1.5); Haemoptysis (183–1.4); Spontaneous pneumothorax (191–1.3); Thyrotoxicosis (194–1.2); Osteochondritis (198–1.2); Febrile convulsions (202–1.1); Corneal ulceration (204–1.1); Down's (205–1.0); Impacted faeces (208–1.0); Small ovarian tumours (213–0.9); Osteitis deformans (215–0.9); Acute glaucoma (221–0.9); Roundworms (225–0.8); Manic depressive syndrome (226–0.8); Imbalance ocular muscles (229–0.8); Pleural effusion (231–0.8); Ischiorectal abscess (232–0.8); Twisted ovarian tumour (240–0.7); Peritoneal adhesions (247–0.6); Thyroid adenoma (243–0.6); Endometriosis (249–0.6); Acute osteomyelitis (252–0.6); Chronic pyelonephritis (254–0.5); Secretory otitis media (256–0.5); Trigeminal neuralgia (260–0.5); Femoral hernia (262–0.5); Incomplete descent of testes (263–0.5); Breast abscess (264–0.5).

Subgroup D. (*Chronic, progressive diseases — many problems*) — 12 entities. Cerebral arteriosclerosis (164–1.7); Prolapsed cervical I.V.

disc (165–1.7); Schizophrenia (167–1.7); Mental deficiency (168–1.7); Senile osteoporosis (205–1.0); Nonspecific urethritis (209–1.0); Arteriosclerotic gangrene (211–1.0); Ulcerative colitis (212–1.0); Achrondroplasia (235–0.8); Spastic colon (238–0.7); Disseminated sclerosis (241–0.7); Mucous Colitis (261–0.5).

Subgroup E. (*Life threatening diseases*) — 14 entities. Meningitis, encephalitis and cerebral abscess (163–1.8); Acute intestinal obstruction (173–1.6); Bronchogenic carcinoma (185–1.4); Attempted suicide (187–1.4); Pulmonary embolism and infarct (195–1.2); Carcinoma of colon (197–1.2); Carcinoma of breast (200–1.2); Cerebral tumour and space occupying lesion of skull (207–1.0); Tuberculous meningitis (210–1.0); Carcinoma of stomach (219–0.9); Carcinoma of rectum (242–0.6); Perforated peptic ulcer (245–0.6); Intussusception (246–0.6); Carcinoma uterine cervix (255–0.5).

Group V (Rank numbers 267–475 (incl); 209 entities, comprising 1% of all diagnoses made)

Subgroup A. (*Minor diseases — few problems*) — 5 entities. Chapped hands (267–0.4); Pediculosis pubis (288–0.3); Excoriation of skin (292–0.3); Brittle nails (341–0.2); Pediculosis corporis (453–0).

Subgroup B. (*Relatively minor — must be watched*) — 50 entities. Scarring alopecia (268–0.4); Incontinence of faeces and urine (271–0.4); Episcleritis (272–0.4); Pilonidal sinus and cyst (275–0.4); Mastitis of puberty in boys (278–0.4); Abscess of Bartholin's glands (279–0.4); Erythema nodosum (281–0.4); Knock knees (282–0.4); Hammer toes (283–0.4); Coccydynia (284–0.4); Olecranon bursitis (285–0.4); Breath holding attacks (295–0.3); Wandering (297–0.3); Stealing (298–0.3); Pseudocyesis (299–0.3); Virus pneumonia (304–0.3); Q fever (305–0.3); Blocked lachrymal duct (306–0.3); Prolapse of rectum (308–0.3); Ringworm of nails (312–0.3); Dermatitis herpetiformis (313–0.3); Lichen planus (314–0.3); Erythema serpens (315–0.3); Granuloma annulare (316–0.3); Semimembranosus bursitis (317–0.3); Dupuytren's contracture (318–0.3); Thumbsucking (323–0.2); Rocking and head banging (in sleep) (324–0.2); Paraphimosis (332–0.2); Papilloma of urinary tract (334–0.2); Ringworm of scalp (336–0.2); Erythema multiforme (337–0.2); Onychogryphosis (340–0.2); Granuloma pyogenicum (342–0.2); Mallet finger (343–0.2); Primary amenorrhea (351–0.1); Spina bifida occulta (352–0.1); Cleft palate and harelip (355–0.1); Epidemic vertigo (361–0.1);

Molluscum contagiosum (368–0.1); Traumatic osteitis of patella (370–0.1); Urethral caruncle (393–.05); Torn ligament of knee (399–.05); Acute infective polyneuritis (405–.025); Epidemic hiccup (406–.025); Orf (436–.025); Baker's cyst (439–.025); Roseola infantum (452–0); Epidemic winter vomiting (474–0); Herpangina infection (475–0);

Subgroup C. (*Early diagnosis and treatment of major importance*) — 82 entities. Acute gonorrhoea (269–0.4); Paranoia (270–0.4); Acute iritis (273–0.4); Acute pulmonary oedema (274–0.4); Acute nephritis (276–0.4); Ectopic pregnancy (280–0.4); Congenital pyloric stenosis (287–0.4); Brucellosis (289–0.3); Erysipelas (290–0.3); Diphtheria (290–0.3); Cretinism (294–0.3); Subarachnoid haemorrhage (302–0.3); Hydronephrosis (310–0.3); Acute salpingitis (311–0.3); Postural deformities of spine (319–0.3); Dislocation of joints (excluding shoulder) (320–0.3); Chorea (321–0.3); Tapeworm (322–0.2); Cerebral emboli (327–0.2); Retinal detachment (328–0.2); Chronic glaucoma (329–0.2); Acute mastoiditis (330–0.2); Acute haemorrhage pancreatitis (331–0.2); Haemolytic disease of the newborn (347–0.2); Dislocation of shoulder (348–0.2); Latent syphilis (349–0.1); Vascular accidents in the eye (350–0.1); Congenital dislocation of hip (354–0.1); Haemorrhagic disease of newborn (356–0.1); Cardiovascular syphilis (357–0.1); Uraemia (358–0.1); Acute retention of urine (359–0.1); Secondary T. B., bones and joints (360–0.1); Toxoplasmosis (362–.07); Staphylococcal and haemophilus pneumonia (363–.07); Carpo-pedal spasm (364–.07); Urethral stricture (367–.07); Anarthritic rheumatism of elderly (369–.05); T.B. of urinogenital tract (371–.05); Lupus vulgaris (372–.05); Tabes dorsalis (373–.05); Typhoid and para-typhoid (374–.05); Malaria (376–.05); Simmond's disease (379–.05); Exophthalmos with obesity (380–.05); Henoch-Schonlein purpura (383–.05); Stokes-Adams attacks (388–.05); Deep femoral vein thrombosis (389–.05); Empyema (390–.05); Pyonephrosis (392–.05); Pemphigus neonatorum (395–.05); Acute septic arthritis (396–.05); Osteochondritis dessicans (397–.05); Reiter's syndrome (398–.05); Miliary tuberculosis (401–.025); Tuberculous endometritis (402–.025); Intestinal tuberculosis (403–.025); Schistosomiasis (407–.025); Amoebic dysentery (408–.025); Pituitary infantilism (409–.025); Chronic iridocyclitis (415–.025); Coeliac syndrome (426–.025); Chronic salpingitis and pyosalpinx (433–.025); Haematocolpos (434–.025); Multiple neurofibromatosis (435–.025); Steroid osteoporosis (440–.025); Primary syphilis (445–0); Secondary syphilis

(447–0); General paralysis of the insane (448–0); Gumma (449–0); Congenital syphilis (450–0); Acute rheumatic fever (457–0); Hyperparathyroidism (459–0); Adrenal medulla tumour (460–0); Addison's disease (461–0); Scurvy (462–0); Rickets (463–0); Plummer-Vinson syndrome (467–0); Regional ileitis (469–0); Perinephric abscess (470–0); Slipped femoral epiphysis (472–0).

Subgroup D. (*Chronic, progressive — many problems*) — 42 entities. Prostatitis (277–0.4); Congenital eye defects (286–0.4); Senile dementia (296–0.3); Homosexuality (300–0.3); Addicts (excluding alcohol) (301–0.3); Healed choroiditis (303–0.3); Portal cirrhosis of liver (309–0.3); Petit mal (325–0.2); Symptomatic epilepsy (326–0.2); Fistula in ano (332–0.2); Dermatitis artefacta (338–0.2); Bedsore (339–0.2); Imperforate anus and megacolon (344–0.2); Major deformities of limbs (345–0.2); Meningomyelocele (346–0.2); Monstrosity (353–0.1); Complete heart block (365–.07); Chronic nephritis (366–.07); Idiopathic laryngeal palsy (375–.05); Bronzed diabetes (377–.05); Anorexia nervosa (384–.05); Narcolepsy (385–.05); Menière's disease (386–.05); Motor neurone disease (387–.05); Hydrocephalus (400–.05); Sarcoidosis (404–.025); Hypertensive encephalopathy (418–.025); Periarteritis nodosa (419–.025); Achalasia (425–.025); Nephrotic syndrome (429–.025); Renal dwarfism (431–.025); Ankylosing spondylitis (438–.025); Sudeck's osteoporosis (441–.025); Microcephaly (442–.025); Congenital polycystic kidney (443–.025); Tuberous sclerosis (444–.025); Presenile dementias (445–0); Acromegaly (455–0); Diabetes insipidus (456–0); Cushing's syndrome (458–0); Raynaud's disease (464–0); Buerger's disease (465–0).

Subgroup E. (*Major life threatening diseases*) — 30 entities. Hypoglycaemic coma (293–0.3); Carcinoma of oesophagus (307–0.3); Large ovarian cyst (335–0.2); Multiple myelomatosis (381–.05); Acute leukaemia (382–.05); Carcinoma of gall-bladder and pancreas (391–.05); Carcinoma of prostate (394–.05); Hodgkin's disease (410–.025); Giant follicular lymphoma (411–.025); Chronic myeloid leukaemia (412–.025); Chronic lymphoid leukaemia (413–.025); Mycosis fungoides (414–.025); Dissecting aneurysm (416–.025); Middle meningeal haemorrhage (traumatic) (417–.025); Valvular (tension) pneumothorax (420–.025); Epithelioma lip (421–.025); Epithelioma tongue (422–.025); Carcinoma of tonsil (423–.025); Mixed parotid tumour (424–.025); Mesenteric infarction (427–.025); Carcinoma of kidney (428–.025); Carcinoma of bladder (430–.025);

Carcinoma of vulva (432–.025); Sarcoma of bone (437–.025); Smallpox (451–0); Diabetic coma (454–0); Carcinoma of larynx (466–0); Volvulus of intestines (468–0); Carcinoma of body of uterus (470–0).

Appendix VIII

Personal assessment of consultations using video tape

Video tapes of consultations are a useful method of teaching consultation to undergraduates.

When used for postgraduate training their most effective use is to enable a doctor to see and criticise his own consultation not that of others.

OBJECTIVE

1. To encourage self awareness and constructive self criticism of consulting techniques.
2. To develop the habit of automatic self-monitoring during every consultation.

METHODS

Real clinics or role play situations can be used. Both methods have advantages and disadvantages.

A. Real clinics are video taped

There are few technical difficulties with modern equipment. Lighting, the smallness of the consulting room and positioning of the camera may cause a few difficulties. These are easily overcome if it is realised that for self criticism, only the audio element requires to be of good quality.

ADVANTAGES

1. Real situations are used. The self criticism that is generated is more likely to be acted on. Also criticisms are likely to be related to realistic consultation practice.
2. The camera can be left in situ for several clinics and camera awareness is greatly reduced.

DISADVANTAGES

1. The patient's permission is required.
2. The awareness of the camera may inhibit both patient and doctor. In practise both parties usually cease to be aware of the video in a few minutes.

B. Role play situations

ADVANTAGES

1. Several doctors can use the same role player and then compare their different handling of the same situation.
2. Complex or emotionally sensitive consulting situations can be created and their handling discussed.
3. A skilled role player can give helpful advice to the doctors concerned.
4. High quality recordings and short excerpts can be obtained which can be used for other teaching purposes.

DISADVANTAGES

1. The feeling that the role play is not real, means that self criticism is less likely to be acted on.
2. Roles and role players have to be prepared and payed for.
3. Special recording rooms, studios may have to be used. These may be upsetting.
4. Role players may not wish to be physically examined.

EQUIPMENT

Video recording equipment is simple and cheap to hire. Often it can be borrowed from postgraduate centres, local medical schools or vocational training schemes.

> NOTE: Adequate audio equipment is essential. Audio recording without video although easy to obtain, rarely generates much self criticism. There are many pauses when it is not certain what is happening. The doctor finds it difficult to remember what he was thinking.

THE VIDEO REPLAY

This can be extremely threatening to the doctor concerned; perhaps this explains why it is such an effective teaching tool.

The following five rules (Pendleton, Ref. 30.6) should be applied in their correct order. If this routine is rigidly adhered to the replay is noticeably more constructive and much less threatening.

Rules for discussing video consultations

1. Briefly clarify any matters of fact.
2. The doctor on the video goes first and must discuss first what he did *well*.
   Ask: What did you do well?
3. Observers then discuss what he did *well*.
   Ask: What did he do well?
4. The doctor on the video then describes what he did not do well *and* recommendations for change.
   Ask: How would you have done it better?
5. Observers then discuss what he did not do well *and* recommendations for change.
   Ask: How could he have done it better?

Another useful method is to ask trainees to view their tapes once or twice on their own and then fill in a report form based on Howard Barrows four outcomes for the consultation:

Video Tape Report Form *Trainee's Name* *Date*
Outcome I *Exploration of the Patient's Problems* ....../..../...... ..../..../..........

Problems I explored well.

Problems I would like to have explored further.

Diagnoses I considered likely.

Other diagnoses which I might have considered.

My assessment of patient's unspoken or subconscious motivations (if any).

My assessment of patient's expectations.

My assessment of patient's personality and likely insecurities.

(Were you aware of any insecurities in yourself as the doctor?)............................
....

Outcome II *Management*

Management areas that were well covered.

Management areas I would like to have covered differently. Describe:

Outcome III *Appropriate use of Time*

Areas in which consultation time was effectively used?

Areas in which time could have been saved or used more effectively?

Outcome IV *Rapport*

Was my explanation appropriate and adequate?

Was rapport adequate?

How could rapport have been improved?

Appendix IX

Graphic recording — the family gram

Graphic methods of recording are under-utilised in medicine. They have great potential for records made during consultation because they are much quicker and more accurate than writing. Any area of medicine where change and stress affect complex structure is amenable to graphic recording. The family gram provides an excellent and useful example. The method was developed for personal use and is included here because trainees and residents over the past 14 years have wanted to learn and use it.

THE FAMILY GRAM

Aims:

1. To facilitate the quick accurate recording of changes in a patient's family structure.
2. To enable the doctor to record those stresses which threaten the security of a particular family.
3. To remind the doctor of any unspoken value judgements about those stresses on a family which have influenced his decisions and choice of management options.

The family gram represents the interaction of two areas vital to general practice which are extremely lengthy to describe in words:

1. The relationship (and interaction) of members of a household.
2. The 'refuge' of emotional security that every family unit builds to protect itself from the cold winds of insecurity in the wider world.

The method and conventions will be described first followed by a discussion of advantages and disadvantages. Finally, all conventions are summarised in Fig. 78 (pp. 742 to 745); these can be duplicated for partners or health visitors who wish to 'read' any family gram.

The summary can also be enclosed with a patients' records if these have to be sent to another practice.

I. THE METHOD AND CONVENTIONS

A. The family structure

1. *The patient* is always indicated by a double thick line.
2. *Sex and partnerships* — usually husband and wife, who own, rent or manage any household are always represented by vertical ·strokes. The woman always being on the right side with sex indicated by a little sloping 'skirt' (dash) at the lower end. This skirt also indicates female sex in other household members.

Example (*Fig. 58*)

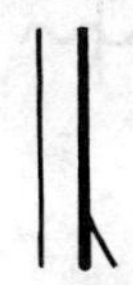

Fig 58

Explanation
— man and wife, the wife being the patient.

3. *The children* of any union lie across the parents. Their age being indicated, if relevant at their right hand and sex at the foot or left hand end. Thus:

Example (*Fig. 59*)

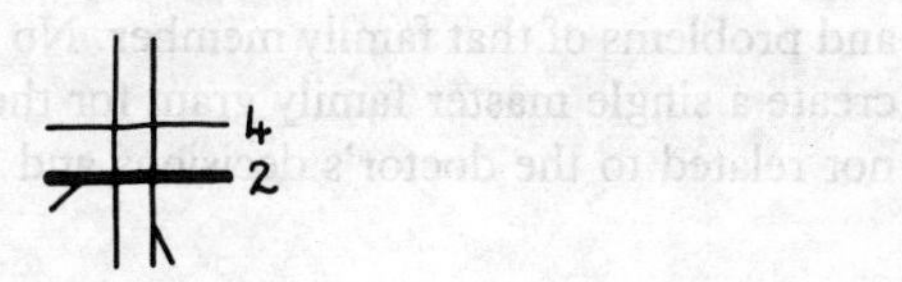

Fig 59

Explanation
— a son of 4 years
a daughter of 2 years, who is the patient.

4. *Adopted children* are indicated by a wavy line:

Example (*Fig. 60*)

Explanation
— an adopted 18 month old son has been added to the family and is now the patient.

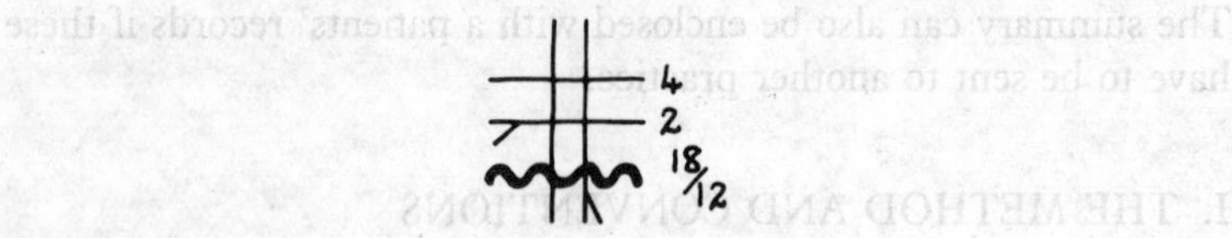

Fig 60

5. *Step children* lie horizontally in relation to their parent but do not cross their step parent.

Example (*Fig. 61*)

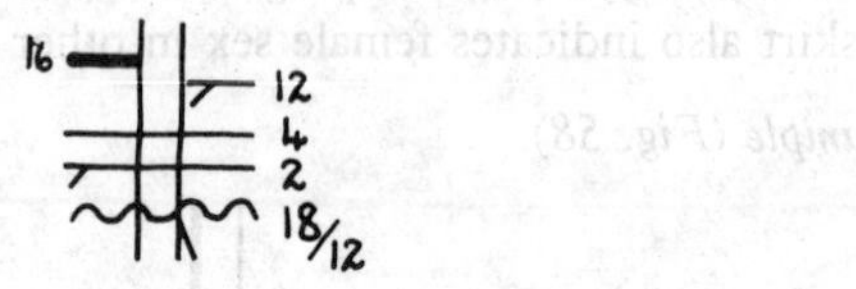

Fig 61

Explanation

— the doctor discovers and adds to the above family gram the presence of the male partner's 16 year old stepson (now the patient) and the 12 year old stepdaughter of the female partner.

Even if the family gram is taken no further the above method provides an accurate, quick way of recording changing family structures. Each family member may collect over the years, similar 'family grams' on their own record card. Each family gram will relate to the stresses and problems of that family member. No attempt should be made to create a single master family gram for the family as a whole, this is not related to the doctor's decisions and soon becomes overloaded.

B. The emotional security areas

The family is enclosed in a 5-sided 'house' each of the 5 sides represent an area of emotional security which may be threatened or under stress, in a variety of recordable ways.

6. *Example* (*Fig. 62*)

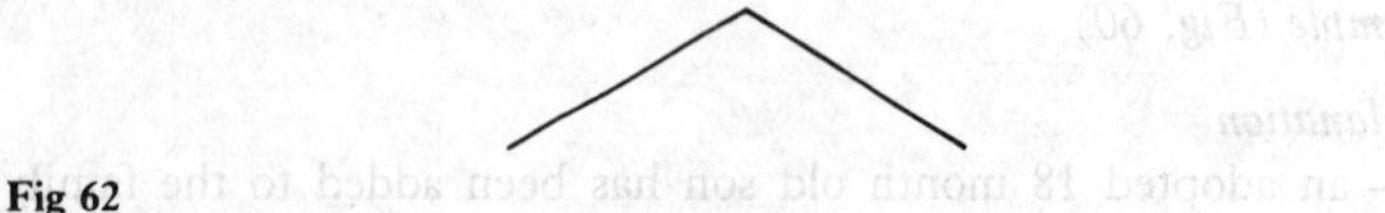

Fig 62

Explanation

— the 'roof' on the male partner's side represents the husband's sexual area; the roof on the female partner's side represents the wife's sexual area.

7. *Example* (*Fig. 63*)

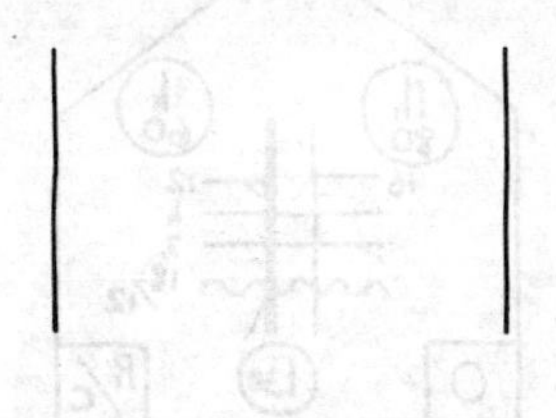

Fig 63

Explanation

— similarly the walls on the male and female partners' sides represent the respective 'community' areas of each partner. i.e. leisure, culture, religion, neighbours, etc.

8. *Example* (*Fig. 64*)

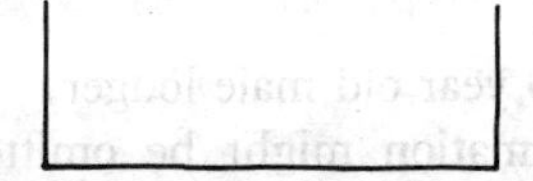

Fig 64

Explanation

— the joint floor of the house represents the joint social foundations of the household, i.e. the job and financial contributions of male and female partners.

9. *Example* (*Fig. 65*)

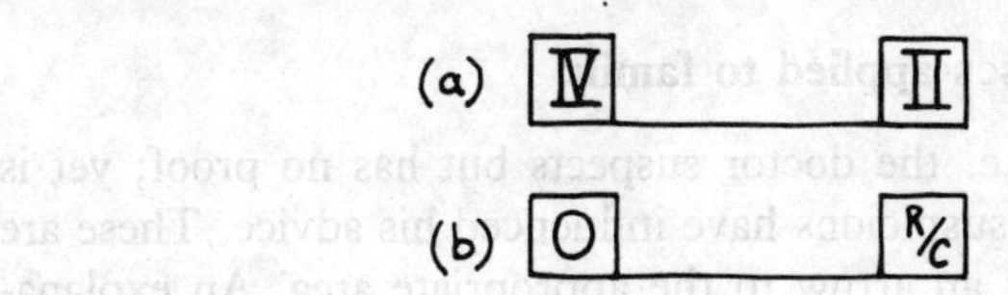

Fig 65

Explanation

— two boxes on either side of the floor can be used to indicate areas of difference between husband and wife which may cause stress, i.e. social class (a), religion (b), culture, etc.

C. Other household members

It is now possible to indicate other members of the household.

10. Example (Fig. 66)

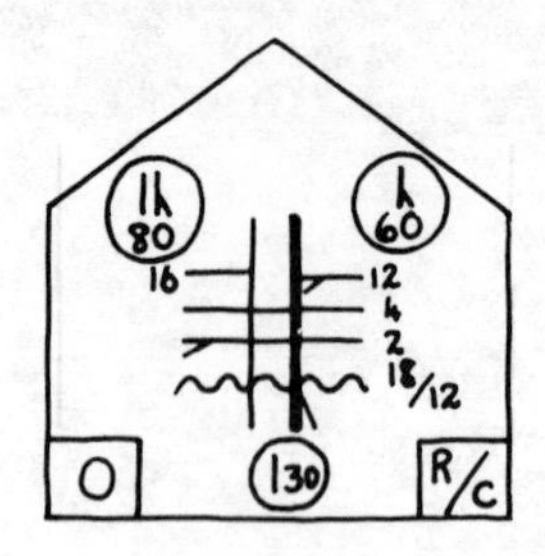

Fig 66

Explanation

— the wife is the patient, the children are the same.

— the wife's mother, aged 60, is living in the same home.

— both the husband's parents are also living in the household (aged 80).

— there is also a 30 year old male lodger.

Some of this information might be omitted, i.e. the ages of adopted child or the lodger if this was not contributing to the patient's problems.

Even if the family gram is taken no further it provides a quick accurate method of recording household structure.

Most family doctors having learnt this simple method of recording family structure quickly now find it useful to add the conventions which indicate common stresses.

D. External stresses applied to family

11. *Covert stress*, i.e. the doctor suspects but has no proof; yet is aware that his suspicions have influenced his advice. These are represented by an arrow to the appropriate area. An explanatory abbreviation may be needed to assist recall. (A list of useful abbreviations is given on p. 736.)

Example (Fig. 67)

Explanation

— 13 years have elapsed and a new family gram is needed.

— the oldest daughter is the patient and wants to go on the pill.

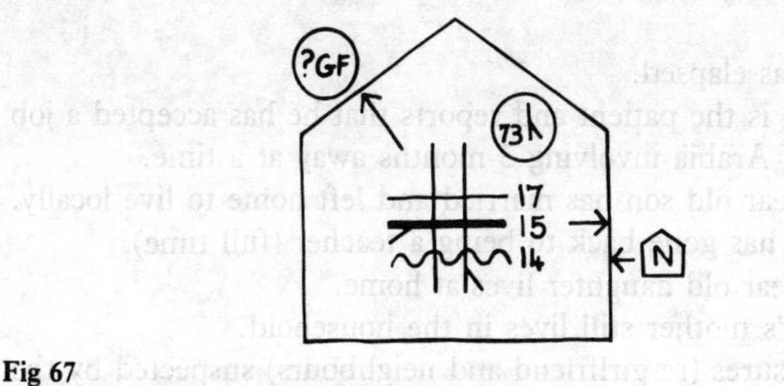

Fig 67

— she is obviously anxious to leave home.
— there is trouble with the neighbours but the doctor is uncertain who is at fault.
— from other sources the doctor wonders if the girl's father has a covert girl friend.
— the husband's parents have either died or are being cared for elsewhere. The lodger has left.
— the two step children have also left the home.
— no more children have been added.

NOTE: This family gram will be recorded on the notes of the daughter who is the patient. No attempt should be made to update the information on the records of other family members.

12. Overt, openly accepted or non-threatening stresses; family security areas may be breached in socially normal or openly accepted ways. These are represented by a single line crossing the relevant wall or security area. An explanatory label or abbreviation may be helpful.

Example (*Fig. 68*)

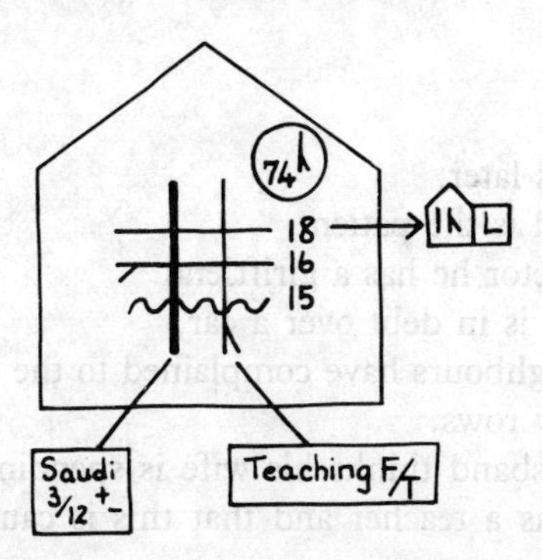

Fig 68

Explanation

- — 1 year has elapsed.
- — husband is the patient and reports that he has accepted a job in Saudi Arabia involving 3 months away at a time.
- — his 18 year old son has married and left home to live locally.
- — his wife has gone back to being a teacher (full time).
- — the 16 year old daughter lives at home.
- — the wife's mother still lives in the household.
- — the pressures (re girlfriend and neighbours) suspected by the doctor a year ago are not mentioned by the husband and do not affect the doctor's decision-making at this time and are not recorded.

13. *Overt (openly admitted) stresses causing problems*
Such threats to family security may affect any of the five main areas and are indicated by an extra line re-inforcing the single line of a non-threatening breach illustrated in (12). The explanatory labels are the same.

Example (a) (Fig. 69)

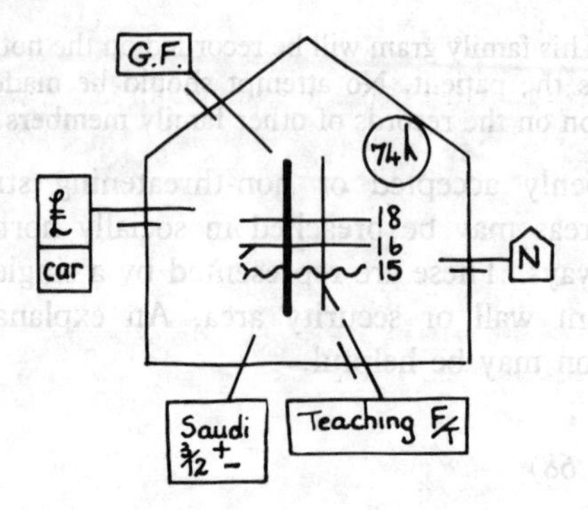

Fig 69

Explanation

- — a few weeks later.
- — the husband is the patient.
- — tells the doctor he has a girlfriend.
- — also that he is in debt over a car.
- — that the neighbours have complained to the council about the noisy family rows.
- — that the husband thinks his wife is spending too much time at her job as a teacher and that this is causing considerable family friction.

At this stage a rapid glance round the 5 security sides of the diagram reminds the doctor instantly of the major overt causes of trouble that have been identified at this consultation. Also it is unnecessary to redraw the whole family gram for the second of the husband's consultations.

Example (*b*) (*Fig. 70*)

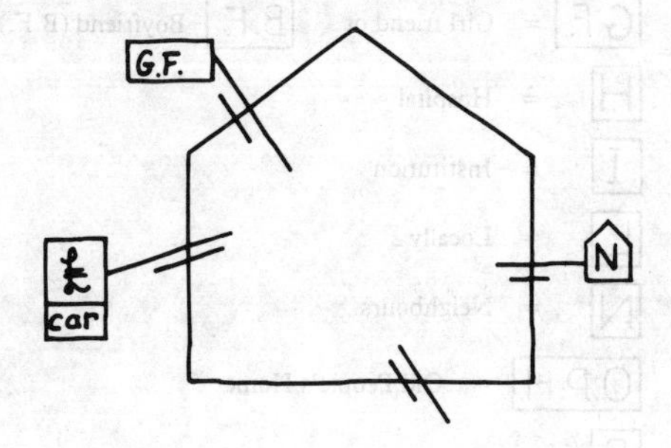

Fig 70

Explanation

— the closeness in time between the family gram in Fig. 69 and that in Fig. 70 enables much of the details in Fig. 69 to be assumed. Much recording time is thus saved.

If the patient had only reported the information about his girlfriend all that would have been needed to indicate this would have been a record of the single area affected, as in Fig. 71(c):

Example (*c*) (*Fig. 71*)

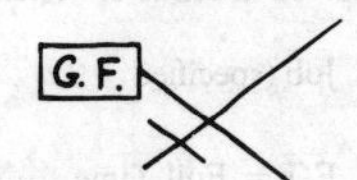

Fig 71

Explanation

— this rapid shorthand has the added advantage of appearing to the patient as a 'doodle'; also confidentiality is not openly broken.

14. The following stressful life events (Fig. 72) are sufficiently common to justify learning a recognised symbol.

Note because many of these life events are confidential, the use of symbols both assists the confidentiality of the family gram and encourages their more general use by the doctor in the written records.

A	=	Alcohol
B	=	Birth
C	=	Chronic disease etc.
D	=	Death
G.F.	=	Girl friend or B.F. Boyfriend (B.F.)
H	=	Hospital
I	=	Institution
L	=	Locally
N	=	Neighbours
O.P.H.	=	Old People's Home
P	=	Prison
R.T.A.	=	Road Traffic Accident
Rx	=	Dependance on Drugs
S	=	Suicide
Sx	=	Sex deviance
W.A.	=	Works Accident
£	=	Debts
☒	=	Involved in crime or violence
nurse	=	Job (specified
F/T	=	F/T = Full Time
P/T	=	P/T = Part Time

Fig 72

Also the routine abreviations for time which are used elsewhere in the history, i.e.

1′	= One second	often used in records but rarely in a family gram.
2″	= Two minutes	
3‴	= Three hours	
④	= Four days	
$\frac{5}{52}$	= Five weeks	
$\frac{6}{12}$	= Six months	
7y.	= Seven years.	The y is omitted when the figure clearly gives the age of the patient.

E. Individual behaviour and internal stresses which affect the doctors' decisions may also usefully be included. No attempt should be made to learn these conventions until the previous 14 have been mastered.

15. Parental dominance in a household. This is usually a value judgement made by the doctor which can change from situation to situation. It is often helpful to record the opinion in a family gram when it has influenced the doctor's choice of options. It might be useful to record this in the family gram of a child with Asthma or in a 15 year old girl who requested the pill.

Example (*a*) (*Fig. 73*)

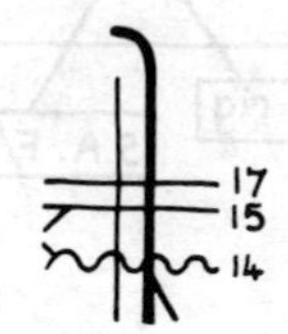

Fig 73

Explanation

— mother is the patient and is likely to be the dominant partner.

Example (*b*) (*Fig. 74*)

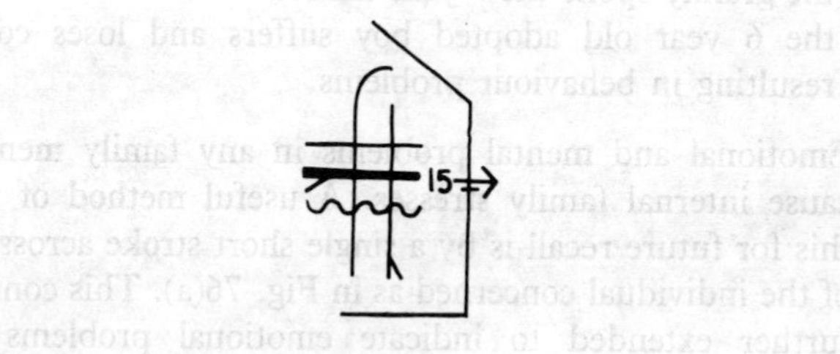

Fig 74

Explanation

— 15 year old daughter is the patient and father is considered to be the dominant parent in relation to the daughter's problems.

This is a useful convention for a factor that is often relevant to primary situations but rarely stated. As a result once learnt it tends to slip into the doctor's wider written recording habits.

16. Imbalances of self confidence, especially in children. These are value judgements which may have considerable influence in our

handling of behaviour problems. The family gram is an ideal way of recording for future recall such judgements, which have affected past decisions.

Example (Fig. 75)

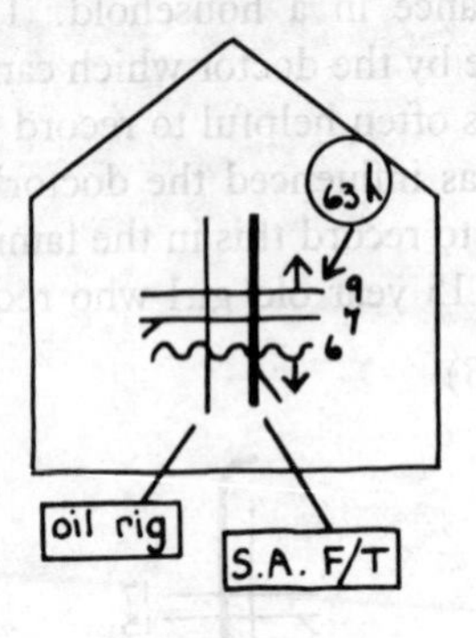

Fig 75

Explanation

— mother of family is the patient.
— mother's mother lives with family.
— mother out as shop assistant all day.
— father works on an oil rig.
— the granny spoils the 9 year old son who is full of confidence.
— the 6 year old adopted boy suffers and loses confidence, resulting in behaviour problems.

17. Emotional and mental problems in any family member may cause internal family stresses. A useful method of recording this for future recall is by a single short stroke across the head of the individual concerned as in Fig. 76(a). This convention is further extended to indicate emotional problems between (dominant) husband and wife, as in Fig. 76(b), or as a thick black line indicating openly reported violence between dominant husband and wife as in Fig. 76(c).

Example (Fig. 76)

Explanation of Fig. 76(a)

— father — authoritarian — dominates.
— wife (and mother) is patient.
— wife anxious, worries dependent on tranquillisers.
— emotional problems in adopted 10 year old son who is insecure

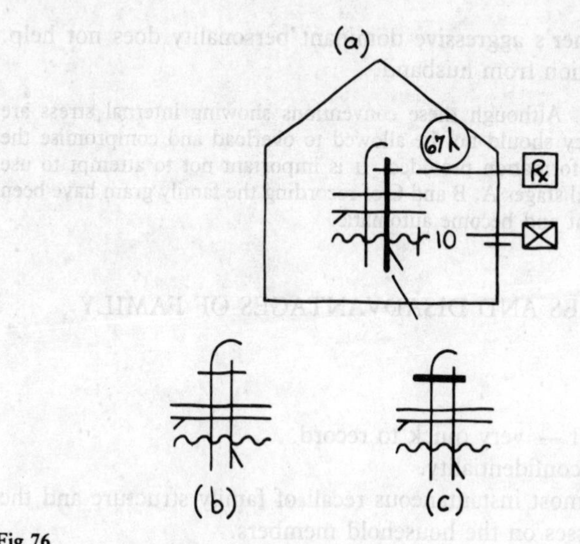

Fig 76

and in trouble with the police.
— wife's mother lives in same household.

18. Physical or disease problems in an individual if they are causing internal stress can likewise be flagged by a stroke across the foot of the individual's line.

Example (*Fig.* 77)

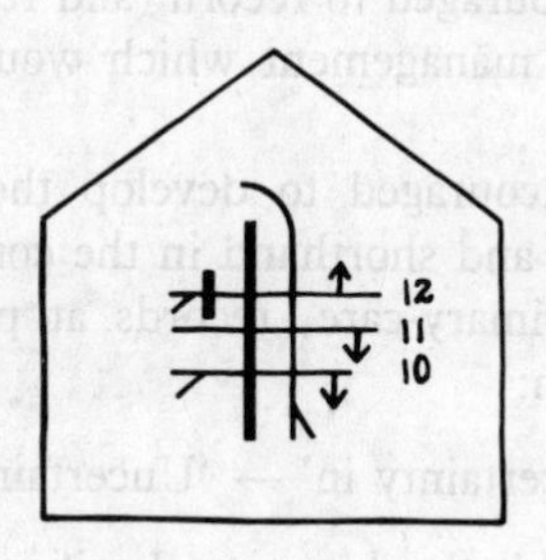

Fig 77

Explanation

— A different family: the family gram reminds the doctor that the chronic illness in the 12 year old daughter (diabetes — the disease is not specified in the family gram because it will be known) is causing over confidence to the detriment of the confidence of both the 11 year old and 10 year old siblings.

— the mother's aggressive dominant personality does not help.
— Information from husband.

NOTE. Although these conventions showing internal stress are useful they should not be allowed to overload and compromise the factual information provided. It is important not to attempt to use them until stages A, B and C of recording the family gram have been well learnt and become automatic.

ADVANTAGES AND DISADVANTAGES OF FAMILY GRAMS

Advantages

1. Once learnt — very quick to record.
2. Maintains confidentiality.
3. Enables almost instantaneous recall of family structure and the major stresses on the household members.
4. Family grams take up very little space and can be repeated when updating is needed.
5. Non-threatening to the patient to record — it looks as if the doctor is merely 'doodling'.
6. Because the relevant information is usually recorded by a single stroke of the pen, this can be performed without interrupting the patient/doctor interaction. Any further details can be filled in later on.
7. The doctor is encouraged to record (and recall) data and judgements that affect management which would not otherwise be recorded.
8. The doctor is encouraged to develop the wider potential of graphic recording and shorthand in the consultation.
9. Computerised, primary-care, records at present have not got much further than:

   'Uncertainty in' → 'Uncertainty out'

   Family grams enable the doctor to classify and label some important uncertainties in a way that can eventually be computerised.

Possible disadvantages

1. The family gram appears to take up valuable consulting time to record. This is incorrect. The rapid recall of patient problems

can be striking. The doctor 'runs an eye' round the 5 sides of the household's security shield and is reminded of all major problems. The doctor is enabled to move with confidence almost instantaneously back into the patient's problems. Time wasting questions which enable the doctor to refamiliarise and reorientate are avoided.

2. The family gram conventions take time to learn. This is not correct. We found that an afternoon seminar combined with this Appendix as a hand out, was sufficient. The seminar had the following structure:

   Step 1 — Appendix IX given to each member before seminar.
   Step 2 — Method explained and clarified.
   Step 3 — Each member of resident or trainee seminar draws their own family gram and passes it to their neighbour for reading.
   Step 4 — Each member recalls and verbally describes a problem family from their own practice. While this is being done all members of the group record the appropriate family gram.
   Step 5 — Recall of the 8–10 family problems is compared, with and without, the aid of family grams
   Step 6 — Participants agree to record one family gram at every clinic during next 2 weeks.
   Step 7 — Report problems back 2 weeks later.

3. Other colleagues and health professionals are confused because they cannot read them. In fact, given the single sheet summarising all conventions (see Fig. 78) they can be read quite easily by interested professionals who have been previously warned.
4. In Britain where records are passed to other doctors when patients change their domicile the new doctor may be confused. The answer to this is that the new doctor should not be dependent of a family gram for such information, he should be collecting the data himself from the patient.
5. Family grams can easily be overloaded. They should not be regarded as a comprehensive data base. Fresh family grams should be redrawn rather than adding to old ones. This avoids confusing previous situations and allows the doctor to see exactly over the years how different family and household stresses and tensions have altered and affected his decisions.

A. Family and household structure

(1) Male head of house — vertical, left side Female head of house — vertical, right side

(Females always have skirt or dash at 'foot end')

(2) Patient is always a double thick line:

here wife is the patient.

(3) Children lie across their parents: with age if relevant at right hand or head and sex at left end:

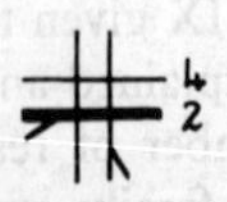

= son of 4 years daughter of 2, who is the patient.

(4) Adopted children — a wavy line

(5) Step-children — horizontal but do not cross their step-parent:

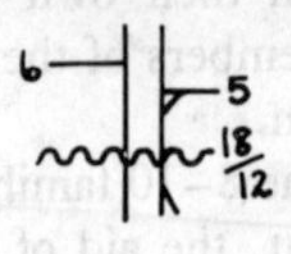

= adopted daughter of 1½ also 2 step children of 6 (male, by father) and 5 female by mother.

B. Emotional security areas

(6) Sexual areas

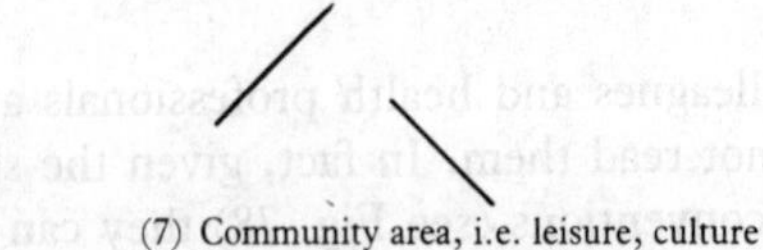

Roof, left side is father's (male partner's) sex area. Roof, right side is mother's (female partner's) sex area.

(7) Community area, i.e. leisure, culture religion, neighbours, etc male partner's is left wall female partner's is right wall

(8) Joint area on 'floor' of house represents joint social foundations, i.e.: job, finance of house hold.

(9) Boxes on either side of floor represent any area of social or cultural difference between partners. e.g. (a) class, race, (b) religion etc.

(a) IV II

(b) O R/C

Fig. 78 List of conventions for family grams and shorthand.

C. Other household members are

(10) enclosed in a circle in the position that shows their relationships

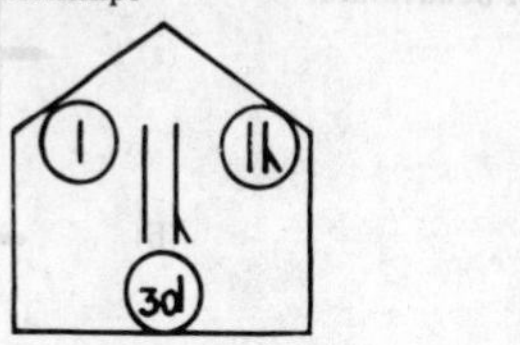

— husband's father — left roof
— wife's parents — right roof
— lodger (male 30) — floor

D. External stresses applied to family

(11) Covert or suspected stresses — an arrow to the appropriate area, an explanatory label helps recall,

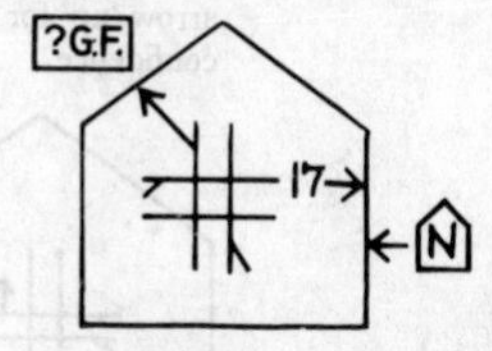

i.e. daughter (17) wants to leave home and father may have a girl friend; also possible trouble with neighbours.

(12) Non-threatening or acceptable stresses — breaching the family security in a normal or acceptable way is represented by a single line that crosses the relevant area:

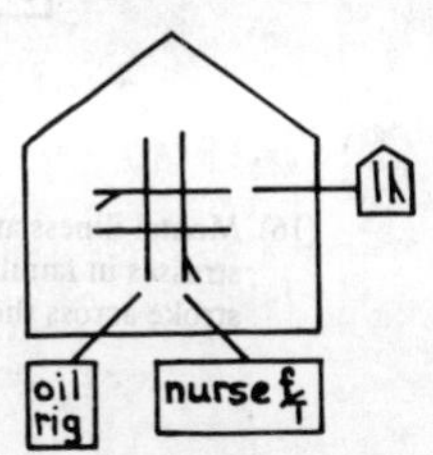

— daughter leaves home to marry.
— wife takes full-time job as a nurse.
— husband away working on an oil rig.

(13) Overt stresses causing problems or threatening household security, an extra line, reinforcing (12) above. i.e. husband (the patient) tells the doctor:

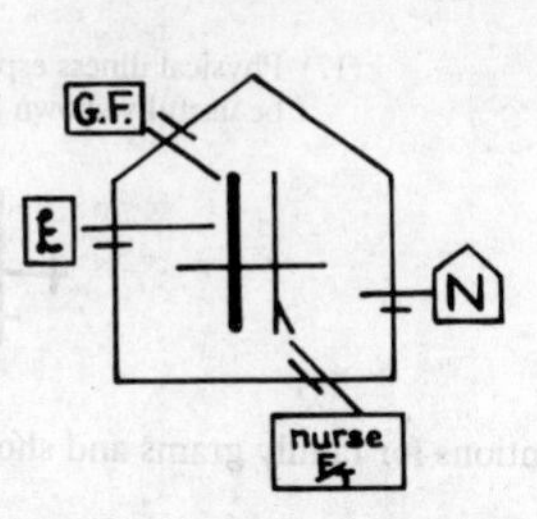

— he has a girl friend.
— he is in debt
— the neighbours are complaining.
— his wife is out all day and too busy.

Fig. 78 List of conventions for family grams and shorthand.

E. Internal stresses due to personality or behavioural influences.

(14) Parental dominence

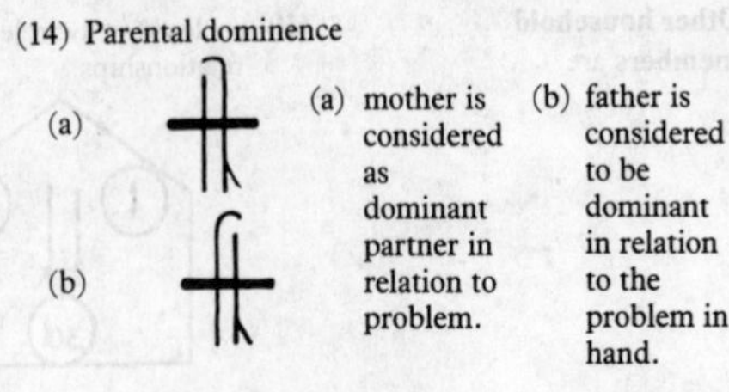

(a) mother is considered as dominant partner in relation to problem.

(b) father is considered to be dominant in relation to the problem in hand.

(15) Imbalances in self confidence in children with behaviour or emotional problems are shown by an arrow 'up' for over confident and 'down' for lack of confidence.

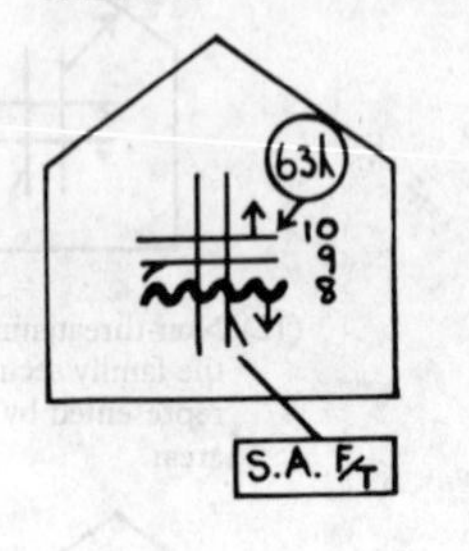

— wife working as shop assistant.
— wife's mother lives with family and spoils 10 year old son.
— 8 year old lacks confidence with behaviour problems.

(16) Mental illness and emotional problem may cause stresses in families and can be represented by a short stroke across the head end of any family member i.e.

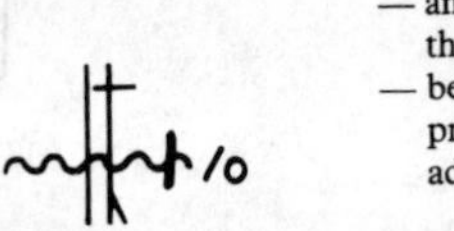

— anxiety in the mothers.
— behaviour problems in adopted son.

(17) Physical illness especially chronic or disabling can also be usefully shown by a similar stroke at the foot.

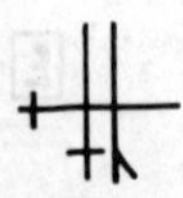

— father and son, both have a chronic illness.

Fig. 78 List of conventions for family grams and shorthand.

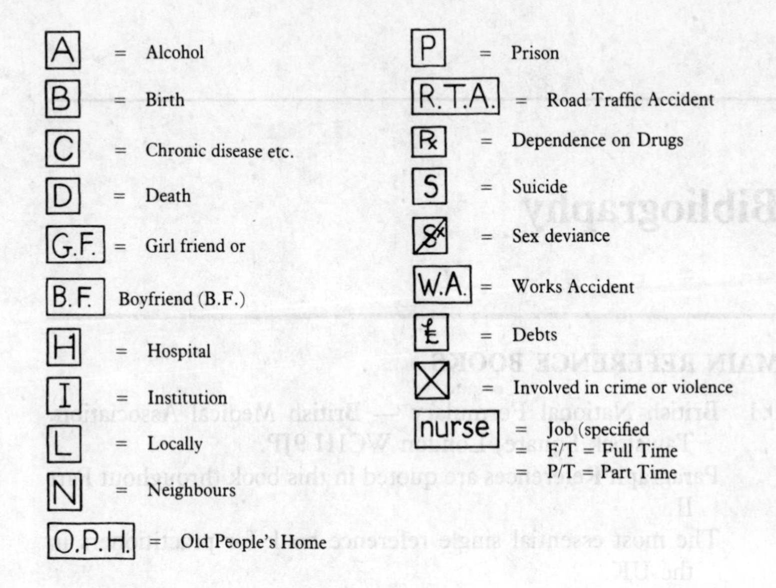

Other abbreviations used by doctor in the records.

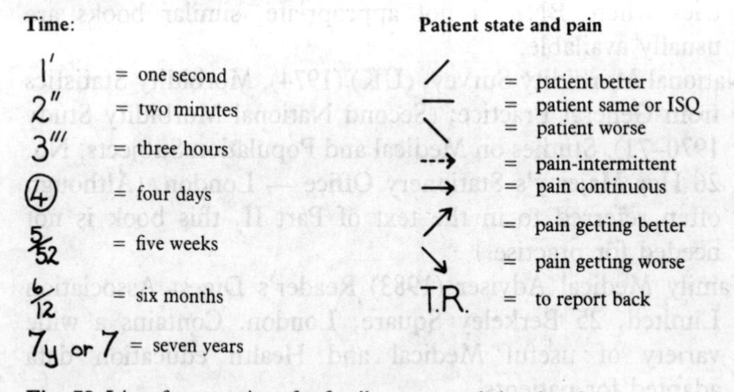

Fig. 78 List of conventions for family grams and shorthand.

Bibliography

MAIN REFERENCE BOOKS

0.1 British National Formulary — British Medical Association, Tavistock Square, London WC1H 9JP.

Paragraph References are quoted in this book throughout Part II.

The most essential single reference book for practitioners in the UK.

Note: The BNF is updated twice a year but paragraph references remain the same for each new edition. In countries where BNF is not appropriate, similar books are usually available.

0.2 National Morbidity Survey, (UK) (1974). Morbidity Statistics from General Practice; (Second National Morbidity Study 1970–71). Studies on Medical and Population Subjects. No. 26 Her Majesty's Stationery Office — London. (Although often referred to in the text of Part II, this book is not needed for practise.)

0.3 Family Medical Adviser (1983) Reader's Digest Association Limited, 25 Berkeley Square, London. Contains a wide variety of useful Medical and Health education data adapted for patients.

0.4 Physifax — A Physician's Pocket Compendium of Normal Values, Tests, Diagnostic Criteria and other useful Data. Geigy Pharmaceuticals, Horsham, West Sussex, England.

0.5 A Guide to General Practice — The Oxford Trainee Group (1981) Blackwell Scientific Publications, Oxford, England. A useful collection of check lists and data suitable for all family doctors but especially those in the UK.

0.6 The General Practitioner's Year Book (Parts I & II) (1983) Winthrop Laboratories. Produced by House Information Services Ltd., 178–202 Great Portland Street, London.

Contains much useful information and a list of addresses of all charity and medical self help groups in the UK; for family doctors in Britain.

0.7 Dermatology an illustrated Guide. Lionel Fry Update Publications — 33/34 Alfred Place, London, WC1E 7DP or Manual of Skin Diseases, Sauer, Gordon. Lippincott — Philadelphia.

REFERENCES FROM CHAPTERS

1.0 Elstein, A. S., Kagan, N., Shulman, L. S., et al (1972) Methods and Theory in the Study of Medical Inquiry. *J. Med. Educ.* **47**, 85

1.1 The Future General Practitioner: Learning and Teaching. RCGP, 14 Princes Gate, London.

1.2 Maxwell, R. (1975) The Growing Dilemma — A McKinsey Report. McKinsey and Co. Inc. 245 Park Avenue, New York, NY 10017.

1.3 Ashton, T.B. (1982) Financial Implications of Medical Practice. *Update* **25** (Nov. 1st), p. 1399.

1.4 Spitzer, W. (1976) Nurse Practitioner in Primary Care. *Can. Med. Assoc. J.*, **114.**, 1099

1.5 McLachlan, G. (1982) *The Public/Private Mix for Health* London: Nuffield Provincial Hospitals Trust.

2.1 Hodgkin, K., Freedman, R., Fuller, I. & Whewell, J. (1970) *British Medical Journal*, **iii**, 368–371.

2.2 Illych. I (1976) *Limits to Medicine. Medical Nemesis.* London: Boyars Publishers Ltd.

3.1 Freedman, R. (1978) *Journal of the Royal College of General Practitioners* **28**, 421–425

4.1 Illingworth R. S. (1980) *The development of the infant and young child* Edinburgh: Churchill Livingstone

4.2 Illingworth R. S. (1981) *Your child's development in the first five years.* Edinburgh: Churchill Livingstone

5.1 Berne, E. (1960) Games People Play. London: Deutsch (Also in Penguin Books.)

5.2 Brown (1975) Social Class and Psychiatric Disturbance in Women in an Urban Population. *Sociology*, **9**, 225

7.1 Mayhew, S. R. (1982) A Computerised Age/Sex Register and Diagnostic Index. *Update* **24** (May 1st), p. 1671.

7.2 While Robin, (1982). An Integrated Computer System. *Update* **25** (Oct. 1st), p. 1033

7.3 Royal College of General Practitioners (1980) Occasional Paper No. 13 Computers in Primary Care. RCGP, 14 Princes Gate, London

8.1 Family Doctor Booklet STD & VD, Dr. Duncan Catterall BMA House, Tavistock Square, London, WC19SR.

10.1 Diabetic Association, 10 Queen Anne Street, London, W1M OBD Telephone: 01-323-1531.
10.2 Farquhar J. W. (1981) The diabetic child. Edinburgh: Churchill Livingstone.
10.3 Farquhar J. W. (1982) Diabetes in your teens. Edinburgh: Churchill Livingstone.
10.4 Tattersall, R. (1981) Diabetes: a practical guide for patients on insulin. Edinburgh: Churchill Livingstone.

12.0 Schizophrenia Assoc. of Great Britain, Llanfair Hall, Caernarvon, Gwynedd LL55 ITT. (Telephone: 0248–670379).
National Schizophrenia Fellowship, 29 Victoria Road, Surbiton, Surrey.
12.1 Alcoholics Anonymous, 11 Redcliffe Gardens, London, SW10 9BQ (Telephone: 01–352–9779).
12.2 Al-Anon Family Groups UK & Eire, 61 Great Dover Street, London, SE1 4YF (Telephone: 01–403–0888).
12.3 Medical Council on Alcoholism, 3 Grosvenor Place, London, SW1X 7EE (Telephone: 01–235–4182).
12.4 British Dyslexia Association, Church Lane, Peppard, Oxon RG9 5JN.

13.1 *Addresses and Aid Centres for Disabled*

Organisations

Disabled Living Foundation, 346 Kensington High Street, London, W14 8NS (Telephone: 01–602–2491). Provides advice, aids, information sheets and books, and will supply a list of provincial aid centres providing similar services. Visits may be made by appointment.

Centre on Environment for the Handicapped, 126 Albert Street, London, NW1 7NE (Telephone: 01–267–6111).

Rehabilitation Engineering Movement Advisory Panel, Thames House North, Millbank, London, SW1P 40G (Telephone: 01–834–4444 ext. 4112).

Exhibition

The Naidex exhibition, organised by the Royal Association for Disability and Rehabilitation, 25 Mortimer Street, London, W1N 8AB (Telephone: 01–637–5400) is held annually in various parts of Great Britain. An extensive display of specialised equipment including the most recently developed.

Aid Centres

There are aid centres with a wide range of aids on display in the following towns: Belfast, Birmingham, Caerphilly, Edinburgh, Glasgow, Liverpool, London, Newcastle-upon-Tyne, Sheffield, Southampton, Stockport and Wakefield. Details from the Disabled Living Foundation (see Organisations above).

Publications

Equipment for the Disabled, 11 separate booklets including Housing and Furniture and Home Management available from 2 Foredown Drive, Portslade, Brighton, BN4 2BB.

Apparatus and Games for the Blind illustrated catalogue available from the Royal Institute for the Blind, 224 Great Portland Street, London, W1N 6AA.

In Touch, printed Braille and tape versions available from BBC Publications, PO Box 234, London, SE1 3TH.

Aids for the Disabled, Department of Health and Social Security Leaflet, HB2. Available from local DHSS offices, libraries and post offices.

Designing for the Disabled, available from RIBA Publications Ltd., 66 Portland Place, London, W1N 4AD.

Fuller details appear in section two of Directory for the Disabled, Third edition, available from Woodhead-Faulkner (Publishers) Ltd. 8 Market Passage, Cambridge, CB2 3PF.

13.2 Multiple Sclerosis Society for Great Britain, 286 Munster Road, Fulham, London SW6 (Telephone: 01–381–4022).

13.3 Parkinson's Disease Society, 36 Portland Place, London WIN 3DG. Telephone: 01.323.1174 (Handbooks: *Parkinson's Disease, Parkinson's Disease Day to Day*)

13.4 Laidlaw, M. V., Laidlaw, J. (1980) *Epilepsy explained*. Edinburgh: Churchill Livingstone.

13.5 British Epilepsy Association, Crowthorne House, New Wokingham Road, Wokingham, Berkshire, RG11 3AY (Telephone: 034–46–3122).

13.6 Medical Aspects of Fitness to Drive (Medical Commission for Accident Prevention).

13.7 Migraine Trust, 45 Great Ormond Street, London, WCIN 3HD (Telephone: 01 278 2676).

13.8 *Update*, (1982). **25**, 1726 Soft Tissue Injections — Goodwill.

16.1 *British Medical Journal* (1984) **i**, 423 Hypercholesterolaemia and coronary heart disease: an answer.

17.1 Foundation for Study of Infant Deaths, 5th Floor, 4 Grosvenor Place, London, SWIx7HD (Telephone: 01–235–1721).

18.1 Colostomy Welfare Group, 38–39 Eccleston Square (2nd Floor), London, SW1V 1PB (Telephone: 01–828–5175).

18.2 Ileostomy Association of Great Britain, Amblehurst House, Chobham, Woking, Surrey, GU 24 8PZ (Telephone: 09905–8277).

21.1 Mastectomy Association, 25 Brighton Road, South Croydon, England CR2 6EA (Telephone: 01–654–8643).

22.1 Family Planning Association, Margaret Pyke House, 27–35 Mortimer Street, London, W1N 7RJ (Telephone: 01–636–7866).

22.2 Catholic Marriage Advisory Council, Clitheroe House, 15 Lansdowne Road, London, W11 3AJ (Telephone: 01–727–0141)

23.1 National Eczema Society, Roger Oliver, Tavistock House North Tavistock Square, London, WC1H 9SR (Telehone: 01–388–4097).

23.2 The Psoriasis Association, 7 Milton Street, Northampton, NN2 7JG 0604–711129).

24.1 British Rheumatism & Arthritis Association, 6 Grosvenor Crescent, London, SW1X 7ER (Telephone: 01–235–0902)

25.1 Royal Society for Mentally Handicapped Children, 117–123 Golden Lane, London EC1Y ORT (Telephone: 01–253–9433).

26.1 National Society for Prevention of Cruelty to Children, 1 Riding House Street, London, W1P 8AA (Telephone 01–580–8812). Branch addresses available also in Ref. 0.6 — Winthrop General Practitioners' Year Book, House Information Services, 178–202, Great Portland Street, London, W1N 6NH.

Appendix IB
30.1 *British Medical Journal* (1983) i, 266.

Appendix II
30.2 Mayhew, S. B. (1982) A Computerised Age/Sex Register and Diagnostic Index *Update* (May 1st) p. 1671.

Appendix III
30.3 Moulds, A. et al. (1983) *Update* (March 15th) p. 1028.

Appendix III
30.4 The Royal Flying Doctor Service, Broken Hill, New South Wales, Australia.

Appendix IV
30.5 Birmingham Research Unit (PAA), R. C. G. P., 54 Lordswood Road, Birmingham B17 9DB.
Fleming, D. (1982) Practice Activity Analysis. *Update* (March 15th). p. 1117.
30.6 Pendleton, D. A., Schofield, T., Tate, P., Havelock, P. (1984) *The Consultation. An Approach to Learning and Teaching*, Oxford University Press.

Index